AF700903

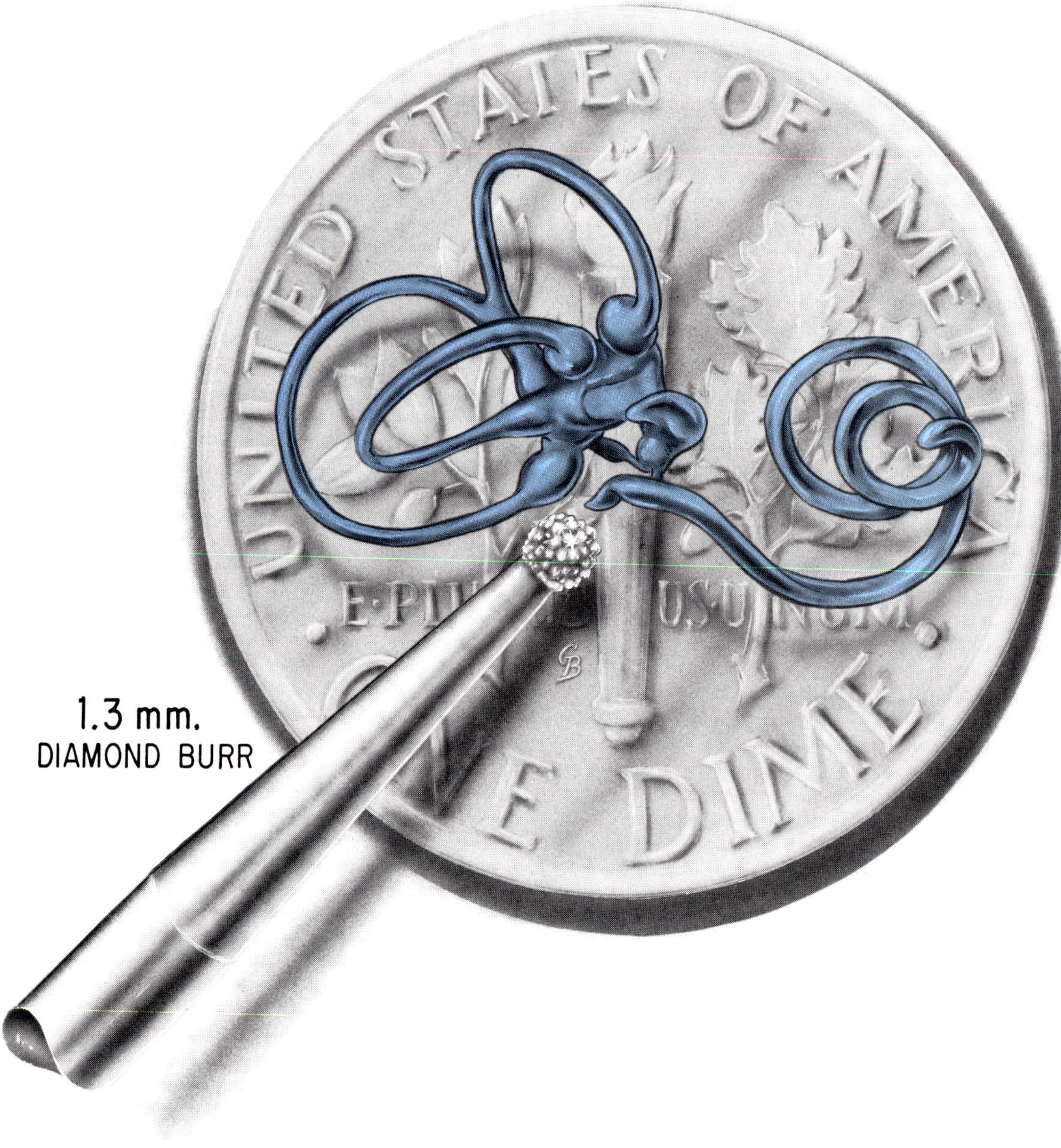

The size of the membranous labyrinth shown in comparison with that of a ten-cent piece. This reconstruction was prepared by the Born wax-plate method.

Barry J. Anson, Ph.D. (Med. Sc.)

Research Professor, Department of Otolaryngology
and Maxillofacial Surgery, College of Medicine,
The University of Iowa, Iowa City, Iowa;
Robert Laughlin Rea Professor Emeritus of Anatomy,
Northwestern University Medical School, Chicago

James A. Donaldson, M.D., F.A.C.S.

Professor and Chairman, Department of Otolaryngology,
School of Medicine, The University of Washington,
Seattle, Washington

SURGICAL ANATOMY OF THE TEMPORAL BONE AND EAR

Second Edition

1973 W. B. SAUNDERS COMPANY · PHILADELPHIA · LONDON · TORONTO

W. B. Saunders Company: West Washington Square
Philadelphia, Pa. 19105

12 Dyott Street
London, WC1A 1DB

833 Oxford St.
Toronto 18, Ontario

Surgical Anatomy of the Temporal Bone and Ear ISBN 0-7216-1291-1

© 1973 by W. B. Saunders Company. Copyright 1967 by W. B. Saunders Company. Copyright under the International Copyright Union. All rights reserved. This book is protected by copyright. No part of it may be reproduced, stored in a retrieval system, or transmitted in any form or by any means, electronic, mechanical, photocopying, recording, or otherwise, without written permission from the publisher. Made in the United States of America. Press of W. B. Saunders Company. Library of Congress catalog card number 72-82800.

Print No.: 9 8 7 6 5 4 3 2 1

Dedication to

THEODORE H. BAST, PH.D.[1]

September 1, 1890–January 23, 1959

Theodore Hieronymus Bast was an active member of the faculty of the University of Wisconsin for thirty-nine years. He was a native son of the State of Wisconsin. The formative years on the farm engendered a love of nature and a disciplined respect for hard work which characterized him as a man. He received the A.B. degree from Ripon College in 1912, and the Ph.D. degree in anatomy from the University of Chicago in 1921.

Dr. Bast was a teacher of the biological sciences throughout his professional life. In the early years of his career he taught science at Tillotson College (1913–1915) and biology at Piedmont College (1915–1919).

Dr. Bast came to the University of Wisconsin in 1920 as assistant professor of anatomy and attained the rank of professor in 1933. In the years at Wisconsin he demonstrated an unusual capacity as a teacher, investigator and counselor of students. His success as a teacher is attested to by the large number of students who returned to his laboratory for advanced study.

Dr. Bast published seventy-eight scientific papers on a variety of subjects, often jointly with students and colleagues. For more than thirty years he studied intensively the development and the detailed structure of the ear. He was joined in this work by the senior author. Dr. Bast's collection of anatomical material for the study of the human ear is unmatched anywhere in the world and it will remain a legacy for future scholars. The accurate large scale models of the ear which Dr. Bast reconstructed from histological sections exemplify an innate manual dexterity which was also expressed in his wood carving and furniture making.

Dr. Bast's achievements won him an international reputation and honorary memberships in the American Otological Society, the Chicago Laryngological and Otological Society, and the Triological Society. In 1947 he was given the "Citation Award" from Ripon College for outstanding work in anatomy. He was "Honorary Medalist" of the American Otological Society in 1951.

Medical history was his true avocation. As a member and leader in the William Snow Miller Medical History Seminar, Dr. Bast published nineteen papers on historical subjects. Biographical sketches predominated, but the history of the University and other cognate subjects were recorded by his pen.

An account of the contributions of Dr. Bast to the University and Medical School would not be complete without reference to his final major extracurricular activity, which was the design and construction of the Bardeen Medical Laboratories. He had drawn many sets of preliminary plans before the opportunity for their realization came.

Dr. Bast was an active participant in community life. He served as trustee of the Village of Shorewood Hills, as Sunday School teacher and deacon of the Congregational Church, and always as a good neighbor.

BARRY J. ANSON

[1]Adapted from Document 1368 of April 6, 1959, Memorial Resolutions of the Faculty of the University of Wisconsin on the Death of Professor Theodore Hieronymus Bast. Memorial Committee: Maxine E. Bennett, O. A. Mortensen (Chairman), H. W. Mossman, H. H. Reese.

THE TRAGEDIE OF HAMLET

The Ghost speaks:

Sleeping within mine Orchard,
My custome always in the afternoone;
Upon my secure hower thy Uncle stole
With juyce of cursed Hebenon in a Violl,
And in the Porches of mine eares did poure
The leaperous Distilment; whose effect
Holds such an enmity with bloud of Man,
That swift as Quick-silver, it courses through
The naturall Gates and Allies of the Body;
And with a sodaine vigour it doth posset
And curd, like Aygre droppings into Milke,
The thin and wholsome blood: so did it mine;
. . . .
Thus was I, sleeping, by a Brothers hand,
Of Life, of Crowne, and Queene at once dispatcht . . .

From the Norton Facsimile of the First Folio
Special Collections Department
The University of Iowa Libraries

In the concept of bodily fabric and function held in Elizabethan and Caroline England, and in centuries backward in time to Graeco-Roman culture, man was an ambulatory sponge, through whose body coursed the humors and the spiritus—by way of thoracic and abdominal organs and cutaneous spiracular pores which both exuded sweat and admitted noxious vapors or elements. When lost inordinately, or depauperated in sustaining quality, the way was open to disease or death; from one body to the other the infectious irradiations could be passed to work their subtle malignity—especially in time of plague.

Thus, "like eager droppings into milk," the poison did curdle the King's once uncontaminated blood.

The way to each organ was open through every aperture, whether pore, meatus or maw. Even in our day, the movement of otologic fluids (in their restricted labyrinthine excursion) still offers problems of exchange whose solutions tend to elude our diligent searching.

PREFACE TO THE SECOND EDITION

An initial plan merely to revise the first edition of this book was supplanted by one more mature that called for the extension of sets of illustrations depicting the adult anatomy of the ear and the addition of a totally new part on development.

In the six-year period since the earlier edition left the press, several pertinent studies in morphology have been completed and reported in part at meetings of the Triological Society and of the American Otological Society, of the American Academy of Ophthalmology and Otolaryngology; these and other, unpublished, phases of the inclusive investigation are represented by picture and text in the present edition.

It has been the continuing experience of the authors that there exists an inalienable cousinage between the content of courses given to residents and the topics in a textbook designed, in part, to direct the professional hand. The purposes are in unity; the only difference lies in chronology.

The senior author has been privileged to use, uninterruptedly, the serially sectioned temporal bones in the Wisconsin Collection brought together by the late Professor Theodore H. Bast. Virtually all of the 117 photomicrographs comprising Part II of the present edition have been taken from sections in this monumental collection. Others from the same source appear in Part III. Dr. Otto A. Mortensen and Dr. James H. Brandenberg have fostered the project in every helpful way. To the list of Project Assistants working in Dr. Mortensen's department, for whose collaboration thanks have been previously expressed, we would now add the name of Michael J. Rensink, M.D.

For this edition and for its predecessor, the drawings, with a few exceptions, were prepared by George Buckley.

The authors, in every one of the variegated phases in the preparation of this edition, have been, as before, dependent upon the talents and zeal of Mrs. Patricia Edberg, Editorial Secretary. While possessing full comprehension of the research-purpose of the inclusive project of which publication of this book is one element, even the minutiae of syntax have never escaped her acute perception. On countless occasions her ability to act as knowledgeable intermediary between author and publisher has proved to be of the greatest aid.

A vote of thanks is due, and is gladly given, to the staff of the W. B. Saunders Company, whose clear-sighted guidance and perennial encouragement have made the preparation of this edition a stimulating endeavor.

The senior author wishes to pay special tribute to the memory of the late J. Gordon Wilson, M.D., Professor of Otolaryngology at Northwestern University Medical School. Dr. Wilson guided the conjoint program at Wisconsin and at Northwestern and secured vital financial aid from the American Otological Society at a time when there was no other source of supportive funds. The present study has been supported by the continuing aid of the Research Fund of the American Otological Society and the National Institutes of Health of the United States Public Health Service Grant No. NS 03855-10.

Iowa City, Iowa BARRY J. ANSON, PH.D. (MED. SC.)

Seattle, Washington JAMES A. DONALDSON, M.D.

PREFACE TO THE FIRST EDITION

The obligation of imparting requisite knowledge of man's anatomy has fallen to the courses in the basic sciences presented at postgraduate level. In the opinion of the present authors, the need for such instruction is nowhere more urgent than in the field of otology. This volume represents an effort to provide information in surgical anatomy needed in residency training and, later, in the practice of this specialty.

Whether offered in a book or as part of a curriculum for residency training, the fundamental purpose is the same. Therefore, the general pattern for the book is related to that of the Basic Science Course in the Department of Otolaryngology and Maxillofacial Surgery planned by Dr. Lierle and administered by Dr. Brain F. McCabe, Chairman of the Department of Otolaryngology and Maxillofacial Surgery. Dr. McCabe has read the proof of the text and examined the illustrations, especially in relation to service in the capacities named. The authors are grateful to him for critical appraisal of their undertaking.

It may be taken as established that a modern textbook of anatomy in a specialty must be preponderantly pictorial. In the present instance new illustrations were prepared from gross specimens and from serially sectioned temporal bones, the latter available in the collection of the late Professor Theodore H. Bast.

Since Dr. Bast's untimely death in 1959, it has been the senior author's privilege to continue the studies pursued in congenial and rewarding cooperation at Madison. Gratitude for this rare opportunity is due, and is hereby happily expressed, to Otto A. Mortensen, M.D., Chairman of the Department of Anatomy and Associate Dean at the University of Wisconsin. In every way possible Dr. Mortensen has aided in the extension of the collaborative program. Five graduate students in Dr. Mortensen's department have served in succession as Project Assistants in the course of this investigation: Shafik F. Richany, M.D.; Gerald P. Stelter, M.D.; Jerome R. Hanson, M.D.; David G. Harper, M.D.; and Thomas R. Winch, the present appointee, now in his fourth year in the College of Medicine.

For many years the senior author and his associates have benefited in their investigation by grants generously provided by the Central Bureau of Research of the American Otological Society. When the Committee on Neurological Diseases and Blindness expanded the initial program to include otological problems, funds were allocated by the U.S. Public Health Service.

The authors wish to express their thanks to Mrs. Patricia Edberg for her meticulous secretarial aid, both in work on the manuscript and in the arranging of engraver's proofs for the guidance of the Production Department at Saunders. For earlier contributory effort in the threefold capacity of secretary, linguist, and co-author, the writers are in equal debt to Mrs. Eycke Strickland.

For the selection of the photomicrographs, the authors are beholden to Thomas R. Winch; and for their preparation, to Mr. Homer Montague, Medical School Photographer, University of Wisconsin. Many of the special dissections of osseous specimens of temporal bones were carried out by Dr. Raymond L. Warpeha of the Department of Anatomy, Northwestern University Dental School. Dr. Warpeha's skilled and ingenious handling of the air-driven dental handpiece made possible the intricate demonstration of the internal structure of the petrous part of the temporal bone.

The successful production of any treatise dealing with morphology, especially one of atlas nature, requires the collaboration of an illustrator of exceptional ability. In the preparation of the present book, the authors were fortunate in having as their artist Mr. George Buckley of the Department of Medical Illustration. All drawings are products of his capable hand.

Many former colleagues and co-workers have contributed, albeit at the time unwittingly, to the fund of information requisite to the preparation of this volume. Any attempt to name them all would only lead to the unhappiness that comes of failing to do justice to those whose aid, however vital, was proffered in the early years of association. One name looms large in the roster of those upon whom the authors have more recently been dependent: Dr. Henry L. Williams, by his constructive criticism and through his stimulating acquaintance with the earlier literature in otology, has been largely responsible for the selection of topics in surgery, the bases of which always rest in structure.

Variegation in the course-work of the medical student spells need for a directive channel, an instrumentality for his burgeoning, somewhat nebulous fund of knowledge. For the authors such guidance was effectually provided by Professor Edward Allen Boyden in his anatomical teaching at Harvard Medical School for one, at the University of Minnesota for the other. The concept of the interdependence of anatomy and surgery would remain an empty maxim were it to lack administrative nurturing. Needed sustentation was provided by Dean M. Lierle, M.D. To Professor Boyden and Dr. Lierle this book is gratefully dedicated.

It is a source of pleasure and satisfaction to broaden an association with the W. B. Saunders Company. To work jointly with the members of their staff is to benefit by the availability of a broad and long-term experience in an honored craft and by gentlemanly discretion in imparting a mature form of bibliophilic guidance.

Iowa City, Iowa BARRY J. ANSON, PH.D. (MED. SC.)

Seattle, Washington JAMES A. DONALDSON, M.D.

CONTENTS

Part I The Temporal Bone

Part II The Ear: Developmental Anatomy

Part III The Ear: Adult Anatomy

Part I

THE TEMPORAL BONE

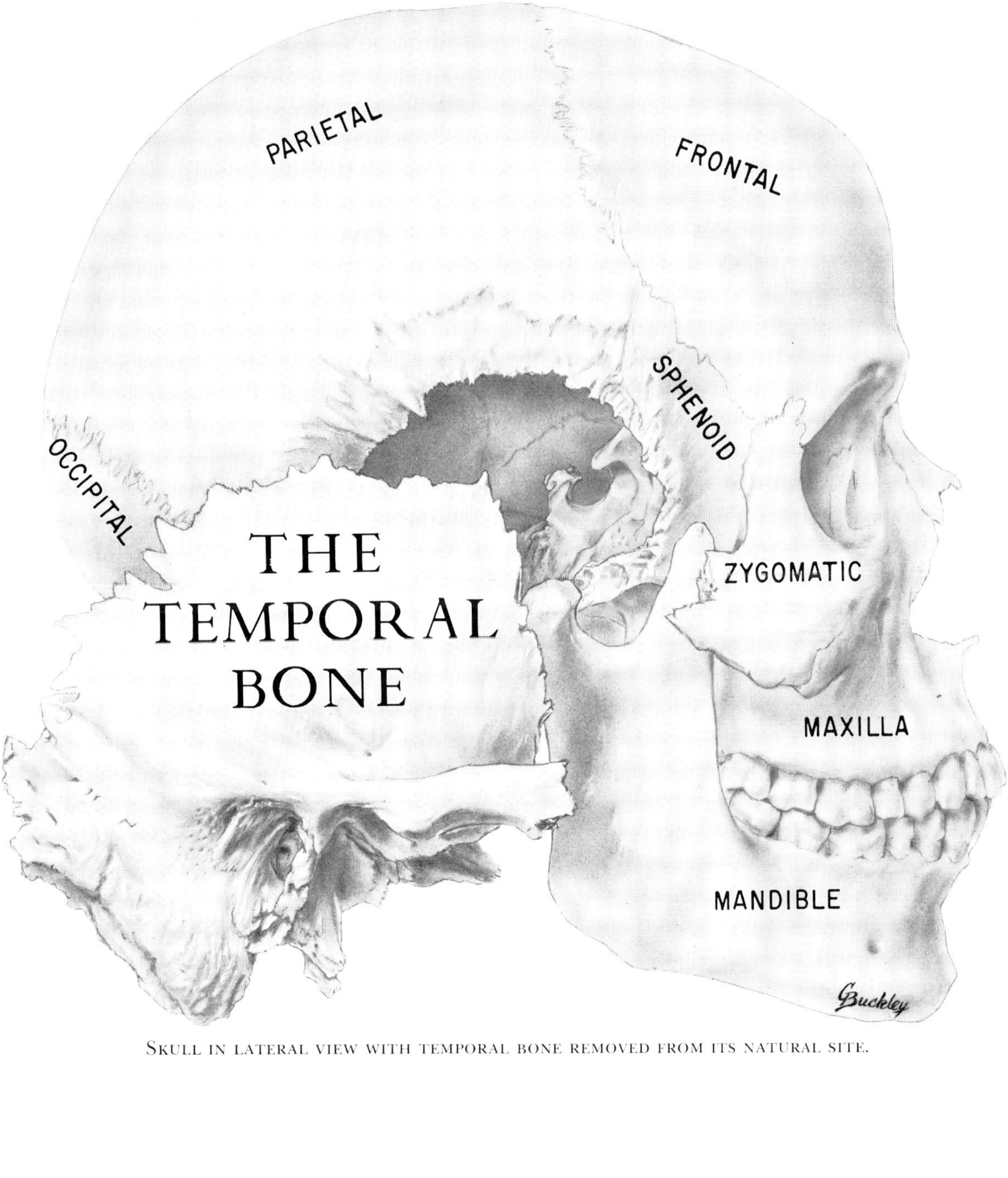

Skull in lateral view with temporal bone removed from its natural site.

The Temporal Bone

The paired temporal bones contribute to both the base and the lateral wall of the skull. For the cranial cavity, each forms part of the middle and posterior fossae.

Each bone is divisible into the following four parts: squamous, mastoid, petrous, and tympanic (Figures I–1 to I–9). When the pore of the external acoustic meatus is taken as a point of topographical reference, the squamous part is directed upward therefrom, the mastoid part backward, the tympanic forward and downward, and the petrous portion medianward. The temporal bone articulates with the sphenoid, parietal, and occipital bones.

SQUAMOUS PART

The squama is a vertical plate, the semicircular free border of which is serrate on the anterosuperior portion and beveled from within (Figures I–1 to I–6).

The *lateral surface*, for attachment of the temporal muscle, is smooth; the zygomatic process, for attachment of the masseter muscle, projects from its lower surface (Figures I–1 and I–5 to I–8). Below the root of the process is situated the mandibular fossa (Figure I–8). The sulcus for the middle temporal artery passes upward on the posterior part of the squama.

The *medial surface*, directed toward the middle cranial fossa, presents ledges and furrows matching the cerebral sulci and gyri, and a deep sulcus for the middle meningeal artery (Figures I–3 and I–4). The floor of the arterial sulcus and of its offsets is perforated at varying intervals; these foramina communicate with the channels of the diploic tissue.

MASTOID PART

This thick, conical projection from the squamous and petrous parts of the temporal bone comes into apposition with the occipital and parietal bones (Figure I–3).

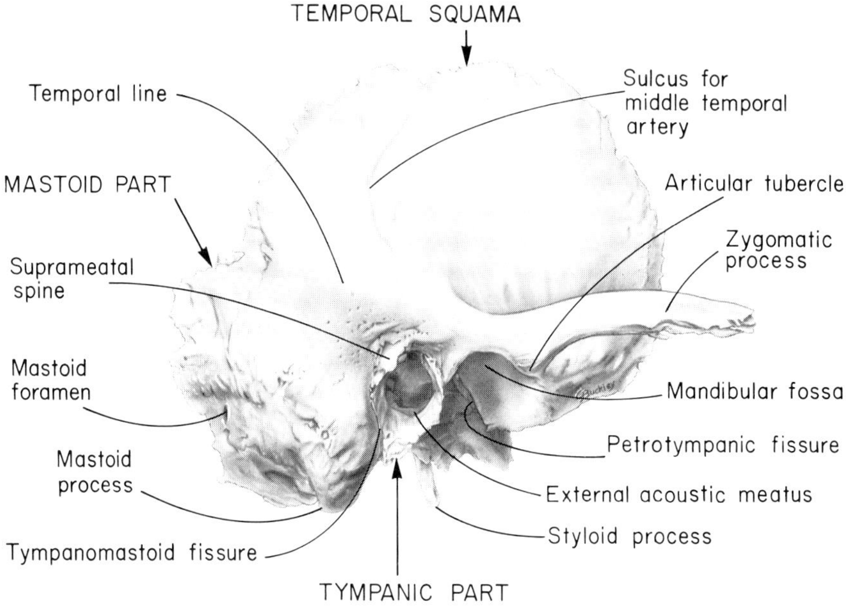

Figure 1–1. RIGHT TEMPORAL BONE. LATERAL VIEW.

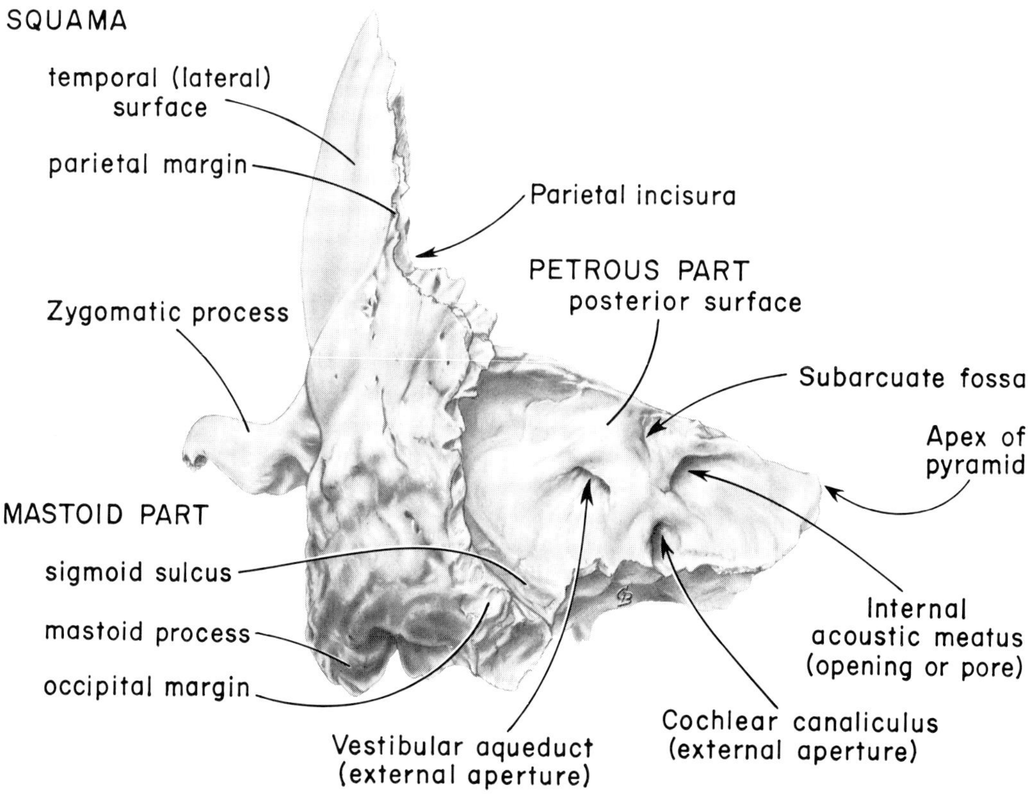

Figure 1–2. LEFT TEMPORAL BONE. POSTEROLATERAL VIEW.

The slightly roughened *lateral surface* gives attachment to the posterior auricular and the occipital muscles. It presents one or more foramina for transmission of the mastoid branch of the occipital artery and the mastoid emissary vein (Figure I–1). A small spur, the suprameatal spine, projects lateralward from the posterosuperior margin of the external acoustic pore (Figure I–1). The slightly depressed surface behind the spine is the mastoid fossa. It is perforated by numerous small foramina for the transmission of blood vessels. A thick, downward-directed portion, the mastoid process, gives attachment of musculature of the shoulder girdle and of the back.

The *medial surface* presents a deep groove, the sigmoid sulcus, for lodgement of the sigmoid venous sinus of the dura mater (Figures I–3 and I–4). Within the process are numerous cavities, the mastoid air cells, lined by mucous membrane that is continuous with that of the tympanic cavity.

PETROUS PART

This part of the temporal bone has been likened to a three-sided pyramid (Figures I–3 to I–8). The base, united with the mastoid part, is inserted into the angle between the occipital and sphenoid bones. A chink of irregular form, the *foramen lacerum,* intervenes between the apex and the sphenoid bone for transmission of the meningeal branch of the ascending pharyngeal artery. The internal carotid artery comes to lie in and partly occupy the foramen, but does not pass through it in a vertical direction. Three surfaces are presented for examination: anterior, posterior, and inferior.

The *anterior surface* is smooth; it forms part of the middle cranial fossa and inclines forward and downward (Figures I–3 and I–4). Laterally it is fused with the squama at the petrosquamosal fissure, where it goes over gradually into the medial (cerebral) surface of the squama (Figure I–5). The anterior margin (termed the anterior angle) is free and roughened; with the large wing of the sphenoid bone it bounds an opening, the musculotubal canal, subdivided by a leaflet of bone into a smaller upper part, the semicanal for the tensor tympani muscle and a larger lower portion, the semicanal of the auditory (eustachian) tube (Figure I–6). Near the middle of the anterior surface is the arcuate eminence, caused chiefly by the underlying superior semicircular canal (Figures I–4 to I–6). In a position lateral and anterior to this eminence a smooth area, the tympanic tegmen, forms a roof for the tympanic cavity (Figure I–5). Further in an anterior direction, toward the apex of the pyramid, two small openings occur, each with a groove running forward from it. The medial opening, termed the hiatus of the facial canal, leads inward to the knee (geniculum) of the facial canal (Figure I–6); it transmits the superficial petrosal branch of the middle meningeal artery and the greater superficial petrosal nerve. The lateral, and smaller, opening is the superior aperture of the tympanic canaliculus; through it

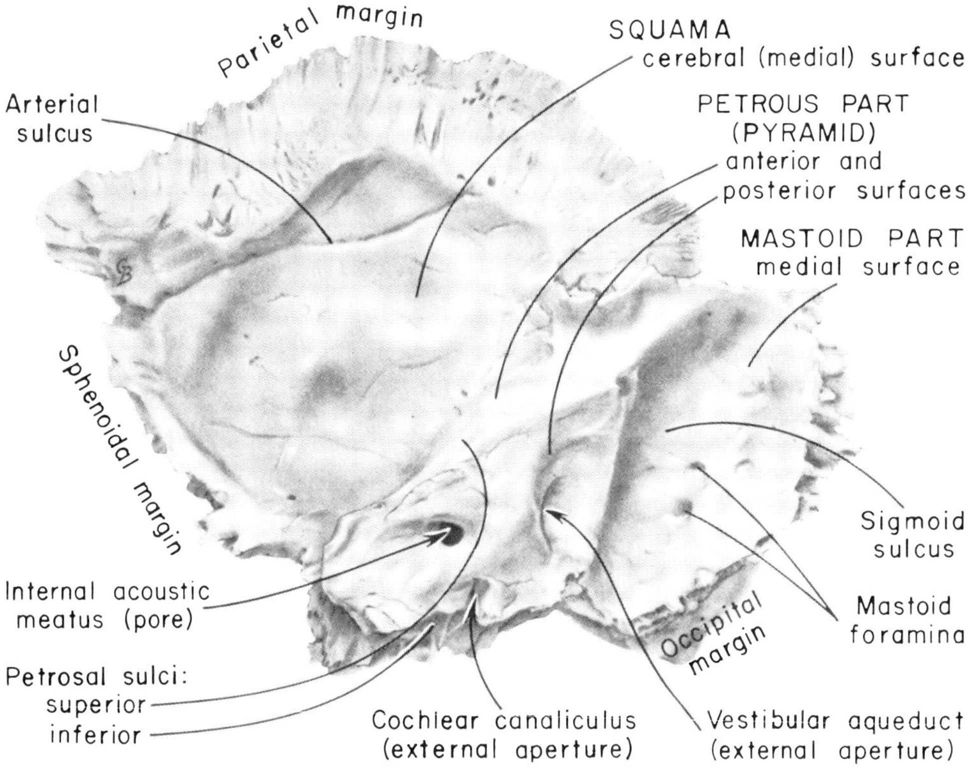

Figure I–3. Right temporal bone. Medial view.

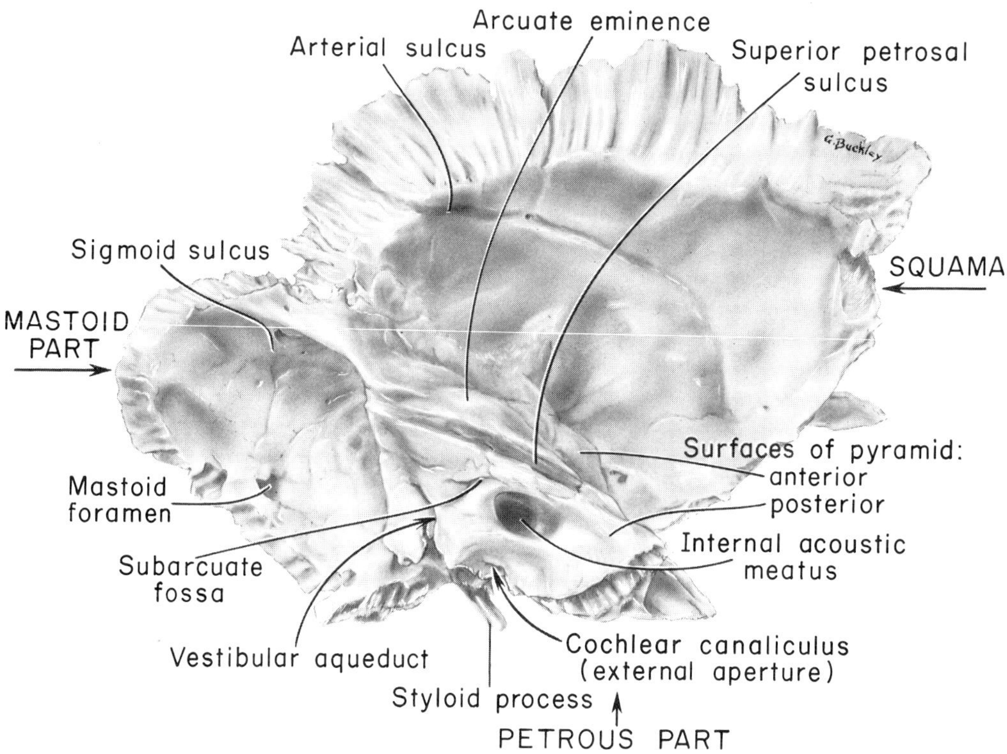

Figure I–4. Left temporal bone. Medial view.

pass the superior tympanic artery and the lesser superficial petrosal nerve. Near the apex is situated the trigeminal impression for the nerve of the same name.

The *posterior surface* lies in an almost vertical plane as it faces the posterior cranial fossa (Figures I–3 and I–4). It is bounded above, at the superior angle, by the sulcus for the superior petrosal sinus, the latter lodged in the attached margin of the cranial dura mater. Below, at the posterior angle, the pyramid unites with the occipital bone, the line of fusion accommodating the sulcus for the inferior petrosal sinus. On this posterior surface, about midway between the base and the apex of the pyramid, is situated the circular opening, or pore, of the internal acoustic meatus (Figures I–3 to I–5; also Figures III–103, III–128, and III–133); the latter is the short canal for the acoustic and facial nerves and the internal auditory blood vessels. Behind the opening of the meatus, between it and the superior petrosal sulcus, a small channel, the subarcuate fossa, passes inward, directed toward the arch of the superior semicircular canal (Figure I–4; also Figures III–111*a*, III–113*a*, and III–115*a*). It is a relatively capacious channel in the midterm fetus, carrying blood vessels into the developing otic capsule. It is minute, even of pinpoint caliber, in the adult, yet may still transmit small veins to the overlying *dura mater*. Further lateralward, downward and usually middistant between the internal acoustic meatus and the sigmoid sulcus, the vestibular aqueduct, for transmission of the endolymphatic duct and sac, opens upon the posterior surface of the pyramid (Figures I–3 and I–4; also Figures III–99, III–102 to III–104, III–106 and III–110 to III–118). This slitlike external aperture is overhung by a thin leaf of bone. The surface of the bone, distal to the aperture, is usually depressed, the foveate impression receiving the intradural segment of the endolymphatic sac.

The *inferior surface* of the pyramid lies in a horizontal plane (Figures I–7 and I–8). Unlike the other two surfaces, it is uneven and roughened for the attachment of muscles. The surface forms, with the occipital bone, the jugular foramen. The lateral part of the foramen contains the sigmoid portion of the transverse sinus; the medial part is occupied by the inferior petrosal sinus, the glossopharyngeal nerve and its superior ganglion, the vagus nerve and its jugular ganglion, and the accessory nerve. Just in front of the lateral compartment lies the broad fossa for the bulb of the jugular vein (Figures I–7 and I–8; also Figures III–110*a*, III–111*a*, III–112*a*, III–113*a*, III–114*a*, III–119, and III–130 to III–132). The mastoid canaliculus, for the auricular branch of the vagus (Arnold's nerve), opens into the fossa. In a median direction from the fossa is seen the funnel-shaped expansion, the external aperture of the cochlear canaliculus, containing the so-called perilymphatic "duct" (Figures I–3, I–4, I–7, and I–8; also Figures III–100, III–119, and III–130). Forward from the jugular fossa is situated a large circular opening, the external carotid foramen (Figures III–119 and III–130). This is the entrance to the canal for the internal carotid artery and its plexus of veins and sympathetic nerves (see internal carotid foramen, Figure I–6).

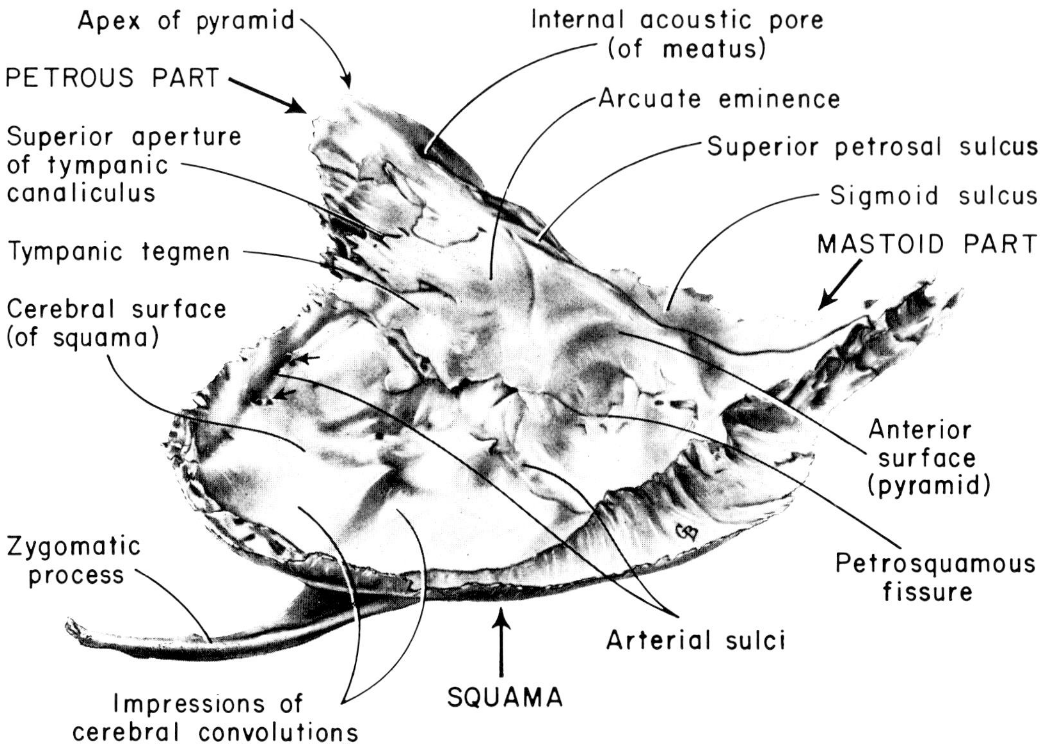

Figure I–5. Left temporal bone. Superior view.

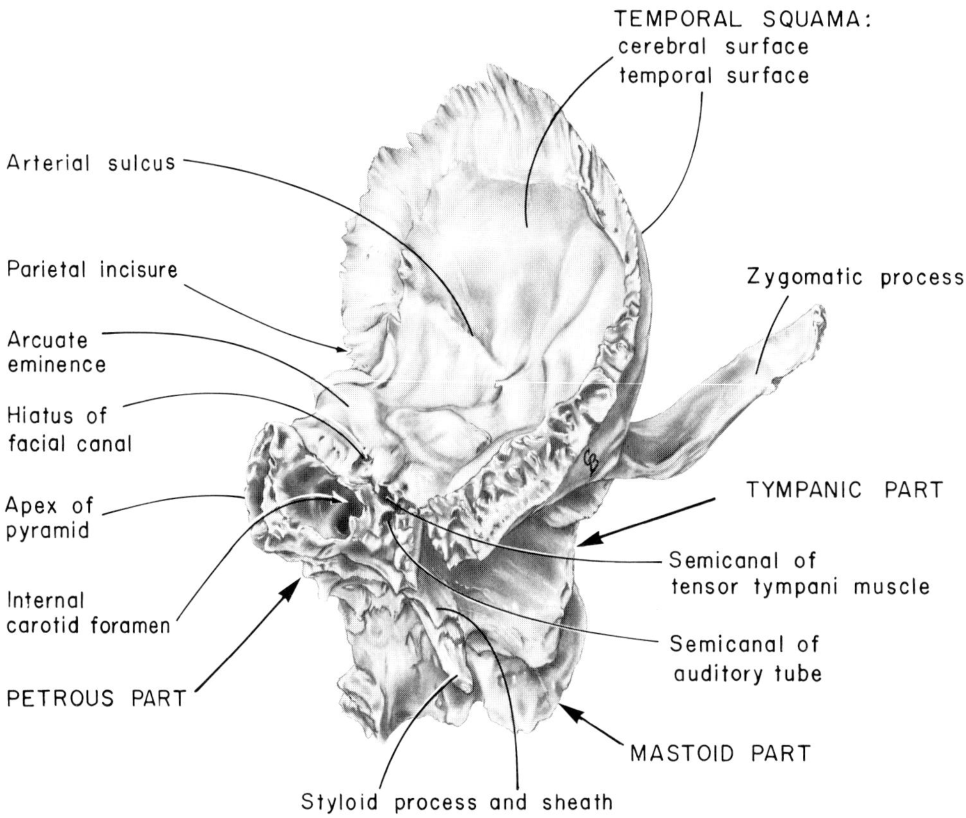

Figure I–6. Left temporal bone. Anterior view.

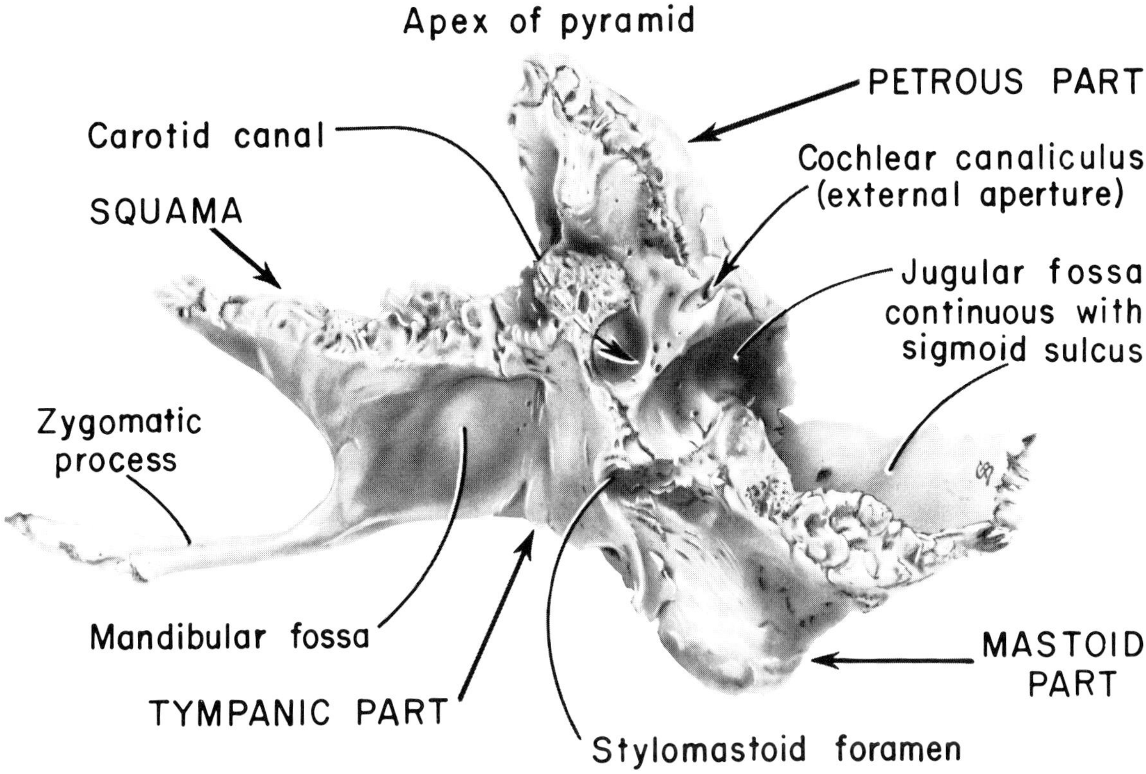

Figure 1–7. RIGHT TEMPORAL BONE. INFERIOR VIEW.

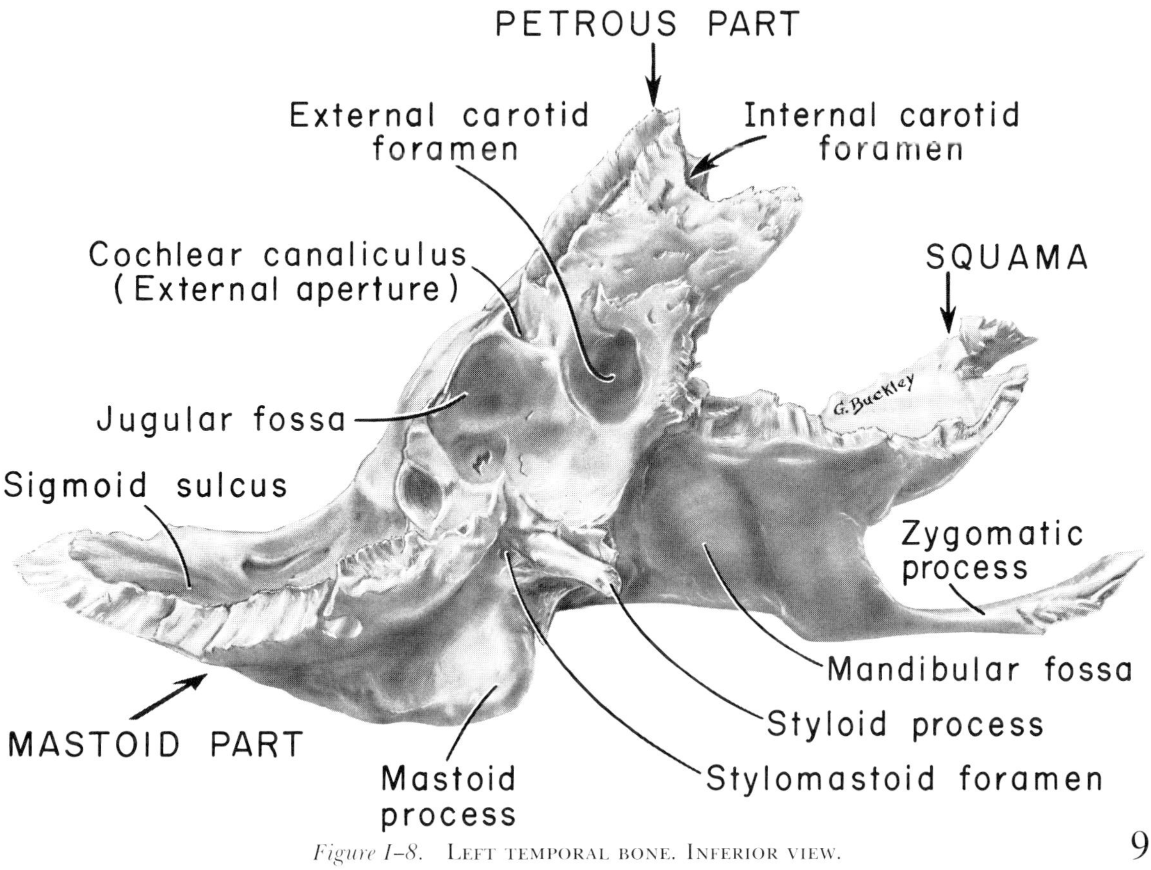

Figure 1–8. LEFT TEMPORAL BONE. INFERIOR VIEW.

Near the external foramen are small openings, the caroticotympanic canaliculi, for transmission of the artery and the nerves of the same name into the middle ear. The inferior aperture of the carotid canal is separated from the jugular fossa by the carotid ridge, on the edge of which is situated the petrosal fossula for lodgement of the petrosal ganglion of the glossopharyngeal nerve. At the bottom of this fossula a minute opening, the tympanic canaliculus, transmits the tympanic branch of the glossopharyngeal nerve (Jacobson's nerve) and the small tympanic branch from the ascending pharyngeal artery. Behind the jugular fossa is situated the rough jugular surface, articulating with the similarly named process of the occipital bone. On the lateral side of this surface is the downward-directed cylindrical spur, the styloid process, with the stylomastoid foramen at its base (Figures I–1, I–4, I–7, I–8, and I–10). It is subject to great variation in size, and sometimes is absent; when long, the process may reach the hyoid bone. The stylomastoid foramen, which is the external orifice of the facial canal, transmits the facial nerve, the stylomastoid artery, and in some cases, the auricular branch of the vagus nerve. A sheath of bone, attached to the styloid process anteriorly, is the lowest portion of the tympanic part of the temporal bone (Figure III–119). In a posterior direction run the mastoid incisure and the temporal groove; the former serves for attachment of the digastric muscle, in the latter courses the occipital artery (Figures I–9 and I–10*d*).

TYMPANIC PART

The tympanic portion of the temporal bone is a thin plate of roughly quadrilateral form (Figure I–1). It is hollowed out above, somewhat concave in front and below; it forms all of the anterior and inferior walls and part of the posterior wall of the external acoustic meatus (Figure I–9). The middle of the anteroinferior surface is thin, sometimes presenting a small foramen (of Huschke) that represents a nonossified portion of the plate (Figure II–13). The posterosuperior surface faces the external acoustic meatus and the tympanic cavity; at its medial end is a narrow groove, the tympanic sulcus, deficient superiorly, which receives the tympanic membrane. The inferior surface is prolonged into the vaginal process which ensheaths the lateral aspect of the base of the styloid process (Figures I–6 and III–119).

SUTURES AND OSSIFICATION

ARTICULATIONS

The temporal bone articulates with the occipital, parietal, sphenoid, and zygomatic bones, and—by a movable joint—with the mandible. Articulations are formed also with the auditory ossicles and the hyoid bone through the intermediation of ligaments. In some instances the squamous portion presents a process that articulates with the frontal (Figure I–11).

OSSIFICATION

Of the triad of parts that constitute the temporal bone at birth, the squama and tympanic parts develop in membrane, the petrous part in cartilage (see pages 79 to 80). The squama is formed from one center that appears as early as the eighth week, ossification extending into the zygomatic process that grows concurrently with the squama. At the outset the inferior border is nearly straight but soon assumes its characteristic concave shape. The postglenoid tubercle is conspicuous at birth, and at the hind end of the squama there is a process that comes into relation with the tympanic antrum and contributes to the mastoid portion of the adult bone. The center for the tympanic part appears from the ninth to the tenth fetal week. At birth it forms an incomplete ring, open above (see pages 32 to 34). The anterior extremity terminates in a small irregular process, and the medial aspect presents, in the lower half of its circumference, a groove for the reception of the tympanic membrane.

Up to the middle of the fifth month the cartilaginous petrous portion is represented by the otic capsule; it then ossifies so rapidly that by the end of the sixth month its chief portion is converted into porous bone. The ossific material appears in 14 centers, each one of which is trilaminar (see pages 79 to 86).

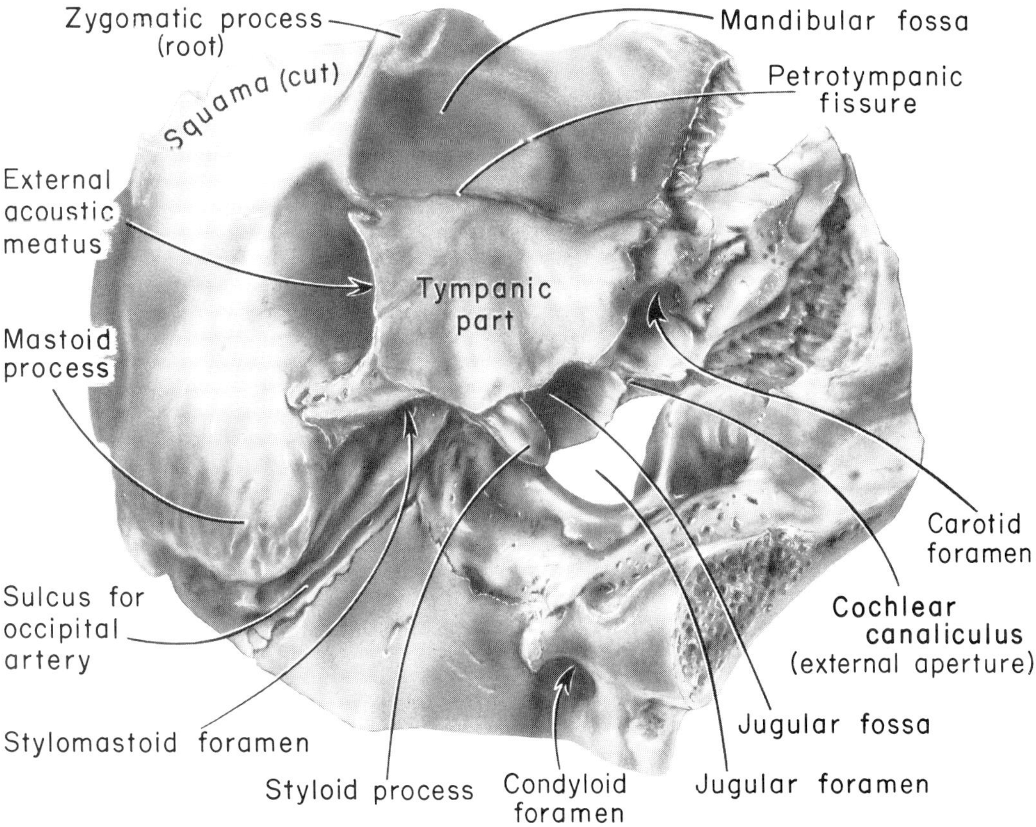

Figure I–9. RIGHT TEMPORAL BONE, INFERIOR SURFACE, WITH RELATED OCCIPITAL BONE.

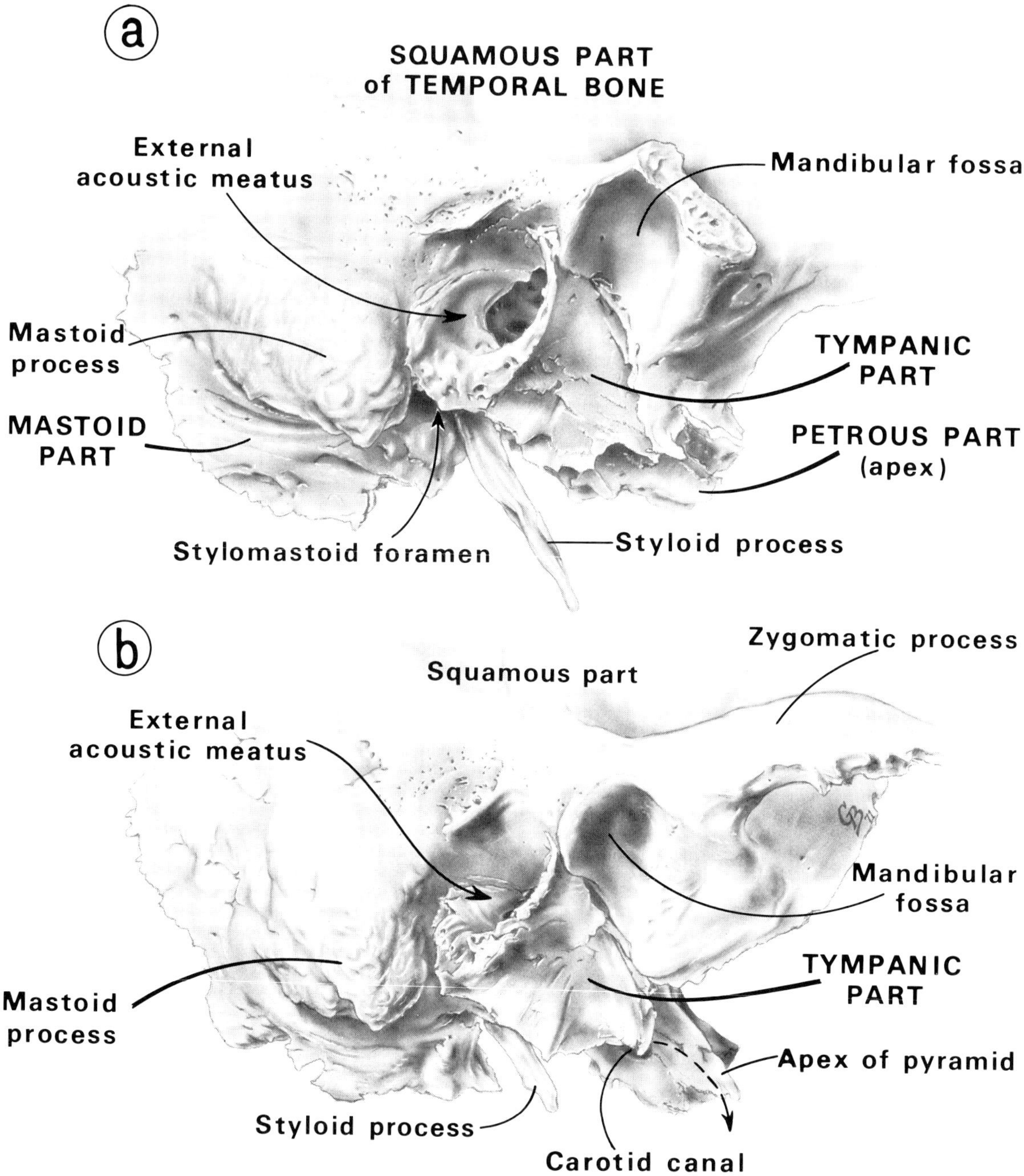

Figure I–10. TEMPORAL BONES, SELECTED SPECIMENS: INFEROLATERAL VIEW. TO DEMONSTRATE ESPECIALLY VARIATIONAL ANATOMY IN THE TYMPANIC AND RELATED PARTS.

a. A specimen with a large styloid process. *b.* A specimen with a styloid process of average prominence. *c.* A specimen sharing an expansive tympanic part with absence of a styloid process. *d.* An example of a small tympanic part, styloid process lacking.

Figure I–10 continues on the opposite page.

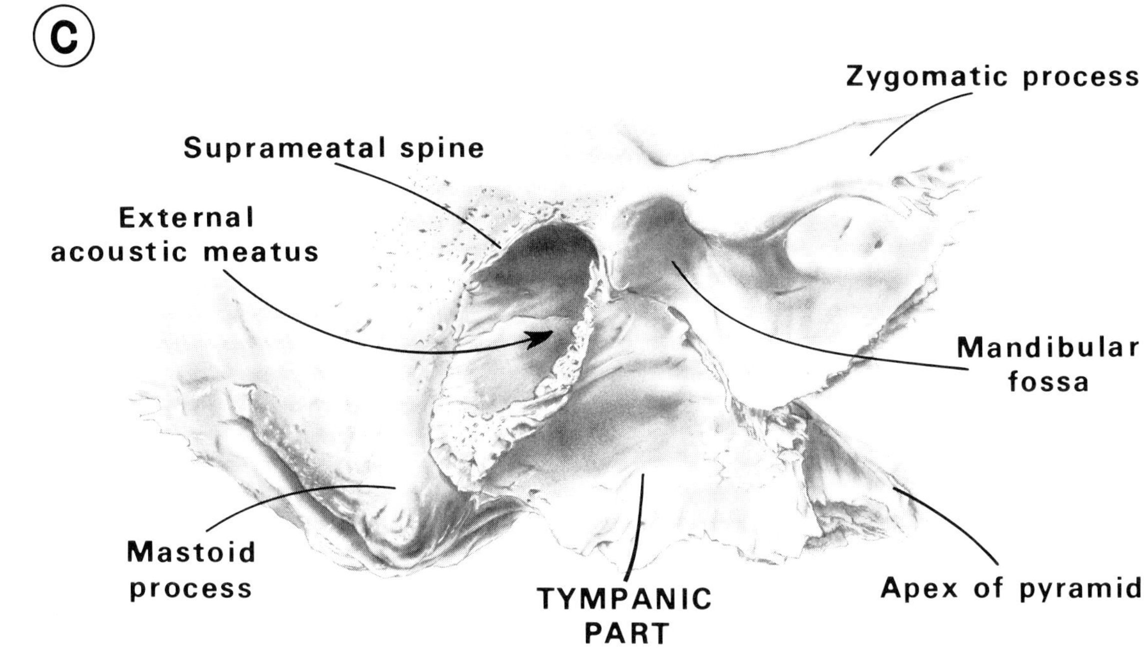

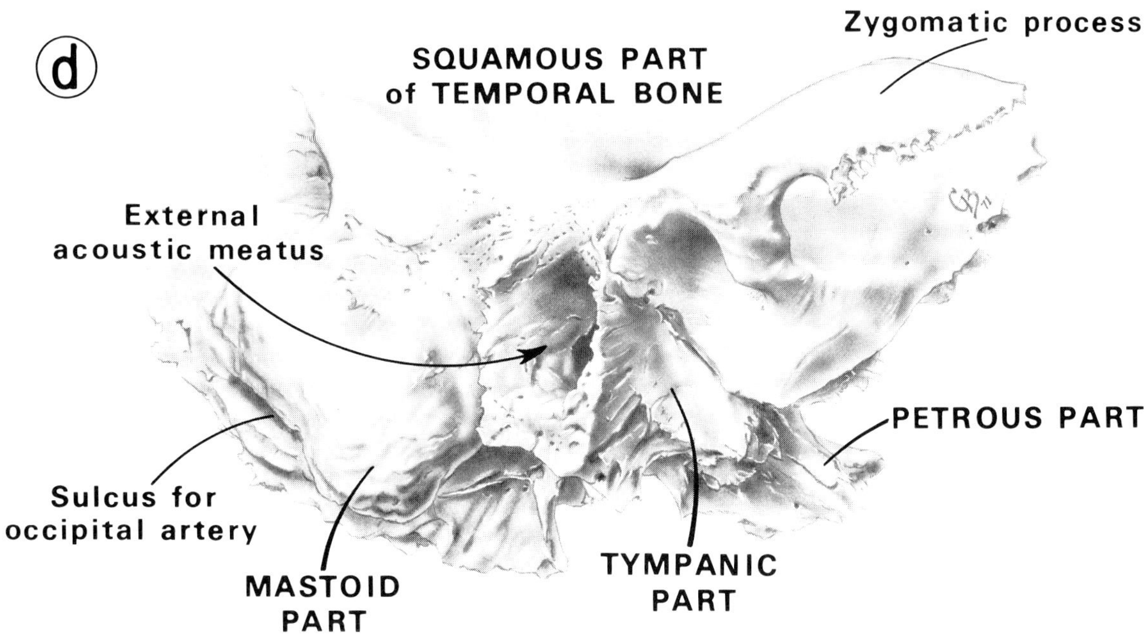

Figure 1–10, Continued.

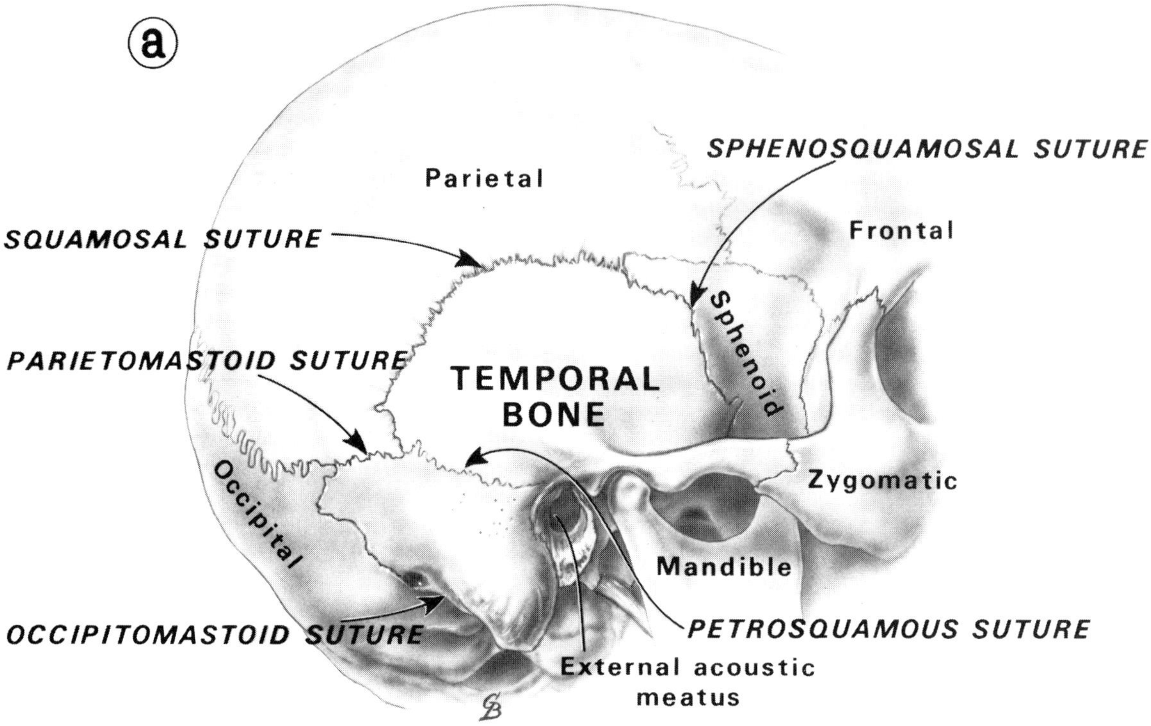

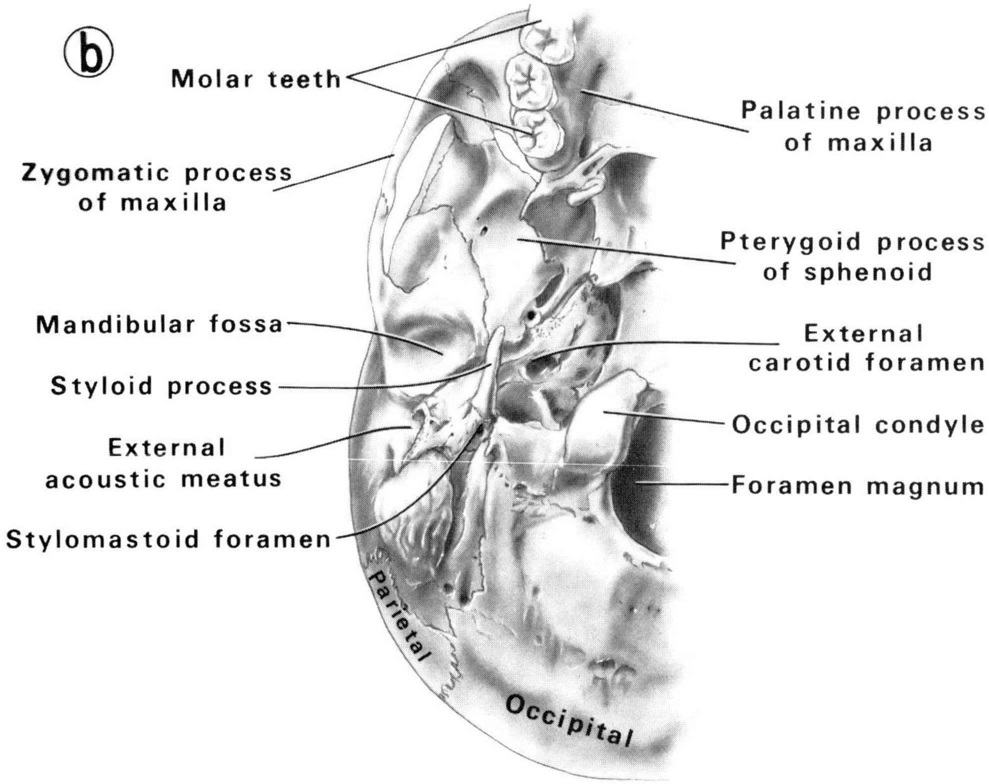

Figure I–11. CRANIUM, EMPHASIZING THE RELATIONSHIP OF THE TEMPORAL BONE TO OTHER SKELETAL ELEMENTS. *a.* SEEN FROM THE RIGHT SIDE. *b.* VIEWED FROM BELOW (RIGHT HALF OF THE CRANIUM).

a. Demonstrating especially the sutures of the squamous, mastoid, and tympanic parts of the temporal bone. *b.* Showing the relationships of the temporal bone to the sphenoid, frontal, parietal, and occipital bones.

Part
II

THE EAR: Developmental Anatomy

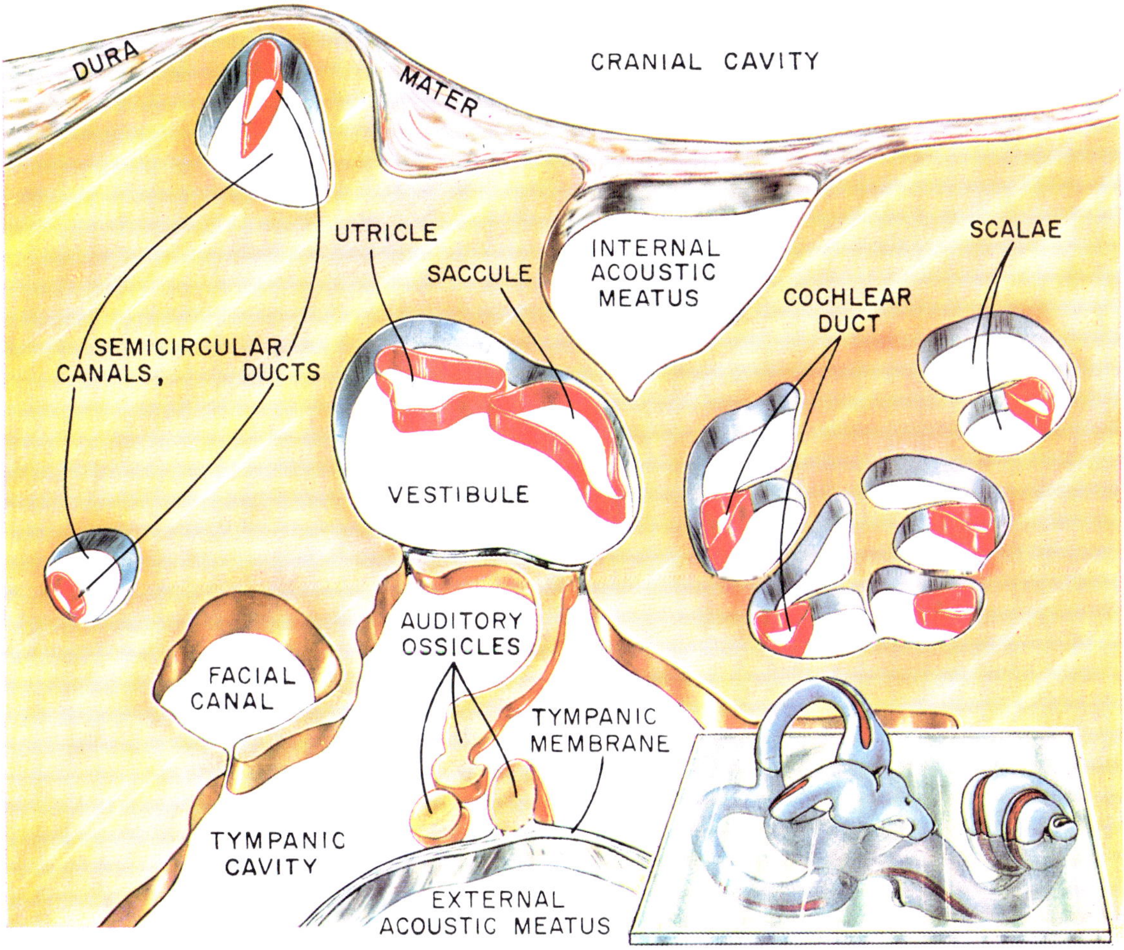

Parts of the ear, shown semischematically. Newborn (4-day premature).

A segment of a reconstruction prepared from a transversely sectioned temporal bone. *Inset.* Recording the plane of section and the approximate thickness of the segment shown in the main figure.

Wisconsin Collection, series 124.

(Adapted from Anson and Bast: Quart. Bull., Northwestern Univ. Med. Sch., 32: 307–325, 1958.)

Clinical Significance of Developmental Anatomy

Appreciation of developmental anatomy is nowhere so important as it is in the study of the structure of the ear and the temporal bone.

This is true for the following reasons: the external ear is a derivative of an embryonic branchial groove; the space of the middle ear is an extension of a primitive pharyngeal pouch; the auditory ossicles are, for the greater part, remodeled segments of the branchial skeleton; although adult dimensions are reached by the labyrinthine spaces and their osseous walls in the fifth month of intrauterine life, the histologic fabric of the investing otic capsule and that of the ossicles remains fetal throughout life.

The ear, like the brain, is a derivative of the outer layer of the embryonic head. But unlike the brain which begins as an elongate axial unfolding, the primordium of the ear is a rotund vesicle. The ear and the brain are alike in their loss of connection with the parental ectoderm. However, they differ profoundly in what happens to them in the course of continuing morphogenesis as the following observations will establish. Whereas the cavity of the neural tube becomes a minute channel of no sensory use, that of the otocyst is all-important, since it will contain the endolymph of the epithelial duct system.

The brain, as it undergoes histogenesis from a simple tube, grows into the second postnatal year; the membranous labyrinth, following precipitate fetal growth and differentiation, retains the dimensions which it attained in the fifth month of intrauterine life. The osseous capsule by which the labyrinth becomes invested – unlike the other bones of the cranium and unlike a typical long bone which grows for more than twenty years – maintains (in its trilaminar structure) a fetal fabric throughout a person's lifetime. In fact, the otic (osseous) capsule, having no areas of "epiphyseal" development, is as large as it will ever be in the fetus of approximately five months. The elements which bring a sequestered labyrinth-within-labyrinth system into functional association with the surrounding air are derived (as elements in a chain) from a branchial apparatus which, in aquatic and amphibious creatures, serves as a respiratory mechanism. In their refashioned state they keep much of the fetal fabric, some even of embryonic source.

The ectoderm which lines the first branchial groove (between the mandibular and hyoid arches) contributes the cutaneous lining of the external acoustic meatus. The two arches which thus bound the groove give rise to the auricle; in the depth of the groove the ectoderm contributes the cuticular layer to the trilaminar tympanic membrane. The entoderm of the primitive pharynx forms a pouch by pressing outward toward the ectoderm at the site of each groove. The groove becomes the elongate auditory (eustachian) tube, the tympanic cavity, and the latter's pneumatic extensions. From the third layer, the mesoderm, arise the remaining elements of the ear, namely, the cartilage and the muscles of the external ear, as well as the auditory ossicles and their associated muscles and ligaments of the middle ear.

The clinical significance of developmental anatomy in otology manifests itself in many ways, both in the field of variational structure and in that of anomalous architecture—medialward from the auricle on the side of the head to the saccus on the wall of the posterior cranial fossa.

Arrested development of the ear may occur in such interrelationship of features as to alert the surgeon. Thus, on the basis of association with an externally evident anomaly he may look for the existence of malformations deeply placed (and therefore out of view). For example, an atrophic auricle or an atretic external acoustic meatus may point to the occurrence of an underdeveloped tympanum and of an aberrant ossicular chain with individual "lines" being incomplete, ankylosed (that is, retaining blastemal continuity), or even totally absent. In this category belongs nonpathological fixation of the stapedial base along the normal site of the annular ligament of the vestibular (oval) window—a circumstance owing to failure in segregation of the footplate from the otic capsule (of which the former was primordially a part).

The highly variegated pattern of pneumatization would be baffling in want of appreciation of the process by which the epithelium of the pharyngeal diverticulum replaces tissue already present—mesenchymal tissue in the middle ear and osseous in the differentiating bone of the *pars petrosa.* This picture accounts for the existence of an endless variety in the types of mastoid pneumatization—increasingly important in surgical progress through an exenterated mastoid part of the temporal bone. Knowledge of the time-sequence of air cell development leads to appraisal (in the infant and the child) of the probable effect of infection on mastoid pneumatization and its relation to capacity for spread of infection.

From the external ear, through the tympanic cavity—with its contents and communications—to the internal ear, a knowledge of developmental anatomy serves to explain surgically important departure from the structural "norm." This statement applies forcibly to the differences in the size, form, and relation of the endolymphatic sac and to variations in the anatomy of the internal acoustic meatus, the jugular fossa, the facial canal, and the canaliculus of the chorda tympani.

The equally consequential applications will come with the widening scope of otologic surgery.

Progression of Development

Figures II–1 to II–7

The human statoacoustic organ rose to present complexity from a humble beginning that is only partly predictive of its service in the human ear. In the shark, a structurally simple aquatic creature, the primordial element (called the *otocyst*) retains its original connection with the parental ectoderm (Figure II–1). Even after the auditory pit has become a vesicle, the contained fluid remains one with the circumambient water of the sea.

In man, ectodermal continuity is lost in the early embryo; the contained fluid thereupon becomes the embryo's very own. Any change in its chemistry will henceforth depend upon processes that are shared with the general physiological economy of the whole body.

The otocyst is now a sequestered epithelial sac. It must undergo profound change so that, on the day of emergence from an "aquatic" habitation in the amnion, new connections will have been made to put its own fluid (the endolymph, not sea water) into physical relationship with the air of the postnatal terrestrial environment (Figure II–2). Thereby the stage is set for a series of remarkable modifications, involving both salvage and alteration. As a result, *air* is brought to act upon *fluid* through the intermediation of an osseous *chain*—parts of a branchial system useless on land. In the course of refashioning, the first visceral (branchial) groove is converted into the external acoustic meatus; the first and second branchial arches into the auditory ossicles; and the first visceral pouch into the auditory tube, tympanic cavity, and related air spaces. A mechanism for aquatic respiration, by these changes, is altered to subserve the function of hearing (Figures II–3 and II–4).

This brief review of phylogenetic salvage suggests that familiarity with the teachings of embryology is nowhere more important than in the study of the structure of the ear and temporal bone. A comparison of the structure of the ear in four crucial stages (Figures II–3 to II–6) will both establish these facts and prepare the way for presentation of adult anatomy.

In the 9-week fetus, the external ear is represented by an elevation marginal to the first pharyngeal groove and by a sulcus anterior thereto (Figure II–4); the elevation will become the auricle, or pinna, while

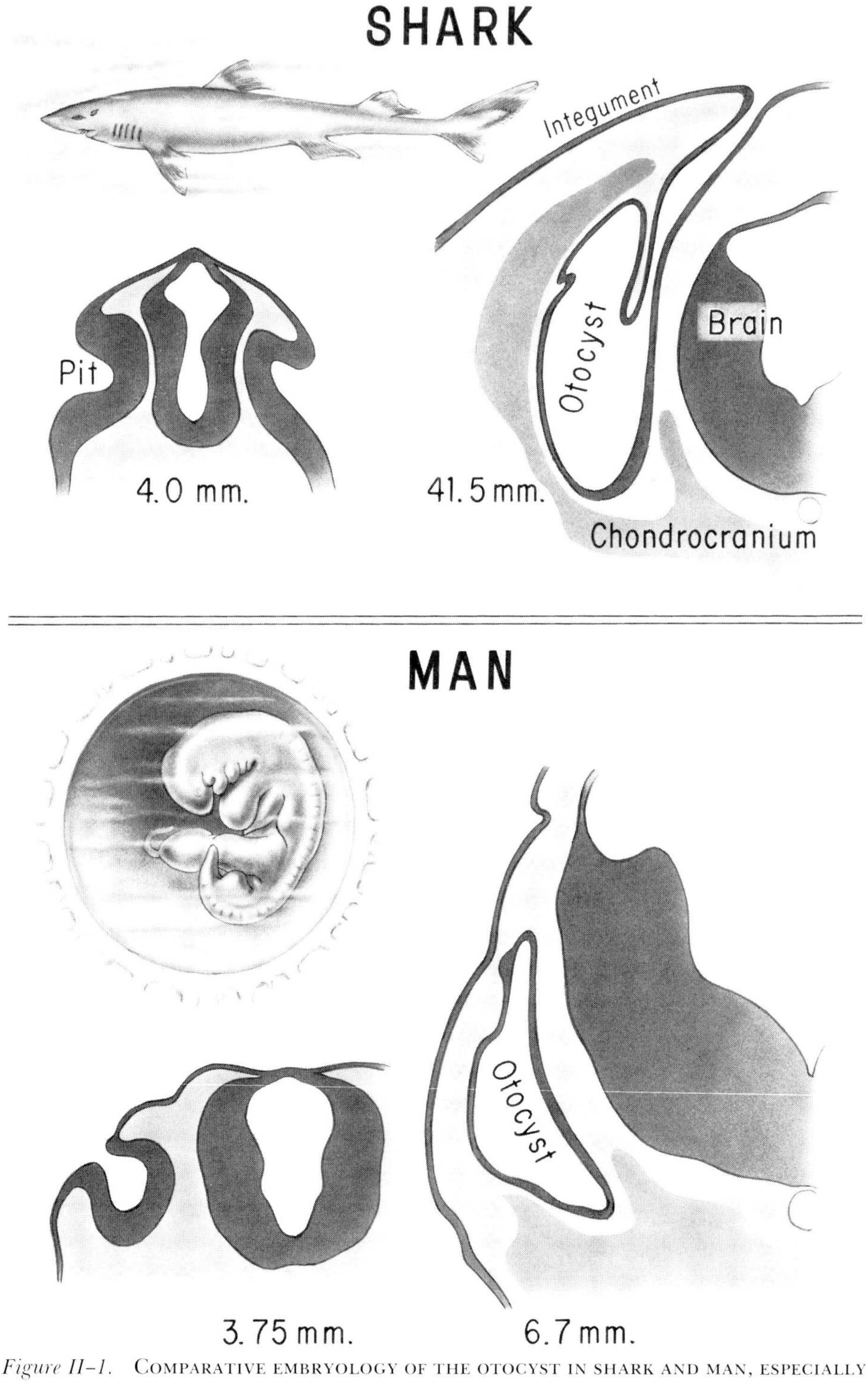

Figure II-1. Comparative embryology of the otocyst in shark and man, especially in relation to environment.

Sections from the Harvard Collection.
(From Anson: Trans. Amer. Acad. Ophthal. Otolaryng., 73:17–38, 1969.)

the sulcus will deepen to form the external acoustic meatus. The middle ear is a slitlike diverticulum of the first pharyngeal pouch which is approaching, and presently will invest, the auditory ossicles. The internal ear is represented by the endolymphatic duct system, lodged in mesenchymal tissue within which early vacuolization predicts the formation of the perilymphatic labyrinth. The cartilaginous otic capsule invests the labyrinth.

In the fetus of approximately 23 weeks, the cochlea has attained full dimensions and the periotic spaces are well formed (Figure II–5). The inner periosteal layer of bone has encircled the labyrinth, except in the territory of the fissula ante fenestram, where cartilage may persist even in the adult temporal bone. Ossification is retarded in the canalicular division of the otic capsule, where cartilage becomes spongy from the activity of invasive buds of vascular tissue; these enter through the subarcuate fossa, which at this stage is a relatively ample excavation. This process makes possible expansion in the arcs of the semicircular ducts. Concurrently, the ossicles are undergoing initial ossification.

In the developmental progress between the sixth and ninth month of fetal life, the internal (periosteal) layer does not change; it remains a thin boundary for the perilymphatic and endolymphatic labyrinthine systems (Figure II–6). The middle layer solidifies, while the outer (periosteal) layer increases rapidly in thickness. The concurrent changes account for the density that is characteristic of the mature bone.

Many of the elements of the ear are derived from the branchial apparatus, which in aquatic and amphibious creatures serves a respiratory function. In the process of conversion to new phylogenic use, the three germ layers contribute to the formation of the embryonic ear (Figure II–7).

The *ectoderm*, which lines the first branchial groove (between the mandibular and hyoid arches), contributes the cutaneous lining of the external acoustic meatus. The two arches which thus bound the depression give rise to the auricle through the production and subsequent fusion of nodular elevations on the facing margins. In the depth of the groove the ectoderm contributes the cuticular layer to the trilaminar tympanic membrane. Ectoderm is also the source layer of the epithelial duct system that is the membranous labyrinth. It begins as a thickening in a position dorsal to the first branchial groove. This placode becomes cup-shaped, then, successively, the following: a vesicle still attached by a stalk to the parent layer; an otocyst independent of the ectoderm; and finally, by growth and differentiation into parts, the labyrinthine (endolymphatic) duct system of the internal ear.

The *entoderm* of the primitive pharynx forms an entodermal pouch by pressing outward toward the ectoderm at the site of the corresponding branchial groove. The groove, situated between the first (mandibular) and second (hyoid) arches and supported, respectively, by Meckel's and Reichert's cartilages, becomes the elongate auditory (eustachian) tube. It also gives rise to the tympanic cavity and the latter's pneumatic extensions—namely, the tympanic antrum, epitympanic recess, the air

(Text continues on page 29.)

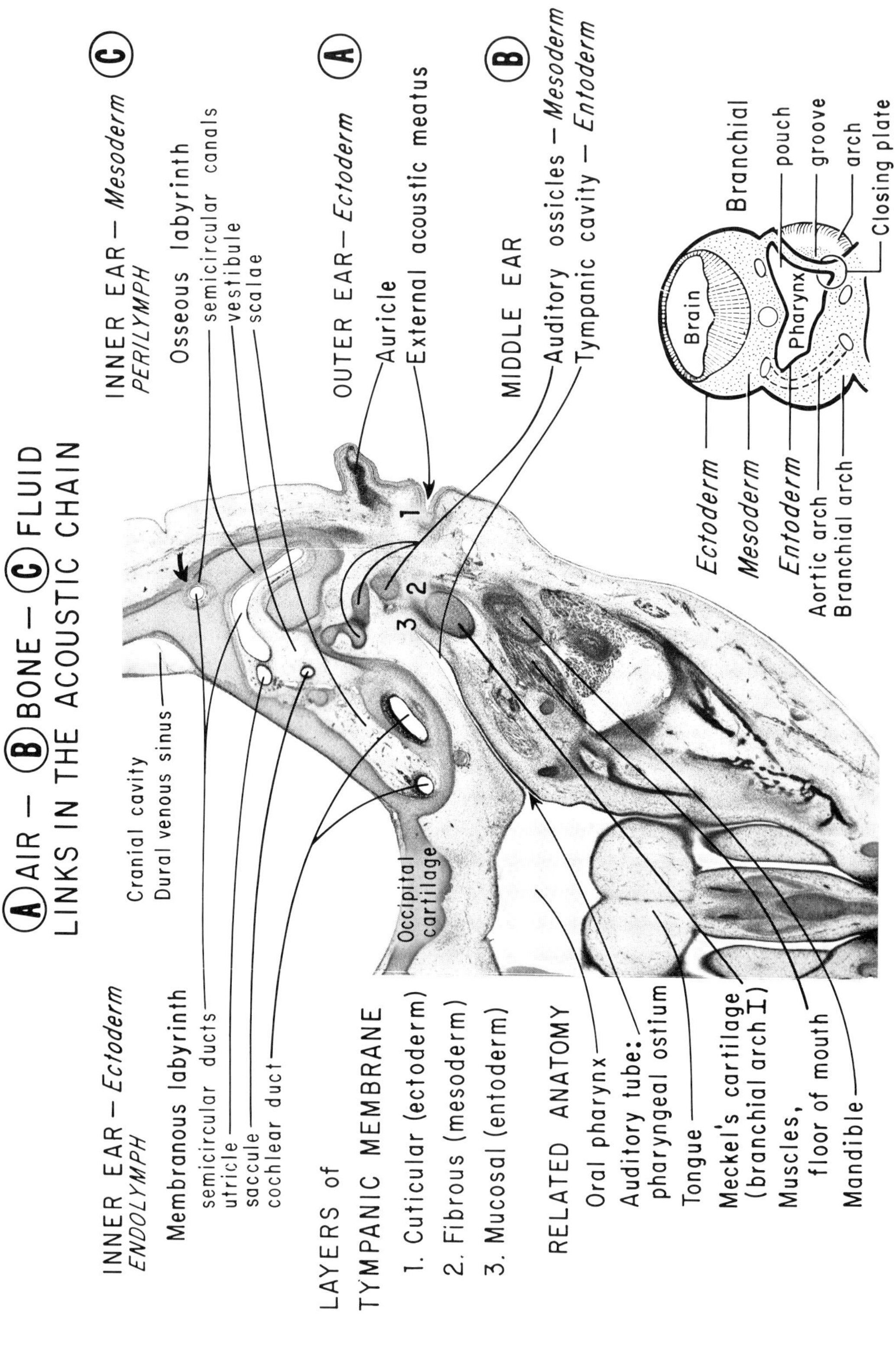
(A) AIR – (B) BONE – (C) FLUID
LINKS IN THE ACOUSTIC CHAIN
INNER EAR – Ectoderm
ENDOLYMPH
Membranous labyrinth
semicircular ducts
utricle
saccule
cochlear duct
LAYERS of
TYMPANIC MEMBRANE
1. Cuticular (ectoderm)
2. Fibrous (mesoderm)
3. Mucosal (entoderm)
RELATED ANATOMY
Oral pharynx
Auditory tube:
pharyngeal ostium
Tongue
Meckel's cartilage
(branchial arch I)
Muscles,
floor of mouth
Mandible
Cranial cavity
Dural venous sinus
Occipital cartilage
1
2
3
INNER EAR – Mesoderm (C)
PERILYMPH
Osseous labyrinth
semicircular canals
vestibule
scalae
OUTER EAR – Ectoderm (A)
Auricle
External acoustic meatus
MIDDLE EAR (B)
Auditory ossicles – Mesoderm
Tympanic cavity – Entoderm
Brain
Pharynx
Branchial
pouch
groove
arch
Closing plate
Ectoderm
Mesoderm
Entoderm
Aortic arch
Branchial arch

Figure II–2. CONVERSION OF THE PARTS OF THE BRANCHIAL SYSTEM AND THE RELATED LABYRINTHS TO ACOUSTIC SERVICE IN A TERRESTRIAL ENVIRONMENT. FETUS OF 9 WEEKS (40 MM.). *Inset.* BRANCHIAL ELEMENTS, SCHEMATIZED.

Air waves, conducted inward by the auricle and the external acoustic meatus, are transmitted to the labyrinthine fluids through the movement of the three bones of the ossicular chain, serving as "intermediaries" in the tympanic cavity between the tympanic membrane and the vestibular fenestra (oval window).

The auricle, the external acoustic meatus and the outer (cuticular) layer of the tympanic membrane are derivatives of the ectoderm of the first pharyngeal groove (*A*). The auditory tube, the tympanic cavity and the inner (mucosal) layer of the tympanic membrane are derived from the entoderm of the first pharyngeal pouch, the latter prolonged toward the corresponding ectodermal groove from the wall of the pharynx (*B*). The auditory ossicles (malleus, incus, and stapes) are refashioned, so to speak, from the cartilaginous branchial arches. Laterally, in the tympanic cavity, the manubrium of the malleus will become attached to the tympanic membrane; medially, the base (footplate) of the stapes will occupy the vestibular window in the lateral wall of the otic capsule. Within the capsule, perilymphatic spaces are forming in the reticulum whose source, like that of the capsule itself, is mesoderm (*C*).

The fundamental element, and the one first to appear, is the otocyst. Primordially a plaque on the ectoderm in the region of the hindbrain, it becomes depressed below the surface as a pit. Next, losing continuity with the parental layer, it attains the form of an otocyst lodged in the mesenchyma (mesoderm). Finally, the originally simple ectodermal vesicle will undergo regional differentiation into the following: the cochlear duct (between the scalae of the perilymphatic system), the utricle and saccule (in the vestibule), the endolymphatic and associated ducts, and the semicircular ducts (in the canals).

Transverse section, Wisconsin Collection, series 168.

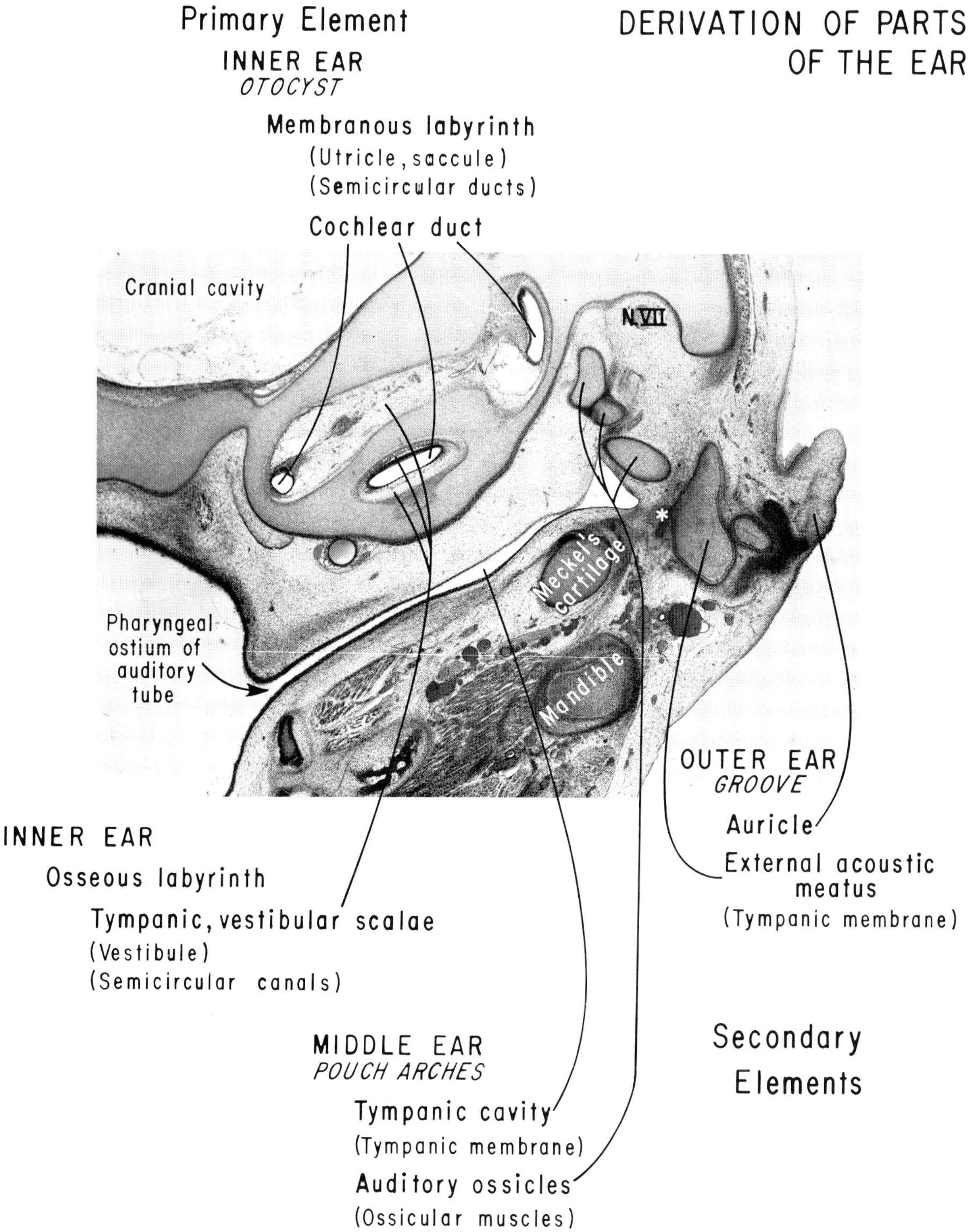

Figure II–3. TRANSFORMATION OF THE BRANCHIAL AND RELATED EMBRYONIC STRUCTURES RESULTING IN PRODUCTION OF AN AUDITORY MECHANISM. FETUS OF 11½ WEEKS (62 MM.).

The fluid (endolymph) in the membranous labyrinth is brought into physical relationship with the surrounding air through the interposition of bones (the auditory ossicles, in a chain), and the fluid (perilymph) in a labyrinthine system external to the membranous labyrinth.

From the integument to the vestibular window, the contributory elements are salvaged from the branchial arch system. These parts and their sources are the following: external acoustic meatus (from the branchial groove); tympanic cavity (from the branchial pouch); and ossicles (from the mandibular and hyoid arches).

Transverse section, Wisconsin Collection, series 16.

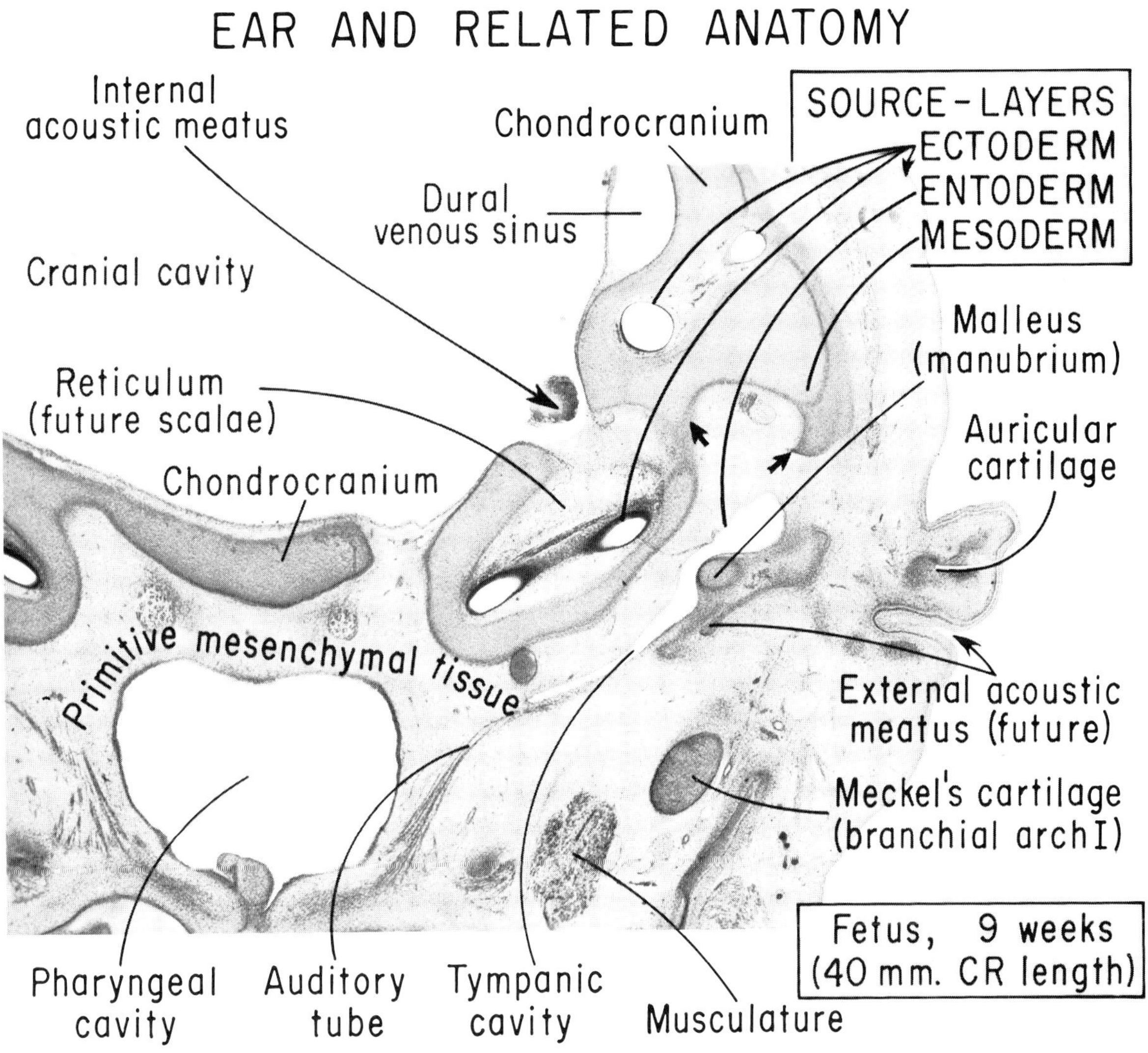

Figure II–4. Parts of the ear: early developmental stage. Fetus of 9 weeks (40 mm.).

The auricle appears as an elevation on the outer surface of the head, the external acoustic meatus as a sulcus (an inpushing of the primordial ectoderm). The tympanic cavity, continuous with the auditory tube, is an entodermal prolongation of the primitive pharynx.

The membranous labyrinth (derived from the ectodermal otocyst) consists, even at this early stage, of the following parts: cochlear and semicircular ducts; utricle and saccule; and the several intercommunicating channels (not sectioned at the level here illustrated).

The membranous labyrinth is lodged in mesenchyma within which the periotic tissue will give way to the spaces of the perilymphatic labyrinthine system. The surrounding cartilage will be transformed into bone. Margins of the facial sulcus are indicated by the unlabeled arrows.

Transverse section, Wisconsin Collection, series 168.

(From Anson: Chapter 1 in Paparella and Shumrick (Eds.): Otolaryngology, Vol. I. W. B. Saunders Co., 1973.)

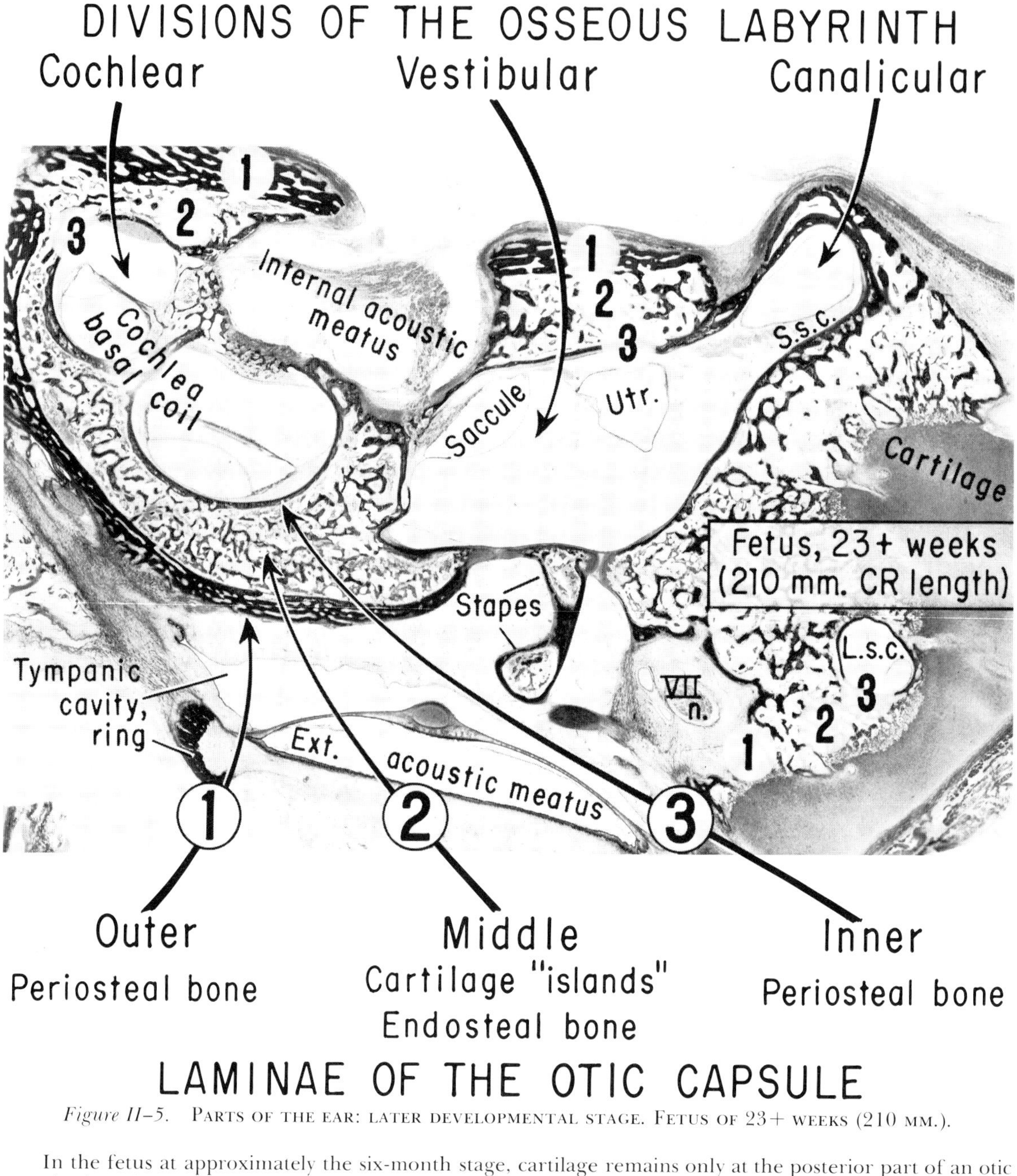

Figure II–5. Parts of the ear: later developmental stage. Fetus of 23+ weeks (210 mm.).

In the fetus at approximately the six-month stage, cartilage remains only at the posterior part of an otic capsule that elsewhere consists of trilaminar bone. Retarded ossification in this canalicular division permits expansion of the canals and their contained ducts after the cochlear part of the capsule, fully formed in bone, has attained adult dimensions (between the fourth and fifth month).

Periotic tissue, a remnant of the original reticulum, persists as anchorage in areas where portions of the membranous labyrinth are closely applied to the facing surface of the inner periosteal layer of the osseous capsule. Abbreviations: *L.s.c.*, lateral semicircular canal; *S.s.c.*, superior semicircular canal; *Utr.*, utricle. The layers of bone are numbered.

Transverse section, Wisconsin Collection, series 47 A.

(From Anson: Chapter 1 in Paparella and Shumrick (Eds.): Otolaryngology, Vol. I. Philadelphia, W. B. Saunders Co., 1973.)

OTIC CAPSULE LABYRINTHS, RELATED ANATOMY

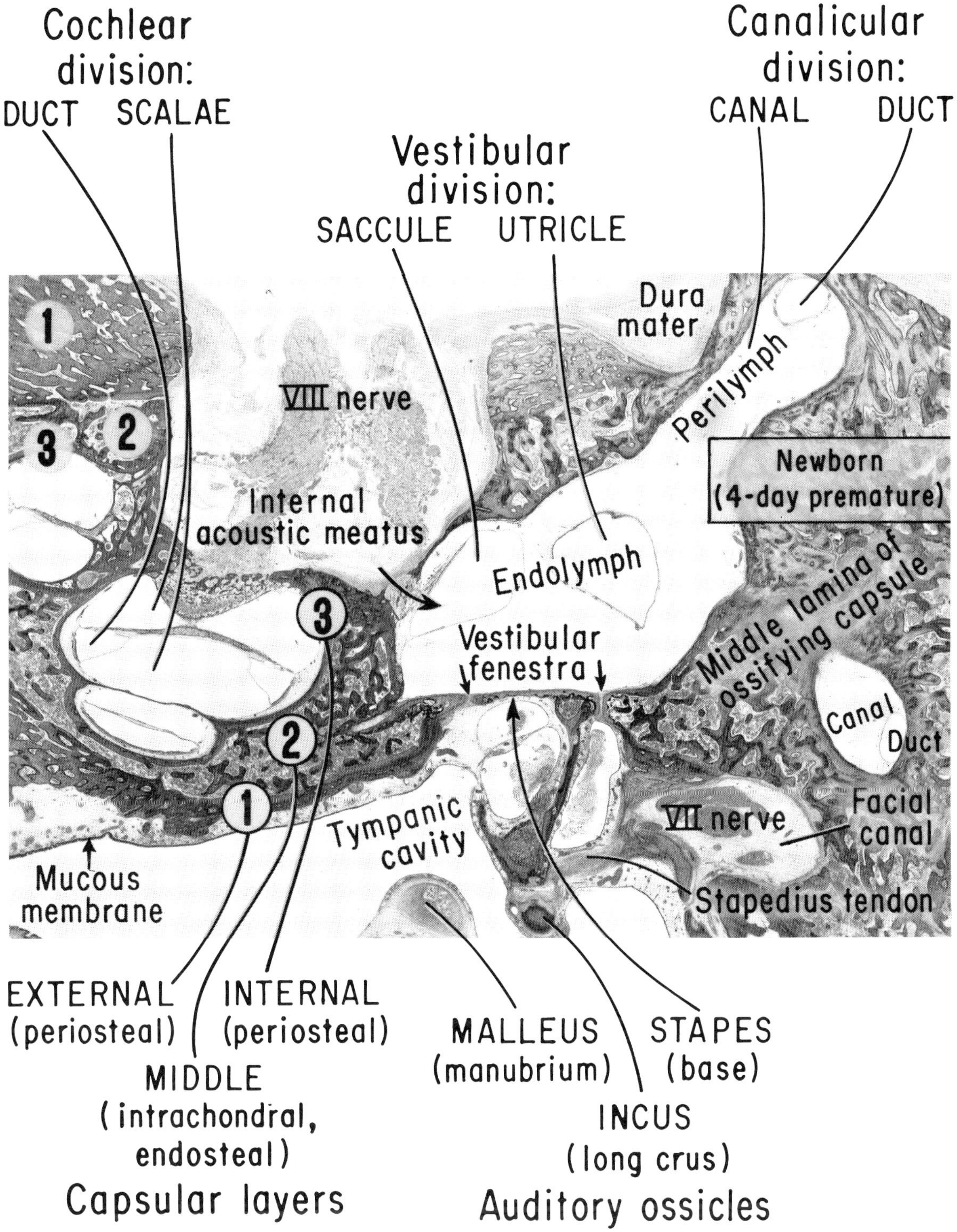

Figure II–6. PARTS OF THE EAR: LATE DEVELOPMENTAL STAGE. NEWBORN (4-DAY PREMATURE).

Developmental progress between the sixth and ninth month of fetal life is virtually limited to slow advance in the process of ossification of the otic capsule and in reorganization of bone of the wall of the vestibular aqueduct around the endolymphatic duct and sac. The long axis of duct and sac changes from straight to curved; concurrently, the sac enlarges (Figure II–24).

Otherwise, the inner (periosteal) layer does not change (3); it remains a thin boundary for the labyrinths. The middle layer (2) solidifies. The outer (periosteal) layer (1) increases in thickness, thus embedding the primordial capsule in the *pars petrosa.*

Transverse section, Wisconsin Collection, series 124.

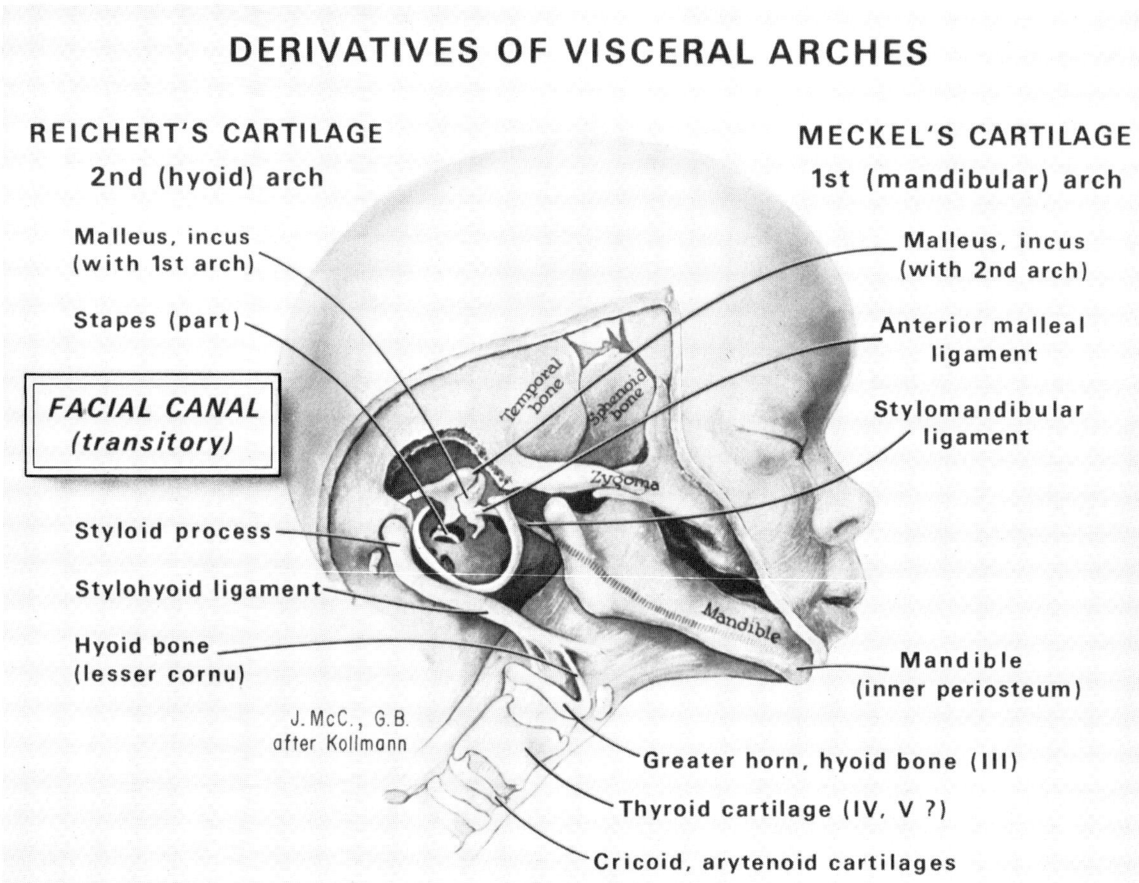

Figure II–7. Derivatives of the branchial arches shown in a dissection of a fetal head (after Kollmann). Demonstrating the outcome of the process of transformation of a skeletal apparatus to a new, functionally different service.

The system of branchial (visceral) arches serving primitively as support for a respiratory system in aquatic creatures (for example, in the selachian fishes) is salvaged, through remarkable transformation, into components of the ossicular chain, mandible, and larynx.

Meckel's cartilage of the mandibular (or first branchial) arch makes a series of contributions to the adult structure of the human head. Beginning at its proximal extremity—and in conjunction with the hyoid arch—it gives rise to the malleus and incus, ending at the distal extremity with tissue incorporated into the mandible in the region of the symphysis. (These tissues are listed in the figure in the order of their derivation from "segments" of the cartilaginous bar.)

Reichert's cartilage of the hyoid (or second branchial) arch makes an equal number of contributions, but to cervical as well as capital anatomy. The most proximally situated element is the stapes, part of which is so derived; the distal element is the lesser horn of the hyoid bone (listed in tabular arrangement by segments of the cartilaginous arch of the embryo). The cartilage serves also as part of the wall of the facial canal in the fetal ear (see Figure II–47*a*, *b*).

(From Anson and McVay: Surgical Anatomy, 5th ed. Philadelphia, W. B. Saunders Co., 1971.)

cells of the mastoid and petrous portions of the temporal bone, and the internal (mucosal) layer of the tympanic membrane.

From the third layer, the *mesoderm,* arise the remaining elements of the ear. These are the following: the auricular cartilage and the muscles of the external ear; the auditory ossicles with their associated muscles and ligaments; the submucosal tissue in which these structures are lodged; the middle (fibrous) layer of the tympanic membrane; and the otic capsule and the periotic tissue of the osseous labyrinth (enclosing the perilymphatic or periotic system of spaces).

The precartilaginous otic capsule develops around the differentiating otocyst. Before the cartilage is converted into bone, reversal in development of the precartilage results in the production of a succession of channels between the epithelial duct system and the capsule. Generally matching the former, but peripheral thereto and more capacious, these spaces will be the tympanic and vestibular scalae, the vestibule, and the semicircular canals of the osseous labyrinth of the adult ear.

The cartilage which encapsulates the perilymphatic system of spaces undergoes rapid ossification, attaining adult dimensions when the fetus has just reached the second trimester of intrauterine life (Figure II–5). Thereupon is initiated the process of ossification, through the operation of which the otic capsule, while retaining fetal dimensions, becomes embedded in the petrous part of the temporal bone.

The External Ear

AURICLE AND EXTERNAL ACOUSTIC MEATUS

Figure II–8

INTRODUCTION

The auricle develops around the first branchial groove. The contributory tissue is thus furnished by both the first (mandibular) branchial arch and the second (hyoid) arch. Six hillocks appear on these arches: three on the facing border of each. These fuse to form the elevations, fossae, and sulci of the adult auricle.

The external acoustic meatus is a derivative of the first ectodermal branchial groove between the mandibular and hyoid arches. The epithelium at the bottom of this groove is in contact with the entoderm of the first pharyngeal pouch. Connective tissue, derived from the mesoderm, is situated between the two epithelial layers. It becomes the fibrous layer of the trilaminar tympanic membrane. The connective tissue around the margin of the membrane begins to ossify at about the third month. This tissue forms the tympanic ring, which serves as the circumferential support of the tympanic membrane.

DEVELOPMENTAL ANATOMY

The arches and groove bounded thereby are clearly seen in the 5-mm. embryo (Figure II–8*a*). Hillocks, present in the 11-mm. embryo (Figure II–8*b*), fuse in the 15-mm. stage (Figure II–8*c*). They are identifiable in the adult ear (Figure II–8*d, e*).

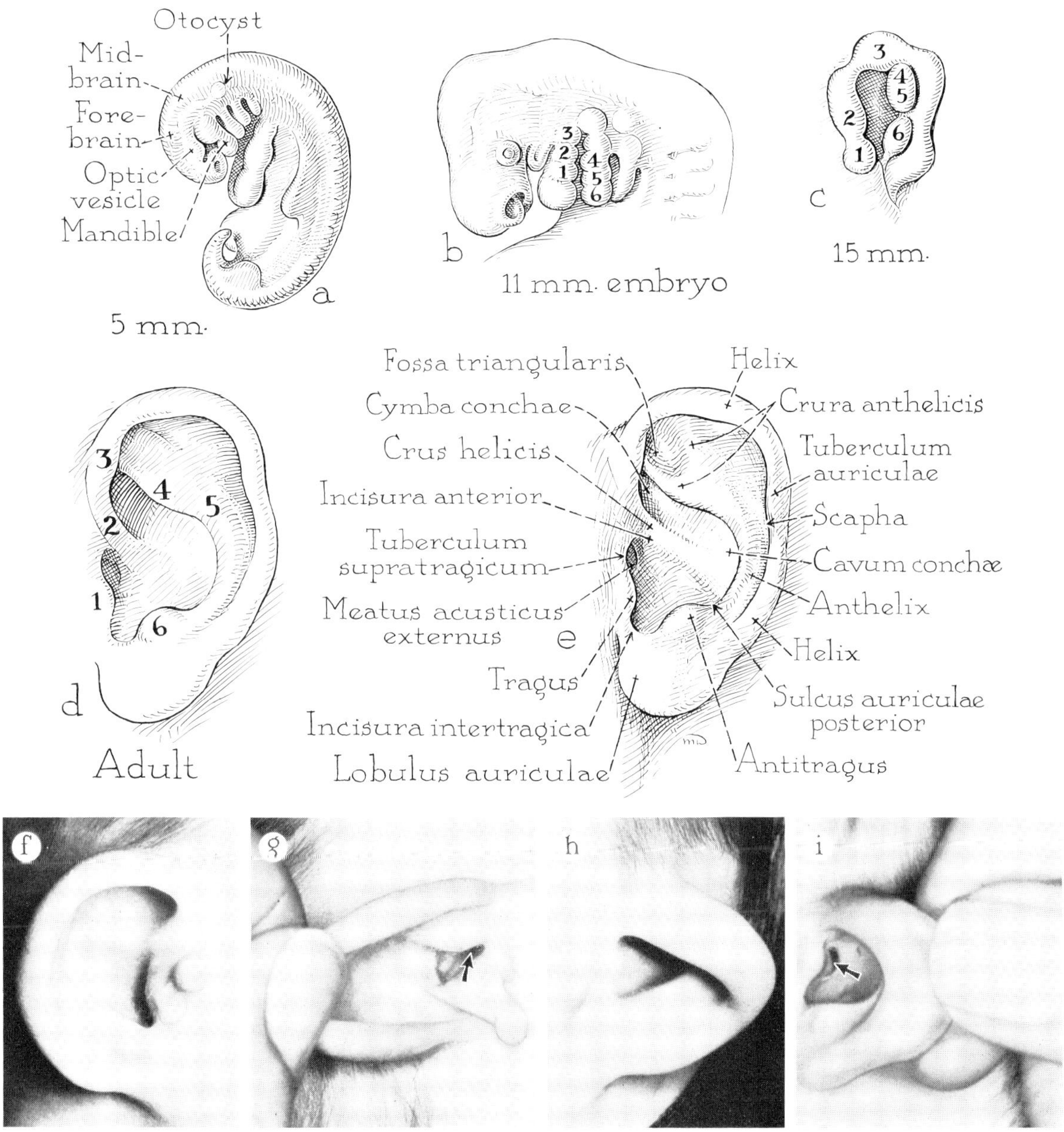

Figure II–8. DEVELOPMENTAL AND ADULT ANATOMY OF THE AURICLE, NORMAL AND ABERRANT.

a. Primordial elevations on the first (mandibular) and second (hyoid) arches.

b to *d.* Progress of embryonic fusion of the hillocks and the adult configuration of the auricle (with corresponding numerals on the derived parts).

e. Adult form of the auricle with parts identified.

f to *i.* Anomalous auricle and external acoustic meatus in a child four and one-half years of age: *f* and *g*, right ear; *h* and *i*, left ear. In *f*, one hillock remains independent, unfused. In *g* and *i*, the auricle is drawn dorsalward in order to reveal the atretic meatus (indicated by arrow). Atresia is the result of failure in splitting of the ectodermal cellular plate which normally occurs during the seventh month of fetal life. The meatus represents the first ectodermal groove of the embryo.

(From Anson and McVay: Surgical Anatomy, 5th ed. Philadelphia, W. B. Saunders Co., 1971. Figures *f* to *i*, courtesy of Leslie Bernstein, D.D.S., M.D.)

ADULT STRUCTURE: Illustrated in Figure III–2.

The Middle Ear

TYMPANIC MEMBRANE

Figure II–9

INTRODUCTION

The three germ layers take part in the formation of the tympanic membrane. The ectoderm, carried inward as the wall of the external acoustic meatus, contributes the cutaneous layer; the entoderm, prolonged from the primitive pharynx, forms the mucosal lamina; from the intervening mesoderm (mesenchyme) comes the fibrous layer. As development proceeds, the last-named stratum becomes compressed into a thin sheet between the other two, so that even in the fetus, the membrane attains an adult appearance.

DEVELOPMENTAL ANATOMY

The external ear is a derivative of the first branchial groove and of branchial arches (mandibular and hyoid) that constitute its boundaries. The external acoustic meatus represents the ectodermal groove. Deeply, the tissue forms a cellular plate that is separated from the entodermal wall of the middle ear by a thin stratum of mesoderm. In the 3-month specimen, splitting of the ectoderm has been initiated (Figure II–9).

The middle ear, with the auditory tube, is a derivative of the first pharyngeal pouch. In the stage illustrated, it has reached the ectoderm plate derived from the corresponding pharyngeal groove. The auditory ossicles develop in the mesenchymal tissue which surrounds the entodermal pouch.

TYMPANIC RING

Figures II–10 to II–13

INTRODUCTION

The tympanic ring is formed from four minute ossification centers of membrane bone. Following fusion of the originally separate centers, growth proceeds rapidly with concurrent increase in overall size. Fixation to the other parts of the temporal bone begins in the posterior part of the annulet. Progressing forward rapidly, anchorage is complete in the newborn.

Considered as a separate skeletal element, the "ring" is never a finished annulus; at the time of fusion with related portions of the temporal bone, it is still open along its cranial segment, the defect being the tympanic incisure (Rivinus). Fixation involves the formation of temporary lines of suture with the squamous and petrous parts of the temporal bone. Concurrently with fusion, two sets of changes are set in motion, *viz*: partitioning of the foramen enclosed by the ring, and growth of the latter along the sides and the floor. The upper, smaller opening is the external acoustic meatus; the lower opening is usually obliterated. In childhood it may persist as the foramen of Huschke. With further growth, that which arose as a partial ring becomes the tympanic part of the temporal bone, contributing largely to the mandibular fossa and forming the sheath of the styloid process. As a result of enlargement, it is as if the attachment of the tympanic membrane were carried deeply into the meatus.

DEVELOPMENTAL ANATOMY

The tympanic ring makes its appearance in the form of four small centers of membrane bone in the fetus of approximately 9 weeks. They have fused in the 10-week specimen. The ring thus formed from the fused centers has become sulcate in the fetus of 16½ weeks (Figure II–10*a*). At this stage bone formation has just been initiated in the otic capsule (as here represented by the occurrence of an ossification center in the basal turn of the cochlea) and the tympanic membrane is a narrow slit; the primordium of the external acoustic meatus is a solid plate of ectoderm already apposed to the mucous membrane of the tympanum.

Within two months, between the 16-week and the 23-week stage, the diameter has increased by almost one and one-half times, and the ring itself has grown wider and thicker (Figure II–10*b*). Maximum growth is attained in the term fetus.

In the 5-month fetus, the anterior limb of the developing tympanic annulus is just beginning to change from rodlike to sulcate form (Figure II–11*a*), a feature which becomes more pronounced as development proceeds. In a specimen approximately a month and a half older, the anterior limb of the ring is definitely sulcate (Figure II–11*b*). The tympanic membrane is approaching the thinned appearance that is characteristic of the adult stage; the ossicles are invested by the advancing mucous membrane. In the fetus at term, the histological structure is similar to that of the annulus in the 25-week specimen, but appreciable growth has taken place in the intervening period (Figure II–11*c*).

The pattern of development is advantageously demonstrated by a comparison of two crucial stages (Figure II–12*a*, *b*). In the fifth month, the ring is represented by several small centers of ossification. In the fetus at term, two prominences (indicated by asterisks in *c*) will, by growth during the first postnatal year, meet and fuse. Thereby, the space enclosed by the primordial annulus will be divided into that of the external acoustic meatus and the foramen of Huschke.

Growth, fixation, and partitioning of the ring may be followed in six stages (Figure II–13*a* to *f*). In the newborn, the presence of a nodular prominence on the free surface of each "arm" of the ring predicts the partitioning of the space originally enclosed by the annulus into that of the future external acoustic meatus and that of the foramen of Huschke (Figure II–13*a*). Toward the close of the first postnatal year, these processes (Figure II–13*b*, at unlabeled arrows) approach each other and fuse. Concurrent growth takes place in the inferior part of the tympanic portion, a process which increases the length of the meatus. The foramen of Huschke (unlabeled arrow in Figure II–13*c*) is a relatively capacious opening, later closed in normal cases. In the adolescent and the adult, the meatal extension of the ring dwarfs the size of the annulus itself (Figure II–13*d* and *e*). Continuing growth has the effect of carrying the tympanic ring inward (Figure II–13*f*).

ADULT ANATOMY

It is important to consider the structures on the medial (labyrinthine) wall of the tympanic cavity as they are seen through the tympanic ring (Figure III–5).

The vestibular (oval) window is situated approximately in the middle of the wall, at the bottom of a fossa (the *fossula fenestrae vestibuli*), plainly visible from the lateral side. Inferior to the window, the wall projects into the tympanic cavity as a promontory produced by the basal turn of the cochlea. A sharp declivity posterior to the promontory leads into a second fossa (the *fossula fenestrae cochleae*) that is bounded superiorly by a smooth projection of bone, the subiculum. At the same time, the subiculum forms the inferior boundary of the tympanic sinus, a (usually deep) fossa that is continuous above with the fossula of the vestibular fenestra (or stapes "niche").

The horizontal segment of the facial canal is seen as it courses posteriorly just below the level of the lesser tympanic spine of the annulus. After a short course lateralward, deep to the ring, the canal turns downward in the mastoid wall of the tympanic cavity to the stylomastoid foramen. In this course it is everywhere closely related to air cells.

The variation in the angular relation of the plane of the tympanic ring to the long axes of the facial canal is a feature of considerable surgical significance (Figure III–6*a*, *b*).

Most frequently the anterior part of the canal is more medial to the ring than the posterior part (Figure III–6*a*).

In some instances the tympanic annulus crosses the facial canal to intersect at an angle as great as 40 degrees, the point of crossing being at the approximate midpoint in the length of the vertical (descending) segment (Figure III–6*b*).

In the adult, the tympanic membrane, or eardrum, is stretched out in the tympanic sulcus and tympanic incisure of the *anulus tympanicus*, thus separating the external acoustic meatus from the tympanic cavity (Figure III–4*a*). It is covered externally by a continuation of the skin and on the inside by mucous membrane. The upper, flaccid portion is pushed forward by the lateral process of the malleus. In the larger inferior tense part it is drawn inward by the tip of the manubrium to produce the funnel-shaped umbo.

On the medial side the tympanic membrane is covered by mucous membrane (Figure III–4*b*). The manubrium of the malleus is imbedded in the membrane, as is also the chorda tympani, as the latter nerve passes from a position between the incus and the malleus to one in which it courses to the iter of the petrotympanic fissure.

TYMPANIC CAVITY

Figures II–14 and II–15

INTRODUCTION

The cavity and lining of the middle ear and of the auditory (eustachian) tube arise from the expanding terminal end of the first (and possibly second) pharyngeal pouches (Figure II–14*a*). The entoderm of the pharyngeal pouch appears early; it is well formed in the embryo of 3 weeks. At the 4-week stage, its terminal end is flattened dorsoventrally against the ectoderm of the infolding first branchial groove. Late in the second month, while the proximal part of the pharyngeal pouch becomes constricted to form the auditory tube, the distal end expands into a flattened sac, the primordial tympanic cavity.

In the 10-week fetus, the tip of this flattened cavity approaches the distal end of the first branchial groove, the latter being the future external acoustic meatus. The ectodermal and entodermal layers of the apposed cavities are now separated by an intervening layer of cellular connective tissue which later condenses to form the fibrous layer of the thin trilaminar tympanic membrane. The distal, expanded part of the auditory tube, which remains a slitlike flattened space up to the fifth month of fetal life, soon begins to expand. In the fetus of approximately 6 months, the loose mucoid connective tissue has given way to the expanding tympanic epithelium. As the enlarging tympanum reaches the ossicles, its epithelium is wrapped around each of them somewhat as the peritoneal mesothelium covers the intestine. Between the eighth and ninth month, pneumatization of the tympanum proper is almost complete. During the last month of fetal life, pneumatization of both tympanum and epitympanum has been virtually completed.

The antrum is a posterolateral extension of the epitympanum, at least when complete. It begins to form when the fetus is about 22 weeks old and is well advanced in the 34-week specimen. Formation of antral and mastoid air cells begins late in fetal life and progresses during infancy and childhood.

Petrous, or so-called apical, air cells occur in varying extent, number, and position. They appear soon after bone is laid down in the otic capsule; that is, about the fetal age of 24 weeks. Similar cells are concurrently formed in the wall of the tympanum and auditory tube, the largest of which is the tympanic sinus.

DEVELOPMENTAL ANATOMY

Even as early as the 9-week stage, the diverticulum from the pharynx has advanced as far as the malleus, which it will soon invest completely with mucous membrane, the entoderm of the first visceral pouch (Figure II–14*a*). As it advances further, the incus and stapes will likewise be invested and cells will be formed, each a cul-de-sac of the cavity proper. Bones of the *pars petrosa* and *pars mastoidea* will be similarly invaded and replaced by pneumatic spaces (see list in Figure II–14*a*). By the sixth month, the malleus and the tympanic membrane on the lateral wall of the tympanic cavity have been invested by mucous membrane. The mucous membrane covers the incus and stapes as it approaches the medial wall of the cavity (Figure II–14*b*); it also forms the tympanic sinus and other similar offsets or extensions of the general tympanic cavity (Figure II–14*c*).

The mechanism of pneumatization is clearly demonstrated in the formation of the cells in the petrous part of the temporal bone; it is one in which bone already formed is replaced by mucous membrane (Figure II–15*a* to *c*).

The tympanic sinus is a well-established feature of the pneumatic spaces of the temporal bone (Figure III–19*a* to *f*). It is a well-formed element of tympanic anatomy in the 5-month fetus when ossification of the capsule is under way (Figure III–19*a*). It is walled by bone, but the sinus is still occupied by primitive mesenchymal tissue in fetuses of 20 and 26 weeks (Figure III–19*a*, *b*). The size of the sinus is subject to considerable variation. Its relationship to other structures is quite constant (Figure III–20*d*, *e*).

ADULT ANATOMY

The mucosal lamina of the tympanic membrane is carried over the manubrium of the malleus and over the chorda tympani, as the latter passes from the canaliculus to the petrotympanic fissure (Figures III–7; III–64*a*, *b*; and III–3*a*, *b*). These and other aspects of its reflections as folds, investments, and the lateral layer of the secondary tympanic membrane, call for special description.

The medial wall of the tympanic cavity presents the fossulae of the vestibular and cochlear fenestrae, the facial canal and numerous air cells (Figures III–17*a*, *b*; III–10*a* to *c*; III–16*a*; and III–18*a* to *c*). The carotid canal and the jugular fossa (like the facial canal) invade its space (Figure III–21*a* to *c*). The cavity is normally subdivided by mucosal septa (Figure III–10*a*), sometimes partially obliterated by cholesteatoma (Figure III–23).

AUDITORY OSSICLES AND OSSICULAR MUSCLES

INTRODUCTION

The small ear bones, refashioned for the greater part from the tissue of the mandibular and hyoid arches (Meckel's and Reichert's cartilages), are first formed as cartilage "models." At the 9-week stage, they have already attained the general configuration that characterizes their appearance in the adult. Two portions have separate origins: the anterior process of the malleus, which forms independently and early in membrane bone; the vestibular portion of the base (footplate) of the stapes, which is primordially a part of the otic capsule.

Growth is rapid: within a 3-week period the ossicles have increased their overall dimensions by three times. Just three months later, in the 15-week specimen, the ossicles have attained maximum size as chondral elements, with clear forecast of the adult morphology.

Bone formation, initiated at the 16-week stage in the malleus and incus, begins somewhat later in the stapes (in one series, at 19 weeks). In the latter stage, periosteal bone is present in the head and in the proximal part of the manubrium of the malleus. On the incus, the periosteal shell is spreading from the body to the short and long crura. In the stapes, ossification is taking place at the basal end of each crus. Endosteal bone is being formed beneath the periosteal lamina of the malleus and incus. Meckel's cartilage undergoes conversion into a ligament, and the anterior process, hitherto free, is attached to the bone of the head of the malleus. Ossification continues at such a rapid pace that the ossicles, except for permanently cartilaginous areas, are essentially adult skeletal elements in the 25-week fetus.

On *a priori* grounds, uniformity in developmental pattern would be expected in the growth and histogenesis of the three ossicles—since they are derivatives of the branchial arches. Such, however, is not the case. Whereas the stapes sacrifices a large fraction of its bulk (as an embryonic element), the malleus and incus attain relative solidity (although canalized by numerous vascular channels).

Stapes

Figures II–16 to II–19

DEVELOPMENTAL ANATOMY

The major steps in the macroscopic development of the stapes are favorably demonstrated by the use of reconstructions. In the embryo of 2 months, the future ossicle is a chondral annulet (Figure II–16*a*). It grows in cartilage through approximately the next 2-month period, changing from annular to stapedial form (Figure II–16*b, c*). The single ossification center appears in the 18-week specimen (Figure II–16*d*). Spreading along the crura toward the head and across the base (footplate), the bone forms a periosteal "collar," internal to which there are scattered spicules of endosteal bone (Figure II–16*e*). No sooner is an osseous shell completed than a process of erosion begins to render it foraminous. Resorption of bone progresses at so rapid a rate that, in the ossicle of the 6-month fetus (Figure II–16*f*), the capital, crural, and basal parts are continuously open toward the obturator foramen. Periosteal bone may persist as a *crista stapedis* on the base (Figure II–16*f*, encircled by arrow). Finally, endosteal bone remains only as a thin lamina on the internal, or obturator, surface of the head and base (Figure II–16*g*).

The preceding account calls for detailed expansion of the histological features which are involved in the process of growth and microscopic differentiation. In the 5-month fetus, periosteal bone is being produced at the basal extremity of each crus (Figure II–17*a*). Foramina, concurrently formed along the obturator surface, transmit blood vessels to the primitive marrow cavity where endosteal bone is transitorily present in the crura, permanently on the internal (obturator) surface of the base (footplate) and head.

As periosteal bone is resorbed on the internal surface of the ossicle, the primitive marrow cavity is opened. Upon being thus exposed, it is invaded by the mucous membrane of the expanding tympanic cavity (Figure II–17*b, c*).

As a result of these changes, the stapes of the adult is a fragile ossicle with a thin bilaminar base (Figure II–17*d*). Cartilage, retained from fetal life, is carried across the vestibular surface to the fenestral margin of the tympanostapedial syndesmosis. The cartilage of the fenestra is continued into the vestibular aperture of the fissula ante fenestram, where it frequently is encountered in late fetal and early postnatal stages and may even persist in the adult.

The special nature of ossicular blood supply warrants, especially, review of the vascular pattern in the stapes. At the very onset of bone formation, the tympanic part of the stapes is lodged in mesenchyma in which small blood vessels of a capillary network are widely distributed (Figure II–18*a*). The vestibular part (base, or footplate) is invested by an excessively thin stratum of periotic tissue in which vessels are both small and numerous. The crura of the stapes, undergoing change from cartilage to bone, are columns of periosteal bone within whose cavity there are still both primitive marrow and remnants of calcified cartilage.

In the 27-week specimen the periosteal layer is well formed. Endosteal bone is being deposited on the internal surface of the base (Figure II–18*b*). In this process vascular channels are formed circumferentially around the footplate.

In late fetal stages, following continued production of endosteal bone, the base of the ossicle becomes two-layered (Figure II–18*c*). In the terminal step in osteogenesis, blood vessels, enclosed by the newly formed bone, occupy vascular channels that are circumferentially arranged. Others cross the base in the mucous membrane; they ascend to the head of the stapes, then continue at submucosal level along the ossicular chain to the tympanic membrane. Offsets are present in the numerous mucosal folds, or septa (see Figures III–67 and III–91).

It is clear from the immediately foregoing accounts that the morphogenesis of the stapes, the establishment of its blood supply as part of the tympanic plexus, and the progress of bone formation in the adjacent part of the otic capsule are closely interrelated processes. To these facets in the composite mosaic of change in and near the labyrinthine wall of the tympanic cavity must be added that of another local area, namely, that of the facial canal (Figure II–18*d*). From the canal, along the stapedius tendon, blood vessels pass to the ossicles. Continuing at submucosal level, the vessels contribute to the tympanic plexus.

The details of anatomy must also be reviewed. In the fetus at approximately the 4-month stage, the stapes, initially annular in form, has attained the form of a stirrup (Figure II–19*a*). The base is flanged, the posterior crus is already bowed more sharply than the anterior, and the head is foveate (to articulate with the lenticular process of the incus) The area of the future vestibular (oval) window is a seam of retrogressively changing precartilage. The facial canal is a sulcate impression on the wall of the canalicular part of the cartilaginous capsule. Although primordial in form, it already houses the facial nerve, stapedius muscle, and numerous blood vessels (veins being more conspicuous than arteries). Mucous membrane of the expanding tympanic cavity has reached the malleus and the incus but has not clothed any part of the stapes. Bone formation has not yet begun in either the otic capsule or the auditory ossicles.

In a specimen one month older the initial step in ossification of the stapes has been taken: the crura have changed from solid rods of cartilage into columns of periosteal bone that contain primitive marrow (Figure II–19*b*). Concurrently bone is being formed in the otic capsule.

In another specimen of the same age, ossification is further advanced. One of the ossification centers forms part of the wall of the developing facial canal (Figure II–19*c*).

Between the 6-month and 7-month stage, the bone of the inner wall of the crura is being removed, the interior of each crus opened on the surface facing the obturator foramen. Both the scattered "spicules" of endosteal bone and the primitive marrow which contains them are being resorbed (Figure II–19*d*). However, the endosteal bone that is formed along the footplate and the head of the stapes (in contact with the original cartilage) will increase to form a permanent layer.

Curiously, production of bone in the middle layer of the otic capsule seemingly comes to a temporary halt (see page 81). Growth of bone is beginning to convert the sulcus into a canal.

Apparent quiescence in bone formation characterizes the middle layer through much of the remainder of the prenatal period. The outer layer, unlike the middle, progressively thickens (Figure II–19*e*). During the same period, the stapes continues to undergo decrease in bulk, expressed chiefly in the loss of the entire obturator wall. The facial canal is now fully formed; the stapedius tendon, passing from canal to stapes, is accompanied by blood vessels which supply the middle ear.

Resorption changes the stapes into an ossicle of striking fragility: each crus consists of a thin layer of periosteal bone; the base and head are composed of a plate of endosteal bone applied to the lamina of the original cartilage (Figure II–19*f*). The bone of the middle layer of the capsule, as if reactivated, converts the "cancellous" fabric into petrous bone. In the facial canal, vascularity of the connective tissue, established in early fetal life, remains a permanent histological feature.

Malleus and Incus

Figure II–20

DEVELOPMENTAL ANATOMY

The incus and malleus, like the stapes, arise in cartilage of the branchial arch system. But differing from the stapes, these two ossicles become relatively dense through continuing deposition of endosteal bone in the course of fetal life. Unlike the stapes, both the malleus and incus thus retain the general form of the cartilage "model."

The malleus and incus in fetuses at approximately the 4-month stage begin to change from cartilage to bone (Figure II–20*a, b*). In a fetus one month older, the tissue in the area of the incudomalleal articulation serves to demonstrate two major steps in the progress of ossification: vascular buds invade the short crus of the incus preparatory to the formation of endosteal bone; in the body of the malleus such bone is being formed internal to the layer of periosteal bone (Figure II–20*c*).

The relationship of the two laminae, periosteal and endosteal, is shown in the incus of a specimen somewhat younger but more advanced in histological change (Figure II–20*b*; compare Figure II–20*a*). In the incus, cartilage is being resorbed beneath a still thin periosteal plate, the latter rendered foraminous to permit the ingress of erosive vascular buds; in the malleus, cartilage has been replaced by endosteal bone and primitive marrow.

In specimens between the 5-month and 6-month stage, both layers are present (Figure II–20*c*). Here two successive phases are demonstrated: whereas the endosteal bone in the long crus of the incus appears chiefly in the form of interconnected spicules, in the malleus it is a true lamina applied internally to the periosteal layer.

The structure of the malleus and incus in the adult ear is one of relative solidity (Figure II–20*d*). The appearance bears some resemblance to that of a typical long bone in miniature, but one in which the marrow cavity of the "diaphysis" is replaced by vascularized endosteal bone.

It is generally accepted that the malleus and incus are derived from the first branchial arch (Meckel's cartilage). Actually, the anterior process of the malleus develops independently in membrane bone (Figure II–20*c*); and in addition to branchial source, the otic capsule contributes to the stapes the medial (vestibular) part of the base, termed the lamina stapedis (Figure II–18*c*).

Each of the branchial arches does much more than contribute the ossicles: from the first (mandibular) arch are derived structures which begin proximally with the ossicles and end distally with the symphysis of the mandible; from the second (hyoid) arch come structures which, again, start proximally with an ossicle and terminate distally (in the neck) with the hyoid bone (Figure II–7).

Tensor Tympani Muscle and Semicanal

Figure II–21

DEVELOPMENTAL ANATOMY

The tympanic tensor muscle is a derivative of the first branchial arch of the embryo. The stapedius muscle comes from the second arch.

In the specimen of approximately 3 months (prior to the onset of capsular ossification), the primordial muscle lies in mesenchymal tissue lateral to the cochlea (Figure II–21*a*). The malleus, to which it will become attached, is—like the incus and stapes—a cartilage "model" of the mature ossicle.

Two months later the histological difference between muscle and tendon is evident (Figure II–21*b*). The latter is attached to the manubrium of the malleus. In a late fetal stage, periosteal bone is forming around the muscle to close the semicanal (Figure II–21*c*).

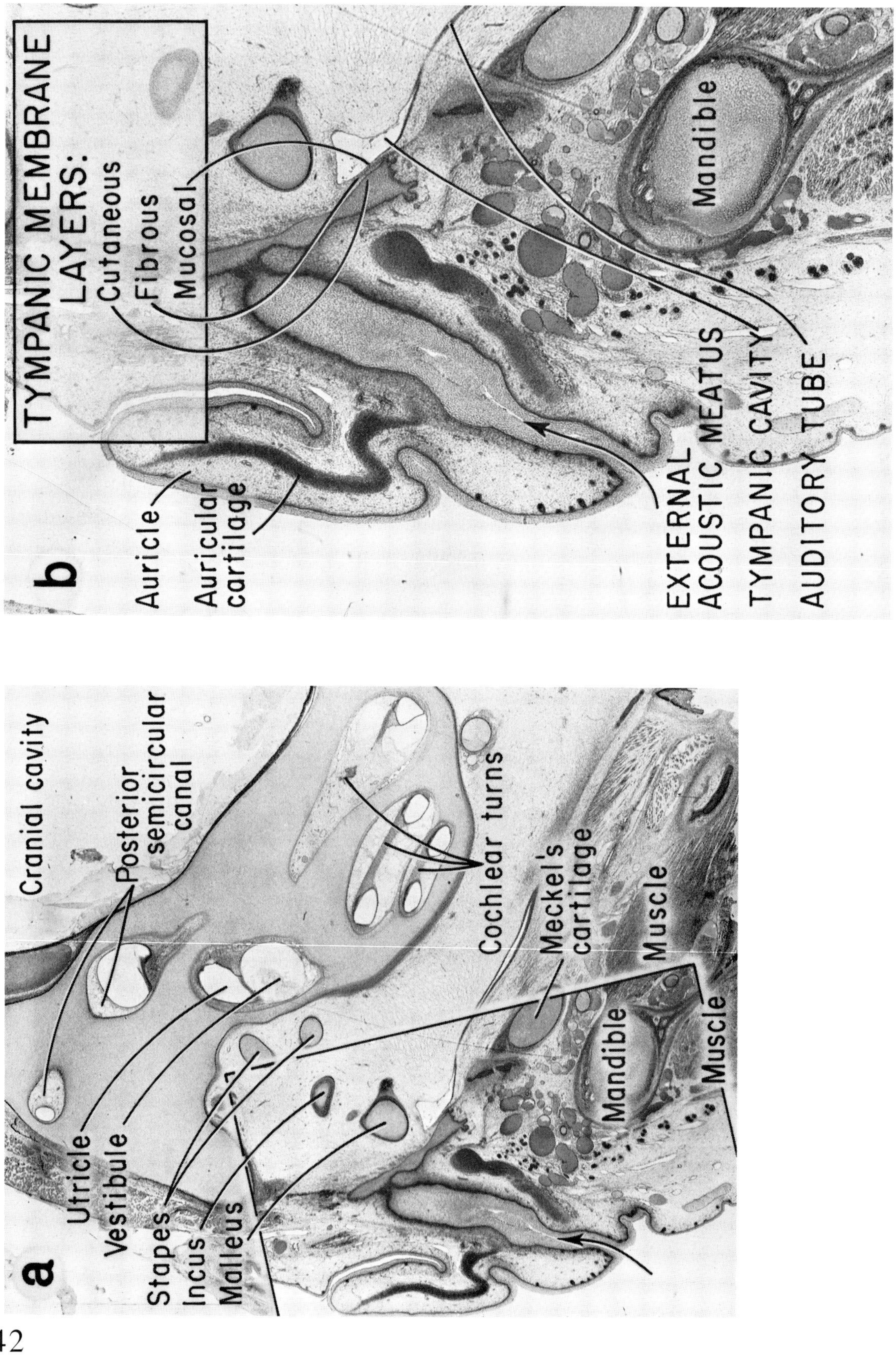
b
Auricle
Auricular cartilage
TYMPANIC MEMBRANE LAYERS:
Cutaneous
Fibrous
Mucosal
Mandible
EXTERNAL ACOUSTIC MEATUS
TYMPANIC CAVITY
AUDITORY TUBE
a
Utricle
Vestibule
Stapes
Incus
Malleus
Cranial cavity
Posterior semicircular canal
Cochlear turns
Meckel's cartilage
Muscle
Mandible
Muscle

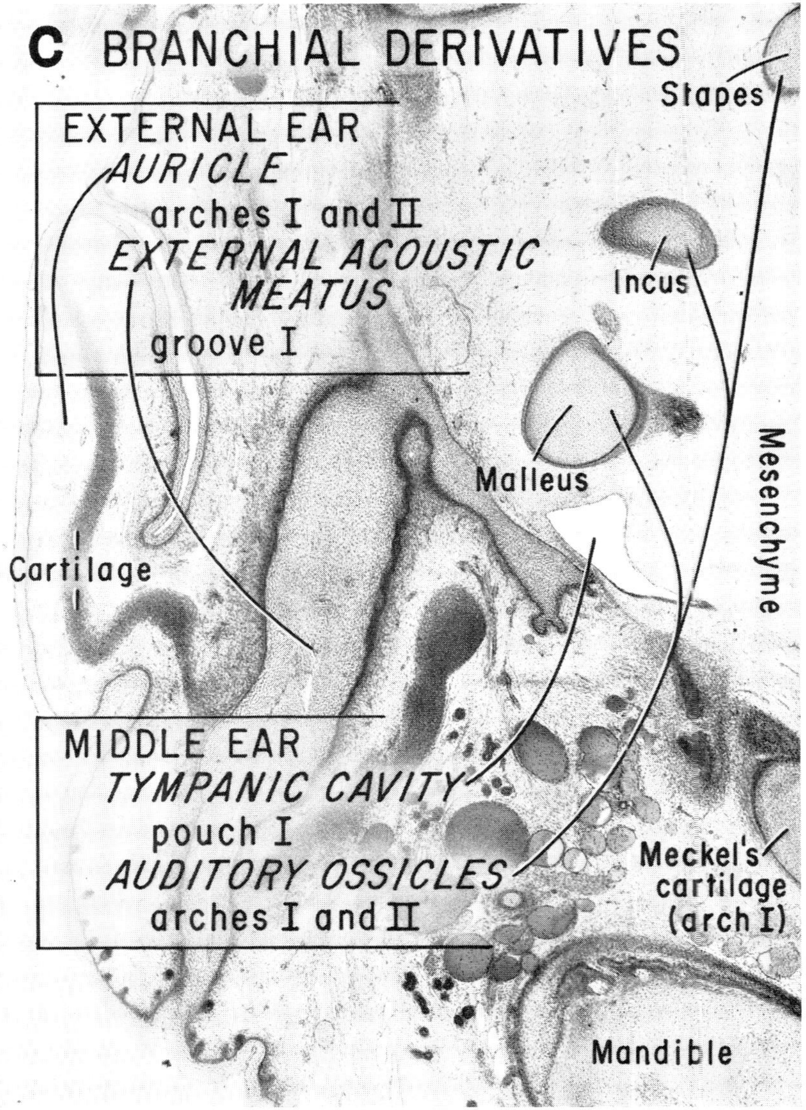

Figure II–9. CONTRIBUTIONS OF THE BRANCHIAL ARCH SYSTEM TO THE ANATOMY OF THE EXTERNAL AND MIDDLE EAR. FETUS OF 12 WEEKS (84 MM.).

a and *b*. Embryology of the tympanic membrane. The area blocked in *a* is shown at higher magnification in *b*. *c*. The derivatives, exclusive of the layers of the tympanic membrane.

The external ear is a derivative of the first branchial groove and of branchial arches (mandibular and hyoid) that constitute its boundaries. The external acoustic meatus represents the ectodermal groove itself. Inward, the tissue forms a cellular plate that is separated from the entodermal wall of the middle ear by a thin stratum of mesoderm. In the 3-month fetal specimen, here illustrated, splitting of the ectoderm has been initiated.

The middle ear (like the auditory tube, with which it is continuous) is a lengthened and expanded derivative of the first pharyngeal pouch. In the stage illustrated, the pouch has reached the ectoderm plate, the latter derived from the corresponding pharyngeal groove.

The entodermal pouch is surrounded by loose mesodermal tissue in which the auditory ossicles develop. They are derivatives of the first and second branchial arches (Meckel's and Reichert's cartilages). In this specimen, the ossicles are still cartilaginous. As they undergo ossification, the ear bones will become invested by the tympanic epithelium (see Figures II–14*b* and II–15). Meckel's cartilage (first branchial arch) is now the major part of the developing mandible (around which bone is beginning to form).

The blind end of the external acoustic meatus meets the wall of the expanding tympanic cavity; the fibrous tissue component intervenes between them. These layers are, respectively, the ectoderm, entoderm, and mesoderm of the embryo. Thus it is clear that the tympanic membrane is a trilaminar structure; that is, of triple germ-layer derivation.

Transverse sections, Wisconsin Collection, series 162. *a*, × 11; *b*, × 25; *c*, × 19.

ADULT STRUCTURE: Illustrated in Figure III–3.

Figure II–10. TYMPANIC RING, TYMPANIC MEMBRANE, AND RELATED STRUCTURES: DEVELOPMENTAL ANATOMY. *a.* FETUS OF 16½ WEEKS (126 MM.). *b.* FETUS, 23 WEEKS (202 MM.).

The tympanic "ring" makes its appearance in the form of four small centers of membrane bone in the fetus of approximately 9 weeks. They have fused in the 10-week specimen. The ring thus formed from the fused centers has become sulcate in the fetus of 16½ weeks (Figure II–12*c*).

The ectodermal plate (at asterisk) of the primitive branchial groove has split; the space (a narrow cleft in sections) is that of the external acoustic meatus. The medial wall thereof is apposed to the entoderm layer of the corresponding branchial groove. The latter space (likewise a cleft in sections) is that of the tympanic cavity. The tympanic membrane, separating the meatus from the tympanum, is a derivative of both layers and of the mesoderm which lies between them (see Figure II–9).

As the tympanic cavity expands, the mesenchyma which now intervenes between the mucosal layer of the tympanic membrane and the perichondrium of the cartilaginous otic capsule will differentiate into the adult connective tissue of the submucosal layer.

The branchial arches give rise to structures which, at this crucial stage, are lodged in the mesenchymal tissue. They are the auditory ossicles and the ossicular ligaments (none of which appear at this horizontal level) and Meckel's cartilage (continuous with the malleus as seen in Figure II–12*b*).

Turning now from consideration of the anatomy of the outer and the middle parts to that of the inner ear, it is seen that Meckel's cartilage is closely related to the stapedius muscle, contributing a partial and transitory wall for a semilunar space that will become the facial canal (see Figures II–44 and II–45).

In this canalicular division of the otic capsule, cartilage is becoming converted into bone. Bone formation is also taking place in the wall of the basal turn of the cochlea (the promontory of the inner ear of the adult). The secondary tympanic membrane is formed, separating the tympanic scala from the future fossula of the cochlear fenestra (round window). The cochlear vein, on the medial wall of the tympanic scala, is sectioned in midcourse between the cochlea and the channel which accompanies the cochlear canaliculus (see Figure II–49).

Ossification progresses less rapidly in the canalicular than in the cochlear division of the cartilaginous otic capsule (see Figure II–5). In the stage here illustrated, the capsule around the semicircular canal is still cartilage. The future perilymphatic space is occupied by a vascular reticulum (compare Figures II–30 and II–31).

Except for the semicircular ducts, the membranous labyrinth has already attained maximum size; they continue to grow after the vestibular and cochlear parts of the duct system are, in respect to dimensions, mature.

The primordium of the membranous labyrinth, namely the otocyst, is the first otologic element to appear. It is followed in the attainment of maturity by the perilymphatic spaces which come to surround it; they are followed in the order of developmental succession by the investing capsule of bone.

These circumstances combine to make a fetal ear from a specimen of this 4- to 5-month period a highly serviceable teaching stage: all constituent parts are present in a transitional form which, while not erasing the rise from genesis, clearly predicts the steps yet to be taken.

Transverse sections, Wisconsin Collection, series 11 and 70, respectively. *a*, × 17; *b*, × 16.

ADULT STRUCTURE: Illustrated in Figures III–3 and III–4.

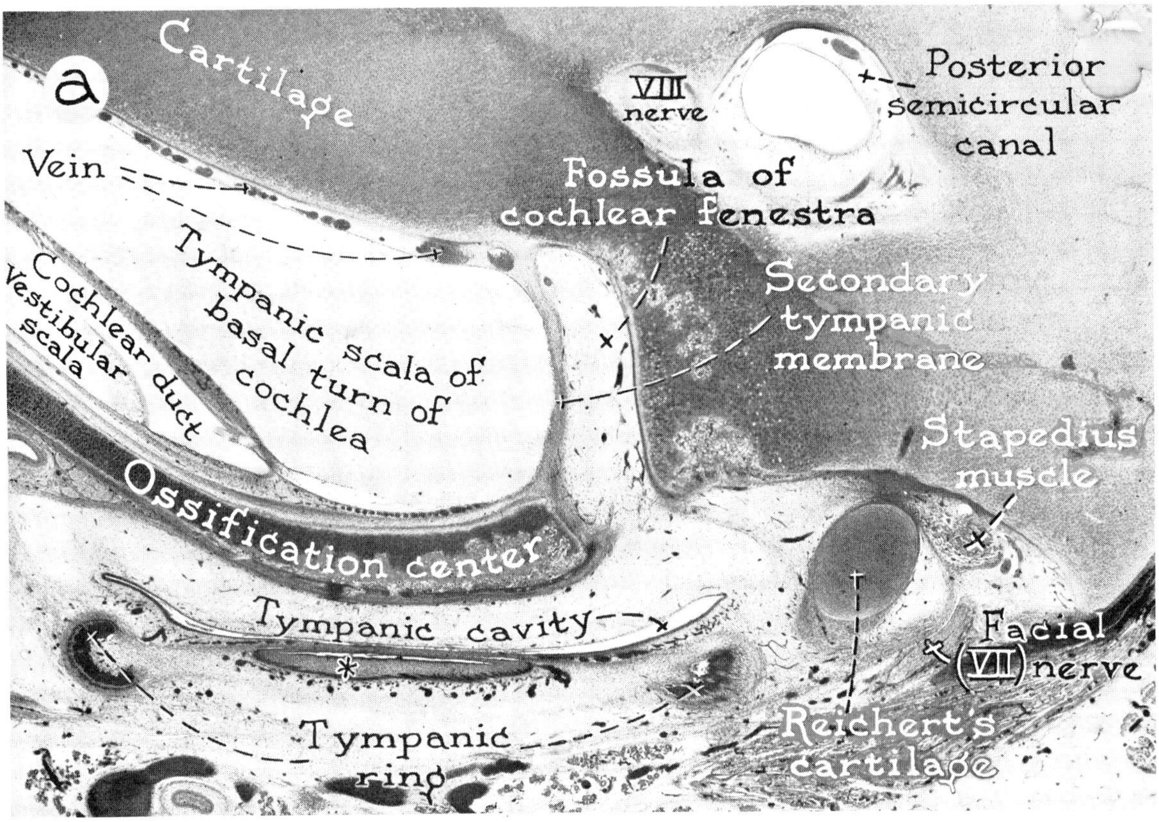

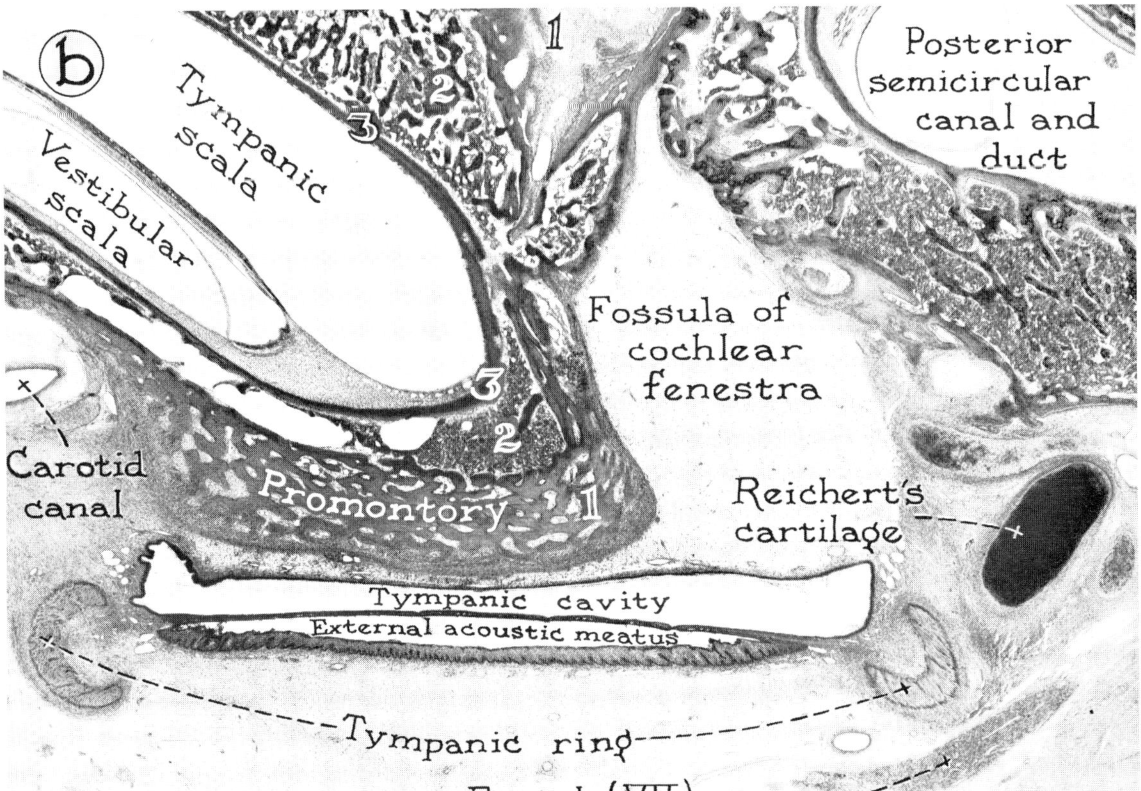

Figure II–10. See legend on the opposite page.

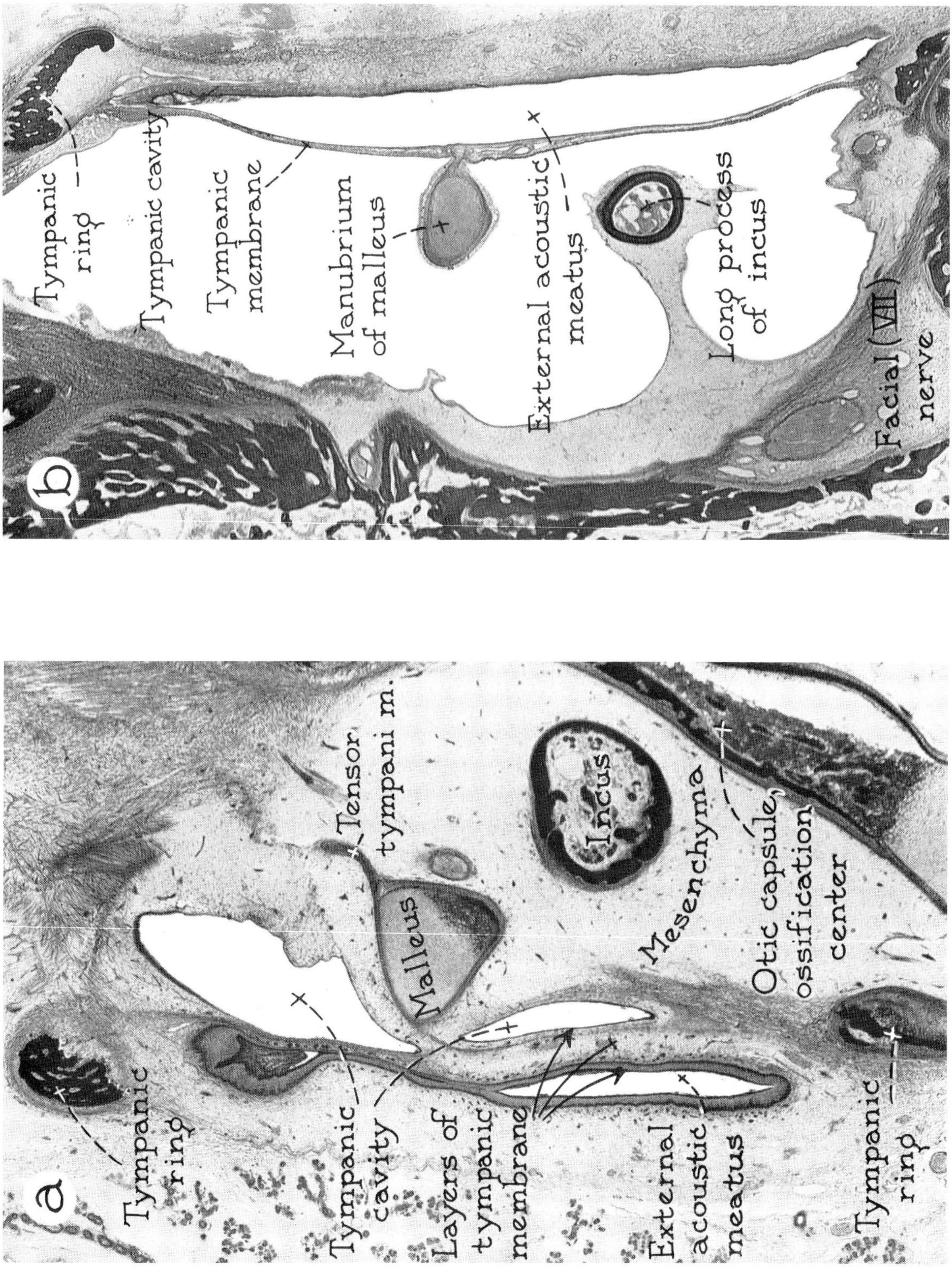
b
Tympanic ring
Tympanic cavity
Tympanic membrane
Manubrium of malleus
External acoustic meatus
Long process of incus
Facial (VII) nerve
a
Tympanic ring
Tympanic cavity
Layers of tympanic membrane
External acoustic meatus
Tympanic ring
Malleus
Tensor tympani m.
Incus
Mesenchyma
Otic capsule, ossification center

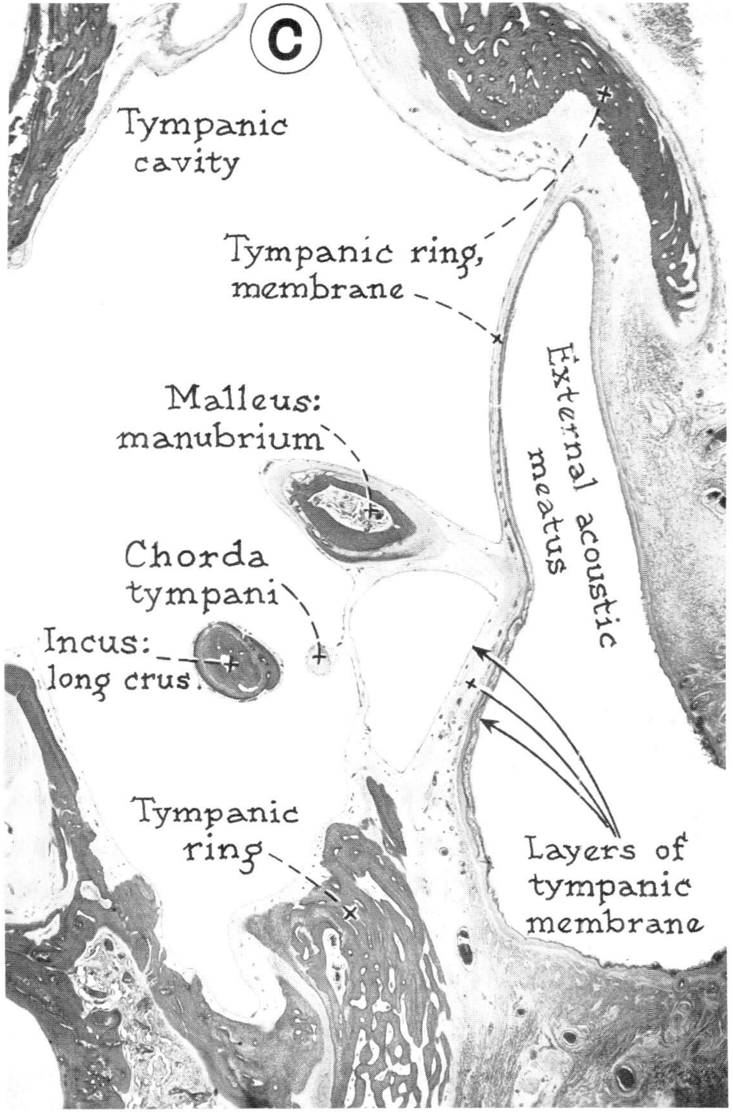

Figure II–11. TYMPANIC RING AND MEMBRANE: DEVELOPMENTAL ANATOMY.

a. FETUS OF 19½ WEEKS (160 MM.). *b.* FETUS OF 25 WEEKS (222 MM.). *c.* TERM FETUS.

a. In the 5-month fetus, the anterior limb of the developing tympanic annulus is just beginning to change from rodlike to sulcate form (see reconstructions, Figure II–12). The laminae of the tympanic membrane are shown. The mucous membrane of the middle ear has not yet invested the auditory ossicles.

b. In a specimen approximately a month and a half older, the anterior limb of the ring is definitely sulcate. The tympanic membrane is approaching the thinned appearance that is characteristic of the adult stage. The ossicles are invested by the advancing mucous membrane.

c. In the fetus at term, the histological structure is still similar to that of the annulus in the 25-week specimen. As demonstrated in a specimen (Figure II–13), the enclosed space is destined to be partitioned.

Transverse sections, Wisconsin Collection, series 41, 46, and 143, respectively. *a*, × 26; *b*, × 17; *c*, × 22.

ADULT STRUCTURE: Illustrated in Figures III–4 to III–7.

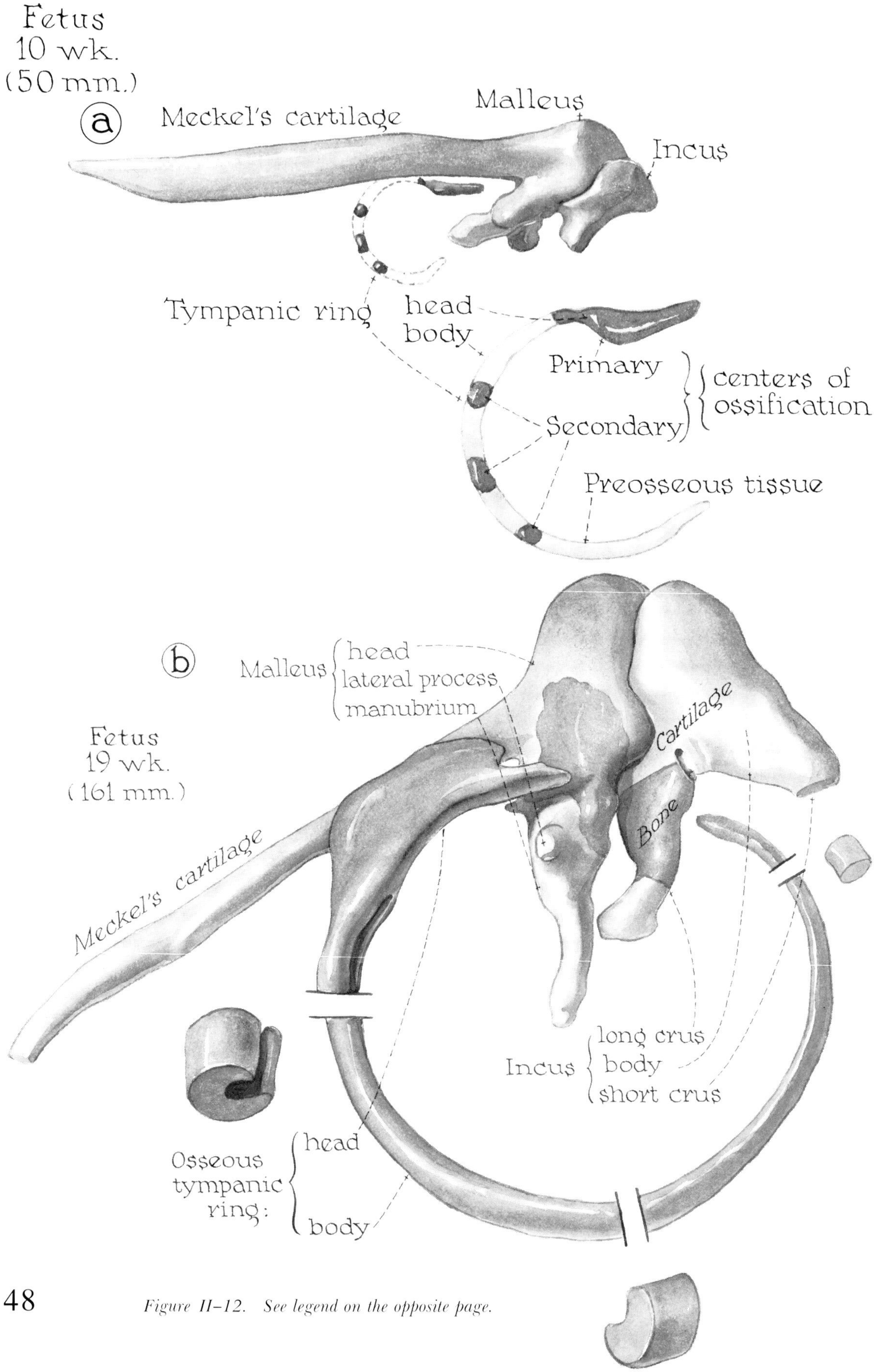

Figure II–12. See legend on the opposite page.

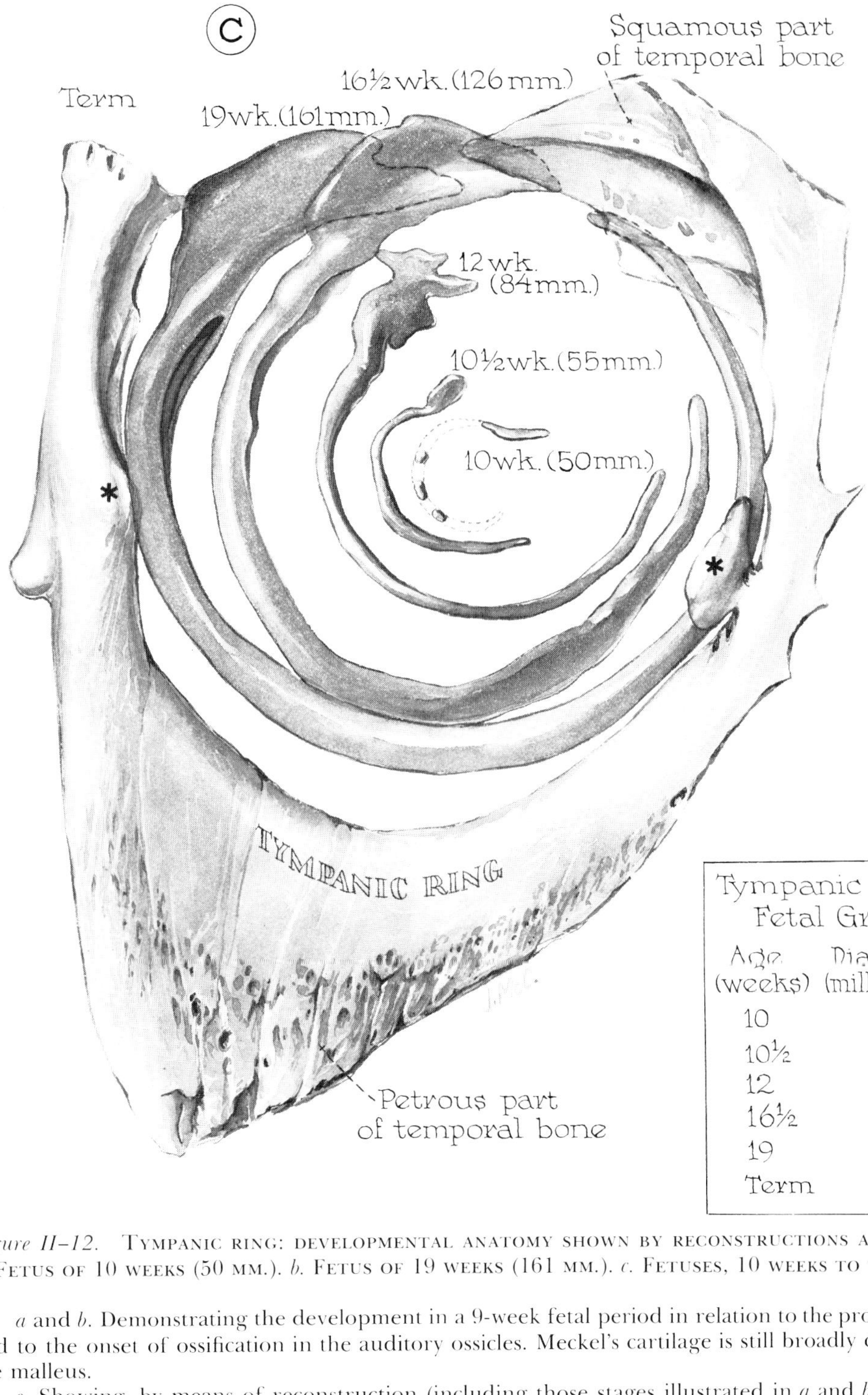

Tympanic Ring Fetal Growth

Age (weeks)	Diameter (millimeters)
10	2.1
10½	2.6
12	4.2
16½	6.4
19	7.4
Term	10.0

Figure II–12. Tympanic ring: developmental anatomy shown by reconstructions and a specimen. *a.* Fetus of 10 weeks (50 mm.). *b.* Fetus of 19 weeks (161 mm.). *c.* Fetuses, 10 weeks to term.

a and *b*. Demonstrating the development in a 9-week fetal period in relation to the progress of growth and to the onset of ossification in the auditory ossicles. Meckel's cartilage is still broadly continuous with the malleus.

c. Showing, by means of reconstruction (including those stages illustrated in *a* and *b*), the course of fetal development of the annulus to the fifth month; as well as the form and size of a specimen from a fetus at term. In the specimen the prominences indicated by asterisks will, by growth during the first postnatal year, meet and fuse. Thereby, the space enclosed by the primordial annulus will be divided into the external acoustic meatus and the foramen of Huschke (see Figure II–13*c*).

a and *b*. Wisconsin Collection, series 194 and 13, respectively. *c*. Reconstructions from Wisconsin Collection, series 194, 185, 162, 11, and 13, respectively.

(From Anson, Bast, and Richany: Ann. Otol., 64:802–823, 1955; Quart. Bull., Northwestern Univ. Med. Sch., 29:21–36, 1955.)

Adult Structure: Illustrated in Figures III–4 to III–7.

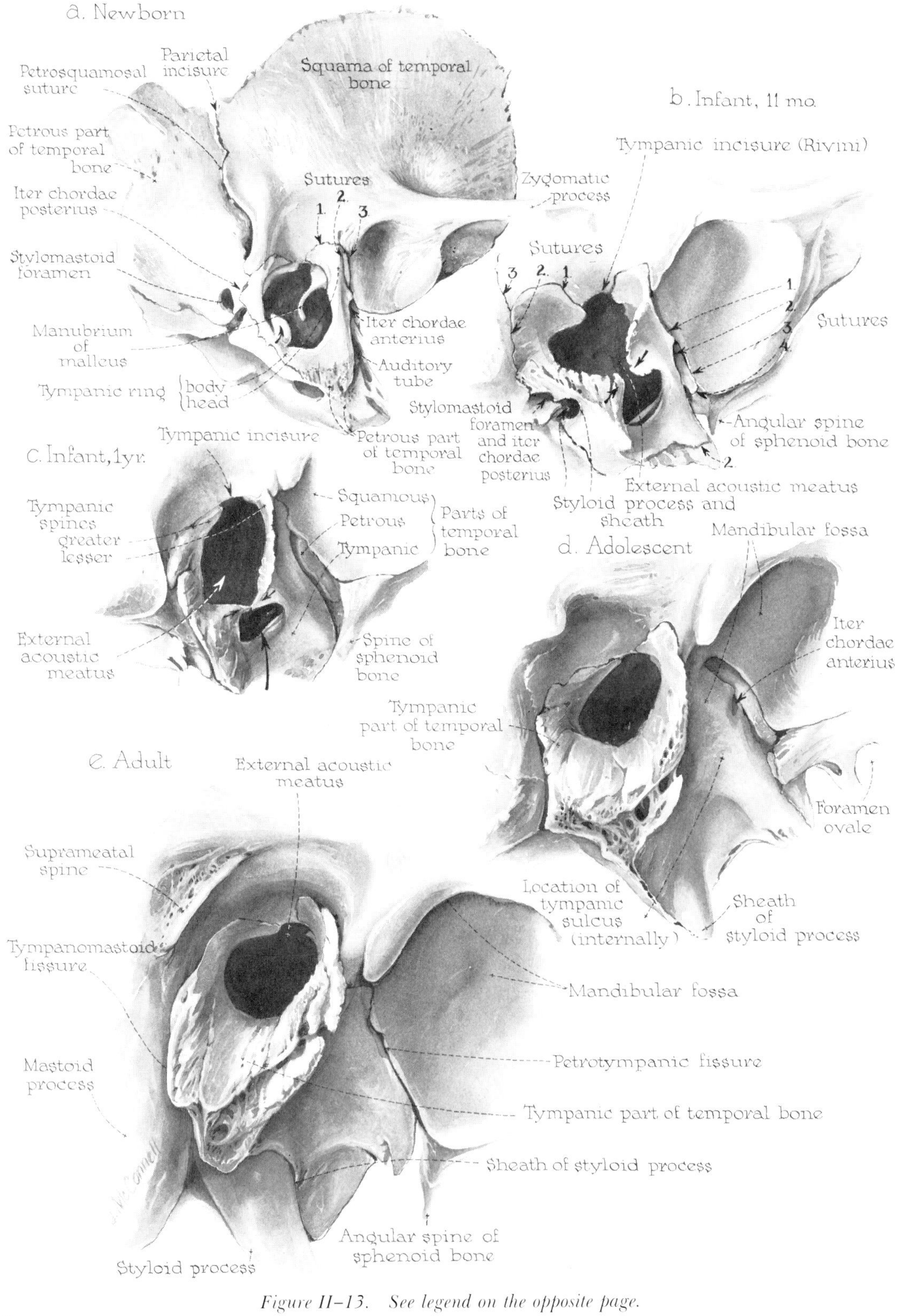

Figure II–13. See legend on the opposite page.

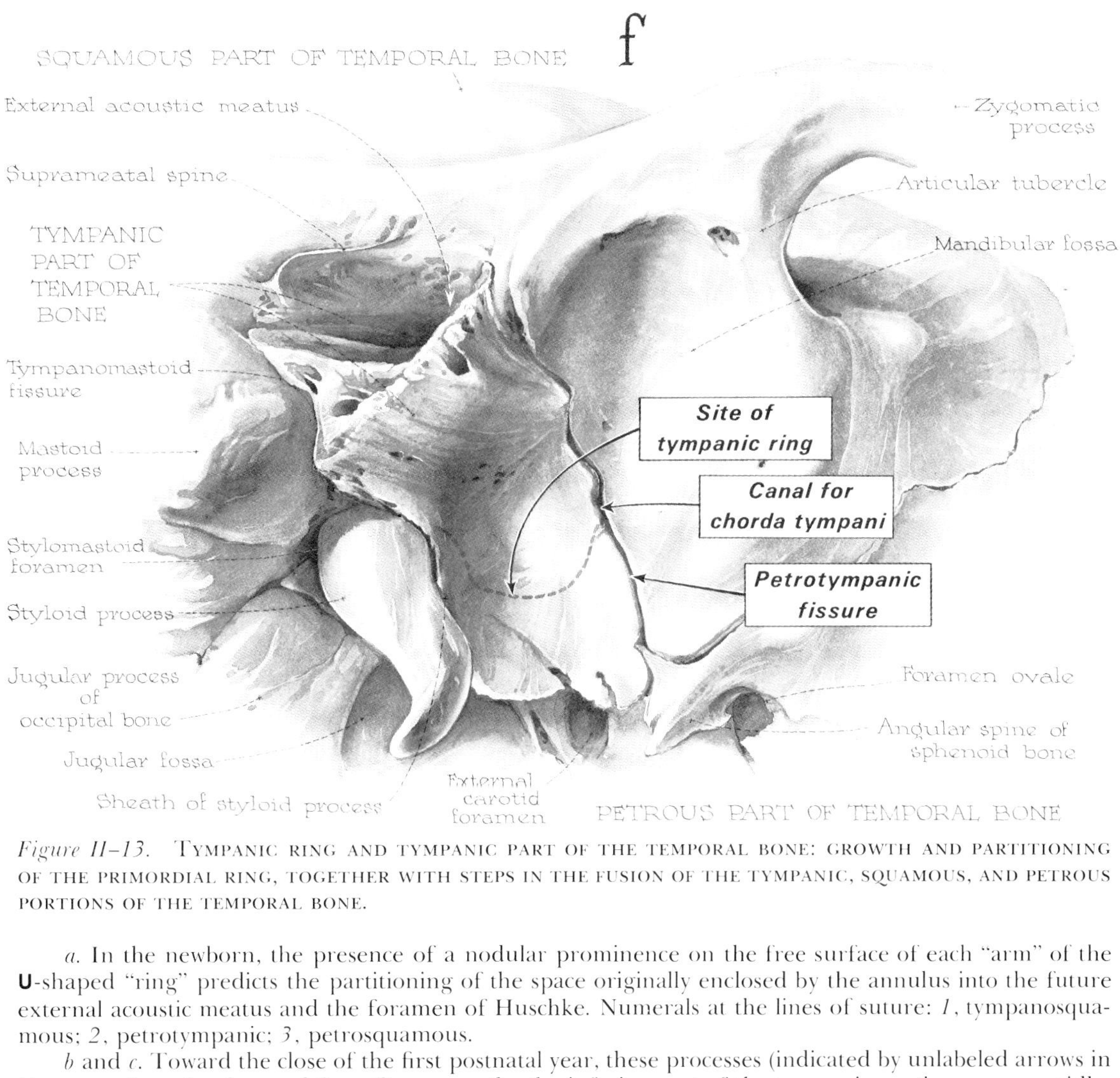

Figure II–13. TYMPANIC RING AND TYMPANIC PART OF THE TEMPORAL BONE: GROWTH AND PARTITIONING OF THE PRIMORDIAL RING, TOGETHER WITH STEPS IN THE FUSION OF THE TYMPANIC, SQUAMOUS, AND PETROUS PORTIONS OF THE TEMPORAL BONE.

a. In the newborn, the presence of a nodular prominence on the free surface of each "arm" of the **U**-shaped "ring" predicts the partitioning of the space originally enclosed by the annulus into the future external acoustic meatus and the foramen of Huschke. Numerals at the lines of suture: *1*, tympanosquamous; *2*, petrotympanic; *3*, petrosquamous.

b and *c.* Toward the close of the first postnatal year, these processes (indicated by unlabeled arrows in *b*) approach each other and fuse. Concurrently, the inferior part of the tympanic portion grows rapidly, thereby increasing the length of the meatus. At this stage, the foramen of Huschke (unlabeled arrow in *c*) is a relatively capacious opening; except in rare instances of agenesis, it is closed by continuing growth of bone. The sphenoid bone is in contact with the petrous part of the temporal bone (at *4*).

d and *e.* In the adolescent and the adult, the meatal extension of the original ring has come to dwarf the size of the annulus. *f.* Showing, in a view of the inferior surface, the form and size of the tympanic part of the temporal bone in the adult. The site of the annulus is indicated by a dotted line.

(From Anson, Bast, and Richany: Ann. Otol., 64:802–823, 1955.)

ADULT STRUCTURE: Illustrated in Figures III–4 to III–7.

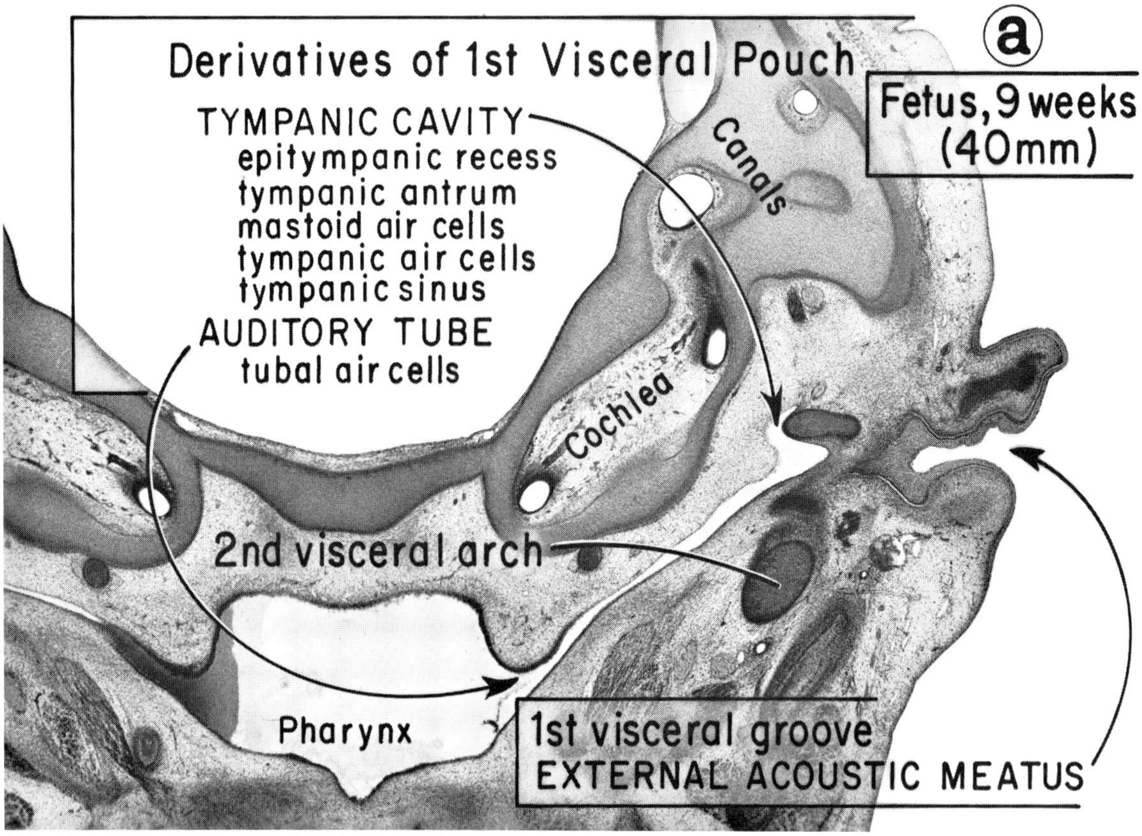

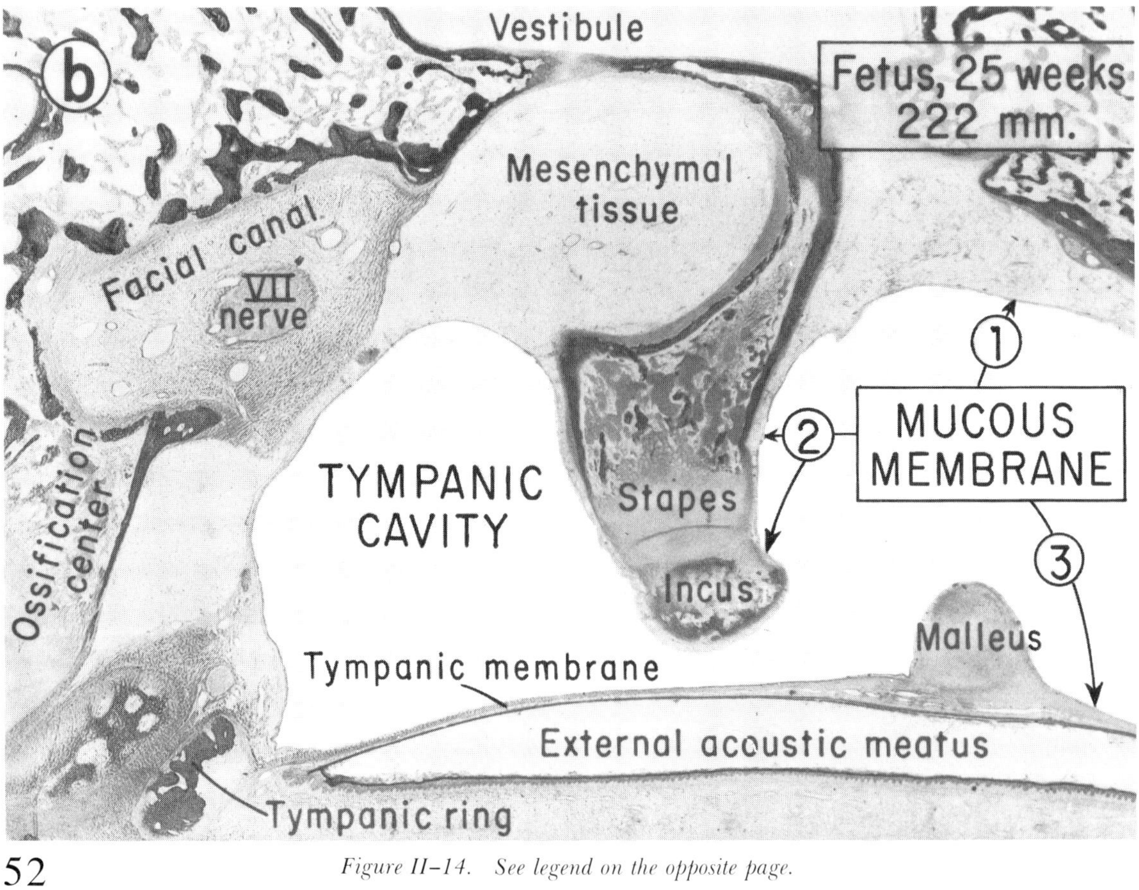

Figure II–14. See legend on the opposite page.

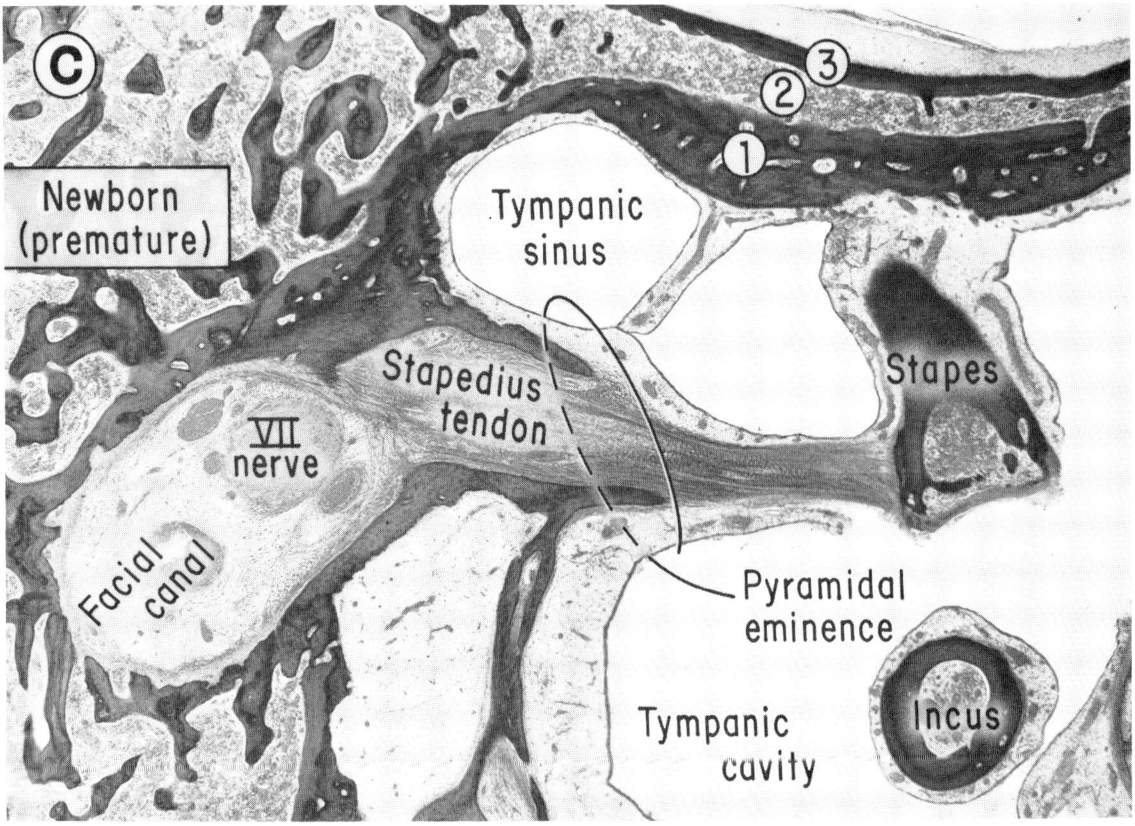

Figure II–14. TYMPANIC CAVITY AND RELATED AIR SPACES OF THE PETROUS AND MASTOID PARTS OF THE TEMPORAL BONE: DEVELOPMENTAL AND ADULT ANATOMY. *a.* FETUS OF 9 WEEKS (40 MM.). *b.* FETUS OF 25 WEEKS (222 MM.). *c.* NEWBORN (4-DAY PREMATURE).

a. In the fetus of 9 weeks the pharyngeal diverticulum has advanced to the primitive malleus, which it will invest with mucous membrane (the entoderm of the first visceral pouch). In further advance, the incus and stapes will be covered and recesses will be formed as offsets of the cavity proper and as pneumatic replacements of bone in the *pars petrosa* and *pars mastoidea* (see list in figure).

b. At the 25-week stage, the mucous membrane has invested the malleus on the lateral wall of the tympanic cavity (at *3*) and has contributed the inner layer of the tympanic membrane. It is being draped over the incus and stapes (at *2*) and is advancing toward the medial (labyrinthine) wall of the cavity (at *1*).

c. Showing the tympanic sinus, situated between the subiculum and the ponticulus. The layers of the capsule are numbered as shown in Figures II–5 and II–6.

Transverse sections, Wisconsin Collection, series 168, 46, and 124, respectively. *a*, × 17; *b*, × 25; *c*, × 25.

(*a* and *b* from Anson: Chapter 1 in Paparella and Shumrick (Eds.): Otolaryngology, Vol. I. Philadelphia, W. B. Saunders Co., 1973.)

ADULT STRUCTURE: Illustrated in Figures III–7 to III–22 and III–32 to III–39.

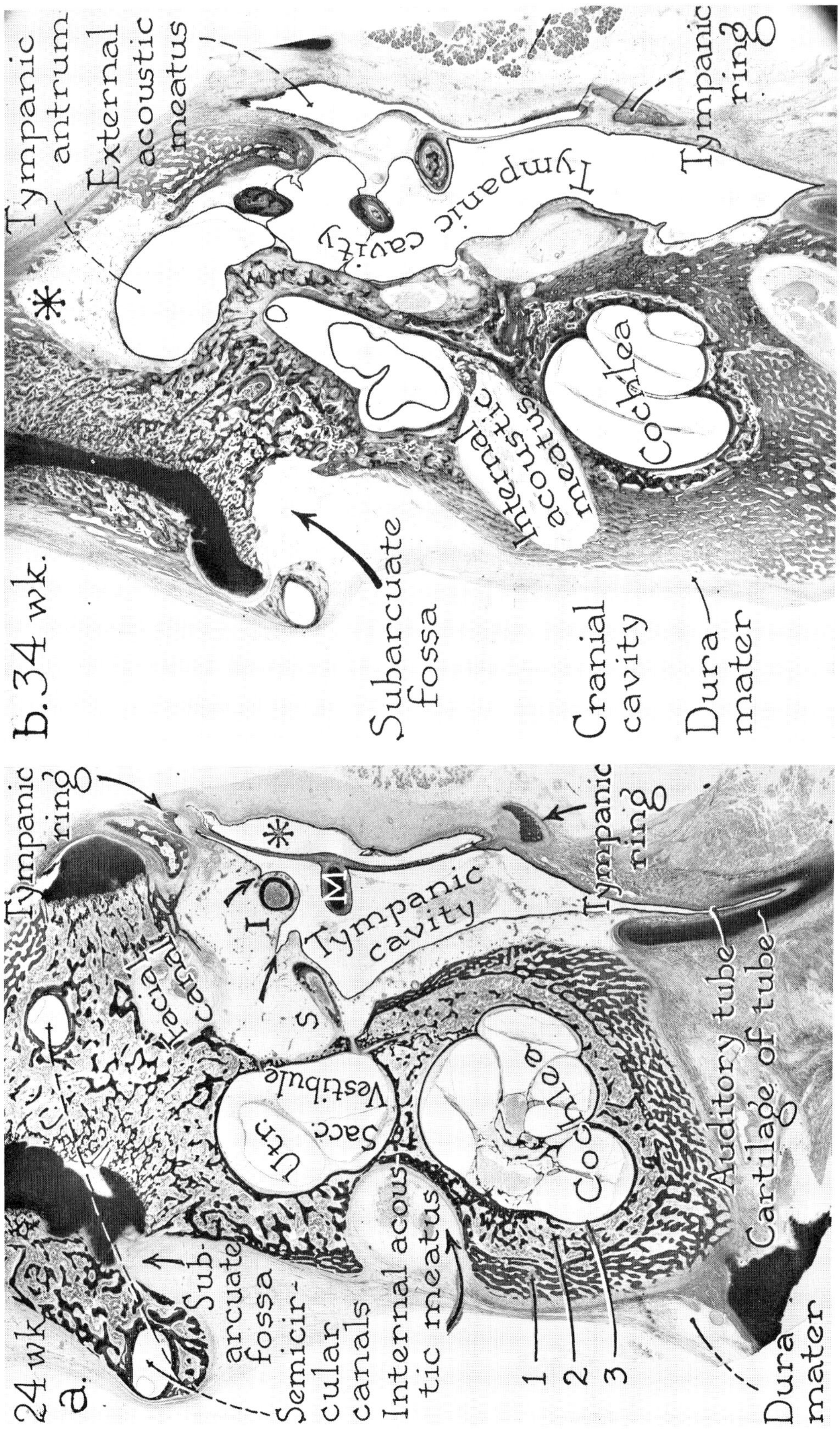

b. 34 wk.
Tympanic antrum
External acoustic meatus
Tympanic cavity
Tympanic ring
*
Cochlea
Internal acoustic meatus
Subarcuate fossa
Cranial cavity
Dura mater
a. 24 wk.
Tympanic ring
Facial canal
Sub-arcuate fossa
Semicircular canals
Internal acoustic meatus
Utr.
Sacc.
Vestibule
Cochlea
I
M
S
Tympanic cavity
Tympanic ring
Auditory tube
Cartilage of tube
Dura mater
1
2
3

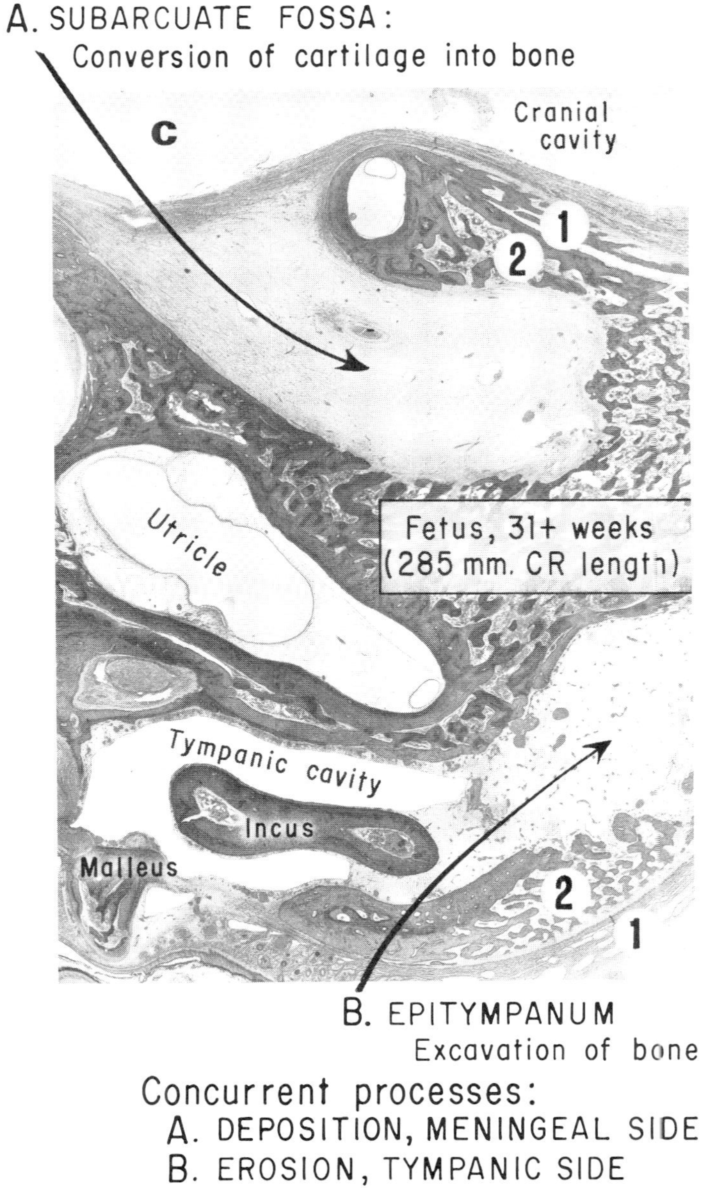

Figure II–15. Tympanic cavity and otic capsule: developmental anatomy. *a.* Fetus of 24 weeks (210 mm.). *b.* Fetus of 34 weeks (310 mm.). *c.* Fetus of 31+ weeks (285 mm.).

a. In the 6-month fetus, the mucous membrane of the expanding tympanic cavity has invested the manubrium of the malleus, has reached the crus of the stapes, and is being draped over the long process of the incus (as indicated by the unlabeled arrows). Abbreviations: *I*, incus; *M*, malleus; *S*, stapes. Numerals: *1*, outer periosteal layer of the ossifying otic capsule; *2*, middle (endosteal) layer; *3*, inner periosteal layer. Asterisk indicates the external acoustic meatus.

b. In a specimen approaching the ninth month of fetal life, epithelial investment of the malleus and incus is almost complete. Continuing expansion of the tympanic cavity has resulted in replacement of recently formed bone of the middle lamina of the otic capsule by mucous membrane (here, in the area of the tympanic antrum). Spicules of intrachondral and endochondral bone undergo resorption (at asterisk) in advance of the mucosal layer.

c. Demonstrating the manner in which concurrent processes, acting on opposite aspects of the otic capsule, reduce the size of the subarcuate fossa and increase that of the tympanic cavity. Numerals as in *a*.

Transverse sections, Wisconsin Collection, series 128, 68, and 108, respectively. *a*, × 12; *b*, × 8; *c*, × 10.

(*a* and *b* from Anson: Section X in Anson (Ed.): Morris' Human Anatomy, 12th ed. Copyright © 1966 by McGraw-Hill, Inc. Used by permission of McGraw-Hill Book Company. *c* from Anson: Trans. Amer. Acad. Ophthal. Otolaryng., 73:17–38, 1969.)

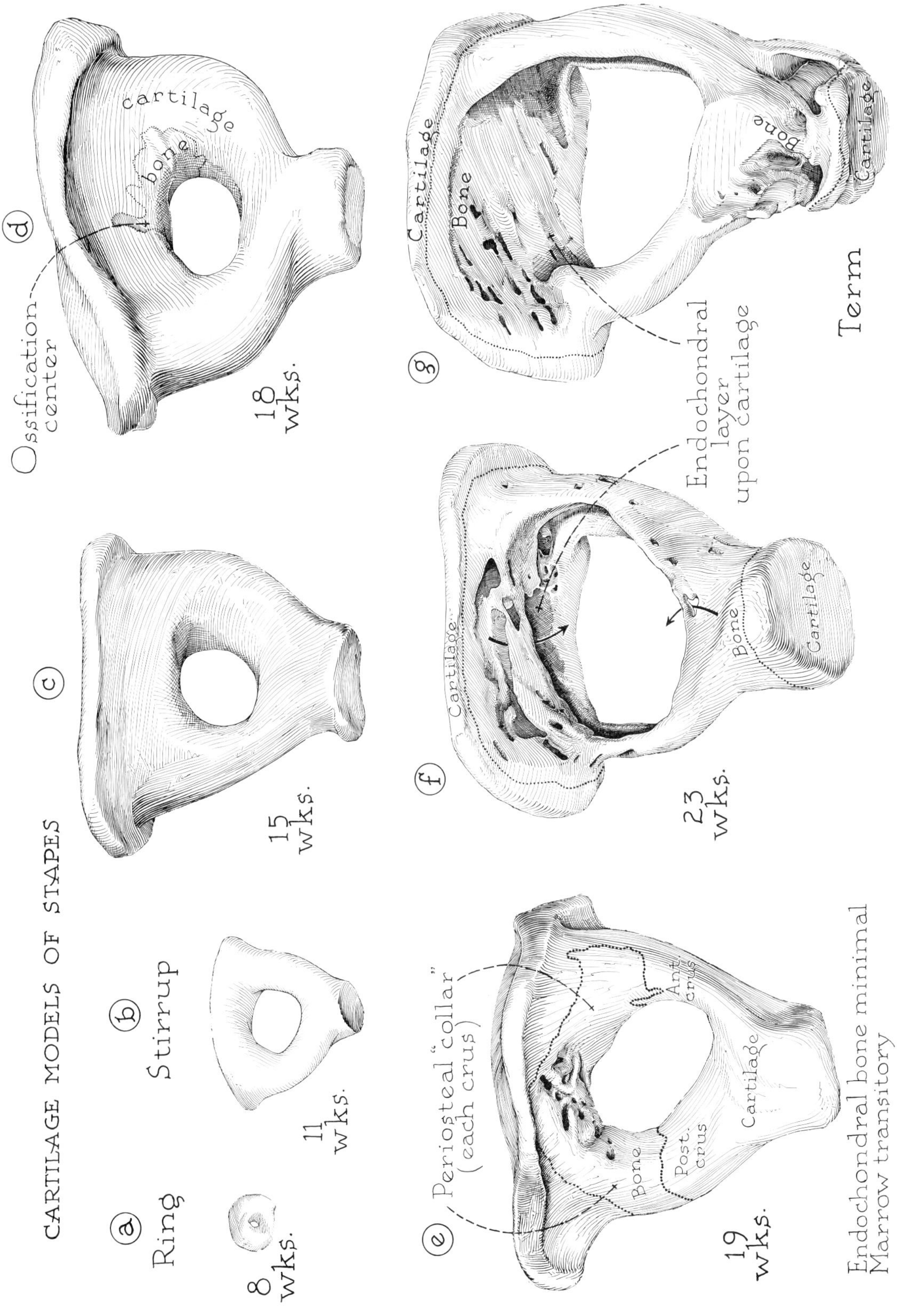
CARTILAGE MODELS OF STAPES
a
Ring
8 wks.
b
Stirrup
11 wks.
c
15 wks.
d
Ossification center
cartilage
bone
18 wks.
e
Periosteal "collar" (each crus)
Ant. crus
Bone
Post. crus
Cartilage
19 wks.
Endochondral bone minimal
Marrow transitory
f
Cartilage
Bone
Cartilage
23 wks.
Endochondral layer upon cartilage
g
Cartilage
Bone
Bone
Cartilage
Term

Figure II–16. STAPES: SEVEN STAGES IN FETAL DEVELOPMENT FROM THE SECOND MONTH TO TERM. SHOWN BY RECONSTRUCTIONS PREPARED BY THE BORN WAX-PLATE METHOD FROM SERIES IN THE WISCONSIN COLLECTION.

a. In the specimen of 2 months, the cartilaginous forerunner of the ossicle is still ring-shaped. *b* and *c.* It grows in cartilage through approximately the next 2-month period, currently changing from annular to stapedial form. *d.* The single ossification center appears early in the fifth month of fetal life. *e.* Spreading along the crura toward the head and across the base (footplate), the bone forms a periosteal "collar," internal to which there are scattered spicules of endosteal bone. No sooner is an osseous shell completed than a process of erosion begins to render it foraminous. *f.* Removal of bone is so rapid that, in the ossicle of the 6-month fetus, the interior of the head, crura, and neck are continuously open toward the obturator foramen. Periosteal bone may persist as a *crista stapedis* on the base (above arrow). *g.* Endosteal bone remains only as a thin lamina on the internal, or obturator, surface of the head and base.

ADULT STRUCTURE: Illustrated in Figures III–24 and III–25.

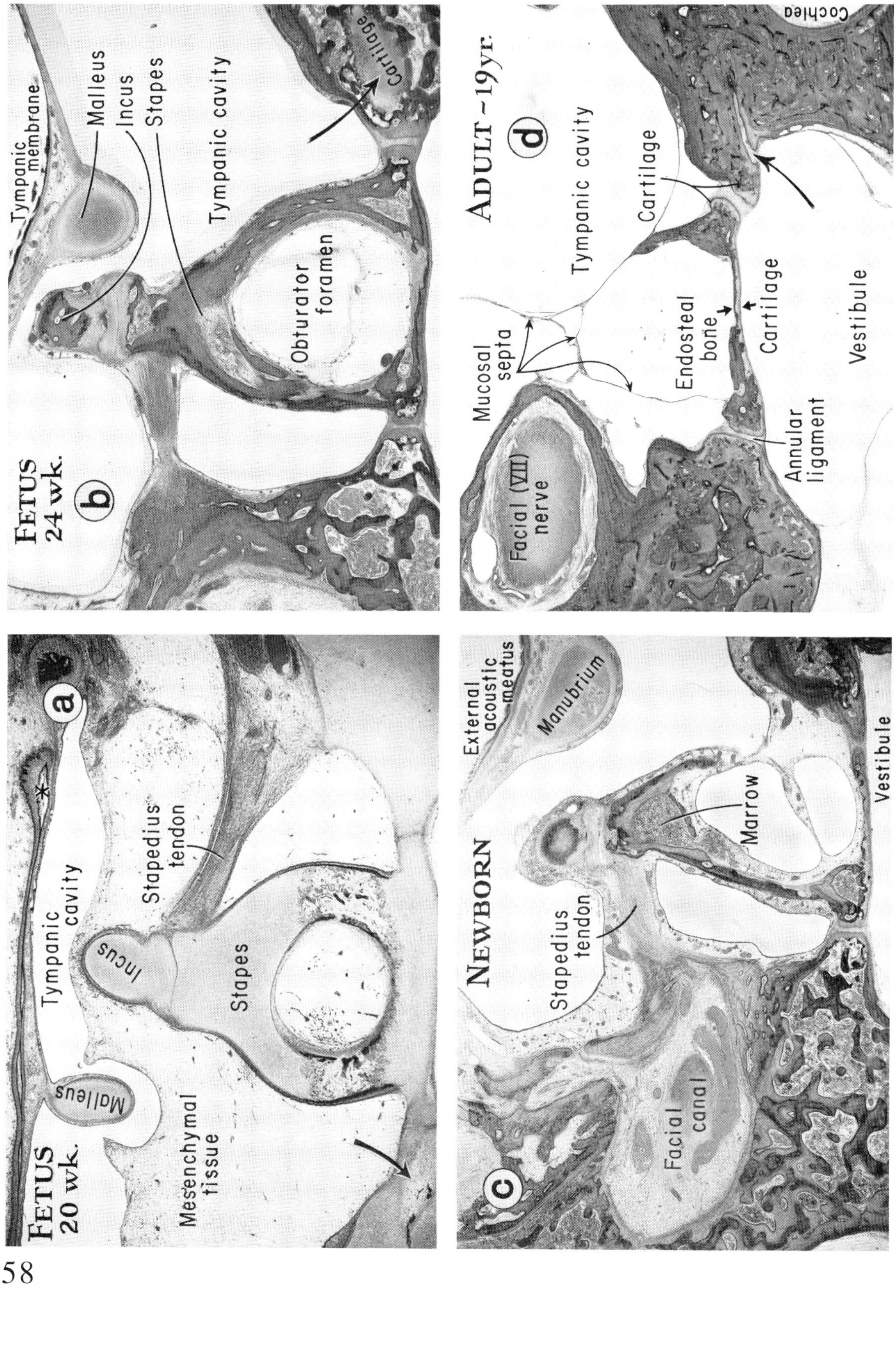
FETUS 20 wk.
a
Malleus
Tympanic cavity
Incus
Stapedius tendon
Stapes
Mesenchymal tissue
FETUS 24 wk.
b
Tympanic membrane
Malleus
Incus
Stapes
Tympanic cavity
Cartilage
Obturator foramen
NEWBORN
c
External acoustic meatus
Manubrium
Marrow
Stapedius tendon
Facial canal
Vestibule
ADULT ~19 yr.
d
Cochlea
Tympanic cavity
Cartilage
Mucosal septa
Endosteal bone
Cartilage
Facial (VII) nerve
Annular ligament
Vestibule

Figure II–17. STAPES: CRUCIAL STAGES IN FETAL DEVELOPMENT AND THE MATURE OUTCOME OF THE PRENATAL CHANGES. SHOWN BY SECTIONS FROM THE OTOLOGICAL SERIES IN THE WISCONSIN COLLECTION.

a. In the 5-month fetus, periosteal bone is being produced at the basal extremity of each crus. Foramina, concurrently formed on the obturator surface, admit blood vessels to the primitive marrow cavity where endosteal bone will be transitorily present in the crura, permanently on the internal (obturator) surface of the base (footplate) and head. Asterisk indicates external acoustic meatus. Arrows in *a*, *b*, and *d* point to the fissula ante fenestram.

b and *c*. Periosteal bone is resorbed on the internal surface of the ossicle; the primitive marrow cavity, thereby opened, is invaded by the mucous membrane of the expanding tympanic cavity.

d. As a result of these changes, the stapes of the adult is a fragile skeletal element whose base is excessively thin despite its bilaminar structure. Cartilage, retained from fetal life, is carried across the vestibular surface to the fenestral margin of the tympanostapedial syndesmosis. The cartilage of the fenestra is continued into the vestibular aperture of the fissula ante fenestram (at arrow), where it occasionally occurs in the form of an aberrant nodule (as in *b*).

Transverse sections, Wisconsin Collection, series 131, 89, 124, and 29, respectively.

ADULT STRUCTURE: Illustrated in Figures III–24 and III–25.

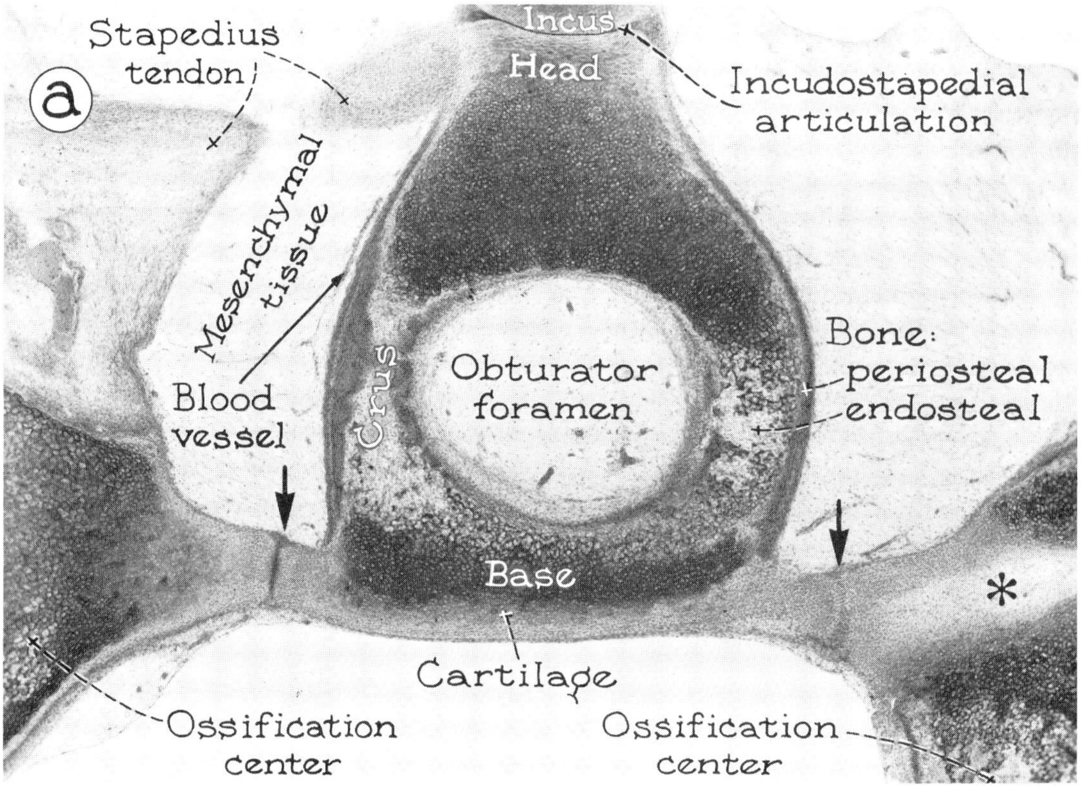

Figure II–18. DEVELOPMENT OF THE STAPES, ESPECIALLY IN RELATION TO BLOOD SUPPLY. *a.* FETUS OF 20 WEEKS (170 MM.). *b.* FETUS OF 27+ WEEKS (243 MM.). *c.* FETUS OF 31 WEEKS (280 MM.). *d.* NEWBORN INFANT (4-DAY PREMATURE).

a. At the onset of ossification, the tympanic part of the stapes is exposed to mesenchyma in which small blood vessels of a capillary network are widely distributed. The vestibular part (base, or footplate) is covered by an excessively thin layer of periotic tissue in which vessels, likewise small, are numerous. The crura of the stapes are undergoing change from cartilage to bone; each is a column of periosteal bone in which the cavity contains both primitive marrow and remnants of calcified cartilage.

Ossification of the otic capsule is in its early stage. The base of the stapes, originally continuous with the capsule, is now being segregated through a process of retrogressive change in the cartilage (at arrows); the reorganized tissue will be the annular ligament. A transcapsular channel, the fissula ante fenestram (at asterisk), is being formed as a result of invasion of the primitive cartilage by periotic tissue (see Figure II–17*a*).

Figure II–18 continues on the opposite page.

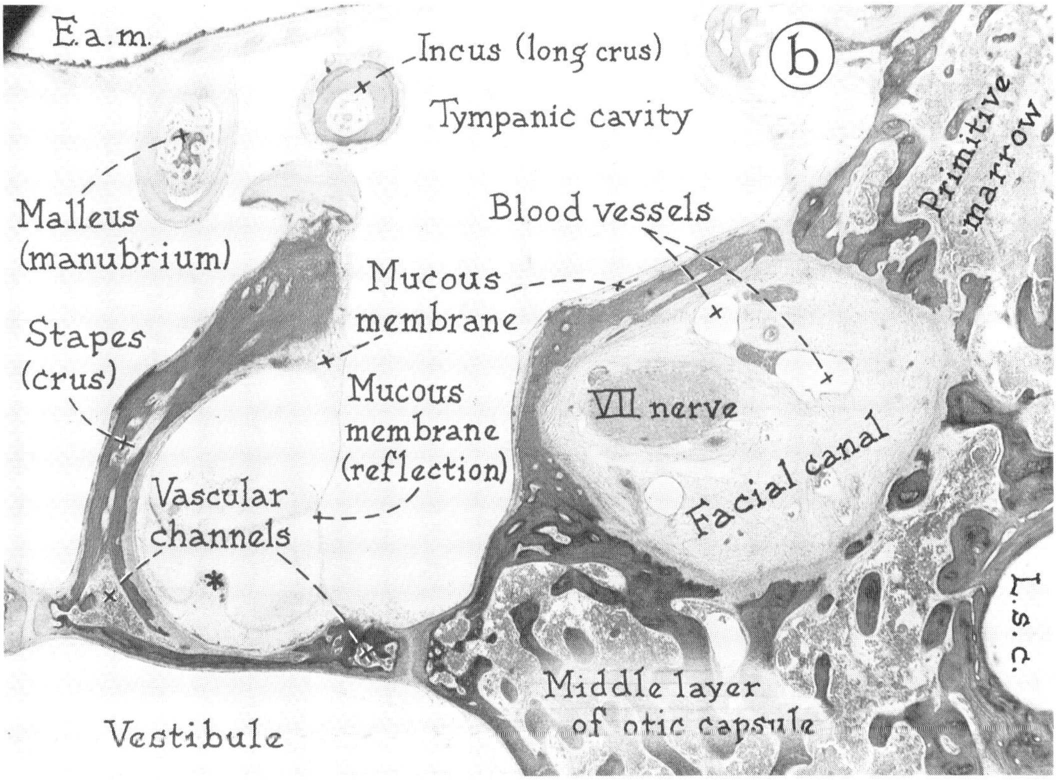

Figure II–18. Continued.

b. In the 7-month stage the stapes is approaching mature form and histological structure; the footplate and the head are now bilaminar and the crura are hollowed on their facing (obturator) surfaces. With the expansion of the tympanic cavity, the mucous membrane comes to form an investment for the ossicles, the stapes being the last member of the ossicular chain to be thus covered. Circumferentially, on the footplate, vascular channels are being formed through the growth of endosteal bone around blood vessels which are already present. Elsewhere, vascular supply is provided by vessels in the newly established submucosal layer (as at asterisk). They are conveyed by reflections of the mucous membrane (see Figures III–65*e* and *f*, III–91*c*, and III–141). These arteries and veins are, at their sources, elements of the general tympanic plexus and of the circumneural arterial plexus in the facial canal (see Figures III–67 and III–69*c*). These vessels communicate, in turn, with those in the middle layer of the maturing otic capsule (see Figure III–75). *Abbreviations: E.a.m.*, external acoustic meatus; *L.s.c.*, lateral semicircular canal.

Figure II–18 continues on the following page.

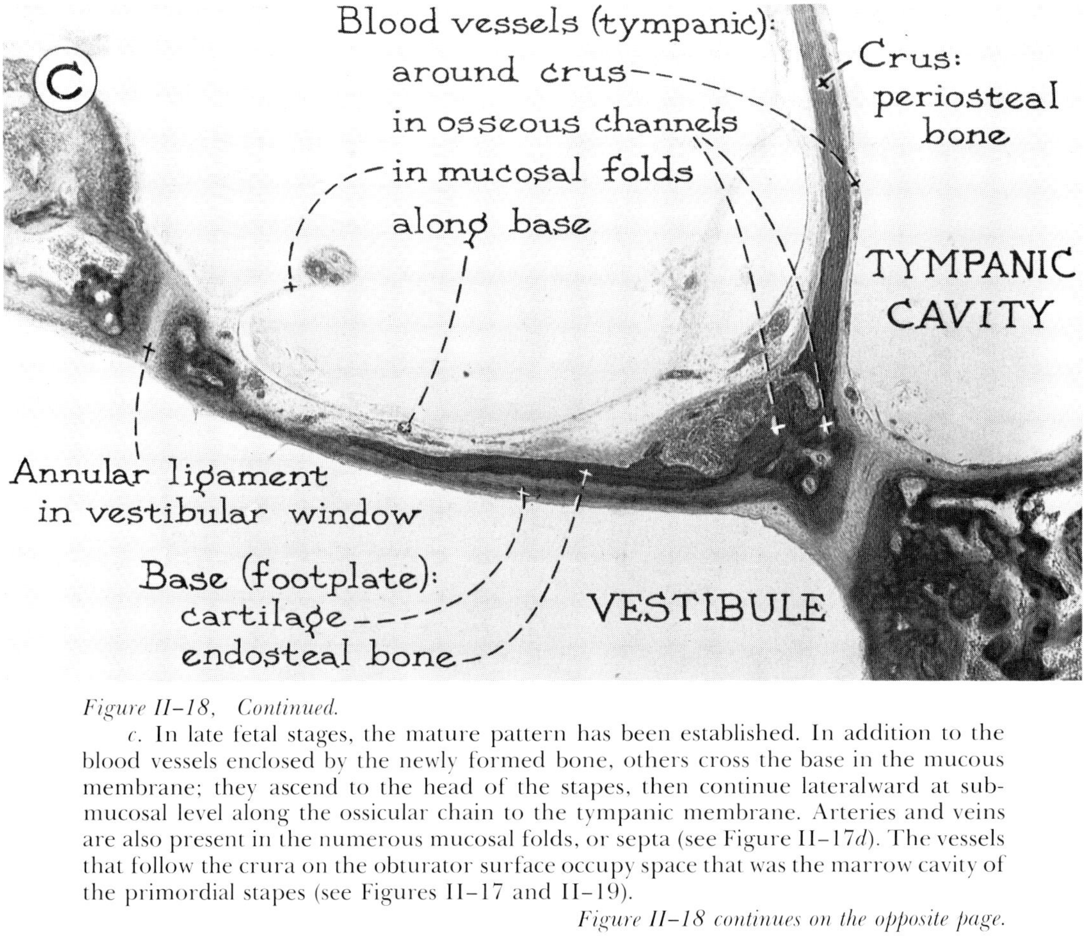

Figure II–18, Continued.

c. In late fetal stages, the mature pattern has been established. In addition to the blood vessels enclosed by the newly formed bone, others cross the base in the mucous membrane; they ascend to the head of the stapes, then continue lateralward at submucosal level along the ossicular chain to the tympanic membrane. Arteries and veins are also present in the numerous mucosal folds, or septa (see Figure II–17*d*). The vessels that follow the crura on the obturator surface occupy space that was the marrow cavity of the primordial stapes (see Figures II–17 and II–19).

Figure II–18 continues on the opposite page.

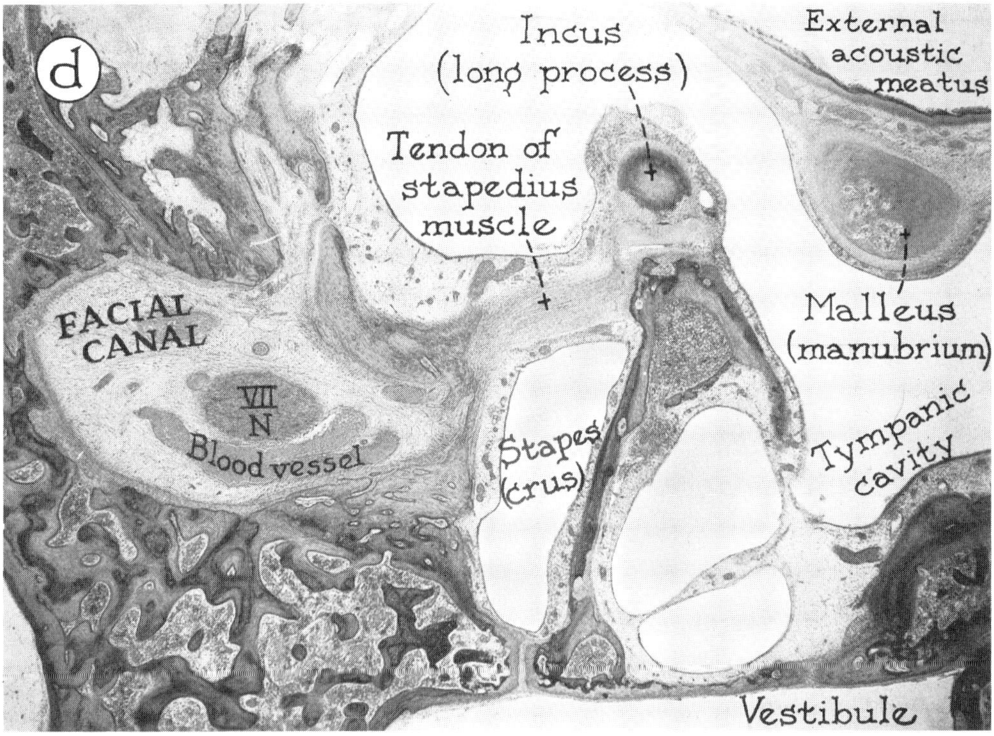

Figure II–18. Continued.

d. The tendon of the stapedius muscle serves as an important means of transmission of blood vessels between the facial canal and the tympanic cavity. They surround the tendon, being in submucosal position; a lesser supply comes through the substance of the tendon itself. The vessels in the canal are branches of the stylomastoid and rami derived from the superficial petrosal branch of the middle meningeal. Within the canal they are elements of the circumneural arterial network and corresponding venous plexus (see Figures III–67 and III–69*c*); in the middle ear they contribute to the richly anastomotic plexus of vessels in the tympanic mucous membrane and to those which occupy the mucosal septa.

Transverse sections, Wisconsin Collection, series 131, 89, 116 A, and 124, respectively. *a*, × 19; *b*, × 21; *c*, × 44; *d*, × 20.

ADULT STRUCTURE: Illustrated in Figures III–24 and III–25.

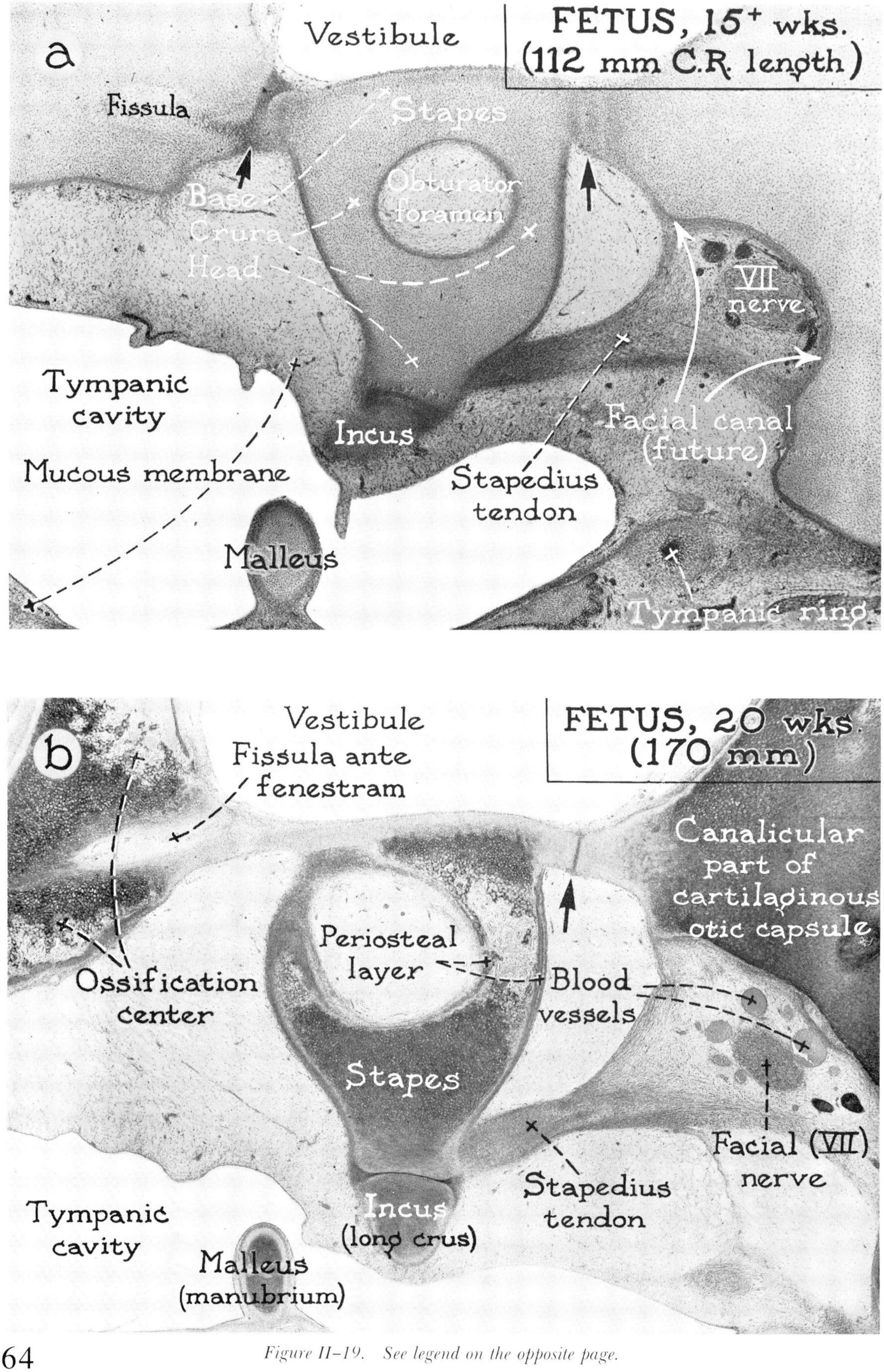

Figure II–19. See legend on the opposite page.

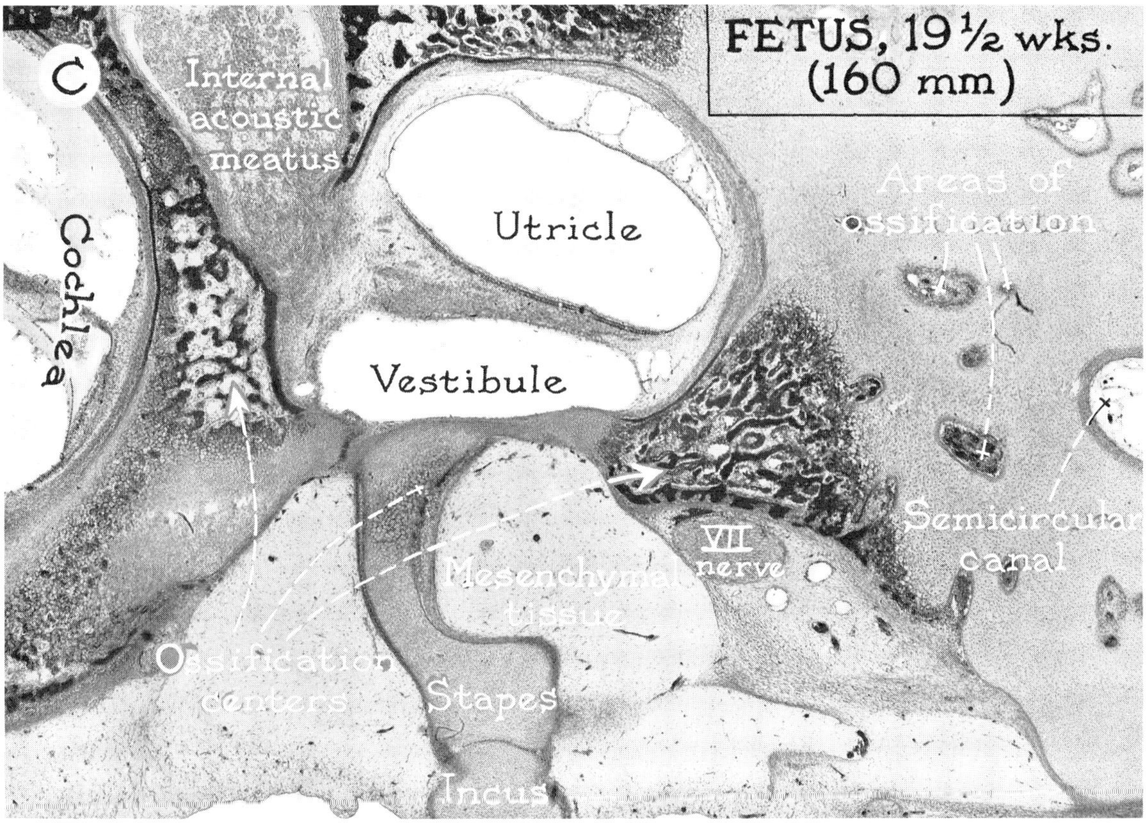

Figure II–19. STAPES, STAPEDIUS MUSCLE, VESTIBULAR (OVAL) FENESTRA, AND FACIAL CANAL: DEVELOPMENTAL AND ADULT ANATOMY. *a.* FETUS OF 15+ WEEKS (112 MM.). *b.* FETUS, 20 WEEKS (170 MM.). *c.* FETUS, 19½ WEEKS (160 MM.). *d.* FETUS, 26 WEEKS (230 MM.). *e.* NEWBORN (4-DAY PREMATURE). *f.* CHILD, 6 YEARS OF AGE.

a. In the fetus at approximately the 4-month stage, the stapes, initially annular in form, has attained the form of a stirrup. The base is flanged, the posterior crus is already bowed more sharply than the anterior, and the head is foveate for reception of the lenticular process of the incus. The area of the future vestibular (oval) window appears as a seam of retrogressively changing cartilage (at unlabeled arrows). The facial canal is a sulcate impression on the wall of the canalicular division of the capsule. Although primordial in form, the canal already houses the facial nerve, the stapedius muscle (inferior to the level of this section), and numerous blood vessels (veins outnumbering arteries). Mucous membrane of the expanding tympanic cavity has reached the malleus (manubrium) and incus (long crus); it has not yet invested any part of the stapes, nor has bone formation begun in either the otic capsule or the ossicles.

b. In the 5-month fetus, the initial step in ossification of the stapes is seen in the conversion of the crura from solid rods of cartilage into columns of periosteal bone that still contain primitive marrow. Concurrently, bone is being formed in the otic capsule.

c. Ossification is further advanced in the otic capsule of this 5-month specimen; one ossification center forms part of the wall of the developing facial canal. Bone formation is in a less advanced stage in the stapes (evidence of independence in speed of differentiation).

Figure II–19 continues on the following page.

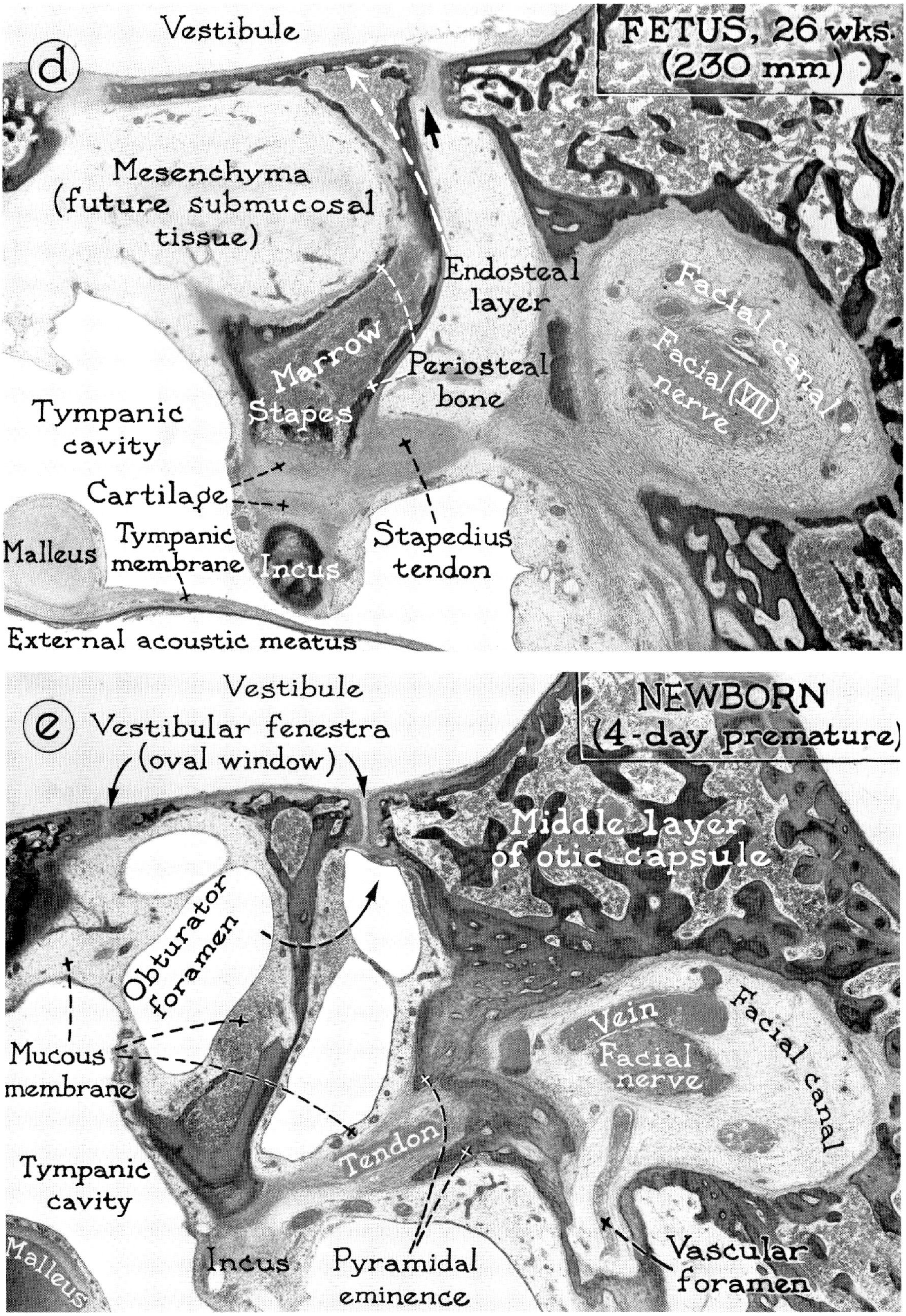

Figure II–19, Continued. See legend on the opposite page.

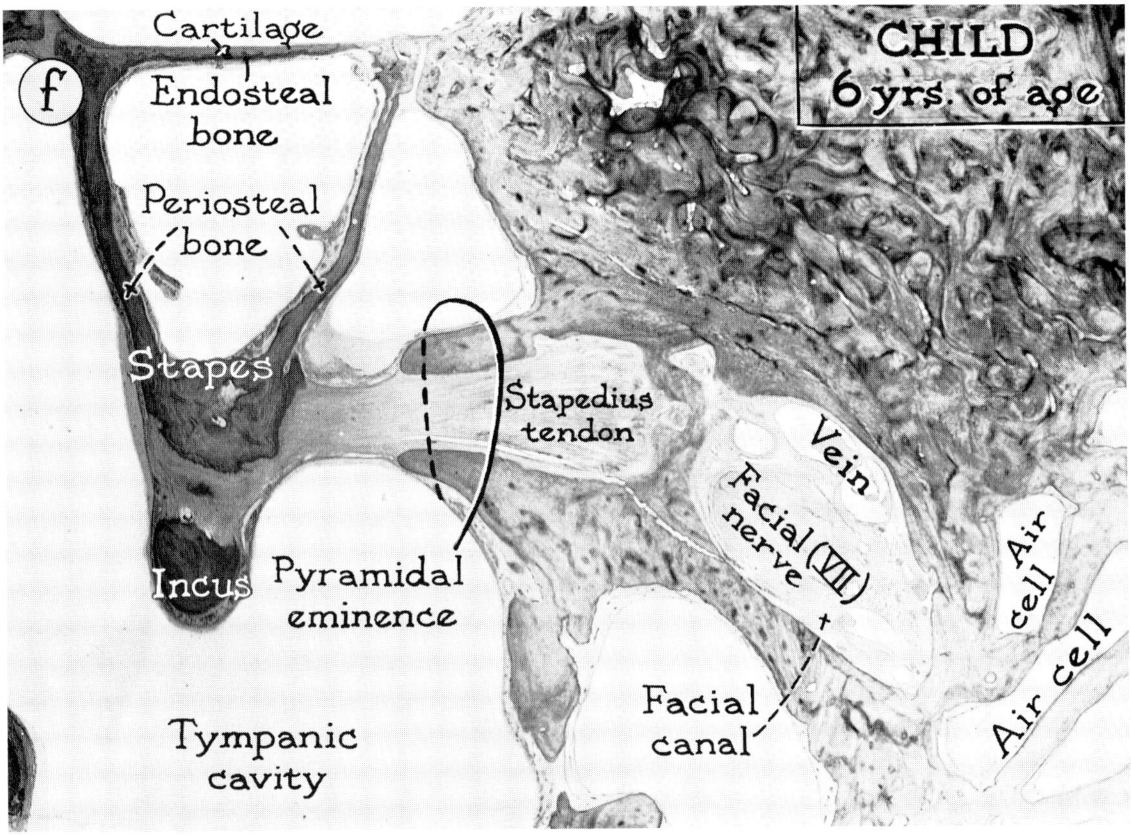

Figure II–19, Continued. STAPES, STAPEDIUS MUSCLE, VESTIBULAR FENESTRA, AND FACIAL CANAL.

d. The inner wall of the crura is being removed. As a result, the interior of each crus will be open on the surface facing the obturator foramen. Scattered "spicules" of endosteal bone are transitorily present in the primitive marrow. Differing from this circumstance, endosteal bone, formed along the base (footplate) and the head of the stapes (in contact with the original cartilage) will become a permanent structural element. In the middle layer of the otic capsule, bone formation has come to a temporary halt. Periosteal bone is beginning to enclose the canal on the anterior aspect.

e. Apparent quiescence in bone formation characterizes the middle layer through the remainder of the prenatal period. Differing from the middle layer, the outer layer of the capsule progressively thickens. During the same period, the stapes continues to undergo decrease in bulk, the outcome being the loss of the entire obturator wall. The facial canal is now fully formed. The stapedius tendon is accompanied by blood vessels which bring the elements of the tympanic vascular plexus into communication with arteries and veins in the facial canal. Additionally, blood vessels pass into the mucous membrane of the middle ear through foramina in the wall of the canal. Together, they vascularize the auditory ossicles, the otic capsule, and the tympanic membrane.

f. The result of the process of resorption in the stapes (seen in figures *d* and *e*) is an ossicle of striking fragility: each crus consists of a thin layer of periosteal bone continuous with equally thin base and head (each composed of a lamina of endosteal bone fused with one composed of the original cartilage). The middle layer of the capsule becomes reactivated whereby endosteal ossification converts the "cancellous" fabric into petrous bone. In the facial canal, the vascularity of the connective tissue, well established in the 4-month fetus, is retained as a permanent feature of the adult *pars petrosa.*

Transverse sections, Wisconsin Collection, series 53, 131, 41, 64, 124, and 81, respectively. *a,* × 33; *b,* × 23; *c,* × 18; *d,* × 26; *e,* × 24; *f,* × 18.

ADULT STRUCTURE: Illustrated in Figures III–24 and III–25.

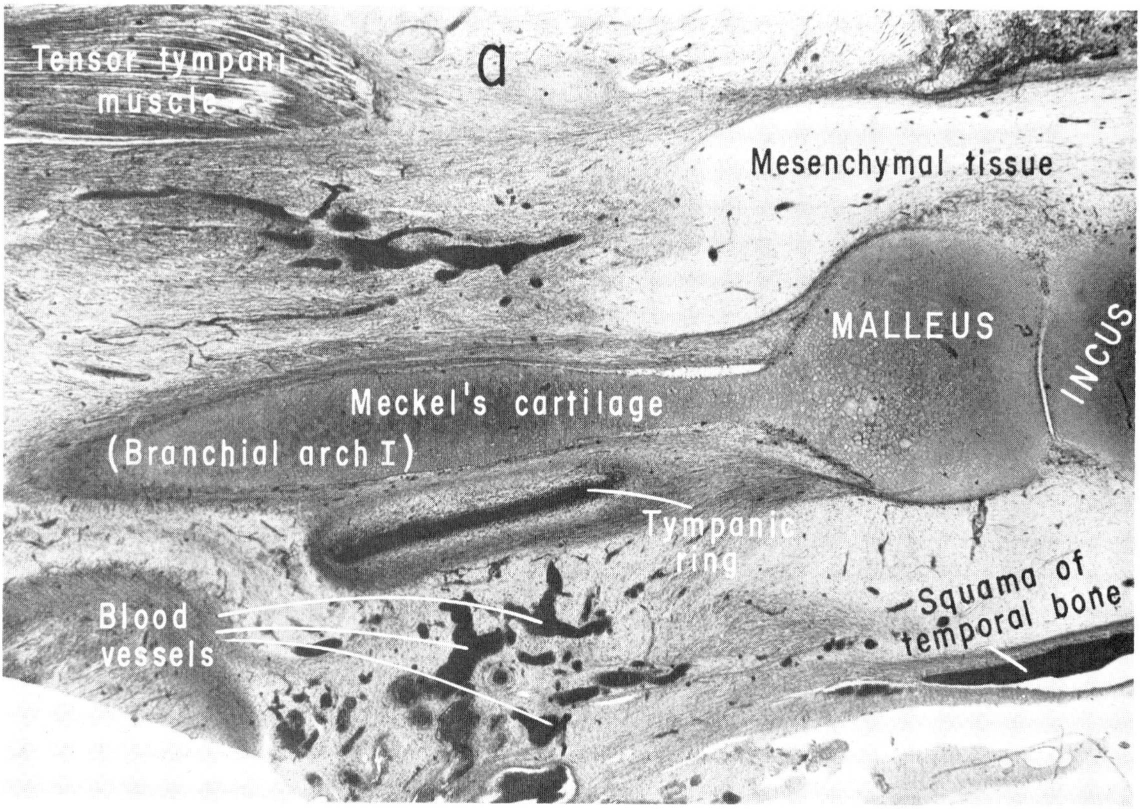

Figure II–20. Malleus and incus: developmental and adult anatomy. *a.* Fetus of 17 weeks (135 mm.). *b.* Fetus, 17 weeks (146 mm.). *c.* Fetus, 22 weeks (193 mm.). *d.* Adult, 19 years of age.

a. In a fetus of 17 weeks both the malleus and the incus are still cartilage "models" of the future ossicles. They are lodged in mesenchyma that will differentiate into submucosal tissue. The malleus is still broadly continuous with Meckel's cartilage.

Figure II–20 continues on the opposite page.

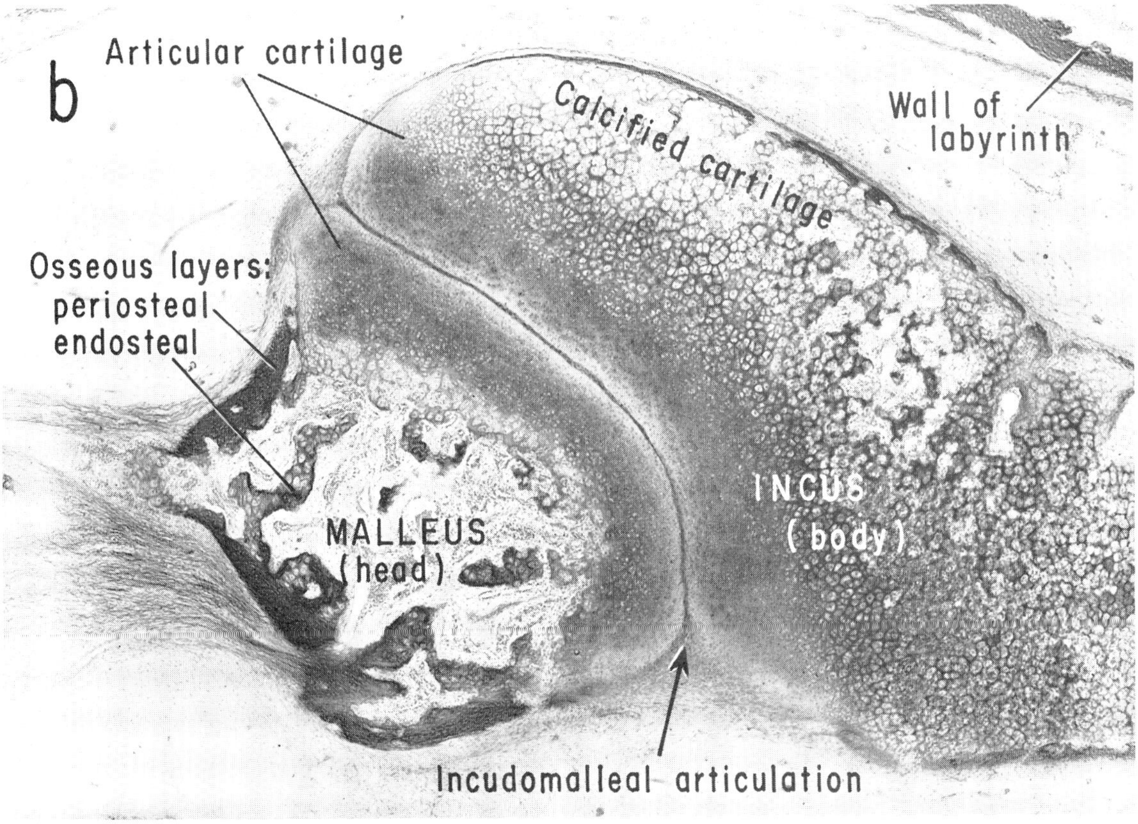

Figure II–20. Continued.

b. In a specimen of the same age but greater crown-rump (CR) length, an ossification center is present in the body of the incus and in the head of the malleus. The two important stages in ossification are illustrated: the initial formation of a periosteal shell (in the incus) and the production of endosteal bone (in the malleus). The cartilage on the facing surface of the two ossicles will remain as the articular cartilages.

Figure II–20 continues on the following page.

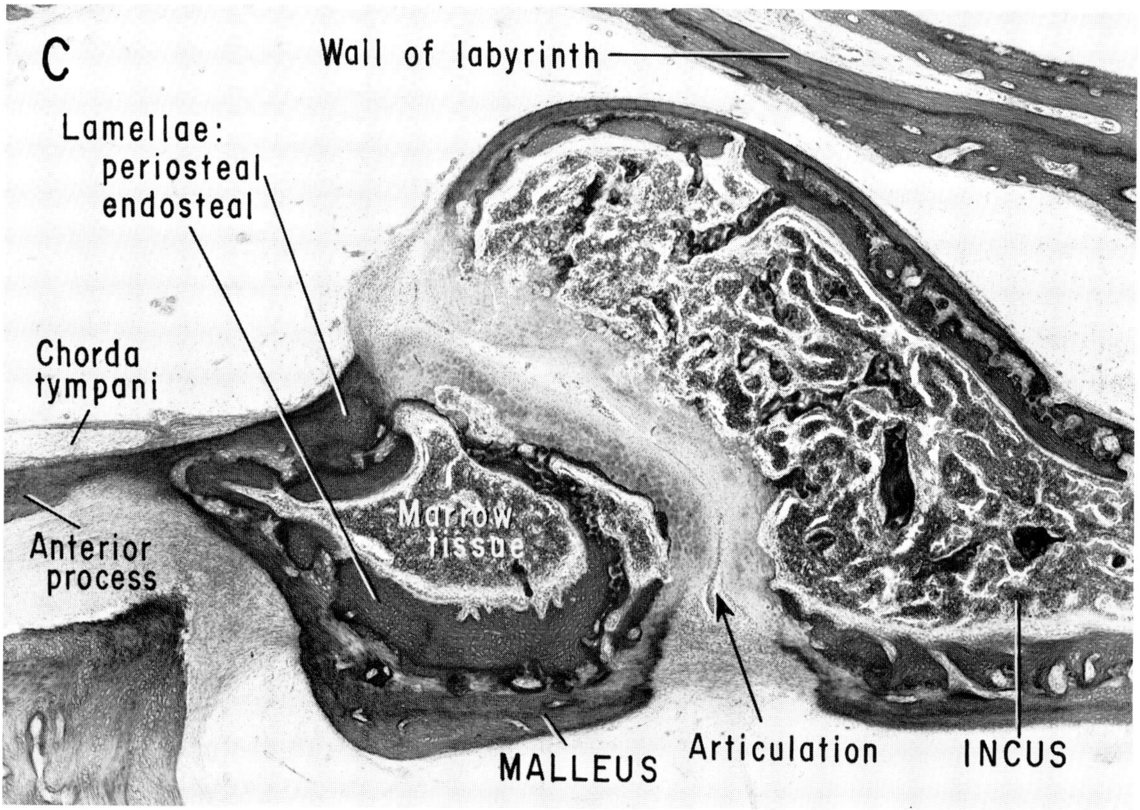

Figure II–20, Continued.

c. Considerable advance is evidenced in a fetal specimen five weeks older. This is especially true in the case of the incus, where endosteal bone is rapidly replacing primitive marrow. The anterior process of the malleus, formed independently in membrane bone, is now attached to the head of the malleus.

Figure II–20 continues on the opposite page.

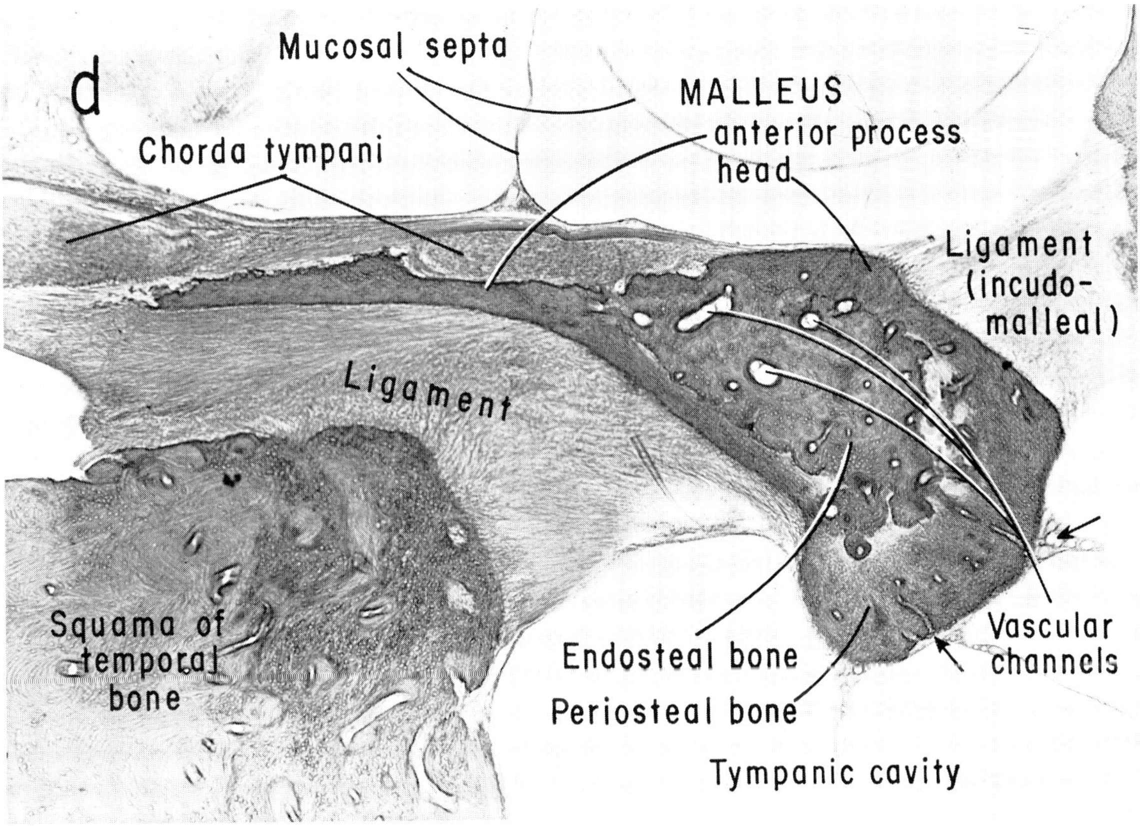

Figure II–20, Concluded.

d. Continued production of endosteal bone results in obliteration of the primitive marrow spaces except where they remain as vascular channels. The contained blood vessels are continuous with those in the investing submucosal tissue and with the small arteries and veins that are transmitted by mucosal septa (see Figure III–141).

Transverse sections at or near the level of the incudomalleal articulation, Wisconsin Collection, series 12, 30, 85, and 29, respectively. *a*, × 35; *b*, × 59; *c*, × 36; *d*, × 36.

(From Guilford and Anson: Trans. Amer. Acad. Ophthal. Otolaryng., 71:398–407, 1967.)

ADULT STRUCTURE: Illustrated in Figures III–26 and III–27.

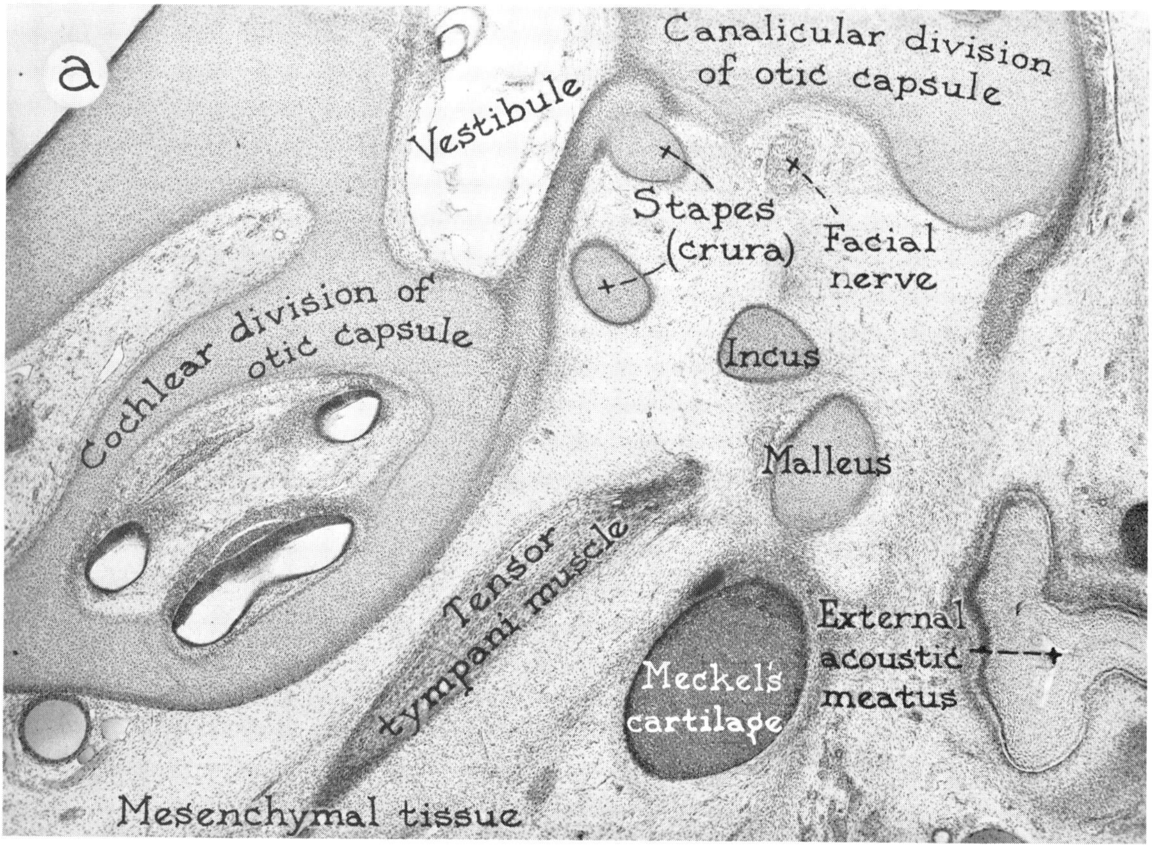

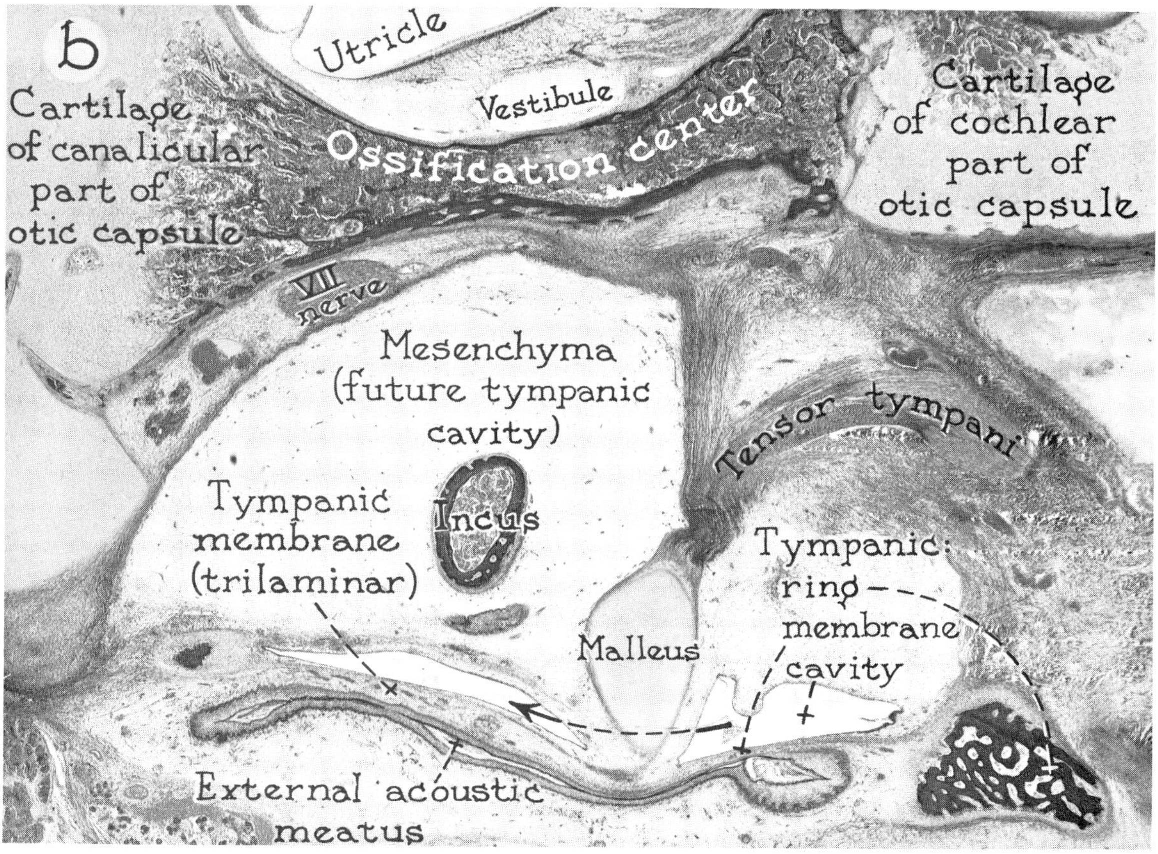

Figure II–21. See legend on the opposite page.

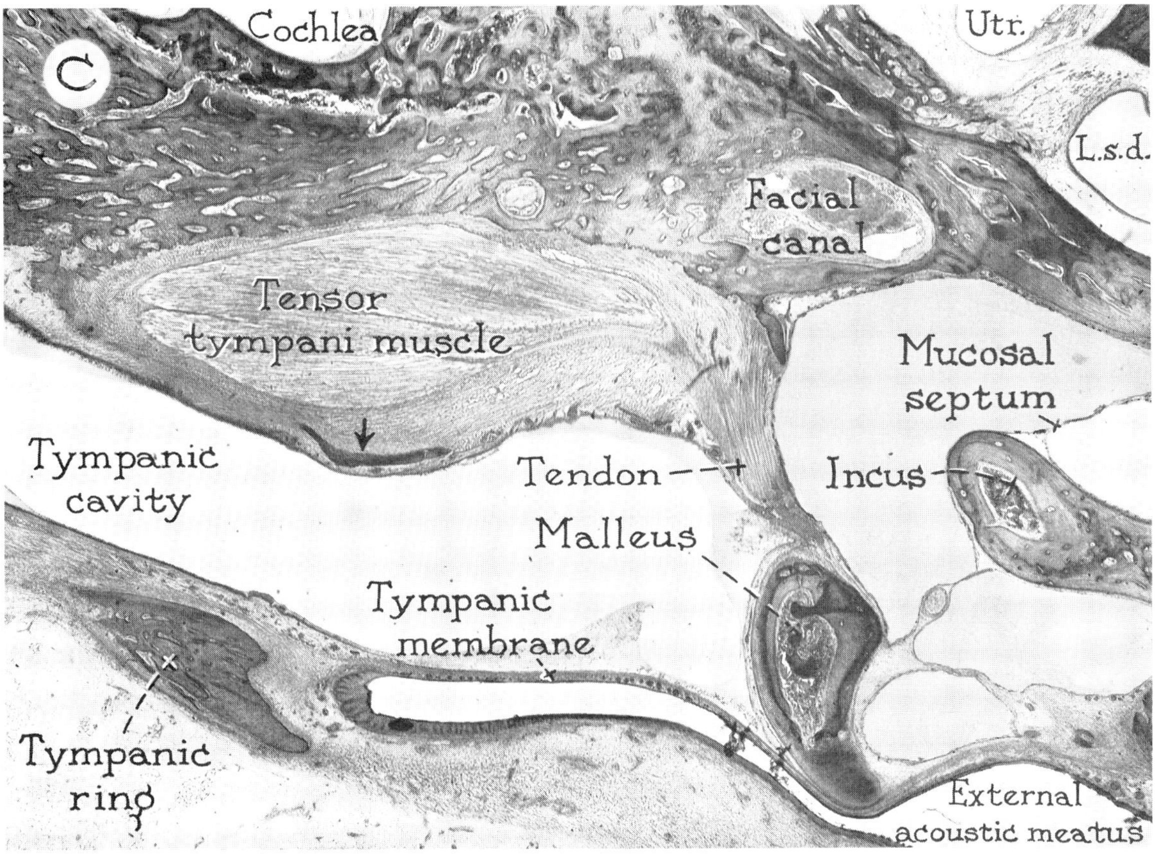

Figure II-21. TENSOR TYMPANI MUSCLE, THE SEMICANAL AND RELATED STRUCTURES: DEVELOPMENT WITHIN APPROXIMATELY FIVE AND ONE-HALF MONTHS. *a.* FETUS OF 11+ WEEKS (62 MM.). *b.* FETUS, 20 WEEKS (170 MM.). *c.* FETUS, 34+ WEEKS (310 MM.).

a. In a 3-month fetus the tensor tympani muscle is lodged in primitive mesenchyma that will differentiate into the submucosal connective tissue of the tympanic cavity. The otic capsule and the ossicles are still composed of cartilage. The future facial canal is a shallow sulcus on the wall of the canalicular division of the capsule. The perilymphatic system of spaces is represented by the capacious vestibular cistern; the external acoustic meatus, by an inpushing of the surface ectoderm (the first visceral groove). Meckel's cartilage. is continuous (in neighboring sections) with the malleus.

b. In the specimen of 5 months all but the last (fourteenth) ossification center are present in the otic capsule. The trilaminar tympanic membrane separates the external acoustic meatus from an expanding tympanic cavity; the space of the latter is interrupted locally by the fixation of the manubrium of the malleus. The tendon of the tensor tympani turns in an even curve from the otic capsule, in which a semicanal has not yet been formed. The tympanic "ring" is now, and will of itself remain, an incomplete annulus. The anterior part is farther advanced in development than the posterior, a gradual decrease in size being evident from the area of the future major tympanic spine to that of the lesser (see Figures II-12 and II-13*a* to *e*).

c. In a specimen approaching the ninth month of fetal life, periosteal bone (at arrow) is spreading as a thin plate from the capsule to complete a semicanal for the muscle (on the wall of the cochlea). The tendon of the tensor tympani muscle turns at almost a right angle to pass lateralward through the tympanic cavity, invested by mucous membrane, to an attachment on the manubrium of the malleus. The incus is now bilaminar, being formed of periosteal and endosteal bone. So also is the malleus, except where it is in contact with the tympanic membrane. Abbreviations: *Utr.*, utricle; *L.s.d.*, lateral semicircular duct.

Transverse sections, Wisconsin Collection, series 160, 170, and 68, respectively. *a*, ×28; *b*, ×18; *c*, ×15.

ADULT STRUCTURE: Illustrated in Figures III-27 to III-29.

The Internal Ear

MEMBRANOUS LABYRINTH

Figures II–22 and II–23

DEVELOPMENTAL ANATOMY

The membranous labyrinth is the fundamental part of the ear. It is the first to form; even before any other part of the internal ear develops, the peripheral processes of the acoustic nerve reach its membranous wall. In these areas the epithelium becomes modified into neuroepithelium for the end organs of hearing and equilibrium.

The primordium of the membranous labyrinth appears in embryos of three weeks as a plaquelike thickening of the ectoderm on each side of the head dorsal to the first branchial groove in the region of the hindbrain. This thickened plate of epithelium, the otic placode, soon invaginates into the mesenchymal tissue to form the otic pit. The invaginated portion then enlarges, and the mouth of the pit narrows by the growing together of the lips. When these meet and fuse, the otic pit is converted into a closed sac, the otocyst, or the otic vesicle (Figure II–22*a*).

The otic vesicle, now divorced from the parent layer, lengthens and changes form (Figure II–22*b*). At first, the vesicle merely enlarges, lengthening faster than it widens. Next, the cranial part becomes marked off as the primordial endolymphatic duct and the caudal part as the primordial extension of the cochlear duct. The intermediate segment will become divided into utricle and saccule. The distal extremity of the endolymphatic appendage becomes the definitive endolymphatic sac. When fully formed, at about midterm, the endolymphatic duct extends from the junction of the saccular and utricular ducts through part of the vestibule just posteromedial and parallel to the common crus, then through the vestibular aqueduct of the otic capsule to terminate as an expanded portion, the endolymphatic sac (Figure II–22*c* to *e*).

In embryos of approximately 5 weeks, three arciform outpocketings appear in the upper lateral (or utricular) part of the utriculosaccular portion of the otic vesicle (Figure II–22*a*). In the embryo of 6 weeks, these ridges are shelflike bays of the utricular part of the differentiating otocyst. At the center of each arched shelf, the opposing epithelial walls meet and fuse, with the result that the cavity is obliterated centrally. The area of epithelial fusion then disintegrates and is replaced by the surrounding mesenchymal tissue. The evaginations are thereby converted into semicircular ducts. In the 6-week embryo, the superior ridge has already been converted into a semicircular duct; the other two protuberances are still ridgelike (Figure II–22*b*). They, too, are soon transformed into semicircular ducts, the posterior preceding the lateral in this phase of development. They attain maximum size in the same order, enlargement of their arcs finally being permitted by the spongy structure of the canalicular part of the otic capsule.

Development of the membranous labyrinth progresses at such a rapid rate that a short period of 5 months intervenes between the stage of early differentiation of the otocyst and the assumption of essentially mature size and form (Figure II–23).

The saccule undergoes considerable expansion in the embryonic and fetal stages. Already in embryos of approximately 5 and 6 weeks, and before the saccule is demarcated from the remainder of the vesicle, it sends out a single ventral evagination, the primordium of the cochlear duct (Figure II–22*b*). This evagination grows in a medial direction and gradually bends to form a coil. At approximately the 8-week stage it has formed one turn (Figure II–22*c*); at 10 weeks, two turns; at the 25-week stage, the cochlear duct has described almost two and one-half turns and has virtually attained the form characteristic of the adult. With the growth of the cochlear duct, the communication of the latter with the saccule becomes constricted, as is already evident in the embryo of 8 weeks. This constricted segment, the *ductus reuniens*, while lengthening, continues to undergo relative narrowing (Figure II–22*d*). In the adult the duct is so attenuated that its patency is sometimes questionable.

All of the sensory end organs of the inner ear develop from epithelial areas of the otic labyrinth into which terminal nerve fibers from the vestibular and cochlear ganglia cells have grown. The cell processes, or nerve fibers, from both these ganglia make up the vestibulocochlear (eighth cranial) nerve. The sensory epithelial areas are divided into two groups; *viz.*, the vestibular end organ, which consists of the cristae and maculae (Figure II–26 and II–27), and the cochlear end organ, or spiral organ of Corti (Figure II–28).

ENDOLYMPHATIC DUCT

Figure II–24

Like the arcs of the semicircular ducts, the endolymphatic duct and sac undergo alteration in form, while the cartilaginous otic capsule begins to change into bone.

The duct remains straight during approximately the first half of fetal life (Figure II–24*a*). Its plane matches that of the common crus of the superior and posterior semicircular ducts. In the late fetal stage the course changes from a straight to a curved course, to establish the configuration observed in the adult; in the mature state, the endolymphatic sac turns downward at an angle of 30 to 60 degrees (Figure II–24*b*).

UTRICULAR DUCT

Figure II–25

The utricle communicates with the sinuslike expansion of the endolymphatic, or otic, duct beneath a fold formed by the epithelial walls of the two chambers. The fold, by projecting into the utricle, forms one boundary of the utricular, or utriculoendolymphatic duct. The long axis of the orifice lies in the vertical plane and measures up to 1200 micra in length; when seen in transverse section, the opening appears slitlike in form (at arrow). The fold was first described by the late Professor Theodore Bast who ascribed to it a valvular function. Its configuration and relationships are well established in the fetus (Figure II–25*a*).

The fold, as usually observed, is in contact with the opposing wall of the utricle, a circumstance suggesting that such closure may occur in the ear of living persons (Figure II–25*b, c*). The sinus of the endolymphatic duct is continuous with the saccule through a narrow communication named for the latter chamber. The saccular duct then expands upon opening into the saccule. An excessively thin conduit, the *ductus reuniens* (see Figure II–22*d*), then serves as intermediary between the vestibulocanalicular and the cochlear sides of the statoacoustic duct system. The tissues of the chambers and of their ducts receive small blood vessels from vascular channels in the walls to which they are adjacent; for example, from canals entering the spherical and elliptical recesses. Additionally, less conspicuous vessels are transported by septa that cross the perilymphatic space. The connective tissue of which they are composed is a remnant of a reticulum present in the fetus. It is continuous, of course, with the fibrous covering of the epithelial structures and with the thin lining of periosteal character that clothes the wall of the osseous labyrinth.

The form of the utriculoendolymphatic duct and the shape of the portions of the utricle and endolymphatic duct are shown by a reconstruction (Figure II–25*d, e*). The change in shape of the passage between them is further recorded by cross-sectional outlines of its lumen. Near the point of communication with the utricle it is chinklike; at the opposite end (continuous with the dilated "sinus") it is roughly oval in form.

MACULAE

Figure II–26

The maculae develop from the epithelium which overlies the areas where the nerves enter the wall of the saccule and utricle. In these zones the epithelium becomes modified into a complex pseudostratified layer (Figure II–26*a*). Two types of cells are present: the sensory cells, which bear bristlelike hairs at their free margin, and the supporting cells. The supporting cells secrete a gelatinous substance which forms a cushionlike membrane, the otolithic membrane (Figure II–26*b, c*); the latter overlies the modified epithelium and bears superficial calcareous deposits, the otoconia. Differentiation begins between the seventh and eighth week of fetal life (Figure II–26*a*). By the tenth to twelfth week, the distinctive types of cells are apparent and the otolithic membrane is being formed (Figure II–26*b*). In fetuses of 14 to 16 weeks, the individual parts of the maculae appear to be well formed and are similar to those seen in the adult (Figure II–26*c*; compare II–26*d*).

CRISTAE

Figure II–27

The vestibular nerve sends a branch to each of the three ampullae of the semicircular ducts. The *crista ampullaris* is that modified and elevated portion of the epithelium of an ampulla into which the terminal fibers of an ampullary nerve extend. Here the epithelium is elevated into a ridgelike fold and its cells are modified in a manner similar to that in which the macula is differentiated. The cristae are already distinguishable in a fetus of 8 weeks as moundlike elevations (Figure II–27*a*). Concurrently with the differentiation of the crista, the surrounding mesenchymal tissue of the fetus of 10 weeks (Figure II–27*b*) becomes the cartilaginous labyrinthine wall and vacuolated periotic tissue of the 15-week stage (Figure II–27*c*). When the crista attains virtually adult structure and size, in the fetus of 23 weeks, the capsular wall is formed in periosteal bone and the periotic labyrinth is well established.

SPIRAL ORGAN

Figure II–28

The sensory end organ in the cochlear duct develops from the epithelium along the posterior wall of the duct where the cochlear nerve fibers enter it (Figure II–28). Like the maculae and cristae, the spiral organ appears in early fetal life and attains adult proportions by midterm. Already in the placodal stage, and also in the vesicle stage, the epithelium is stratified. In the cochlear duct this stratification is still marked in the 8-week fetus; in the anterior wall of the duct, however, it is much thinner than in the posterior and lateral walls. The other parts of the cochlea start to differentiate at the beginning of the eighth week; these elements are the surrounding otic capsule, the centrally placed modiolus, and the tympanic and vestibular scalae. The diameter of these scalae is greater than that of the cochlear duct.

As a result, a spiral shelf (*lamina spiralis ossea*) extends from the modiolus between the *scala vestibuli* and *scala tympani* to the posterior wall of the *scala media*. With the growth of these structures, the cross-sectional form of the cochlear duct changes from rounded (Figure II–28*a, b*) to oval (Figure II–28*c*), and finally to triangular, so that it comes to have three walls—the anterior, posterior, and outer (Figure II–28*d*). The anterior wall fuses with the wall of the scala vestibuli to form the vestibular membrane. The posterior wall merges with the wall of the scala tympani to form the basilar membrane; the outer wall rests on the spiral ligament; the inner angle of the cochlear duct is attached to the anterior surface of the osseous spiral lamina near the free margin of the latter.

With further growth of these structures, the epithelial duct becomes gradually modified. Along the anterior wall, in the area of the future vestibular membrane, it loses its stratification and becomes a simple columnar epithelium in the 11-week fetus. At 14 weeks this epithelium is cuboidal. Soon thereafter it flattens into a simple squamous type and continues so throughout life. The epithelium along the outer wall becomes modified in such a way as to resemble a glandular epithelium. The epithelial layer covers a vascular connective tissue, the *stria vascularis*, which in turn rests on the spiral ligament. The epithelium of the posterior wall, which is the basilar membrane, becomes highly modified into the spiral organ of Corti and the tectorial membrane.

The epithelium of the organ of Corti does not differentiate into its definitive parts in all turns until after midterm. It is more rapid in the basal turn, slowest in the apical turn. The epithelium of the apical turn in a fetus of 11 weeks appears as a thickened, pseudostratified layer (Figure II–28*a*). But along the free surface of this epithelium there is an ill-defined gelatinous membrane, the tectorial membrane, in the lower turn (Figure II–28*b*). In the lower turn the epithelium already shows a bulging and loosening of its cells in the region of the outer hair cells. In the 16-week embryo this condition is more marked, but in the apical turns differentiation has not yet taken place (Figure II–28*c*). The tunnel of Corti is beginning to appear in the basal turn (Figure II–28*d*) but not in the apical turn (Figure II–28*c*). During the succeeding month, the organ progressively completes its development toward its apical end, so that in a fetus of 21 weeks, the tunnel of Corti is present in all turns. At this age or shortly thereafter, the internal ear attains its maximum size and becomes completely encased in its bony capsule. In the fetus of 25 weeks, the organ resembles that of the adult.

OSSEOUS LABYRINTH

Figures II–29 to II–32

DEVELOPMENTAL ANATOMY

The perilymph- containing labyrinth consists of the tissue and tissue-fluid spaces of mesodermal origin which surround most of the membranous labyrinth and, thereby, occupy the interval between the latter and the surrounding inner periosteal layer of the otic capsule (Figure II–29).

Development of this labyrinthine system is rapid, being completed in approximately a 4-month period, beginning near the second month of intrauterine life (Figure II–30). The process is similar in the three parts of the labyrinth: cochlear, vestibular and canalicular.

The several parts of the perilymphatic labyrinthine system owe their formation to a retrogressive change in which precartilage, already formed, is sacrificed to make way for fluid-containing, intracapsular space. This process may be very clearly demonstrated as it progresses in the canalicular division of the otic capsule.

In the 8-week stage the tissue that immediately surrounds the semicircular duct begins to undergo resolution (Figure II–30*a*). At 12 weeks, cartilage has been replaced by a reticulum (Figure II–30*b*). In the 24-week specimen, the reticulum, in turn, has virtually disappeared (Figure II–30*c*).

Formation of the perilymphatic spaces occurs first in the region which will become the vestibule. Next, similar spaces appear around the cochlear duct, those of the scala tympani before those destined to be the scala vestibuli. The appearance of the latter is, in turn, followed by the development of perilymphatic (periotic) spaces which, in surrounding the epithelial semicircular ducts, will be the corresponding semicircular canals. Soon all of these spaces fuse with one another to form a tortuous, but uninterrupted, fluid-containing channel, the perilymphatic labyrinth.

In the ampullary part of each semicircular canal, the schema of development matches that by which the nonampullated portion attains maturity (Figure II–31*a* to *c*). The cochlear division differs from the vestibular and the canalicular in being separated into chambers, the scalae, above and below the cochlear duct. Like them, however, the perilymphatic space is produced through the resorption of the cartilage that immediately surrounds the membranous duct system.

Even as early as the 9-week stage, the future scalae are occupied by a vascular mesenchymalike tissue in which conversion to reticulum is just beginning (Figure II–32*a*). Three weeks later definite spaces have been formed (Figure II–32*b*). They first appear near the cochlear duct of the membranous labyrinthine system, to become the vestibular scala (at asterisk) and the tympanic scala. Development is farthest advanced in the basal turn, least at the apical turn. The perichondrium is in active growth (and will continue to be until ossification begins in the 4-month or 5-month stage). In late stages the remaining periotic tissue is a thin layer on the inner wall of the cochlear turns, except where it becomes part of the spiral ligament or of tenuous "septa" that, in crossing the space of the tympanic and vestibular scalae, transmit minute blood vessels to the cochlear duct (Figure II–32*c*).

OTIC CAPSULE

Figure II–33

DEVELOPMENTAL ANATOMY

The bony capsule around the labyrinthine systems develops rapidly from a cartilage model. It may, therefore, be classified as cartilage bone, although in certain limited and special regions membrane bone takes part either in the initial process of ossification or in some phase of subsequent remodeling (in the modiolus, the tympanic wall of the lateral semicircular canal, the external ostium of the vestibular aqueduct, and the osseous spiral laminae).

During the period of rapid growth, the internal ear is encased in a cartilaginous capsule. This cartilaginous forerunner of the osseous capsule grows in some areas and is deorganized in others to accommodate the enlarging labyrinthine system. Here a comparison between a typical skeletal element and the *pars petrosa* will serve to establish the exceptional developmental course and the retention of fetal structure of the otic capsule (Figure II–33).

Resembling a long bone of the human skeleton (Figure II–33*a*), the capsule begins as a cartilage "model." But differing therefrom, it grows with astonishing rapidity to attain adult dimensions in the fifth month of intrauterine life (Figure II–33*d*; compare Figure II–33*b*). Furthermore, the capsule develops from many (in fact, 14) ossification centers, each of which is trilaminar and without areas of epiphyseal growth. The first center appears at the basal cochlear turn (Figure II–33*c*).

The mesenchyme that surrounds the expanding otic vesicle changes into precartilage at about the 7-week stage. It will become true cartilage in embryos of 8 weeks. Up to the sixteenth week of intrauterine life, it consists entirely of cartilage. Cartilage does not give way to bone until the underlying parts of the internal ear have attained their adult dimensions. In the canalicular region, where growth of the semicircular canals continues to approximately the twenty-first week, the capsule will remain cartilaginous until such growth is complete. The earliest fusion takes place between Center One and Center Two, with the aid of Center Four to form the arch over the cochlear window; this occurs in the fetus of approximately 16 weeks. In a fetus of 19 weeks, all but one of the centers (which appears about the 20-week stage) has fused with one or more adjacent centers to form a unified skeletal element. The last center, Center Fourteen, is present in the fetus of 21 weeks. At the 23-week stage, all centers have fused to form a complete bony capsule in which "suture lines" have been obliterated. There exists no histological mechanism to permit epiphyseal growth between centers.

Otic Capsule: Cochlea

Figures II–34 and II–35

Bone formation in the otic capsule has not yet begun in the 4-month stage. However, the pattern of blood supply to the membranous labyrinth and to the perilymphatic spaces is already established; branches of the internal auditory vessels pass from the meatus and therefrom to the contents of the cochlear coils (Figure II–34*a*).

Within two months, the capsule has reached the midpoint in the course of its change from cartilage to bone of petrous density. The outer periosteal layer is thickening; the inner periosteal layer remains excessively thin and apparently inactive; the middle layer consists of sparsely distributed "spicules" of intrachondrial and endosteal bone lodged in primitive marrow (Figure II–34*b*, *c*). The three layers develop on independent timetables and on a distinctive pattern of histological differentiation.

At term the outer layer has increased in thickness and is assuming petrous character. The inner layer thickens only through deposition of endosteal bone on its external aspect. The middle layer, like the outer layer, is approaching petrous consistency (Figure II–34*d*, *e*). Following a 5-month period of relative inaction, the capsule rapidly attains petrous character (Figure II–34*f*). The marrow spaces of the middle layer, originally capacious, are reduced to minute vascular channels.

In the 5-month specimen, the three layers of bone are present in the ossification centers of the developing cochlear capsule (Figure II–35*a*). They are representative of all the centers, 14 in number, of which the mature capsule is composed. In the cochlea, encapsulation of the coils progresses from base to apex; the apical part is still cartilaginous in the specimen illustrated. The outer periosteal layer, when it first appears, is made up of platelike portions, each one layer thick. The inner periosteal stratum, unlike the outer, is complete, yet thin. The middle layer, differing from the other two, consists of scattered islands of intrachondrial bone. Each of the "osseous globules" is a small area of cartilage on the interior of whose lacunae osteocytes have deposited a thin layer of bone. Concurrently, endosteal bone is laid down by osteoblasts on the exterior of these islands of combined tissue. The middle layer is latent until about the time of birth; a surge in osteogenesis results in precipitate attainment of petrous fabric (Figure II–35*b*). Despite general change, islets of intrachondrial bone remain identifiable throughout life, seemingly unaltered in their histological structure (Figure II–35*c*).

The complexity of morphogenesis warrants review, also. Each constituent ossification center and, therefore, the otic capsule as a unit, is composed of three layers of bone. The outer, or periosteal, stratum is formed from the cambium layer of the periosteum around the cartilaginous capsule. It is similar to the periosteal layer of long bones. The inner periosteal bone, immediately surrounding the labyrinthine spaces, is always thin and uniform in structure; it is derived from the inner periosteum. The middle layer is composed of combined intrachondrial and endochondral bone. The intrachondrial tissue of the middle layer consists of irregular areas of calcified hyaline cartilage which contains true bone within the original cartilage lacunae. It forms the framework upon which endochondral bone is gradually deposited. Ultimately, through the increase of the latter, bone marrow is almost completely replaced; the originally capacious space is reduced to relatively small vascular channels.

Bone formation in the otic capsule is under way in the fifth fetal month, advancing more rapidly in the cochlear than in the canalicular division. In the latter portion, cartilage becomes spongy to permit expansion of the semicircular ducts; even in the 6-month stage, the canalicular capsule has not yet changed to bone and the middle layer of the entire capsule is still "cancellous" in structure. Solidification of this middle stratum is slow, being completed in early postnatal weeks. Replacement of marrow by endosteal bone takes place with precipitate speed. The pattern then established is largely—sometimes totally—retained in the adult capsule.

The dense, or stony, nature of the otic capsule is largely due to the compactness of the bone of the original centers of ossification. Density is not, however, a characteristic of the apical, antral, and mastoid portions of the temporal bone. These regions might reasonably be regarded as extracapsular. The extracapsular part (composed of a late fetal and early postnatal extension of the outer periosteal layer) is not likely to remain petrous; rather it is usually pneumatic. The air cells (whose presence accounts for the "cancellous" nature of the bone) spread from the auditory tube and the tympanic cavity into the periosteal layer, and then into the endochondral bone.

The histogenesis of the middle layer is additionally noteworthy because it finds no counterpart in the human skeleton. The cartilage of the primordial capsule begins to undergo change at the fetal stage of approximately 17 weeks. This initial step in bone formation is marked by invasion of the chondral tissue by osteogenic buds of vascular connective tissue. Some cartilage remains in the form of bars in which the lacunae, opened and invaded by osteoblasts, are converted into cartilage islands, or intrachondrial bone. Osteoblasts begin immediately to deposit endosteal bone on the outer surface of each such island. The intervening spaces that contain primitive marrow are thereby reduced to relatively small vascular channels. As a result of these concomitant phases of development, the bone of the middle layer attains petrous character.

The blood vessels in the vascular channels of supply to the otic capsule and to the immediately surrounding bone communicate mostly with arteries of the tympanic plexus located in the mucous membrane on the medial, or labyrinthine, wall of the tympanic cavity. Differing from the pattern of parietal supply, that of the sensory elements (cochlea, utricle, saccule, and semicircular ducts) comes through the internal acoustic meatus to the spiral organ, acoustic maculae, and cristae. This schema is established even before ossification of the capsule begins and, once formed, is retained.

It is thus made clear that the otic capsule is the most unusual skeletal element in the human body. The following developmental features are unique: origin, despite its small size, from 14 ossification centers which appear within a period of six weeks, beginning with the fifteenth week and ending with the twenty-first; fusion of the centers peripherally without intermediate zones of epiphyseal growth; trilaminar structure of each center, and consequently of the entire capsule; independent timetable of growth for each layer of a center of ossification; self-governing, separate schema in attaining mature histological architecture. The fetal architecture is kept throughout life, in the absence of those processes that elsewhere convert fetal into haversian bone.

Speed of growth is an equally arresting feature. A typical skeletal element (for example, the tibia), arising as a cartilage "model," attains adult dimensions in about 22 years; the otic capsule is as large as it will ever be in the 21-week fetus.

Transcapsular Channels

Considered as a space within an osseous box, the interior of the osseous labyrinth may be said to have nine channels of communication with the exterior: the internal acoustic meatus, subarcuate fossa and vestibular aqueduct on the medial surface; the cochlear aqueduct (or canaliculus) on the inferior surface; the two fenestrae, the fissula ante fenestram and fossula post fenestram on the lateral surface; the facial canal on the medial (labyrinthine) wall of the tympanic cavity.

INTERNAL ACOUSTIC MEATUS

The wall of the meatus is formed around the eighth nerve[1] and the internal auditory blood vessels. It is still a channel in cartilage in the 4-month specimen. Ossification centers are present at 5 months. In the 6-month specimen (at which time the otic capsule has become trilaminar), periosteal bone is spreading along the wall of the meatus. The fetal dimensions of the channel are retained in the adult. (See description under "Blood Supply," page 87.)

SUBARCUATE FOSSA

Figures II–36 to II–38

Like the internal acoustic meatus, the subarcuate fossa of the adult temporal bone is a channel for blood vessels (usually of small size). However, there the similarity ends: the fossa in the fetus is a route for erosive vascular buds (from the internal auditory vessels) which cause the cartilage of the canalicular division of the capsule to become spongy. The resulting porosity permits increase in the arcs of the semicircular canals after growth has ceased in the vestibular and cochlear divisions of the capsule. The capacity of the fossa is reduced after the fifth month of fetal life.

As viewed in gross specimens, reduction in size is slow. In the 31-week specimen, the caliber of the subarcuate fossa exceeds that of the internal acoustic meatus (Figure II–36*a*). Despite growth and change

[1] The statoacoustic, now called the vestibulocochlear, nerve of the *Nomina Anatomica.*

in form of the parts of the temporal bone, the size-relation between fossa and meatus is but slightly altered in the 37-week stage (Figure II–36*b*). In the 40-week specimen, the capacity of the fossa has been appreciably reduced (Figure II–36*c*). The fossa in the temporal bone of the adult is subject to great variability in respect to size, form, and location (see Figures III–115 and III–117). Not infrequently, the aperture is reduced to pinpoint dimensions. The fossa is usually a minute channel in the adult. However, variations do occur; some of them are striking. Departure from the anatomic "normal" may be of surgical consequence where, for example, the fossa approaches or actually occupies the customary site of the external aperture of the vestibular aqueduct (Figure III–115).

A study of sections establishes the fact that in the 21-week specimen, the subarcuate fossa approaches maximum size; the process of erosion of the cartilage between the semicircular canals is at the most active stage, and the erosive vascular buds now extend deeply into the cartilage (Figure II–37*a*). Ossification spreads slowly. In the depths of the fossa, cartilage still remains as a relatively bulky mass in the 23-week specimen (Figure II–37*b*) and is still a prominent feature in late fetal stages as well as early postnatal stages (Figures II–37*c* and II–38*a* to *c*).

VESTIBULAR AQUEDUCT

Figure II–39

The vestibular aqueduct is formed around the endolymphatic duct and sac. At birth its wall still consists, in part, of endosteal bone, and the shape of the external aperture is undergoing alteration in accommodation to the change in position of the endolymphatic sac. In the mature state the external aperture appears in typical cases as an oblique slit on the posterior surface of the pyramid, but variations are frequently encountered (Figures III–102 to III–106).

At approximately the 17-week stage pictured in Figure II–39*a*, only four of the total of fourteen ossification centers have appeared in the cartilaginous otic capsule. In the area of the aqueduct, the capsule remains unaltered cartilage (Figure II–39*a*), and the cartilage of the canalicular part is being rendered into a spongy consistency through the ingrowth of vascular connective tissue from the subarcuate fossa (Figures II–37*a* and II–38*a*). Approximately one month later bone formation has come to involve the area of the aqueduct (Figure II–39*b*). Here the fifth and second centers meet and fuse over the endolymphatic duct and proximal portion of the sac.

In the fetus at the middle of the eighth month, bone surrounds the aqueduct (Figure II–39*c*). The outer periosteal layer is undergoing thickening; the middle layer remains virtually unchanged where it forms part of the wall of the aqueduct. Even in the newborn infant, the middle layer of the capsule has not yet attained petrous structure (Figure II–39*d*; compare adult, Figure II–39*e*).

COCHLEAR AQUEDUCT

Figure II–40

The cochlear aqueduct (or canaliculus) appears in the 4-month fetus as an area of resorption of precartilage on the medial wall of the basal turn of the cochlea, just internal to the developing cochlear (round) window (Figure II–40*a*). Therefrom it crosses the capsule to the meningeal side on the inferior surface of the pyramid (Figure II–40*b*). Its tissue is being separated from the cochlear vein in the 5-month stage (Figure II–42*c*, *d*). Segregation is soon complete (Figure II–40*e*, *f*).

FISSULA ANTE FENESTRAM

Figures II–41; II–42; and II–43a, b

Like the cochlear aqueduct, the fissula ante fenestram is a transcapsular channel formed by resorption of precartilage (Figure II–41). In the fetal and infantile stages it is frequently the site of a cartilage mass (Figure II–42*a*, *b*). In the adult it is the predilected site of otosclerotic bone formation (Figure II–126).

FOSSULA POST FENESTRAM

Figure II–43c

The fossula post fenestram is the counterpart, posteriorly, of the prefenestral fissula and is also an evagination of the periotic tissue (Figure II–43*c*; compare Figure II–43*a*, *b*). It is similar to the fissula in development, in general form, and in content. However, it is inconstant in occurrence and, when present, usually lacks a tympanic communication.

FACIAL CANAL

Figures II–44 to II–47

The form and position of the facial canal are forecast in the chondrocranium of the fetus by the presence of a sulcus on the lateral (tympanic) wall of the canalicular division of the otic capsule (Figure II–44*a* and II–45*a*). The facial nerve, stapedial muscle, arteries, and veins are already grouped in the primordial canal.

In specimens slightly older, bone formation is under way in the area of the facial "canal" and in the auditory ossicles (Figure II–44*b*). In the late fetus and in the newborn, the structures are enclosed in a true canal (Figures II–44*c* and II–45*b*, *c*). The stapedius tendon passes from the tip of the pyramidal eminence to insertion into the head of the stapes.

The facial "canal," while still a sulcus on the canalicular part of the capsule, houses the structures that are its contents in the adult: the blood vessels, the facial nerve, and the stapedius muscle. Even at this early stage, blood vessels are exchanged between the capsule and the future canal (Figure II–46*a*).

In late fetal stages vessels are prominent contents of the canal (Figure II–46*b*). Their presence in the late fetus is predictive of the richness of supply in the adult, where they communicate with others which traverse vascular channels in the bone and with vessels in the submucosal tissue of the middle ear (Figure II–46*c*). The latter vessels reach the ossicles in thin mesenterylike reflections of the mucous membrane (Figures III–10*a* and III–65*e, f*).

The facial canal may retain features of its developmental course, either in the retention of the proximal extremity of the second visceral arch (Reichert's cartilage) as its tympanic boundary (Figure II–47*b*; compare II–47*a*) or in dehiscence of its wall (Figure II–47*c*). The latter condition is an example of congenital failure to complete the regular succession of developmental steps.

VESTIBULAR FENESTRA

Figure II–48

In the 9-week fetus the future site of the vestibular (oval) window is indicated by the area in the lateral wall of the preosseous otic capsule where the basal part of the annular stapes impinges on the wall of the vestibule (Figure II–48*a*).

Through the alteration of its precartilage, the portion of the capsule against which the annular stapes now rests (that is, the *lamina stapedis*) becomes part of the base of the ossicle. Peripheral to the oval zone thus demarcated, the tissue undergoes further change to become the annular ligament (Figure II–48*b*). The rim of the stapedial base and the facing aspect of the fenestra retain their cartilage (Figure II–48*c*).

COCHLEAR FENESTRA

Figure II–49

In the 4-month fetus, ossification is taking place in the basal turn of the cochlea (Figure II–49*a*). However, the wall of the fenestra remains cartilaginous. Periosteal bone, spreading from the ossification center, begins to replace cartilage at the 5-month stage (Figure II–49*b*) and soon thereafter forms a complete rim (Figure II–49*c*). Concurrently, the cochlear aqueduct (containing the so-called perilymphatic duct) is separated from the channel that transmits the cochlear vein.

When fully formed, the fenestra is situated in a declivity, the fossula of the cochlear fenestra, that leads into the tympanic scala of the basal turn of the cochlea. The opening in the bone is closed in the fresh state by the secondary tympanic membrane.

Blood Supply

Figure II–50

It is clear that the above-described arteries and accompanying veins that are transmitted by the facial canal contribute importantly to the tympanic plexus of vessels, and thereby to walls and contents of the tympanic cavity (Figures II–44 to II–47*b*). Thus, to a considerable degree, branches of the stylomastoid vessels (regionally of cervical service) reach the petrous part of the temporal bone—the primordial "core" of which is the otic capsule.

Differing from this pattern, in respect both to the source and to the structures chiefly supplied, is the schema by which the internal auditory artery and vein, entering the internal acoustic meatus from the cranial cavity, reach the membranous labyrinth to include its sensory elements (the spiral organ of Corti, the acoustic maculae of the saccule and utricle, and the cristae of the semicircular ducts).

The labyrinthine schema is established early. In the 4-month fetus the internal auditory blood vessels may be traced into the internal acoustic meatus and their branches followed as the latter course through the area of the developing modiolus to the osseous spiral lamina and the partition between cochlear turns (Figure II–50*a*, *b*). The cochlear branches course through the periotic tissue on the wall of the scala and the cochlear duct; in the vestibule the main vessels are lodged in the periotic tissue on the attached surface of the saccule and utricle.

Blood vessels are present in the cochlea at the onset of ossification (in the 5-month fetus). They are traced from the internal acoustic meatus, through the modiolus to the attached extremity of the osseous spiral lamina, to the walls of the vestibular scala and the tympanic scala.

As development progresses, the independence of osseous and membranous supply becomes a more striking feature (Figure II–50*c*, *d*). Vascular channels pass through the external periosteal layer from the mucous membrane of the labyrinthine (medial) wall of the tympanic cavity (Figure II–50*d*, *e*). They continue through the middle layer to the outer (deep) surface of the internal periosteal layer. So far as is discernible at the present magnification, they do not penetrate the latter stratum. This means that the membranous labyrinth (with its sensory elements) and the periotic connective tissue must be supplied wholly or chiefly by the vessels that enter the capsule through the internal acoustic meatus.

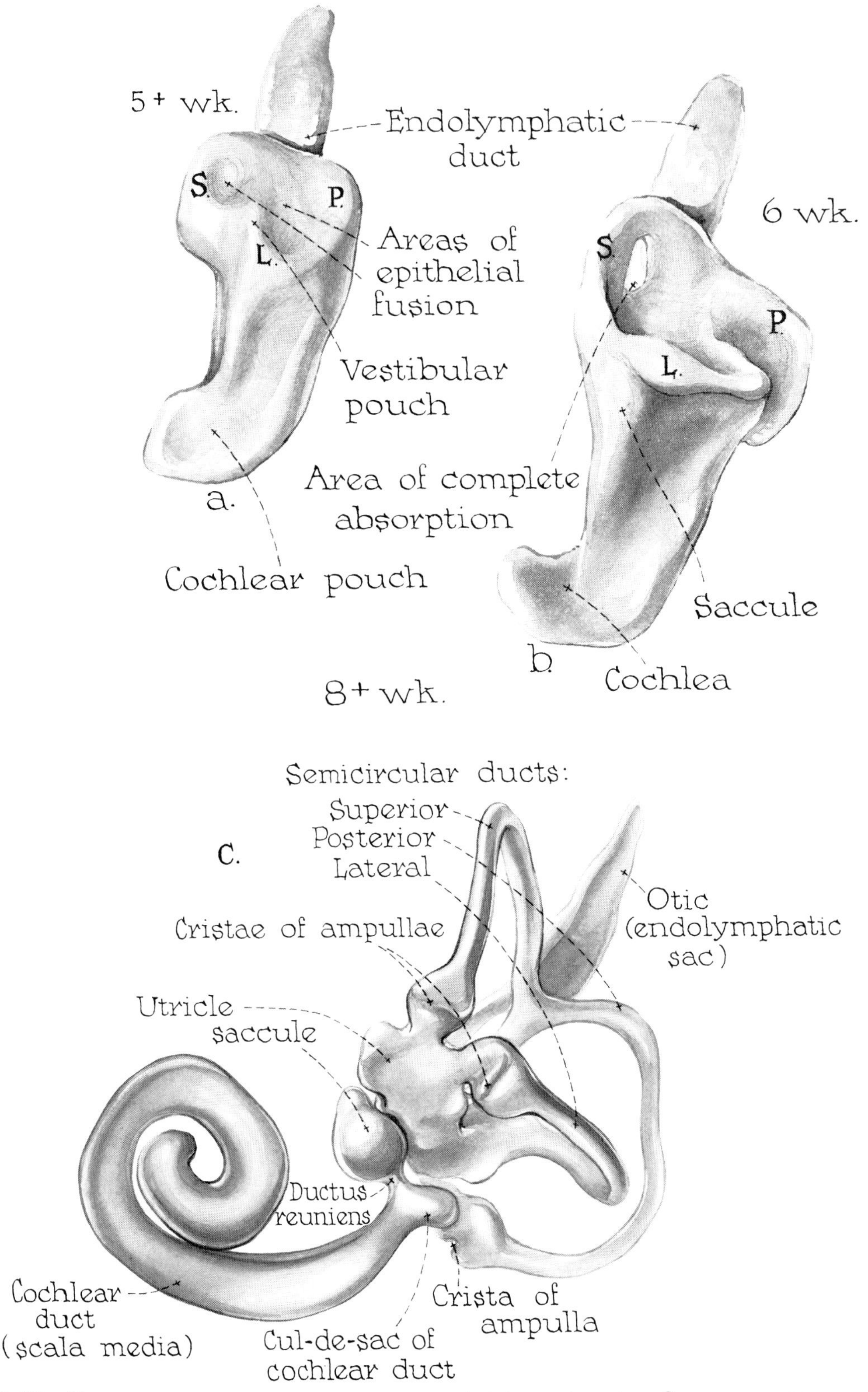

Figure II–22. Membranous labyrinth: developmental and adult anatomy. Shown by reconstructions and by a semidiagram.

a. Differentiating otocyst in the embryo of 5 weeks (8 mm. CR length).

b. Appearance of the primordia of the semicircular ducts, utricle, saccule, and cochlear duct in the embryo of 6 weeks (13 mm.). Abbreviations for the semicircular ducts: *L*, lateral; *P*, posterior; *S*, superior.

c. The membranous labyrinth at the early definitive stage, in the fetus of 8 weeks (30 mm.).

Figure II–22 continues on the opposite page.

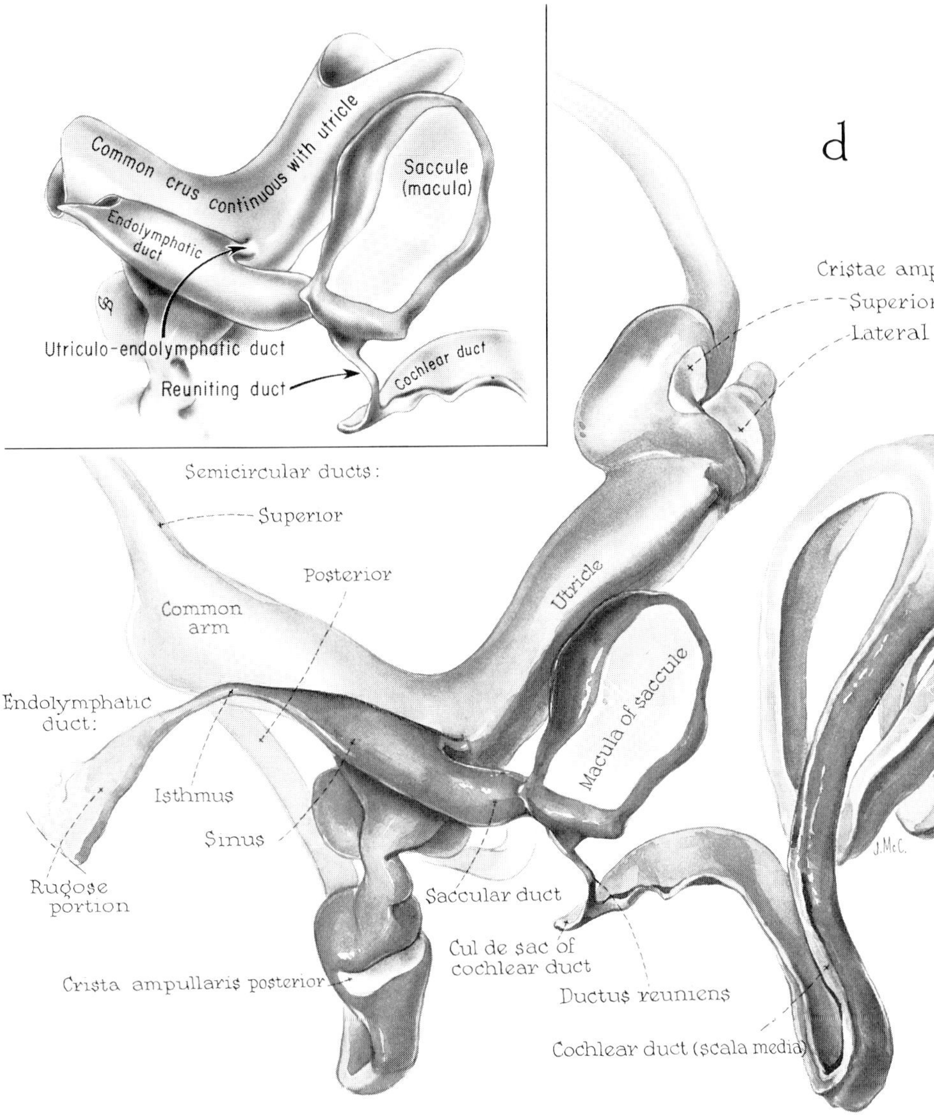

Figure II–22. Continued.

d and *inset*. The membranous labyrinth is a continuous epithelial duct system invested by an excessively thin layer of connective tissue and containing a clear fluid, the endolymph. These membranous ducts lie within the osseous labyrinth, to the form of which they roughly correspond. Their walls are regionally modified to become the terminations of the vestibulocochlear (acoustic) nerve that supply the maculae, the cristae, and the spiral organ (of Corti).

In the vestibular division of the surrounding osseous labyrinth, the membranous elements are the utricle and the saccule. They are not droplet-shaped, characterless vesicles; on the contrary, these chambers actually possess highly distinctive form. The utricle is widely continuous with the common arm of the superior and posterior semicircular ducts; together they have the form of an open V. The utricle, lodged in the elliptical recess of the vestibule, is continuous with the three semicircular ducts. It is anchored to the wall of the recess by connective tissue and by the fibers of the utricular division of the vestibular nerve (Figure III–50*b*); except for this local attachment, it is separated from the vestibular wall by the perilymphatic space. On its anterolateral surface is situated the utricular acoustic macula.

The saccule is an elongate oval whose long axis parallels that of the utricle, to which vesicle it is closely related. Differing from the utricle (which opens widely into its canalicular ducts), the saccule is continuous with the cochlear part of the system by narrow intermediary conduits; namely, the saccular and reuniting ducts. These ducts enter and leave the saccule on the latter's inferior surface; this means that the saccule is set off from its dependent communications. The acoustic macula of the saccule is situated on the anteromedial surface. Like the utricle, the saccule is held firmly to the wall of the vestibule by connective tissue and by bundles of nerve fibers (Figure III–57*c*). The saccule is connected with the utricle indirectly through the saccular and the utricular (or utriculoendolymphatic) ducts; in the opposite direction (that is, toward the cochlea) the connections are the reuniting duct (*ductus reuniens*) and the vestibular cecum, the latter being a cul-de-sac of the cochlear duct proper.

Figure II–22 continues on the following page.

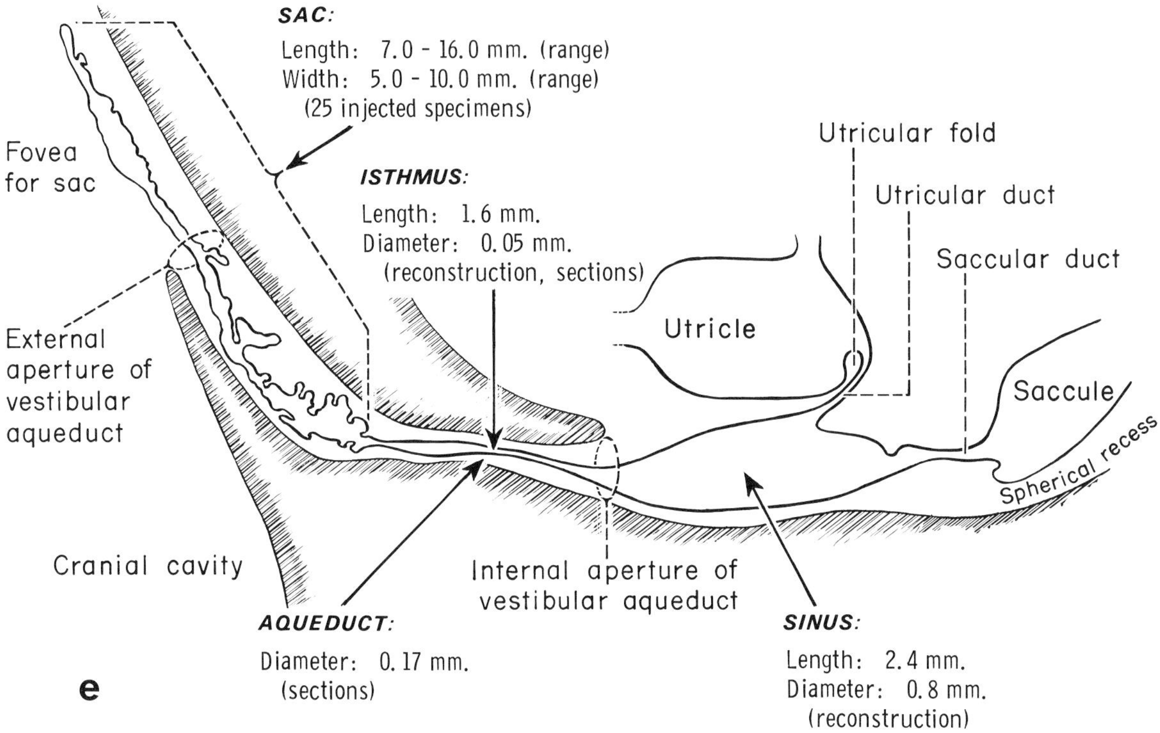

Figure II–22, Continued. MEMBRANOUS LABYRINTH: DEVELOPMENTAL AND ADULT ANATOMY. SHOWN BY RECONSTRUCTIONS AND BY A SEMIDIAGRAM.

e. The endolymphatic duct has been regularly pictured as a quill-like tube with a bulbous terminal expansion. In truth, it is regionally modified in a striking way: the opening into the utricle, for example, is slitlike in form, with an orifice bounded by a folding of the apposed walls of the utricle and the endolymphatic duct. The proximal part of the latter duct is a sinuslike expansion that occupies the internal aperture of the vestibular aqueduct (see *d*). Continuing toward the external aperture of the aqueduct, the duct narrows into an isthmus. While still within the aqueduct, the duct becomes a flattened dilatation, the endolymphatic sac (incomplete in the reconstruction; compare Figure II–24*b*). The *saccus* is prolonged beyond the aperture to rest in encephalic *dura mater* in a shallow saucer-shaped impression on the posterior surface of the pyramid.

The cochlear division of the membranous duct system is formed by the cochlear duct. It begins in a recess of the vestibule, extends within the osseous spiral canal, through basal, middle, and apical turns, where it ends blindly in the cupular cecum. The cochlear duct is in large part triangular in cross section. Its outer wall is held by connective tissue to the osseous cochlea. It contains the spiral organ (*Cortii*), a highly differentiated neural epithelium that contains the endings of the cochlear nerve. The histological details are pictured in Figures III–55 and III–56.

(From Anson and McVay: Surgical Anatomy, 5th ed. Philadelphia, W. B. Saunders Co., 1971.)

ADULT STRUCTURE: Illustrated in Figures III–40 to III–48.

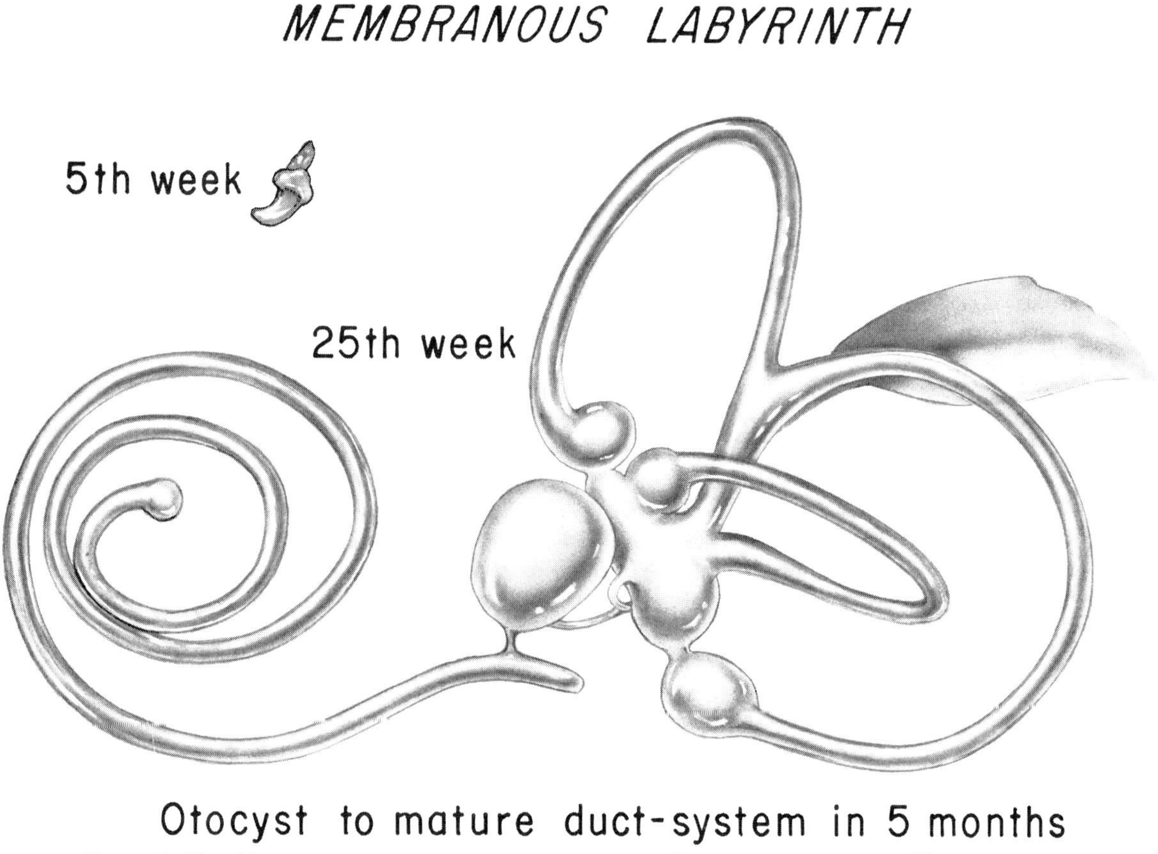

Figure II–23. MEMBRANOUS LABYRINTH: DEVELOPMENT. STYLIZED DRAWING OF 25-WEEK STAGE.

In the 5-week specimen, the future membranous labyrinthine system is represented by an otocyst in which the parts have but lately become definitive. The future endolymphatic duct is a simple dorsally-directed appendage of a common utriculosaccular chamber; the cochlea is a curved projection directed downward. The semicircular ducts appear as a ledgelike eminence on that portion of the chamber that will become the utricle.

The developmental course whose progress is predicted in the 5-week stage has been virtually completed in the ensuing 5-month period. (Semischematic: compare Figure II–22*d*, which demonstrates detail. Intermediate steps and the adult form are also depicted in Figure II–22.)

(From Anson: Trans. Amer. Acad. Ophthal. Otolaryng., 73:17–38, 1969.)

ADULT STRUCTURE: Illustrated in Figures III–40 to III–48.

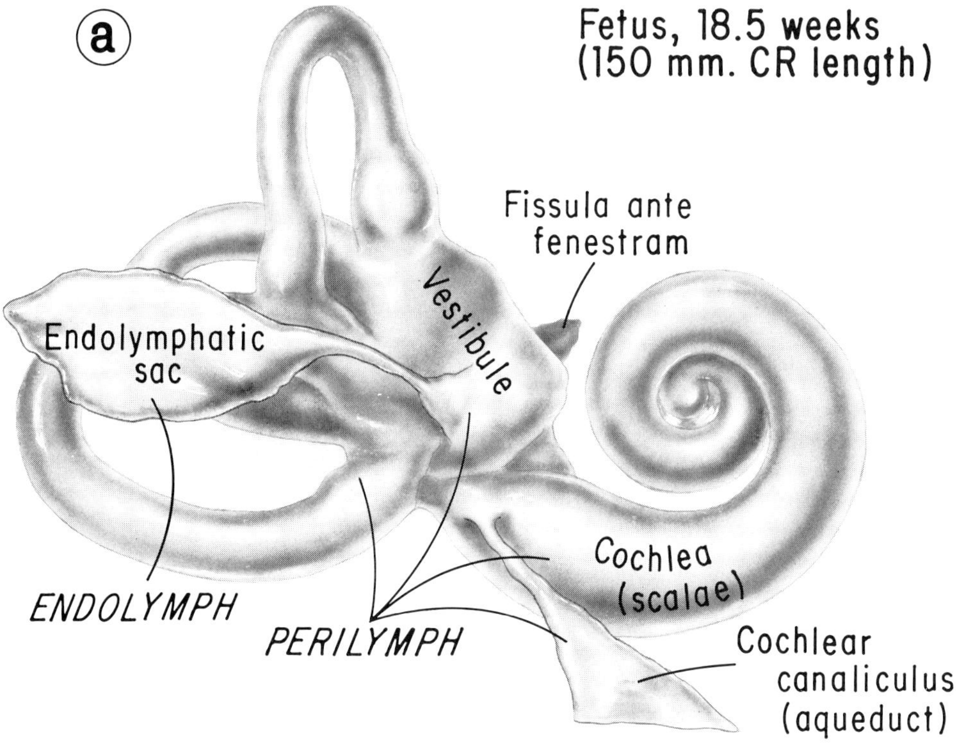

Figure II–24. ENDOLYMPHATIC DUCT AND SAC: DEVELOPMENTAL ANATOMY. *a.* FETUS OF 18½ WEEKS (150 MM.). *b.* ADULT, 65 YEARS OLD.

Demonstrating the result of growth and concurrent change in plane. Drawings of reconstructions prepared by the Born method. The osseous labyrinth is shown in order to demonstrate its continuity with the space of the cochlear aqueduct. The parts of the membranous labyrinth, except for the endolymphatic duct and sac, are lodged within the osseous labyrinth (hence, not seen here).

a. The endolymphatic duct remains straight (as here pictured) during the first half of fetal life, the plane matching that of the common crus.

Figure II–24 continues on the opposite page.

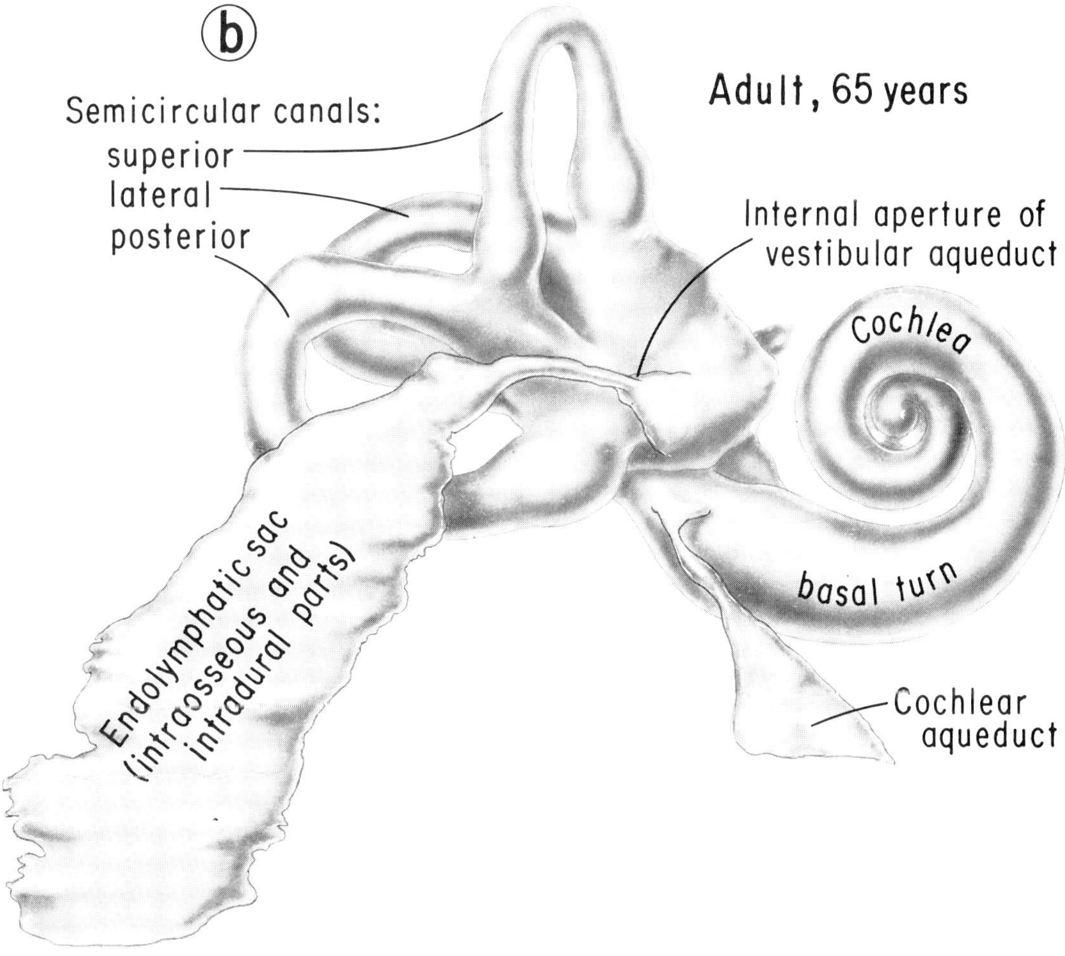

Figure II–24. Continued.

b. In the late fetus the duct changes from a straight to a curved course, turning downward at an angle of 30 to 60 degrees.

Wisconsin Collection, series as follows: *a*, 39; *b*, unknown.

(Adapted from Anson and Bast: Chapter 1 in Coates, Schenck, and Miller (Eds.): Otolaryngology, Vol. I. Hagerstown, Md., W. F. Prior Co., 1955.)

ADULT STRUCTURE: Illustrated in Figures III–60 to III–62.

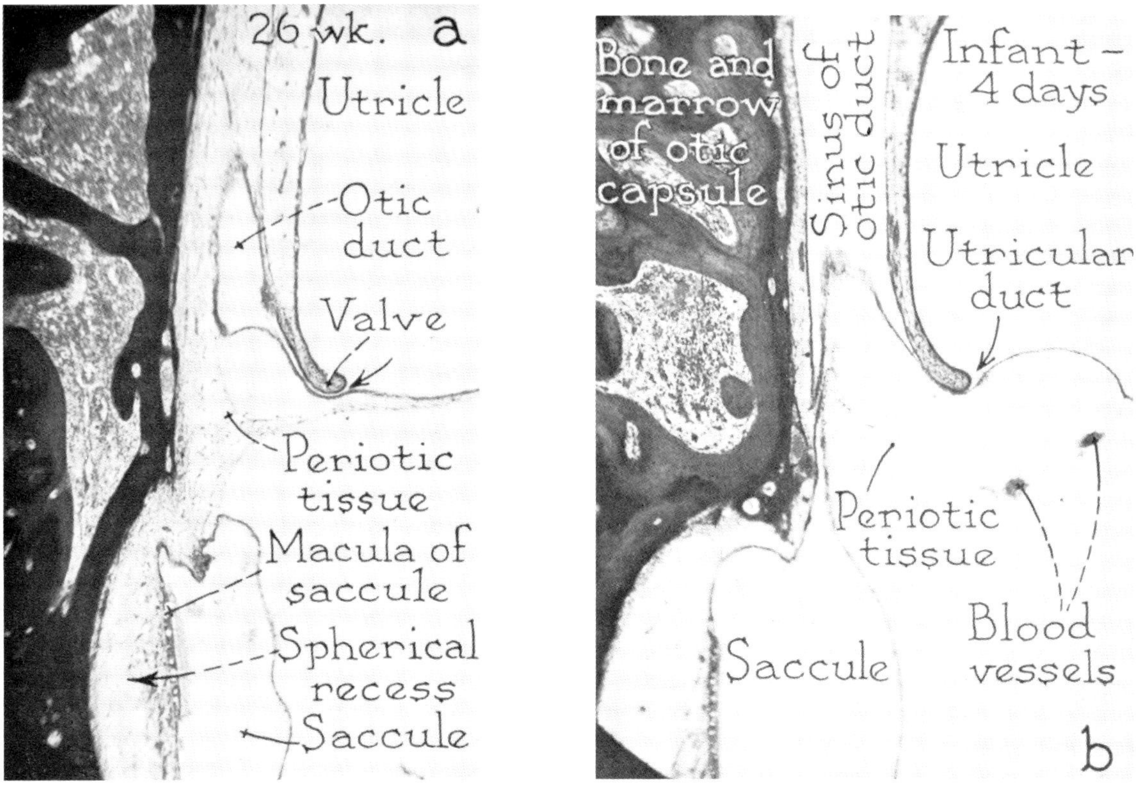

Figure II–25. Utricle, endolymphatic (or otic) duct, related chambers, and interconnecting ducts of the membranous labyrinth. *a*. Fetus, 26 weeks. *b* and *c*. Newborn infant (4-day premature). *d* and *e*. Child, 3 years of age.

a. Demonstrating the establishment of form in the fetus.
b and *c*. Similar form, retained in early infancy.

Figure II–25 continues on the opposite page.

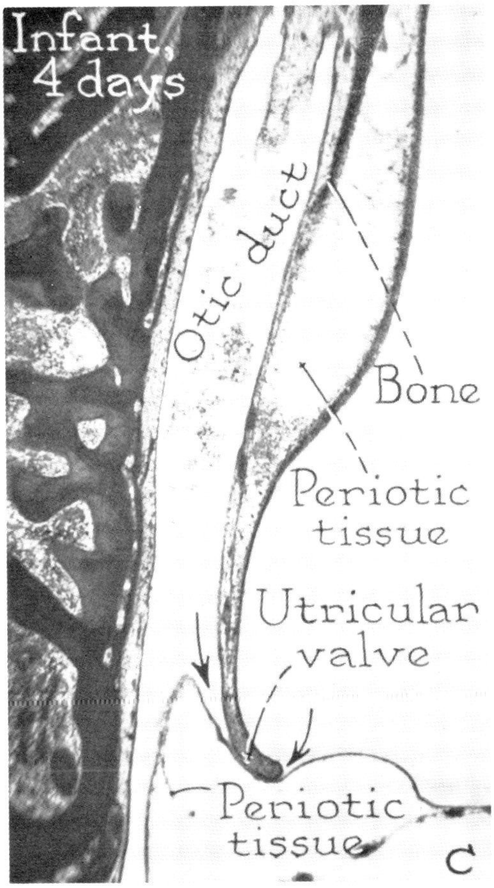

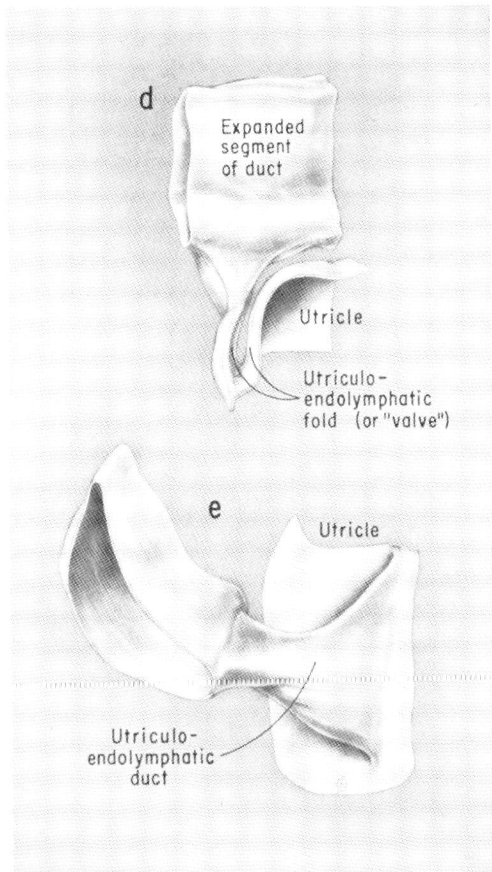

Figure II–25. *Continued.*

d and *e*. Showing, by reconstruction, the narrow, cleftlike form of the communication between the utricle and the endolymphatic duct.

a to *c*, Transverse sections, Wisconsin Collection, series as follows: *a*, 114; *b* and *c*, 124. *d* and *e*, Northwestern Collection, series 12.30.28. *a*, × 40; *b*, × 40; *c*, × 40; *d*, × 56; *e*, × 56.

(Adapted from Bast and Anson: The Temporal Bone and the Ear. Springfield, Charles C Thomas, 1949.)

Adult Structure: Illustrated in Figures III–60 to III–62.

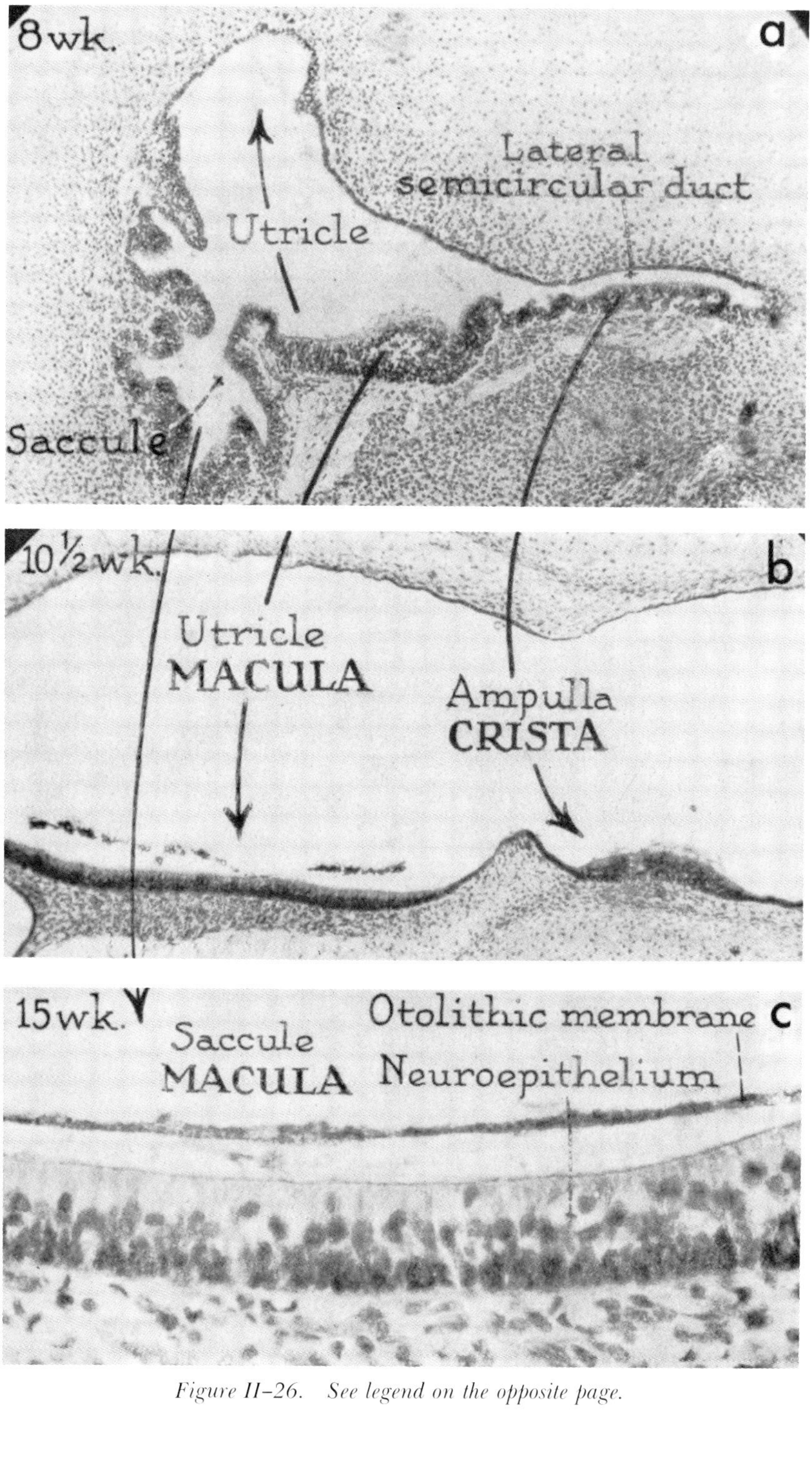

Figure II–26. See legend on the opposite page.

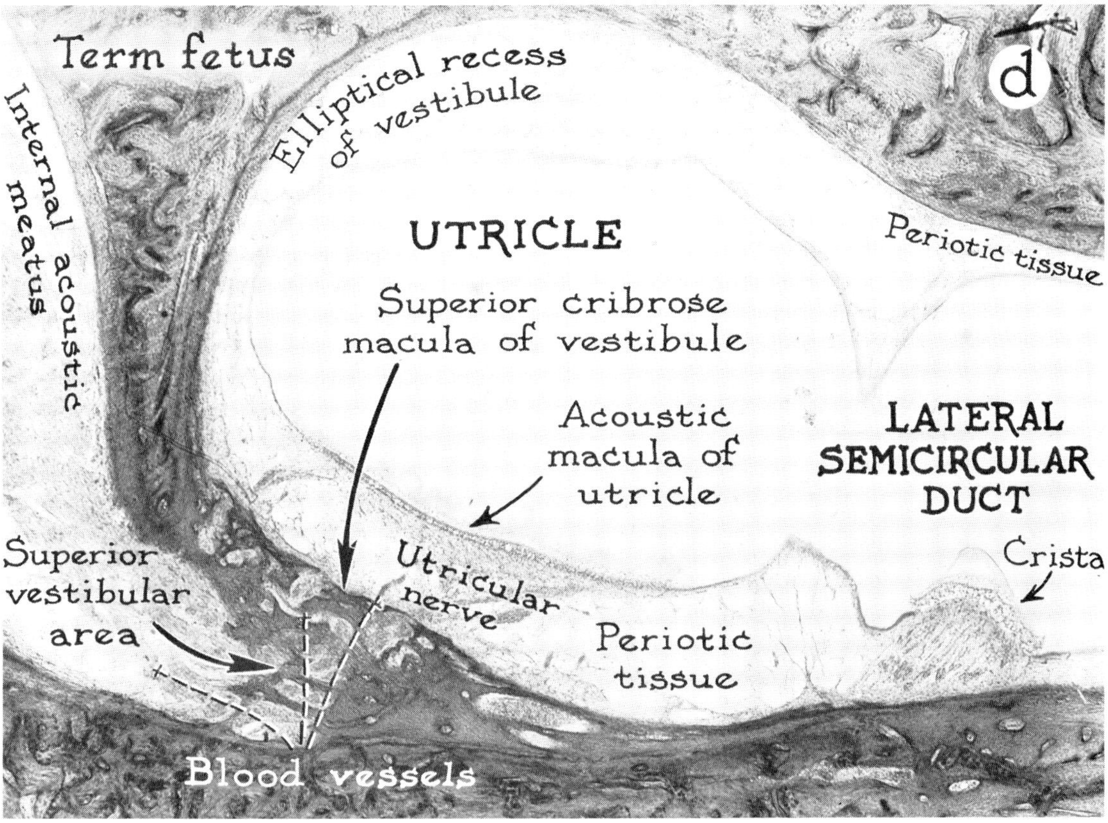

Figure II–26. CRISTA AND MACULA: DEVELOPMENTAL AND ADULT ANATOMY. *a.* FETUS OF 8 WEEKS (25 MM.). *b.* EMBRYO OF 10½ WEEKS (50 MM.). *c.* FETUS OF 15+ WEEKS (115 MM.). *d.* FETUS AT TERM.

a. Showing the early stage in differentiation of the acoustic macula of the utricle and of the crista of the lateral semicircular duct. The change from simple to neural epithelium occurs in those portions of the wall of the membranous labyrinth where the sensory nerves enter. Differentiation is initiated between the seventh and eighth week.

b. By the tenth to twelfth week, the typical cells are present: sensory cells, which bear bristlelike hairs at their free margin, and supporting cells. Already the otolithic membrane is being formed. The ampullae of the semicircular ducts are widely continuous with the utricle and will remain so.

c. In fetuses of fifteen weeks, the individual parts of the maculae and cristae are well differentiated. They appear to be similar to those seen in the adult. However, ossification has not yet been initiated; the surrounding otic capsule still consists of cartilage.

d. Demonstrating, in the fetus at term, the virtually mature form of the utricle and duct and the structure of the surrounding system of perilymphatic spaces and investing osseous capsule. Fibers of the upper terminal division of the vestibular nerve, accompanied by branches of the internal auditory blood vessels, are here shown as they pass from the superior vestibular area of the internal acoustic meatus to the acoustic macula of the utricle. Fibers of similar origin innervate the crista of the lateral membranous ampulla (following figure) and the crista of the superior ampulla (not sectioned at this level).

Transverse sections, Wisconsin Collection, series 87, 86, 54, and 123, respectively. *a* and *b*, × 99; *c*, × 397; *d*, × 35.

(From Anson: Chapter 1 in Paparella and Shumrick (Eds.): Otolaryngology, Vol. I. Philadelphia, W. B. Saunders Co., 1973.)

ADULT STRUCTURE: Illustrated in Figures III–50, III–51, III–53, III–54, and III–57 to III–59.

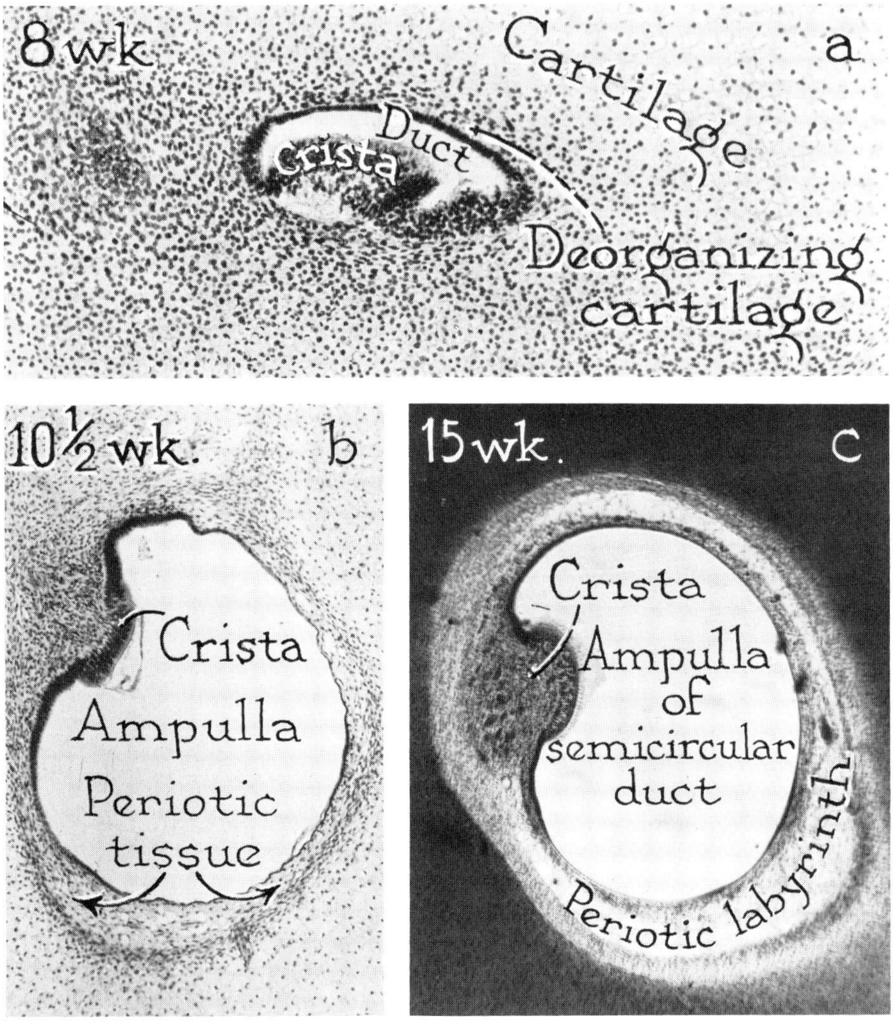

Figure II–27. Crista of ampulla: early development. *a.* Fetus of 8 weeks, lateral semicircular canal. *b.* Fetus of 10½ weeks (50 mm.), lateral canal. *c.* Fetus of 15 weeks (100 mm.), posterior canal.

a. The crista of each membranous ampulla develops as a cushionlike elevation on the side of the ampullary wall where the sensory nerve enters. This corresponds to the convex side of the future semicircular canal (of the osseous labyrinth). At this stage, the perilymphatic space of the bony labyrinth is represented by slight rarefaction of the cartilage in which the membranous ampulla is lodged.

b. As the ampulla enlarges, cartilage undergoes resorption, changing into a reticulum.

c. At the beginning of the fourth month, the crista has attained sickle-shaped form. The primordial reticulum is giving way to space; this is the canalicular part of the perilymphatic labyrinthine system (or osseous labyrinth). In the 5-month stage (not illustrated) the surrounding cartilage has changed to bone.

Each membranous semicircular duct lies eccentrically on the convex side of the osseous canal. The three ampullae are dilatations of the ducts; unlike the latter, they almost fill the corresponding expansion of the surrounding perilymphatic space. Each ampulla presents on the surface that corresponds to the convex side a transverse groove, the sulcus of the ampulla in which the nerve of supply enters, and the shelflike ridge, or crista, which projects into the lumen.

Transverse sections, Wisconsin Collection, series 87, 86, and 22, respectively. *a*, × 126; *b*, × 84; *c*, × 38.

(From Anson: Chapter 1 in Paparella and Shumrick (Eds.): Otolaryngology, Vol. I. Philadelphia, W. B. Saunders Co., 1973.)

Adult Structure: Illustrated in Figures III–50, III–51, III–53, III–54, and III–57 to III–59.

Ex Libri
J. Dennis Branger

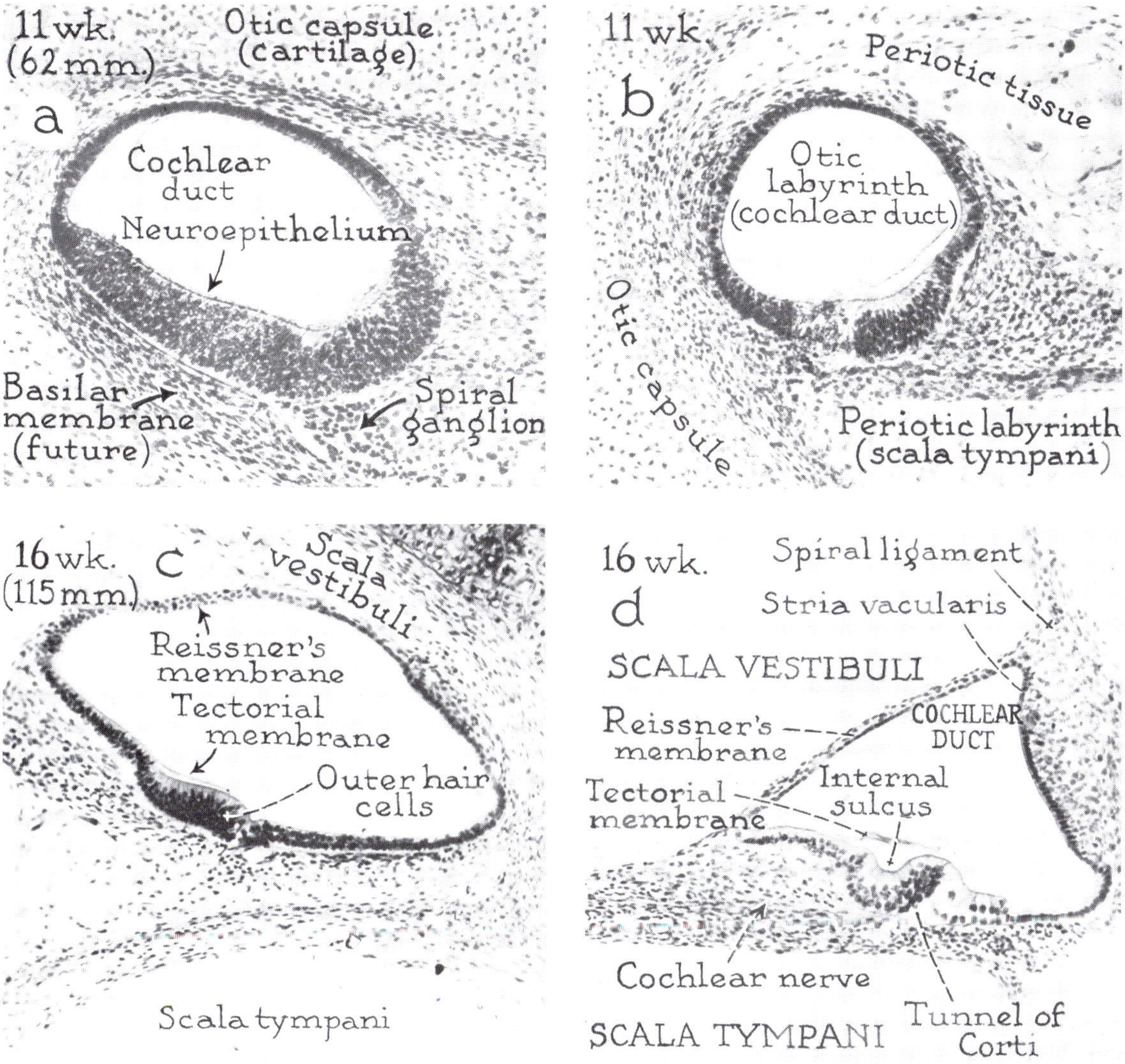

Figure II–28. Regional development of the cochlear duct: progress in a 5-week period. *a.* Fetus of 11 weeks (62 mm.); right ear, apical turn. *b.* Same specimen, middle part of basal turn. *c.* Fetus of approximately 16 weeks (115 mm.); left ear, apical turn. *d.* Same specimen, middle part of basal turn.

a. In the apical turn of the cochlear duct of the 11-week fetus, the spiral organ (of Corti) is in a very early stage of development. The neuroepithelium is a simple stratified thickening of the primitive duct.

b. In the basal turn of the same cochlea, elements of the future spiral organ are identifiable.

c. In a specimen five weeks older, the apical turn of the cochlear duct is in a stage advanced beyond that of the corresponding segment in the younger fetus (*a*). The cochlear duct is set off from the scalae, the latter perilymphatic spaces being formed through resorption of the periotic reticulum (see Figure II–32).

d. In the basal turn of the same cochlea, all structures of the future duct are identifiable: internal sulcus, outer hair cells, vestibular (Reissner's) membrane, vascular stria, tunnel of Corti, and tectorial membrane. The cochlear nerve courses through tissue that will be contained in the osseous spiral lamina.

Transverse sections, Wisconsin Collection, series as follows: *a* and *b*, 160; *c* and *d*, 54. *a*, × 134; *b*, × 142; *c*, × 127; *d*, × 128.

(From Anson: Chapter 1 in Paparella and Shumrick (Eds.): Otolaryngology, Vol. I. Philadelphia, W. B. Saunders Co., 1973.)

Adult Structure: Illustrated in Figures III–52, III–55, and III–56.

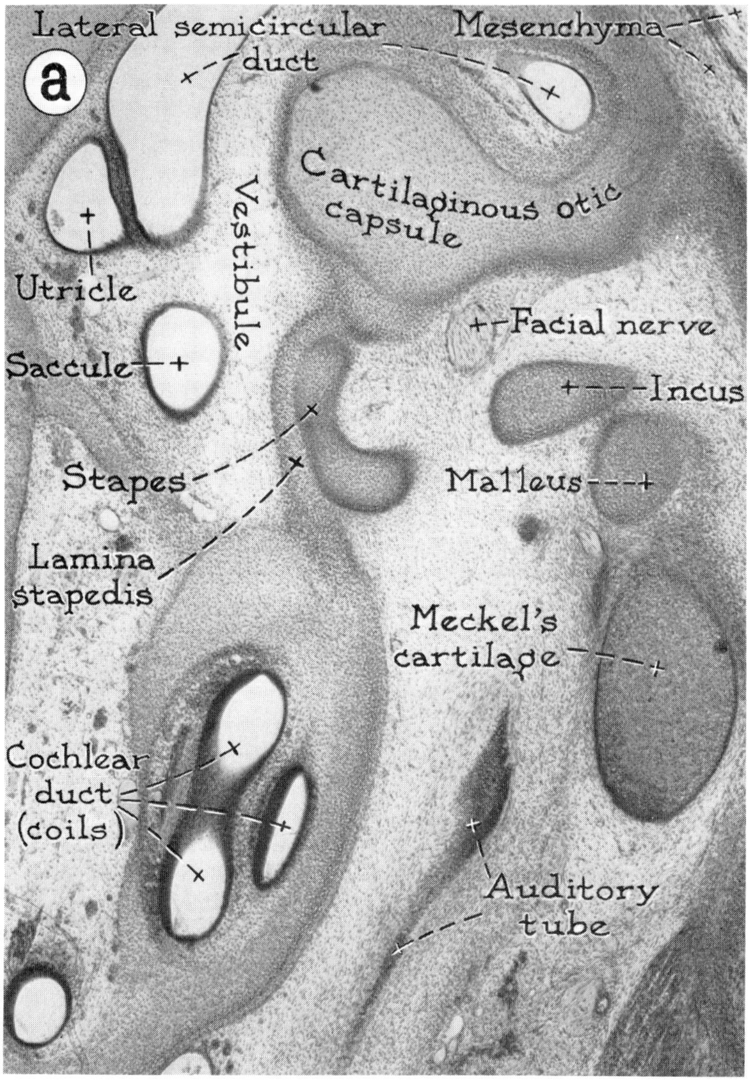

Figure II–29. Development of the osseous labyrinth: vestibular division. *a.* Fetus of 9 weeks (40 mm.). *b.* Fetus of 10 weeks (48 mm.). *c.* Fetus of 27+ weeks (243 mm.).

a. In the fetus of 9 weeks, the future perilymphatic space of the vestibule, like that of the canalicular and cochlear divisions, is occupied by a tissue of reticular type.

b. Within the period of a week thereafter, vacuolated spaces appear in the reticulum. Unlabeled arrows point to the future position of the vestibular window.

c. As early as the 27-week stage, the perilymphatic cistern has been formed around the saccule and utricle.

Transverse Sections, Wisconsin Collection, series 168, 202, and 89, respectively. *a,* × 38; *b,* × 27; *c,* × 16.

Adult Structure: Illustrated in Figures III–46 and III–86 to III–88.

Figure II–29 continues on the opposite page.

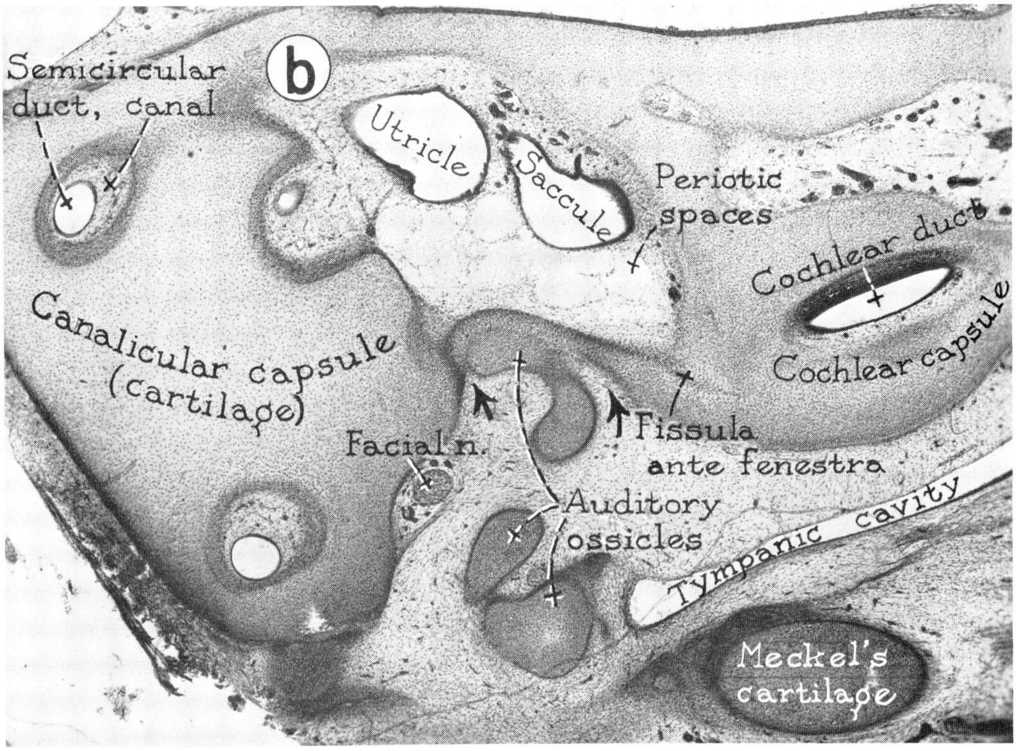

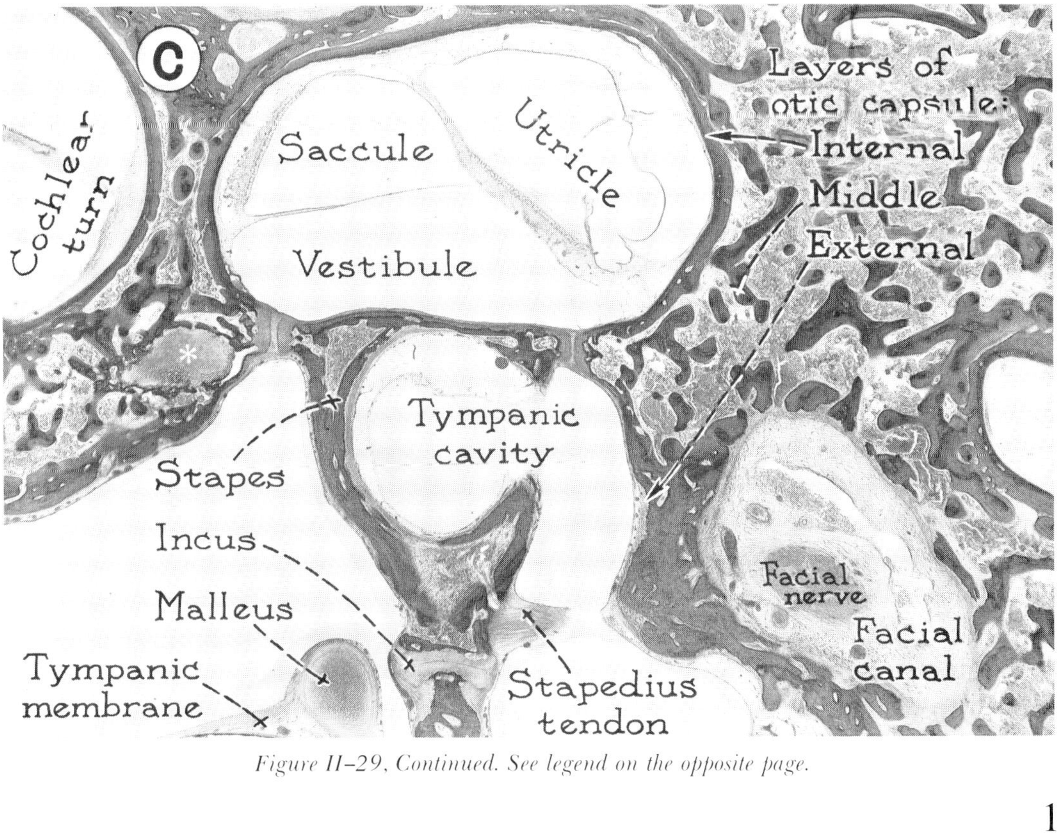

Figure II–29, Continued. See legend on the opposite page.

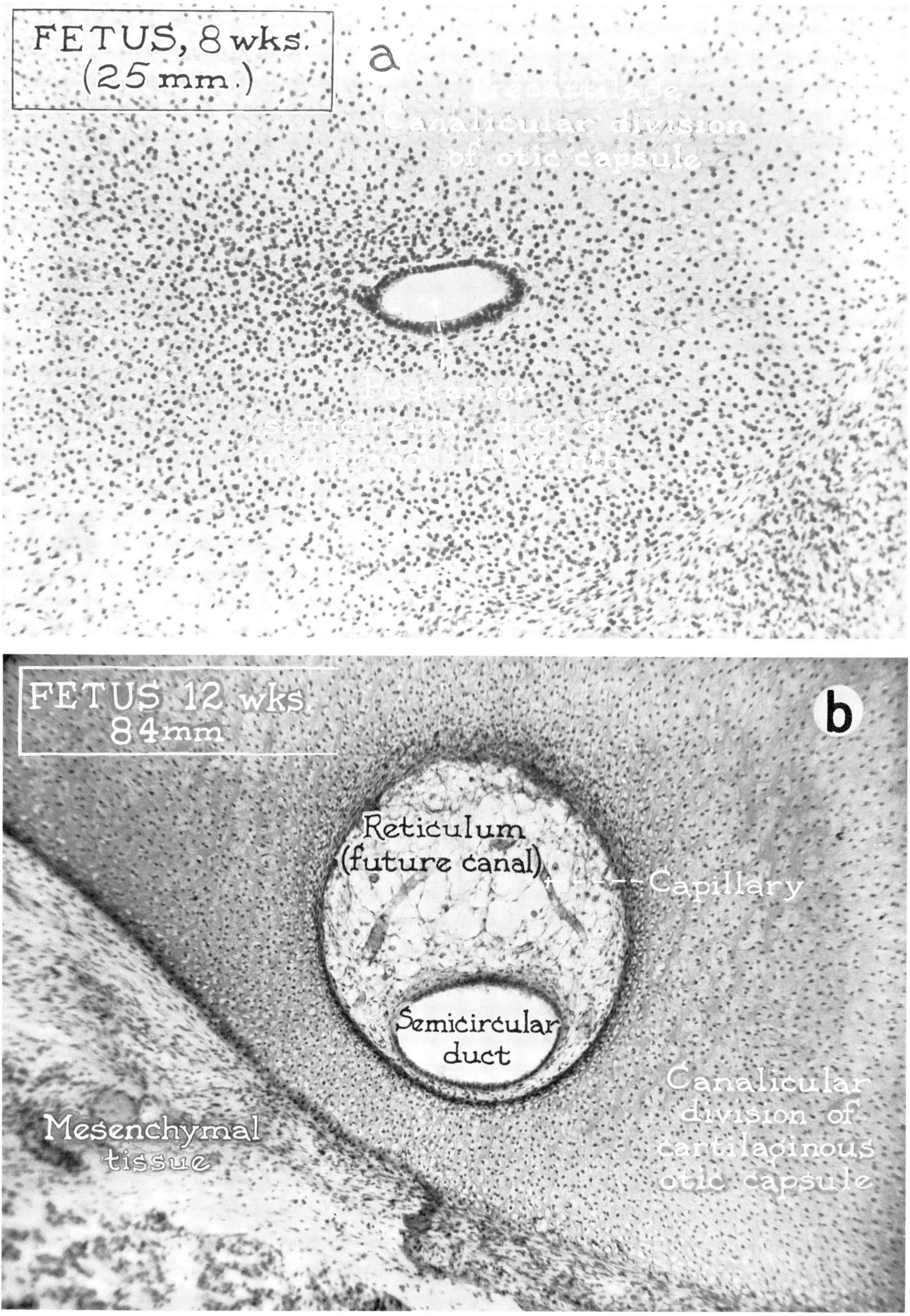

Figure II–30. See legend on the opposite page.

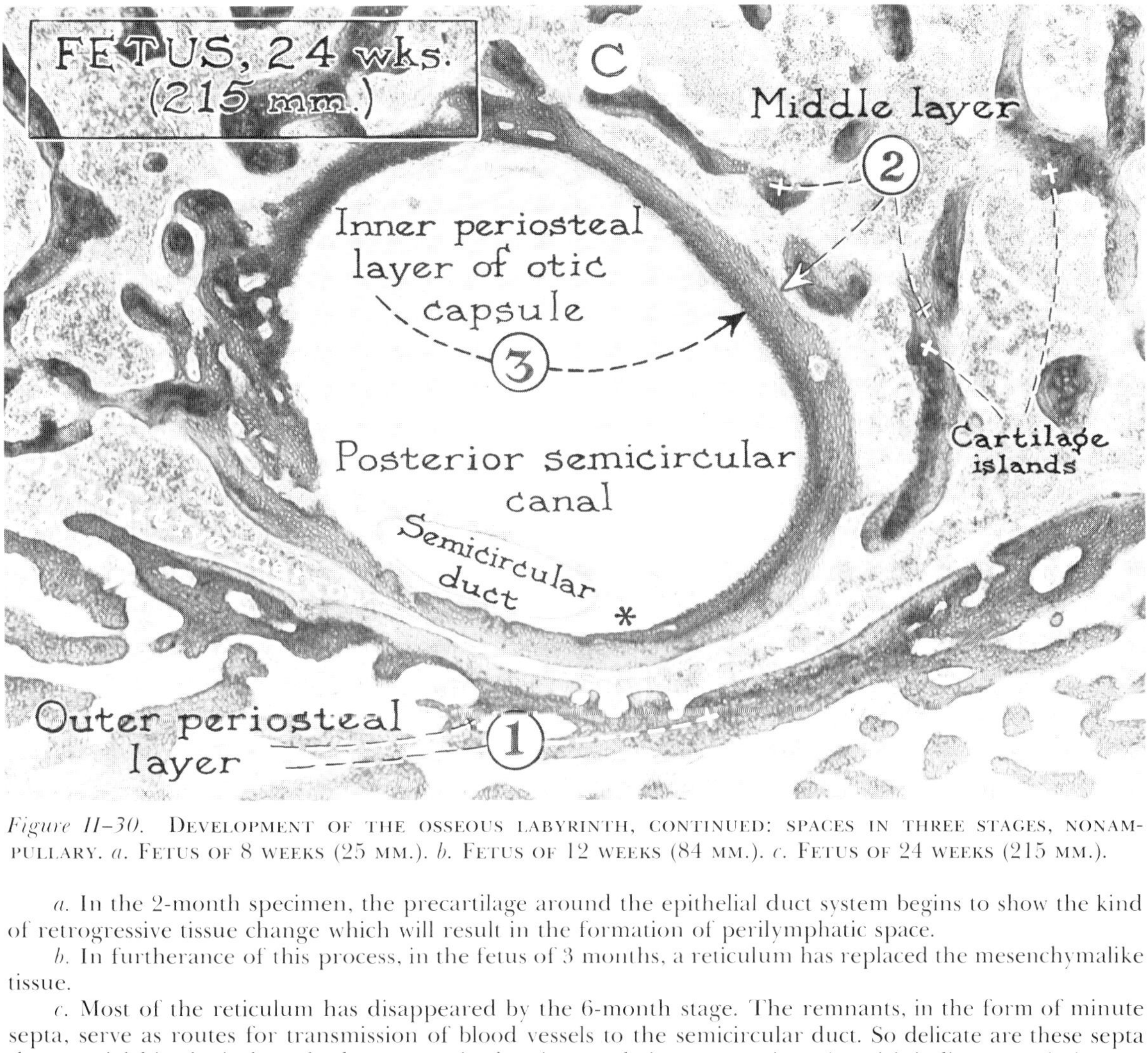

Figure II–30. DEVELOPMENT OF THE OSSEOUS LABYRINTH, CONTINUED: SPACES IN THREE STAGES, NONAMPULLARY. *a*. FETUS OF 8 WEEKS (25 MM.). *b*. FETUS OF 12 WEEKS (84 MM.). *c*. FETUS OF 24 WEEKS (215 MM.).

a. In the 2-month specimen, the precartilage around the epithelial duct system begins to show the kind of retrogressive tissue change which will result in the formation of perilymphatic space.

b. In furtherance of this process, in the fetus of 3 months, a reticulum has replaced the mesenchymalike tissue.

c. Most of the reticulum has disappeared by the 6-month stage. The remnants, in the form of minute septa, serve as routes for transmission of blood vessels to the semicircular duct. So delicate are these septa that special histological methods are required to insure their preservation. Asterisk indicates periotic connective tissue.

Transverse sections, Wisconsin Collection, series 87, 162, and 62, respectively. *a*, × 173; *b*, × 105; *c*, × 41. (From Anson: Trans. Amer. Acad. Ophthal. Otolaryng., 73:17–38, 1969.)

ADULT STRUCTURE: Illustrated in Figures III–46 and III–86 to III–88.

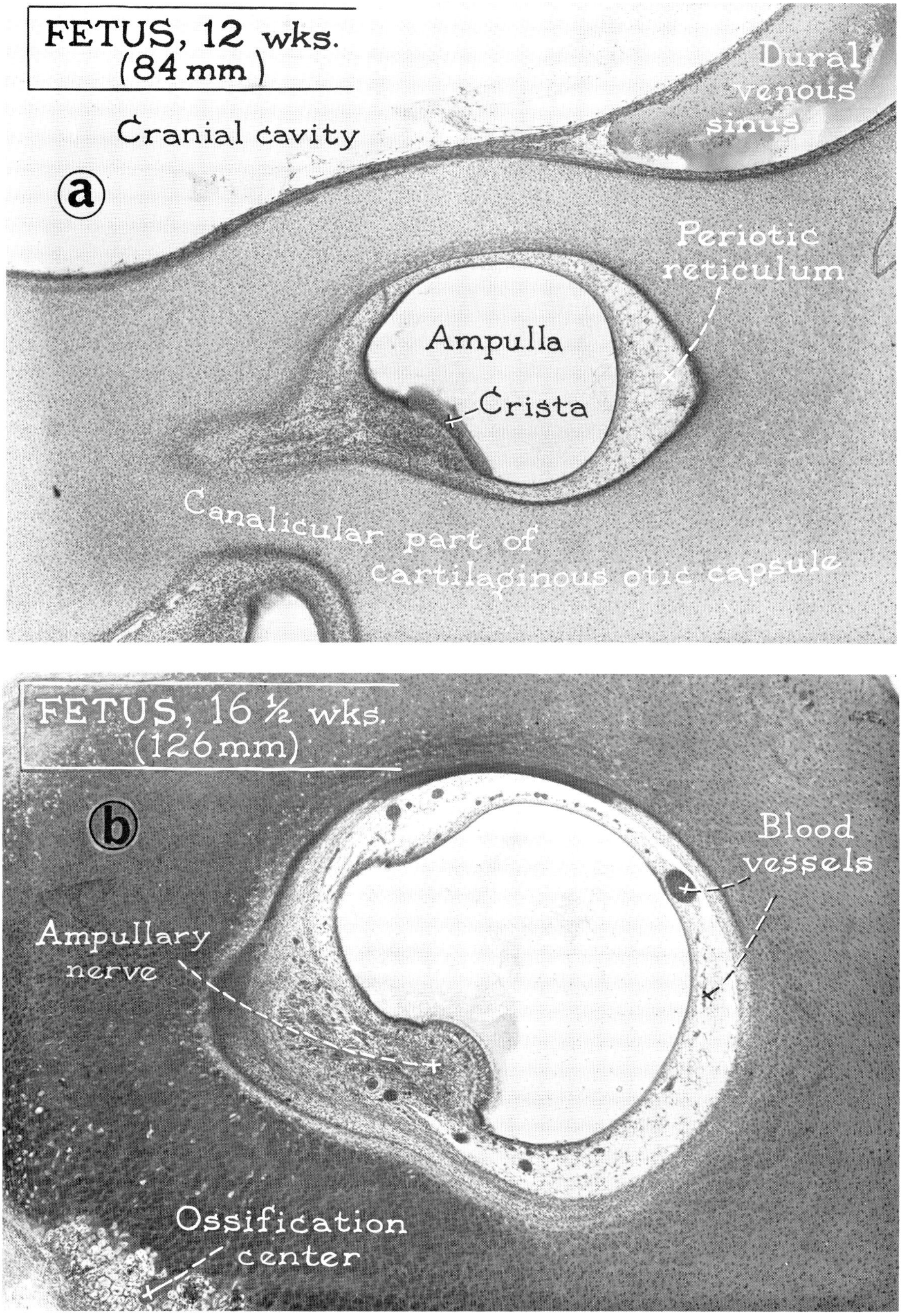

Figure II–31. See legend on the opposite page.

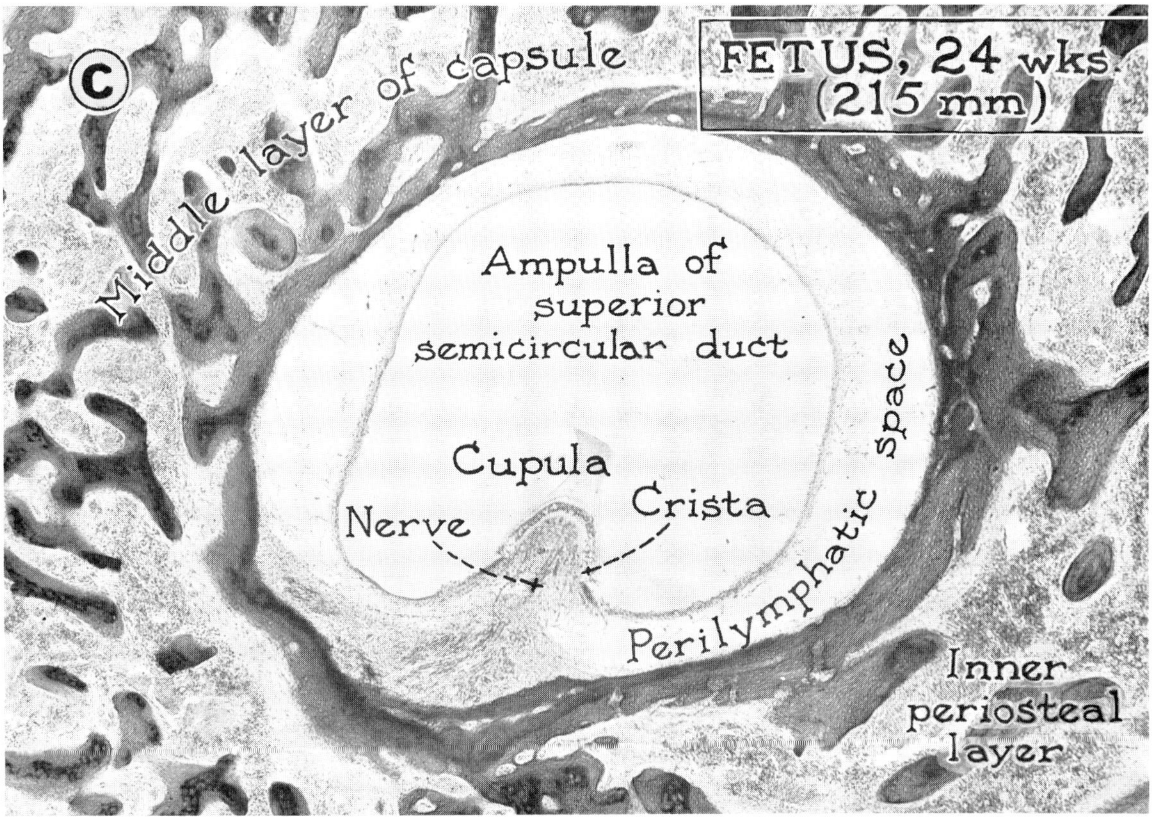

Figure II–31. DEVELOPMENT OF THE OSSEOUS LABYRINTH, CONTINUED: CANALICULAR PART, AMPULLARY. FETUSES OF 3, 4, AND 6 MONTHS (84, 126, AND 215 MM.).

a. In the 2-month specimen (not illustrated) the cartilage around the endolymphatic duct system begins to undergo retrogressive change. This process results in the formation of the system of intercommunicating spaces of the semicircular canals. In the fetus of 3 months, as here shown, the precartilage has given way to a reticulum. Minute blood vessels are present among the fibrils.

b. In the 4-month specimen at the beginning of capsular ossification, the fibrillar reticulum is undergoing further resorption. It will largely disappear, except where it is destined to remain around the nerves of supply to the crista of each ampulla in the form of anchorage and, sparsely, in support of the persistent arteries and veins. At this stage the vascular supply is a prominent feature of the reticulum.

c. Two months later, the reticulum is fragmentary. Special methods are required to preserve the strands and the vessels which they transmit. The capsule is now trilaminar, being composed of the layers that will remain histologically identifiable in the adult *pars petrosa* (see Figures II–5 and II–6).

Transverse sections, Wisconsin Collection, series 162, 11, and 62, respectively. *a*, × 40; *b*, × 45; *c*, × 34.

ADULT STRUCTURE: Illustrated in Figures III–46 and III–86 to III–88.

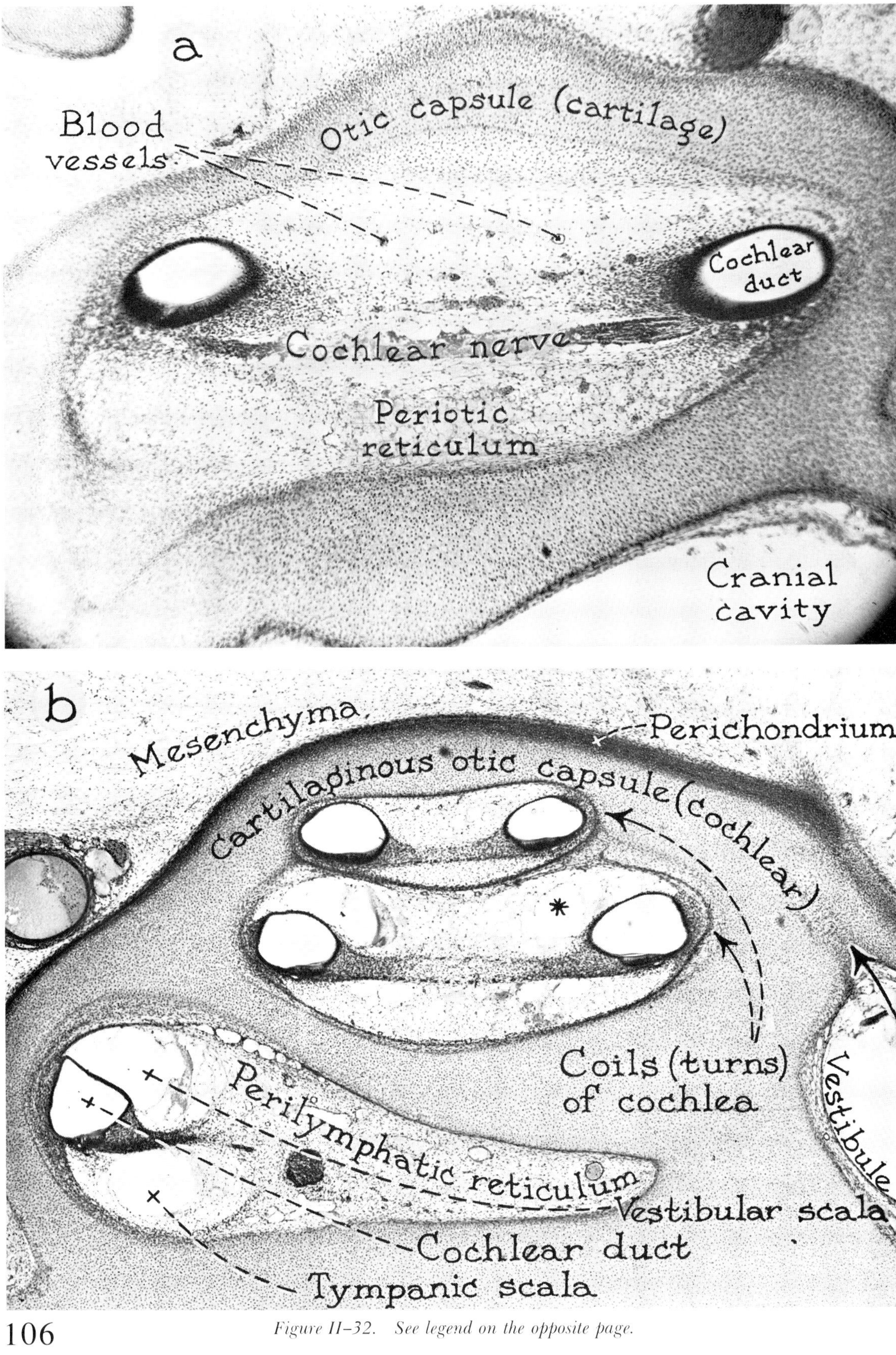

Figure II–32. See legend on the opposite page.

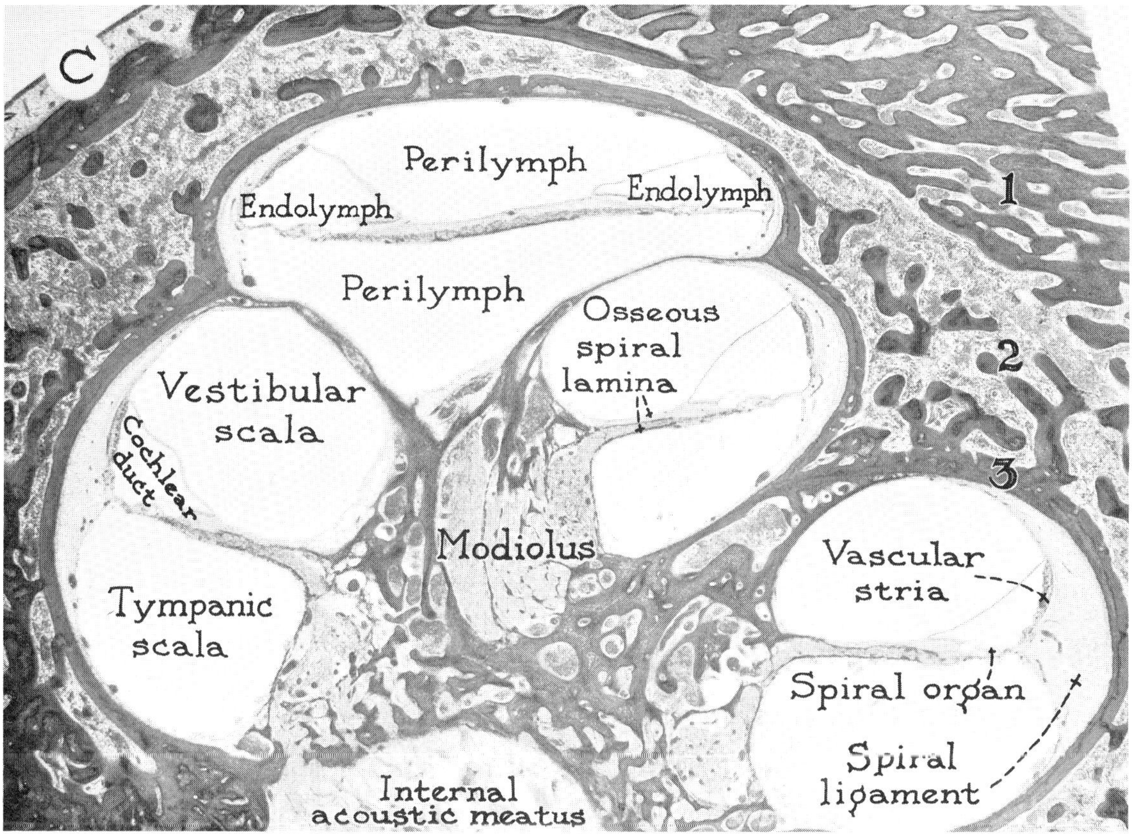

Figure II–32. Development of the osseous labyrinth, concluded: cochlear part. *a.* Fetus of 9 weeks (40 mm.). *b.* Fetus, 12 weeks (84 mm.). *c.* Newborn (4-day premature).

a. In the 9-week fetus, the future perilymphatic space of the cochlear is occupied by a vascular mesenchymalike tissue in which change to reticulum is just becoming evident.

b. At 12 weeks, definite vacuoles have appeared. They first occur near the cochlear duct of the membranous labyrinthine system, to become the vestibular scala (at asterisk) and the tympanic scala. Development is farthest advanced in the basal turn, decreasing as the apical turn is approached. The perichondrium is in a state of active growth (and will continue to be until ossification begins in the 4-month or 5-month stage). The fissula ante fenestram (at arrow) is being formed through retrogressive change in the cartilaginous capsule.

c. In late fetal stages, the periotic tissue (in regular preparations) appears as a thin layer on the inner wall of the cochlear turns, except where it becomes part of the spiral ligament or as tenuous "septa" that, in crossing the space of the scalae, carry minute blood vessels to the cochlear duct.

Transverse sections, Wisconsin Collection, series 168, 162, and 124, respectively. *a,* × 68; *b,* × 33; *c,* × 23.

Adult Structure: Illustrated in Figures III–46 and III–86 to III–88.

Figure II–33. OTIC CAPSULE: DISTINCTIVE DEVELOPMENTAL FEATURES IN COMPARISON WITH THE FAMILIAR STEPS IN FORMATION OF A TYPICAL LONG BONE.

In the reconstruction of the 16-week fetus, the ossification centers are shown in relation to the perilymphatic labyrinthine system. In the "model" of the 21-week fetal specimen, the incomplete area at the right is cartilage in the specimen (see Figure II–5).

The following five features in development of the otic capsule are unique: (1) origin from 14 ossification centers, appearing within a period of 6 weeks, beginning with the fifteenth week; (2) fusion of the centers peripherally without intermediate zones of epiphyseal growth or suture lines; (3) trilaminar structure of each center and, consequently, of the entire capsule; (4) independent timetable of growth for each layer of every center and individual pattern of histogenesis; (5) lifelong retention of fetal architecture in the total absence of those processes that elsewhere convert fetal into haversian bone.

A typical long bone of the human skeleton attains adult dimensions in about 22 years; the otic capsule is as large as it will ever be in the 21-week fetus. The typical bone arises from three centers: one diaphyseal, two epiphyseal; the otic capsule, about $1/150$ as long as a tibia, arises from 14 centers (none of them epiphyseal).

(From Anson: Trans. Amer. Acad. Ophthal. Otolaryng., 73:17–38, 1969.)

ADULT STRUCTURE: Illustrated in Figures III–87*a* and III–88.

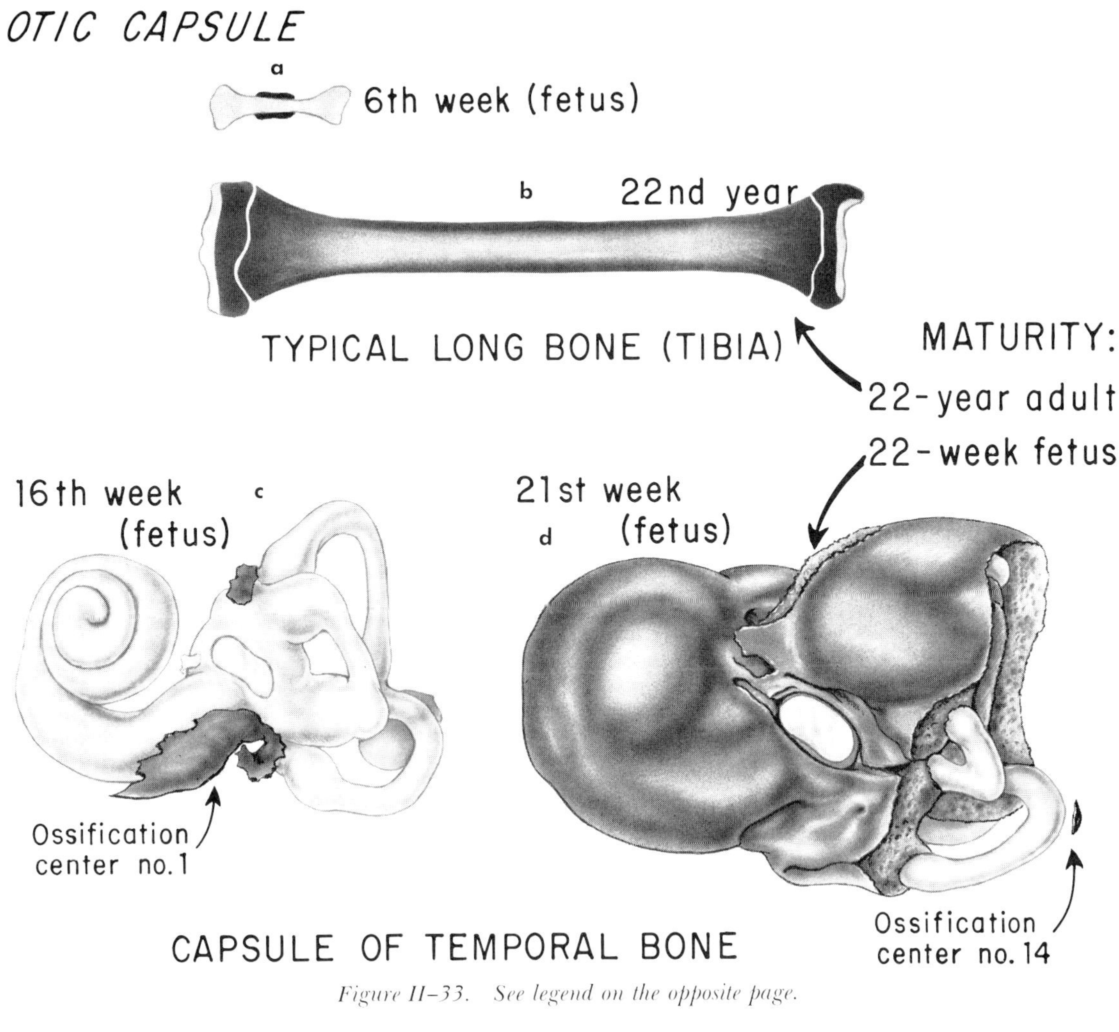

Figure II–33. See legend on the opposite page.

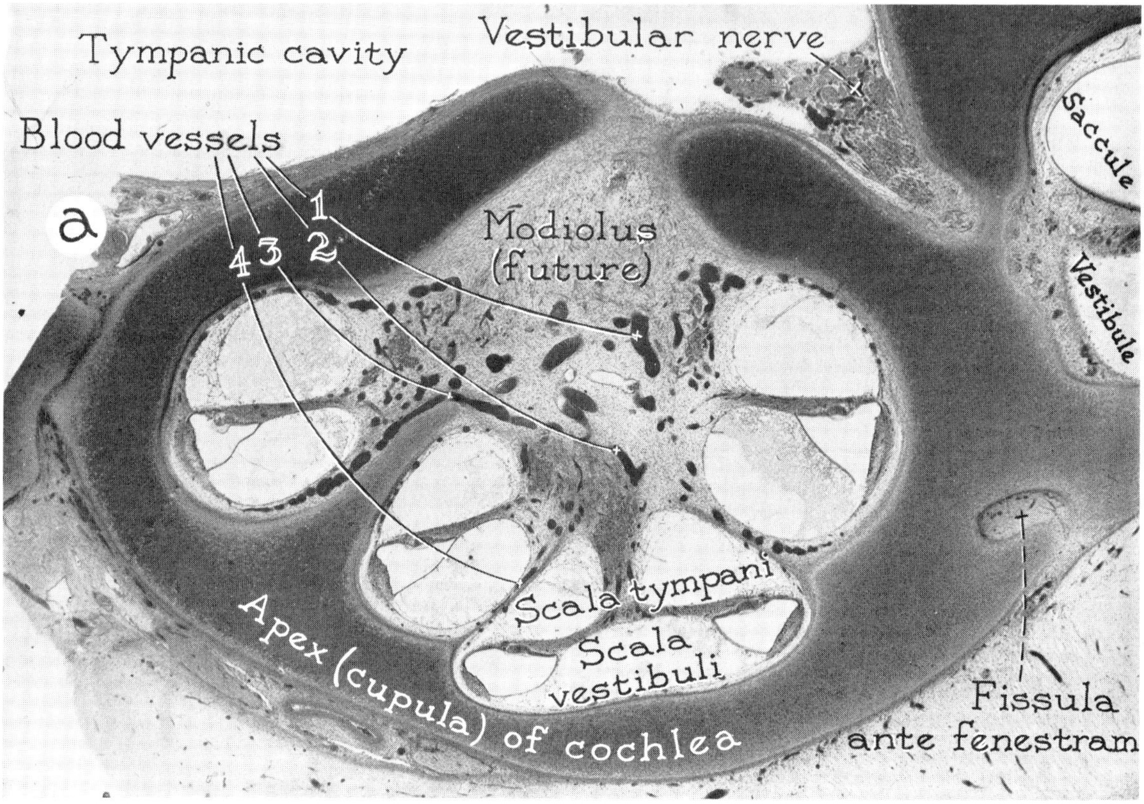

Figure II–34. DEVELOPMENT OF THE OTIC CAPSULE. *a*. FETUS OF 16½ WEEKS (126 MM.). *b* and *c*. FETUS OF 24 WEEKS (210 MM.).

a. In the 4-month fetus the otic capsule is still composed of cartilage. At this early stage the pattern of blood supply to the membranous labyrinth and to the perilymphatic spaces is already established. Branches of the internal auditory vessels pass from the meatus into the modiolus (see *1* and *2*), therefrom along the walls of each scala (*3*), through the partition between cochlear turns (*4*), and within the developing osseous spiral lamina (not numbered) to the spiral organ.

b and *c*. In the 6-month specimen, the fundamental histological structure of the osseous capsule is at the midpoint in the course of its change from cartilage to bone of petrous density. The outer periosteal layer (at *1*) is undergoing rapid thickening; the inner periosteal layer (at *3*) remains excessively thin; the middle layer (at *2*) consists of sparsely distributed "spicules" of intrachondrial bone upon which endosteal bone is being slowly deposited. In this "layer," primitive marrow tissue heavily outbulks bone. It is demonstrated that the layers of the otic capsule develop on different timetables and that each is histologically distinctive.

Transverse sections, Wisconsin Collection, series as follows: *a*, 11; *b* and *c*, 51. *a*, × 18; *b*, × 12; *c*, × 25.

ADULT STRUCTURE: Illustrated in Figures III–87*a* and III–88.

Figure II–34 continues on the opposite page.

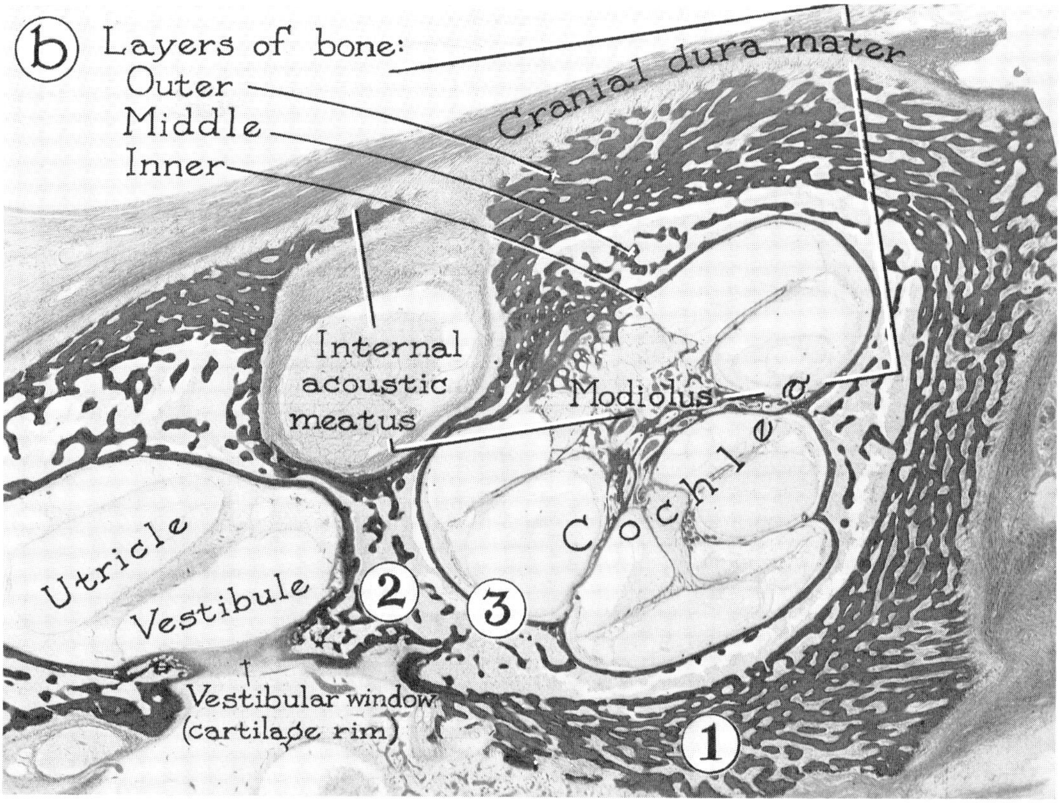

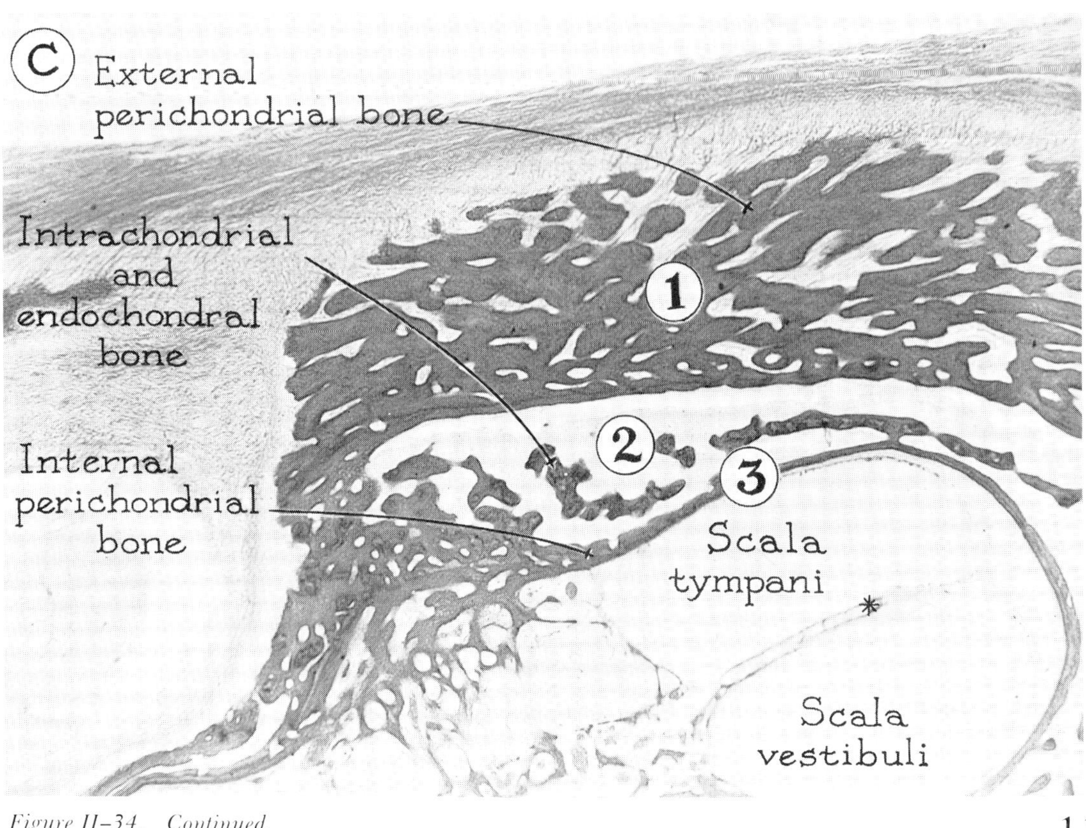

Figure II–34, Continued.

Figure II–34 continues on the following page.

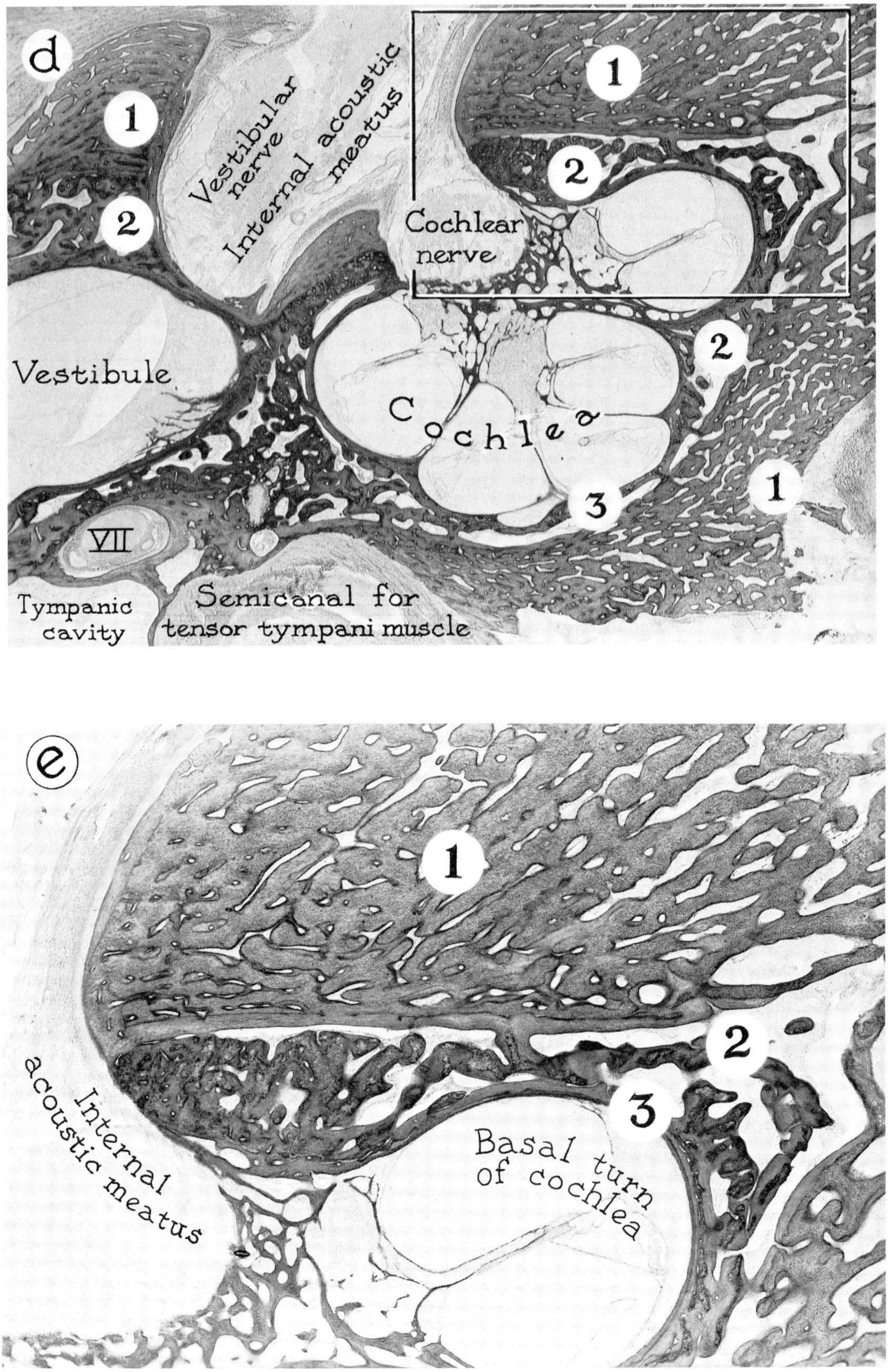

Figure II–34, Continued. See legend on the opposite page.

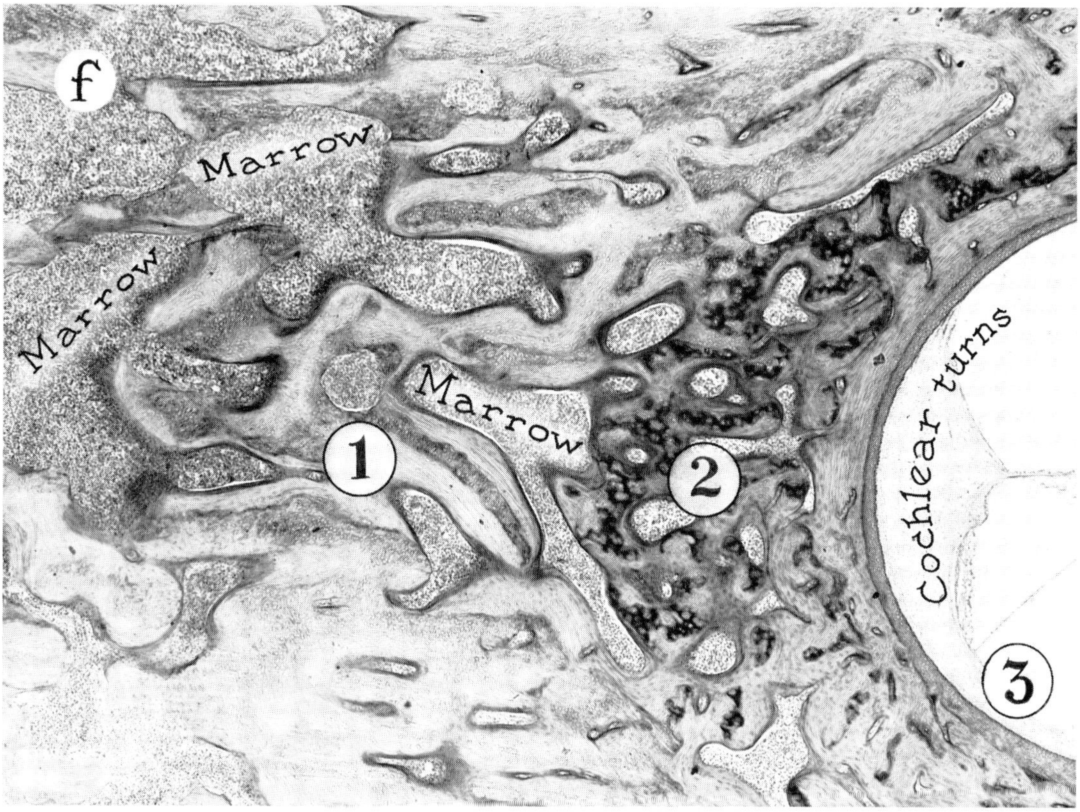

Figure II–34, Continued. DEVELOPMENT OF THE OTIC CAPSULE. *d* and *e*. FETUS AT TERM. *f*. INFANT, 10 WEEKS OLD.

d and *e*. In the term fetus the outer layer (*1*) has increased in thickness; concurrently it is approaching petrous character owing to deposition of periosteal bone on the constituent laminae. The inner layer (*3*) does not, of itself, thicken; however, endosteal bone is deposited thinly on its external aspect. The middle layer (*2*), as a result of the sudden onset of renewed osteogenesis, is, like the outer layer (*1*), approaching petrous consistency. The area blocked in *d* is shown at higher magnification in *e*.

f. Following a period of relative inactivity during the five prenatal months, the capsule rapidly attains petrous character. The marrow spaces of the middle layer (*2*) are reduced in size, ultimately being represented by minute vascular channels. The external layer (*1*), beyond the area of the primordial capsule, may either undergo early postnatal pneumatization or may retain the character of an adult marrow tissue. In some specimens the layer passes through a slow process of rebuilding, the outcome of which is the formation of bone of a gnarly texture. The internal layer (*3*) remains thin. It is readily identifiable as a lamina, being histologically different from the bone of the middle layer, spicules of which were applied early to its outer (or deep) surface. In this way, the otic capsule becomes imbedded in, and part of, the *pars petrosa* of the temporal bone.

Transverse sections, Wisconsin Collection, series as follows: *d* and *e*, 122; *f*, 23. *d*, × 11; *e*, × 21; *f*, × 41.

ADULT STRUCTURE: Illustrated in Figures III–87*a* and III–88.

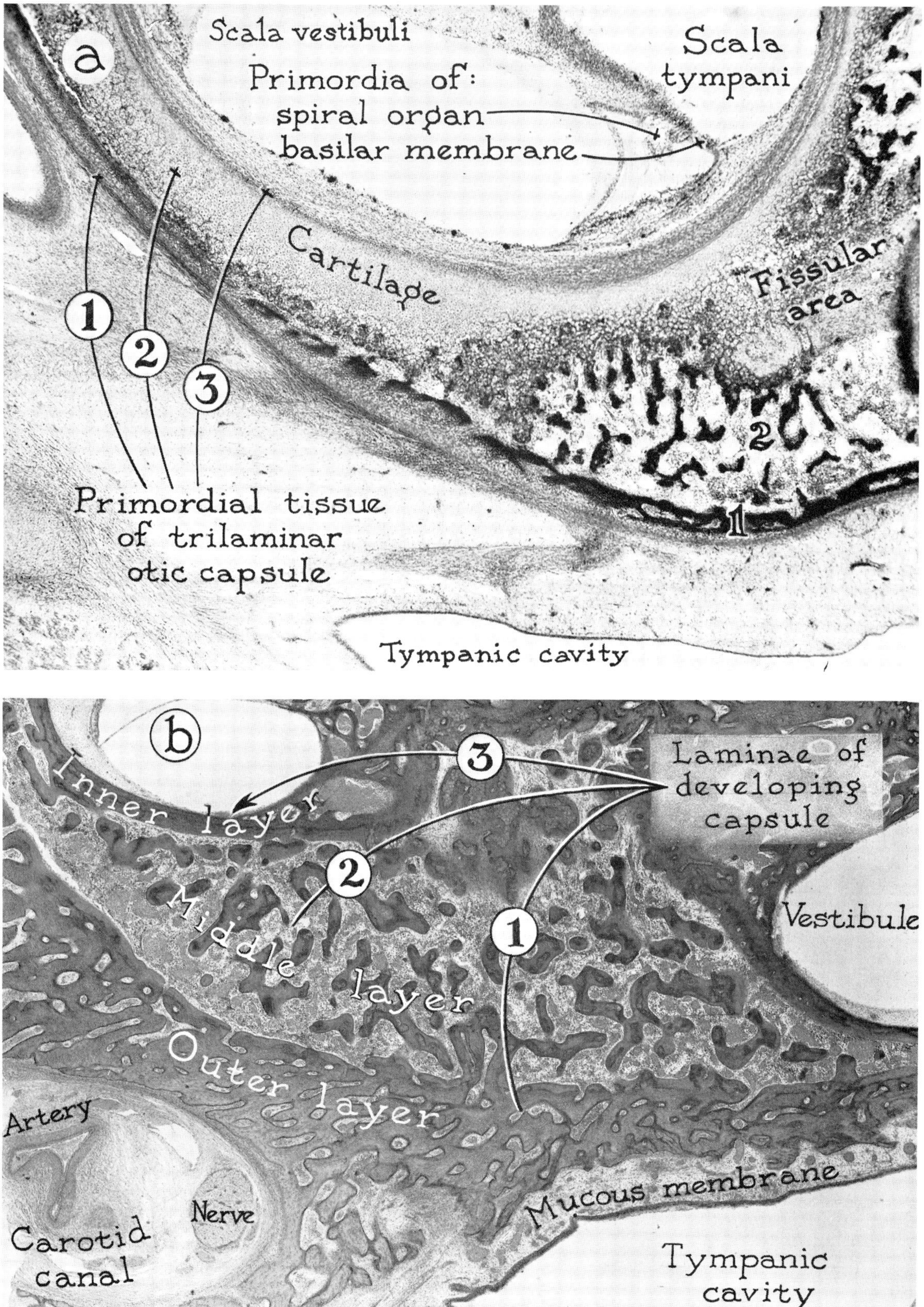

Figure II–35. See legend on the opposite page.

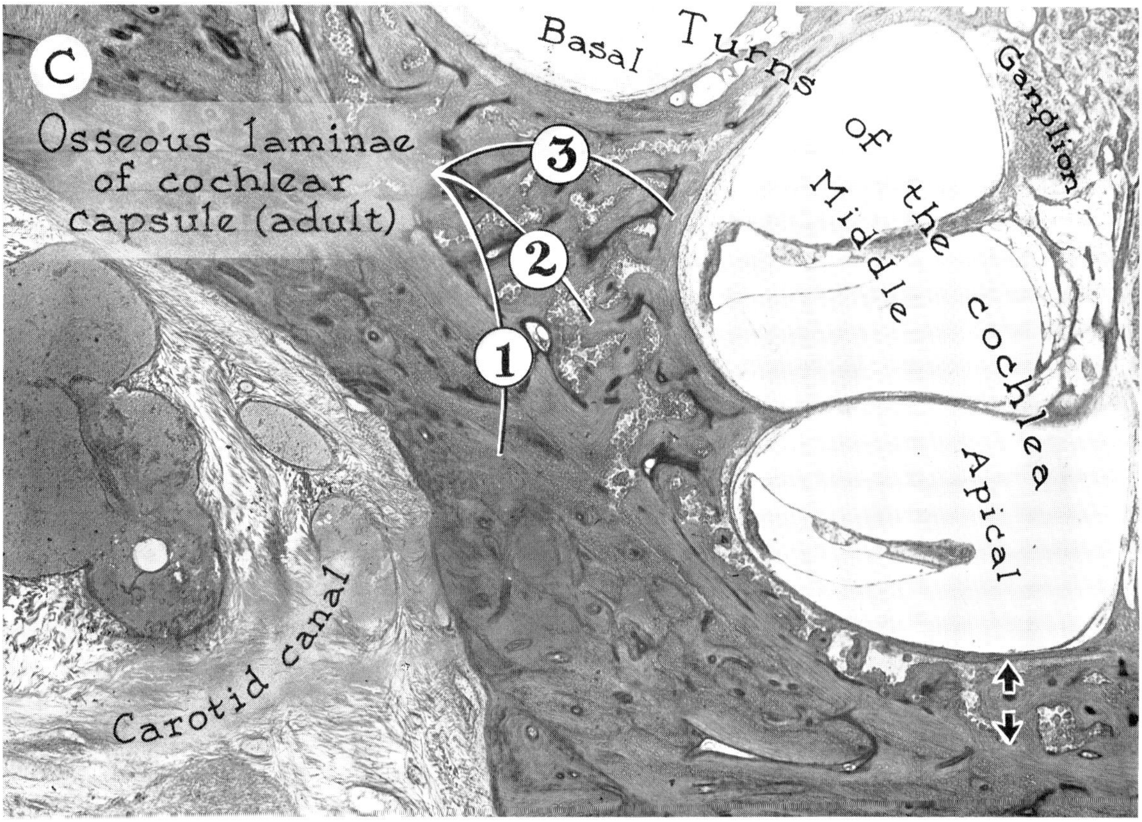

Figure II–35. Developmental and adult structure of the otic capsule in the cochlear region. *a.* Fetus of 19½ weeks (160mm.). *b.* Newborn (4-day premature). *c.* Adult, 19 years of age.

a. In the fifth month of intrauterine life, the three typical layers of bone are present in the ossification centers of the developing cochlear capsule. Those here shown are representative of all the centers, 14 in number, of which the fully formed capsule is composed. In the cochlea, encapsulation of the coils progresses from base to apex; the apical part is still cartilaginous in the specimen illustrated. The outer periosteal layer (at *1*), when it first appears, is made up of platelike portions, each one layer thick. The inner periosteal stratum (at *3*), unlike the outer, is complete, yet thin. The middle layer (at *2*), differing from the other two, consists of scattered islands of intrachondrial bone. Each constituent of the "osseous globules" is a small area of cartilage on the interior of whose lacunae osteocytes have deposited a thin layer of bone. Concurrently, endosteal bone is laid down by osteoblasts on the exterior of these islands of combined tissue.

b. The outer layer rapidly increases in thickness; the inner remains unchanged. In the middle layer, deposition of endosteal bone is slow—latent until about the time of birth. Then a surge of activity results in rapid attainment of petrous fabric.

c. The islets of intrachondrial bone remain identifiable throughout life, seemingly unaltered in their histological structure. None of the layers is resorbed and rebuilt into true haversian bone. The limits of the middle layer are indicated by unlabeled arrows.

Transverse sections, Wisconsin Collection, series 41, 124, and 29, respectively. *a*, × 31; *b*, × 22; *c*, × 30. (*a* and *c* from Anson: Trans. Amer. Acad. Ophthal. Otolaryng., 73:17–38, 1969.)

Adult Structure: Illustrated in Figures III–87*a* and III–88.

Figure II–36. SUBARCUATE FOSSA: FETAL DEVELOPMENT DURING A 10-WEEK PERIOD, MEDIAL ASPECT OF THREE BONES. SPECIMENS DRAWN TO SCALE.

a. In the 31-week specimen the caliber of the subarcuate fossa exceeds that of the internal acoustic meatus.

b. The size-relation between fossa and meatus is but slightly altered in the 37-week stage.

c. Three weeks later, in the 40-week specimen, reduction in the capacity of the fossa is appreciable. Typically, the aperture in the adult temporal bone is of pinpoint dimensions.

Preparations by Dr. Gordon P. Holt.

ADULT STRUCTURES: Illustrated in Figures III–127 and III–128.

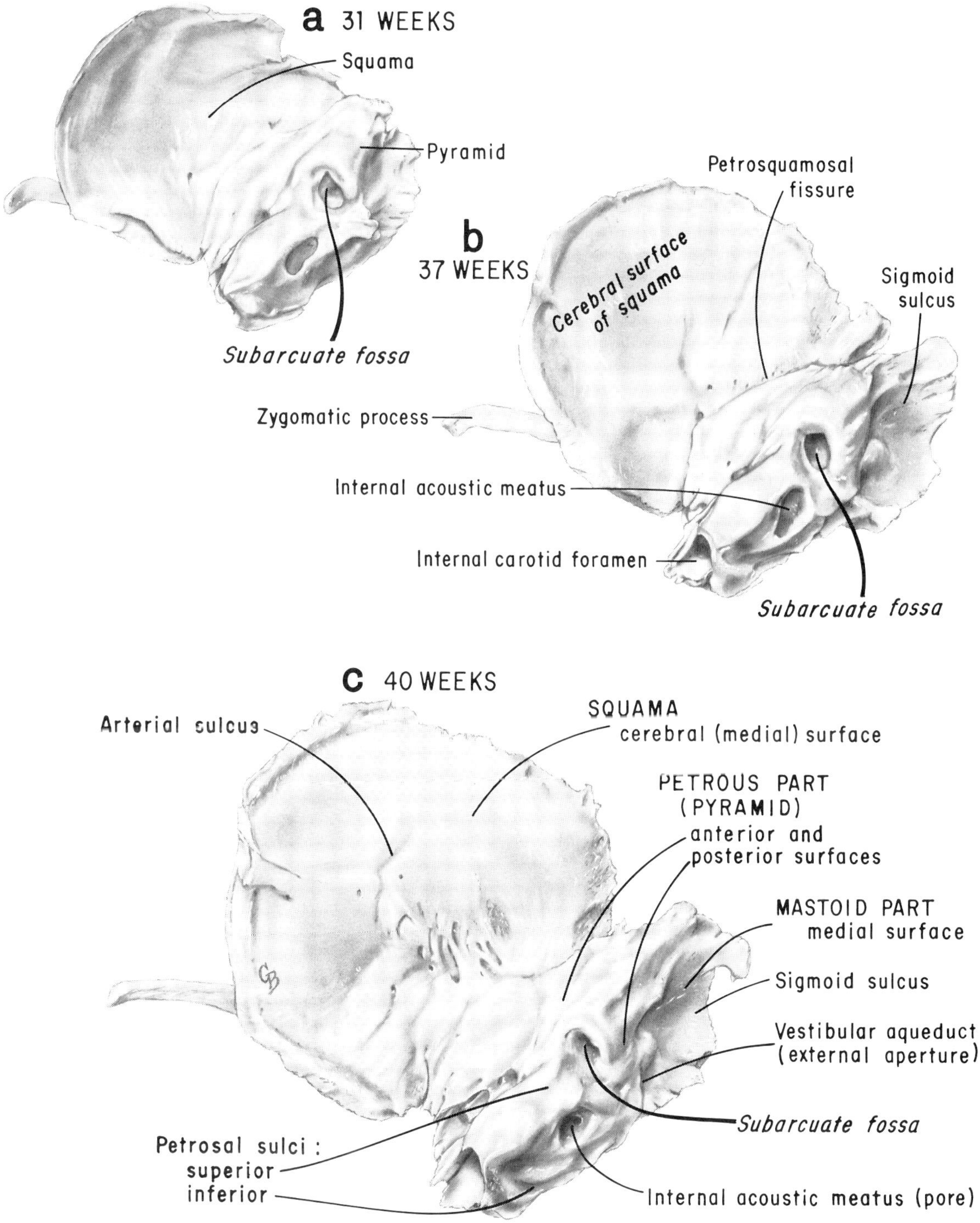

Figure II–36. See legend on the opposite page.

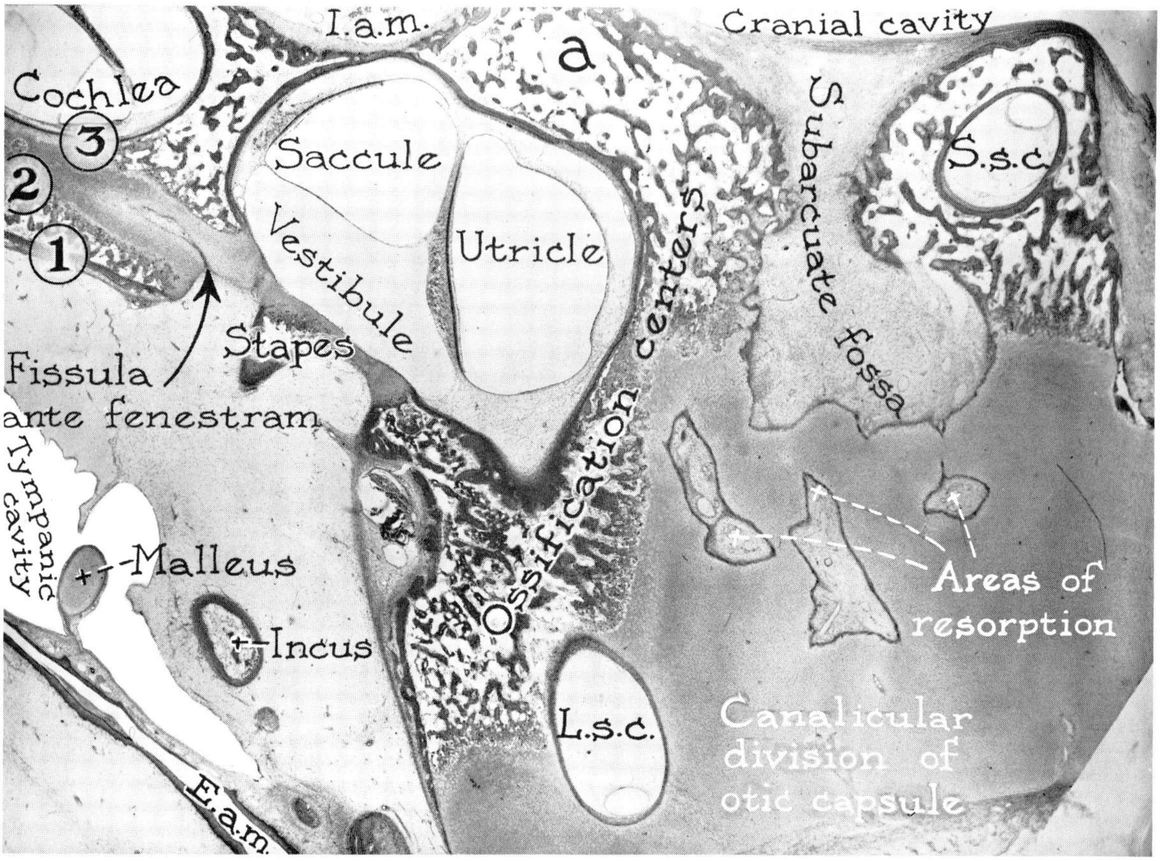

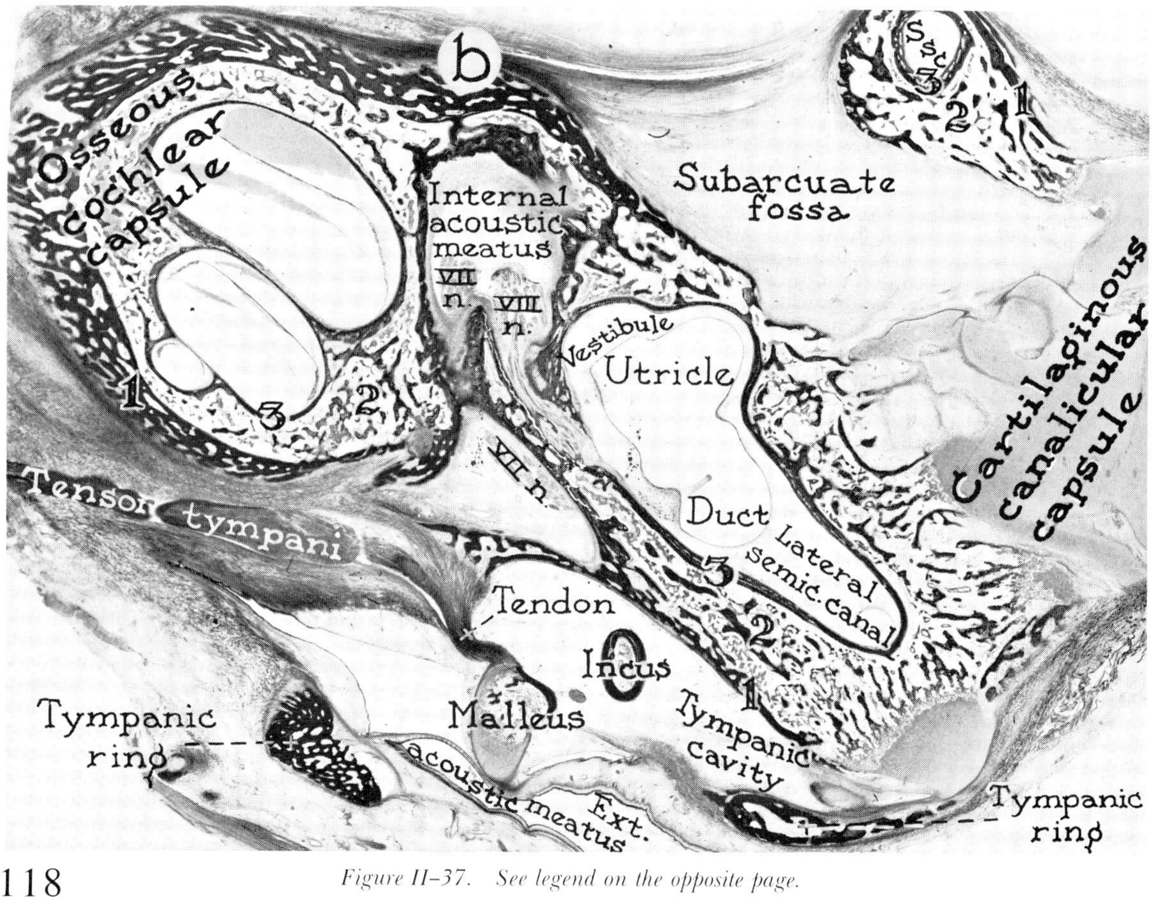

Figure II–37. See legend on the opposite page.

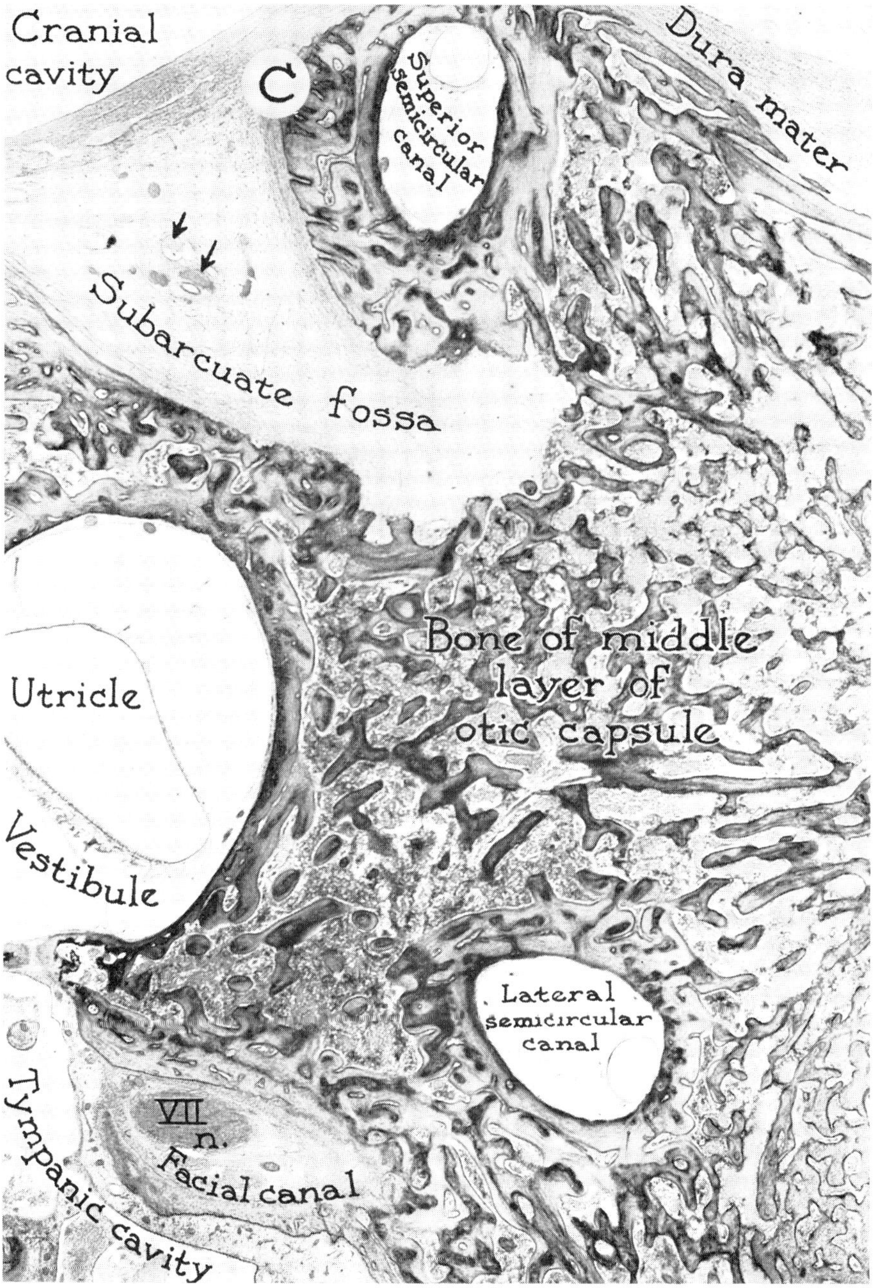

Figure II–37. SUBARCUATE FOSSA: DEVELOPMENTAL ANATOMY. *a.* FETUS OF 21 WEEKS (183 MM.). *b.* FETUS, 23 WEEKS (210 MM.). *c.* NEWBORN (4-DAY PREMATURE).

a. In the 21-week specimen, the subarcuate fossa approaches maximum size, the process of erosion of the cartilage between the semicircular canals being at the most active stage. Cartilage remains around the lateral semicircular canal (*L.s.c.*); it has been replaced by bone of the trilaminar osseous capsule around the superior canal (*S.s.c.*). The erosive vascular buds extend deeply into the cartilage, the coalescent areas of excavation appearing as digitiform prongs from the "floor" of the fossa.

b. In a specimen approximately 2 weeks older, ossification has spread to envelop the lateral semicircular canal. However, in the depths of the fossa, cartilage still remains as a relatively bulky mass. This is the area of the fourteenth (and last) ossification center (see Figure II–33).

c. The fossa is still a prominent feature in late fetal and early postnatal stages. In the adult, although it persists usually as a channel of pinpoint dimensions, the fossa may be relatively large and of varying form. The arrows point to blood vessels.

Transverse sections, Wisconsin Collection, series 21, 47 A, and 124, respectively. *a*, × 12; *b*, × 9; *c*, × 18.

ADULT STRUCTURE: Illustrated in Figures III–127 and III–128.

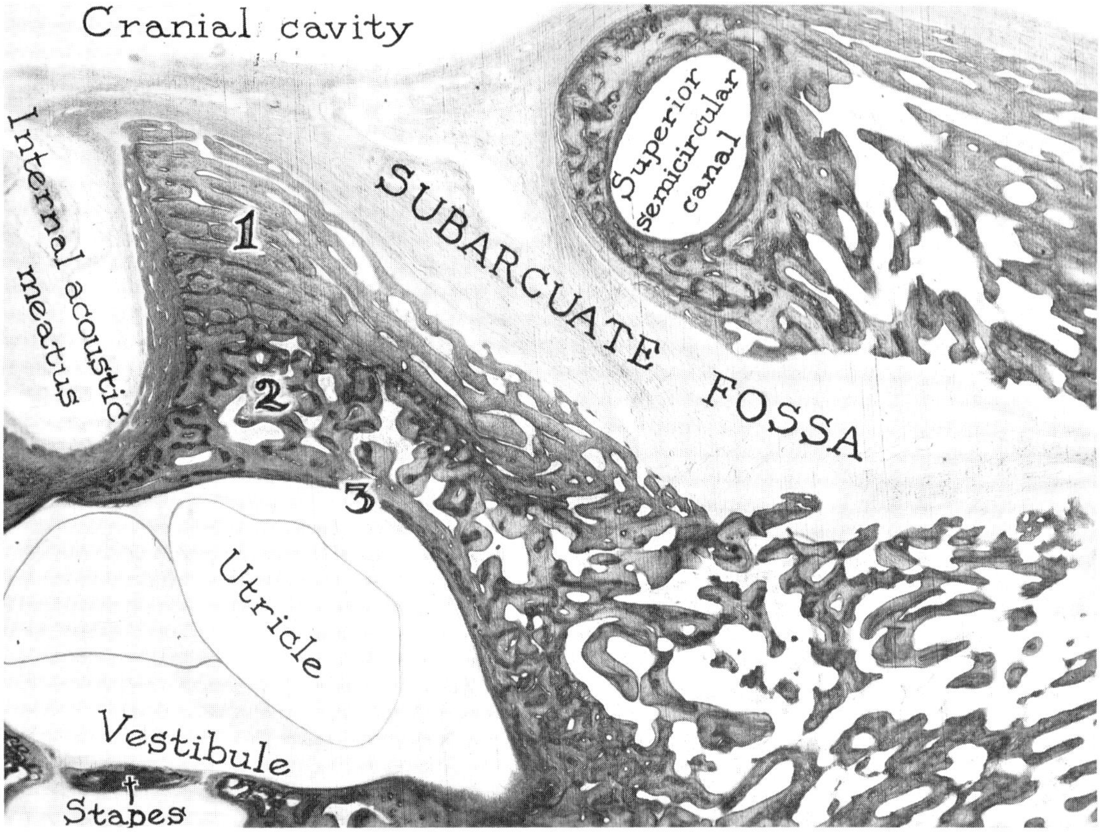

a

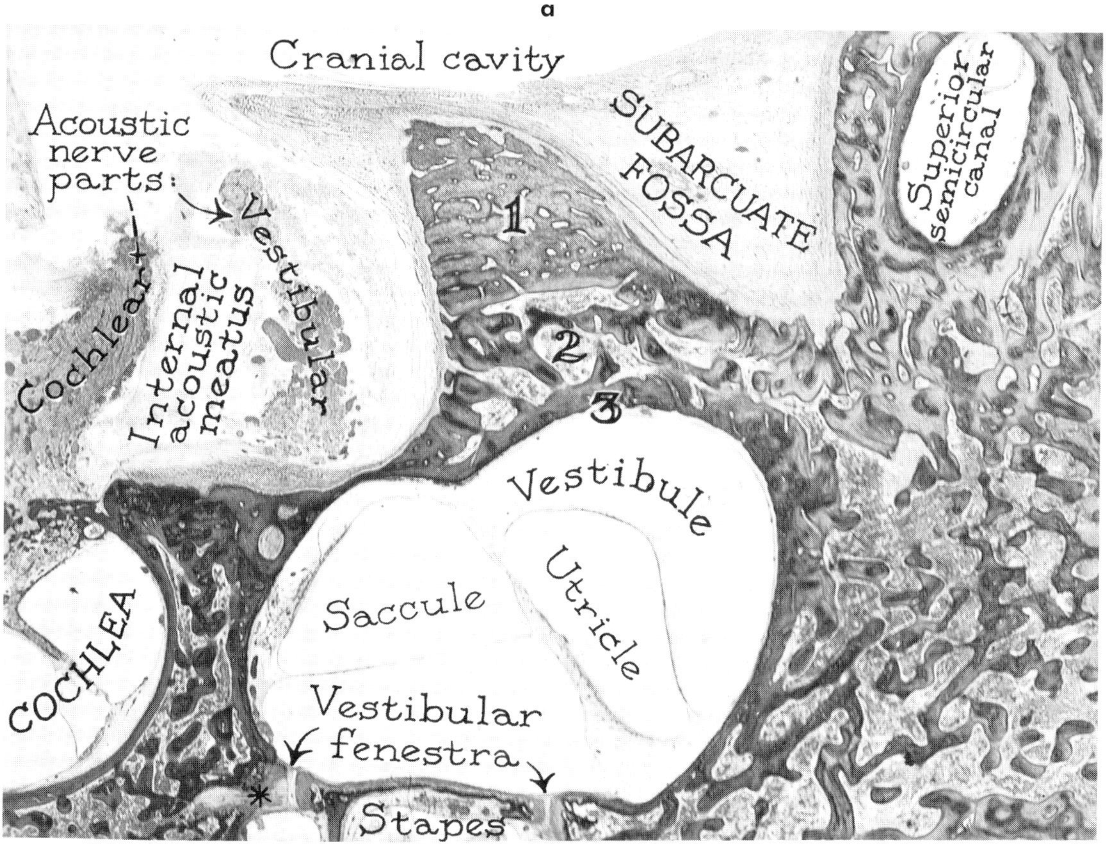

b

Figure II–38. See legend on the opposite page.

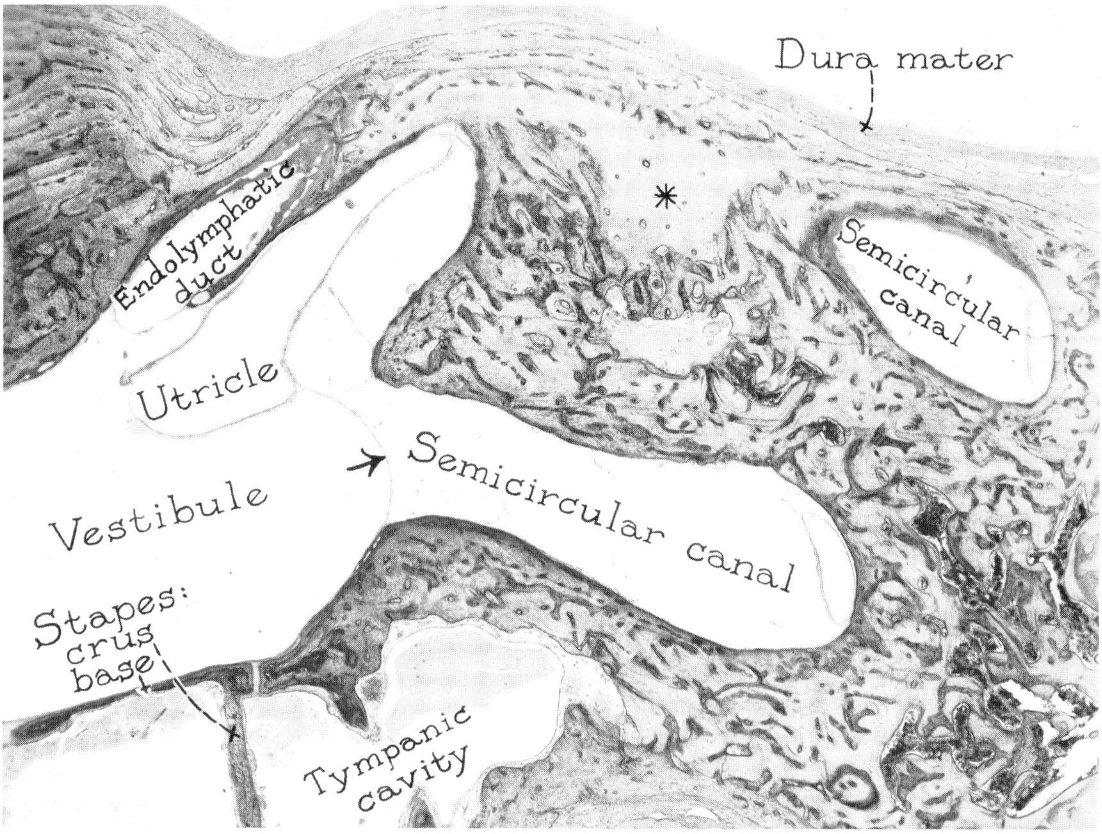

Figure II–38. SUBARCUATE FOSSA: CHANGES IN FORM AND SIZE; RELATION TO VESTIBULAR AND CANALICULAR ANATOMY. *a.* FETUS OF 38+ WEEKS (350 MM.). *b.* NEWBORN INFANT (4-DAY PREMATURE). *c.* FETUS AT TERM.

a. Showing the extent of the fossa and the nature of the contained tissue in a late fetal stage. The channel lies subjacent to the arch of the superior semicircular canal, hence its name. As here encountered, the fossa is undergoing reduction in capacity after having reached maximum size in the fetus of 21 weeks. At the latter stage, vascular buds of the developing meninges make the cartilage of the canalicular part of the otic capsule spongy and thereby permit expansion of the arcs of the semicircular ducts. Numerals indicate the layers of capsular bone.

b. The subarcuate fossa is still represented by a relatively large aperture in the newborn infant. Regularly some of the original vessels persist and thus contribute permanently to the blood supply of the petrous pyramid.

c. In rare instances the fossa is completely closed by the growth of surrounding bone (at asterisk). Obliteration of the channel is seemingly due to activity of the outer periosteal lamina accompanied by invasion from the middle (endosteal) layer—a process which, in the capsule as a whole, changes the texture from trabecular to petrous. As observed in gross specimens, the fossa sometimes terminates on the posterior surface of the petrous pyramid in several openings or in unexpected locations (Figure III–115). It may be situated near the ostia of diploic communications along the course of the superior petrosal sulcus (Figure III–128*b*). Within the substance of the otic capsule the fossa is regularly related to the petromastoid canal (Figure III–68).

Transverse sections, Wisconsin Collection, series 122, 124, and 127, respectively. *a*, × 20; *b*, × 20; *c*, × 20.

ADULT STRUCTURE: Illustrated in Figures III–127 and III–128.

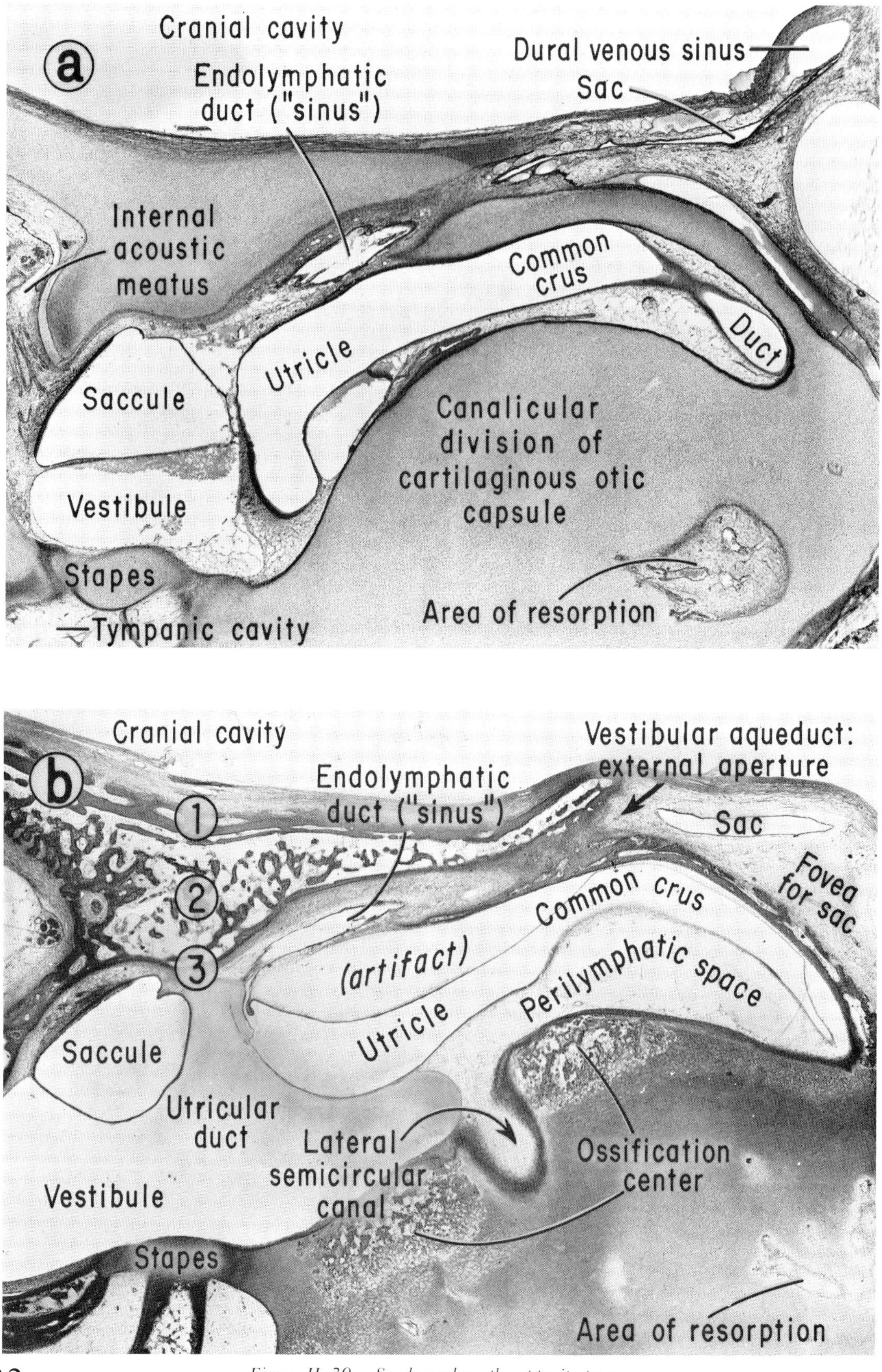

Figure II–39. See legend on the opposite page.

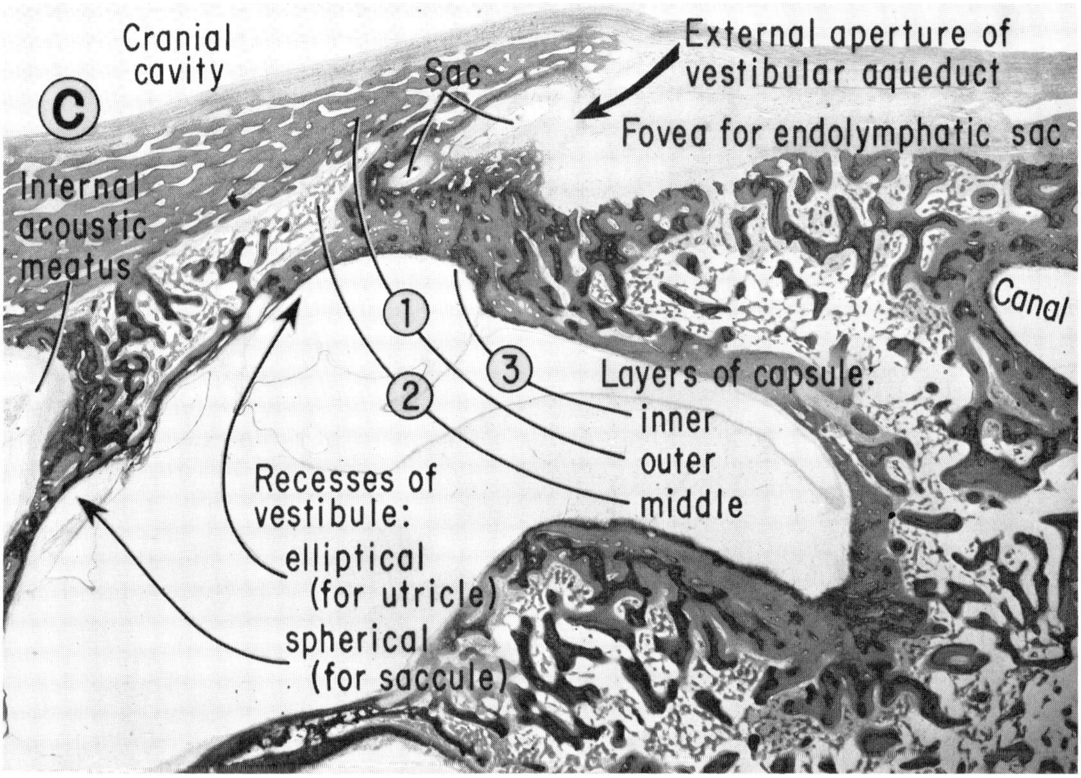

Figure II–39. Vestibular aqueduct and related structures: development in the course of three fetal months. *a.* Fetus of 17 weeks (133 mm.). *b.* Fetus of 21 weeks (183 mm.). *c.* Fetus of 29 weeks (260 mm.). *d.* Newborn (4-day premature). *e.* Adult, 37 years old.

a. At approximately the stage here pictured, four of the total of fourteen ossification centers have appeared in the cartilaginous otic capsule. They are located at the beginning of the first (basal) turn of the cochlea (Center One), at the ampulla of the posterior canal (Center Two) and the ampullae of the superior and lateral canals (see also Figure II–33). In the area of the aqueduct, the capsule remains unaltered cartilage. The cartilage of the canalicular part is being rendered spongy through the ingrowth of vascular connective tissue from the subarcuate fossa (see Figure II–42).

b. During the fifth fetal month, the process of ossification has come to involve the area of the aqueduct. Here the fifth and second centers meet and fuse over the endolymphatic duct and proximal portion of the sac. Each center is trilaminar (see Figures II–5 and II–6, demonstrating the layers in the cochlear division of the capsule).

c. In the fetus at the middle of the eighth month, bone surrounds the aqueduct. The outer periosteal layer (at *1*) is undergoing thickening while the middle layer (at *2*) remains virtually unchanged. It forms part of the wall of the aqueduct; at the external aperture the bone will undergo remodeling.

Figure II–39 continues on the following page.

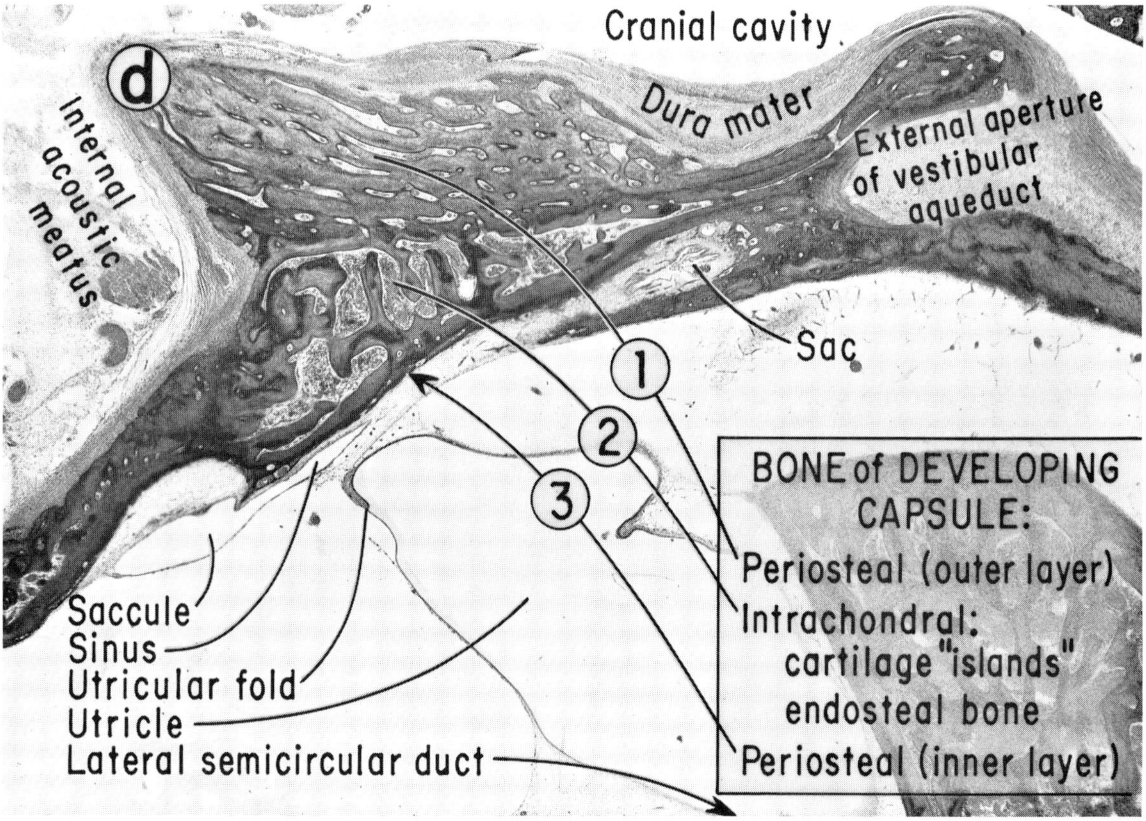

Figure II–39, Continued. VESTIBULAR AQUEDUCT AND RELATED STRUCTURES: DEVELOPMENT IN THE COURSE OF THREE FETAL MONTHS. *a.* FETUS OF 17 WEEKS (133 MM.). *b.* FETUS OF 21 WEEKS (183 MM.). *c.* FETUS OF 29 WEEKS (260 MM.). *d.* NEWBORN (4-DAY PREMATURE). *e.* ADULT, 37 YEARS OLD.

d. In the newborn infant the middle layer (at 2) of the capsule has not yet attained petrous structure. Early postnatal growth of endosteal bone will obliterate the primitive marrow spaces, leaving minute vascular channels of "canaliculi" (see *e*). The section includes both apertures of the aqueduct.

Figure II–39 continues on the opposite page.

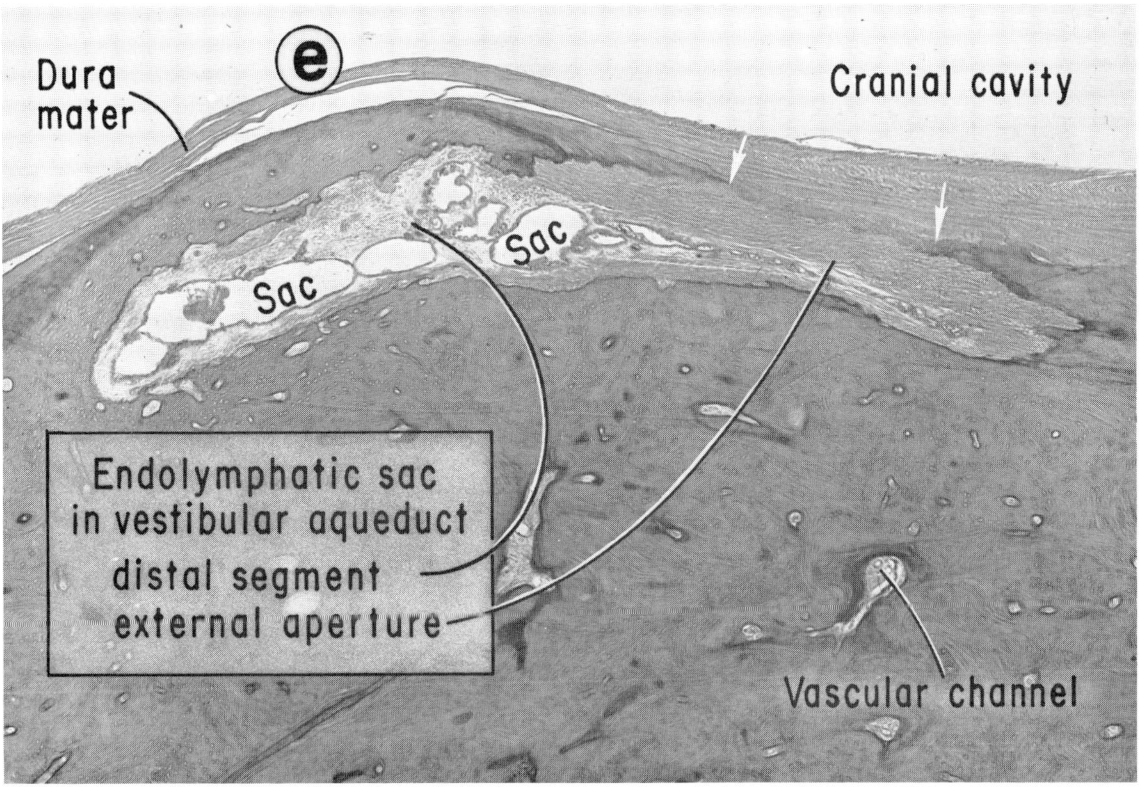

Figure II–39, Concluded.

e. Demonstrating the adult structure of the bone. The section passes through the external aperture (margins indicated by arrows).

Transverse sections, Wisconsin Collection, series 183, 21, 45 A, 124, and 21, respectively. *a*, × 16; *b*, × 15; *c*, × 16; *d*, × 17; *e*, × 44.

ADULT STRUCTURE: Illustrated in Figures III–60 to III–62 and III–98 to III–118.

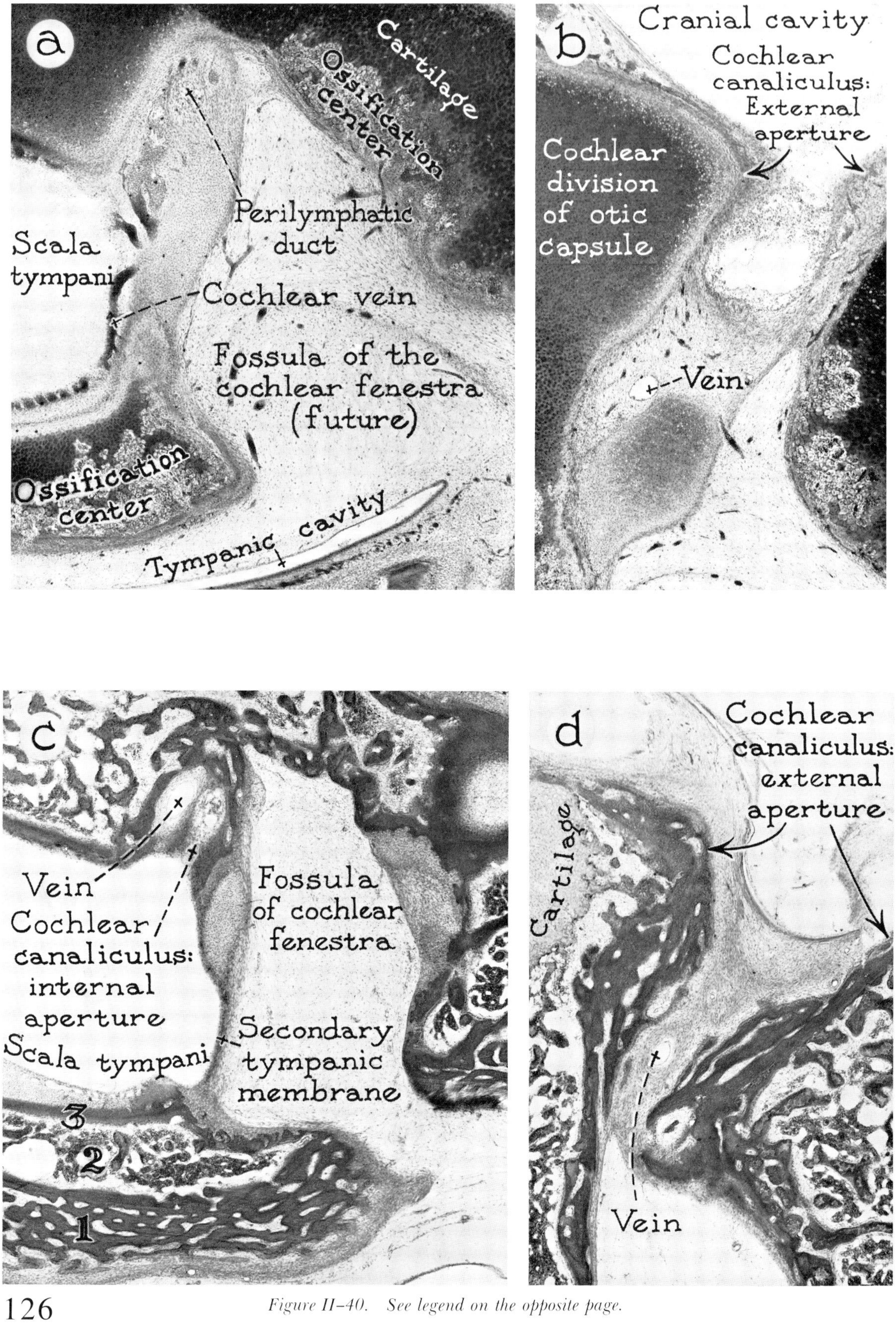

Figure II–40. See legend on the opposite page.

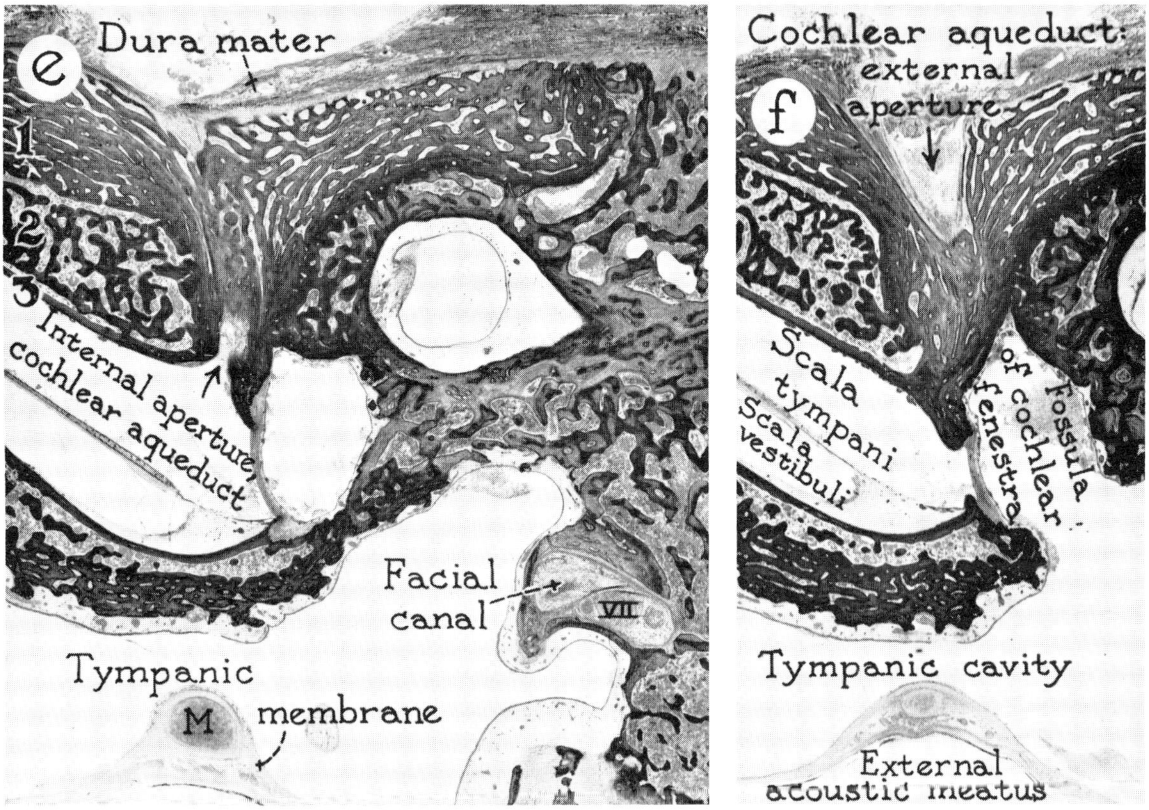

Figure II–40. COCHLEAR AQUEDUCT AND ITS CONTENTS: DEVELOPMENTAL ANATOMY DEMONSTRATED IN THREE STAGES. *a* and *b*. FETUS OF 16+ WEEKS (126 MM.). *c* and *d*. FETUS OF 21 WEEKS (183 MM.). *e* and *f*. NEWBORN INFANT (4-DAY PREMATURE).

a. In the 4-month fetus, at the beginning of bone formation in the otic capsule, the cartilage on the internal wall of the developing cochlear (round) window undergoes resolution by a process matching that by which the semicircular canals were formed (see Figures II–30 and II–31). This change marks the genesis of the perilymphatic "duct" in the cochlear aqueduct.

b. Toward the opposite extremity, the cochlear vein is in the mesenchymal tissue that occupies the primordial canaliculus (aqueduct).

c and *d*. In a specimen five weeks older, the growth of bone on the wall of the tympanic scala has resulted in segregation of the space for the vein from that of the aqueduct. At the opposite extremity they are not yet separate.

e and *f*. In the newborn, the canaliculus traverses the wall of the otic capsule, which is now trilaminar (see numbered layers in Figures II–5 and II–6).

Transverse sections, Wisconsin Collection, series as follows: *a* and *b*, 11; *c* and *d*, 21; *e* and *f*, 124. *a*, × 26; *b*, × 26; *c*, × 24; *d*, × 26; *e*, × 10; *f*, × 10.

(*a* to *d* from Anson, Donaldson, Warpeha, and Winch: Laryngoscope, 74:945–966, 1964; *e* and *f*, adapted from Anson, Donaldson, Warpeha, and Winch: Laryngoscope, 75:1203–1223, 1965.)

ADULT STRUCTURE: Illustrated in Figures III–98 to III–102 and III–119 to III–122.

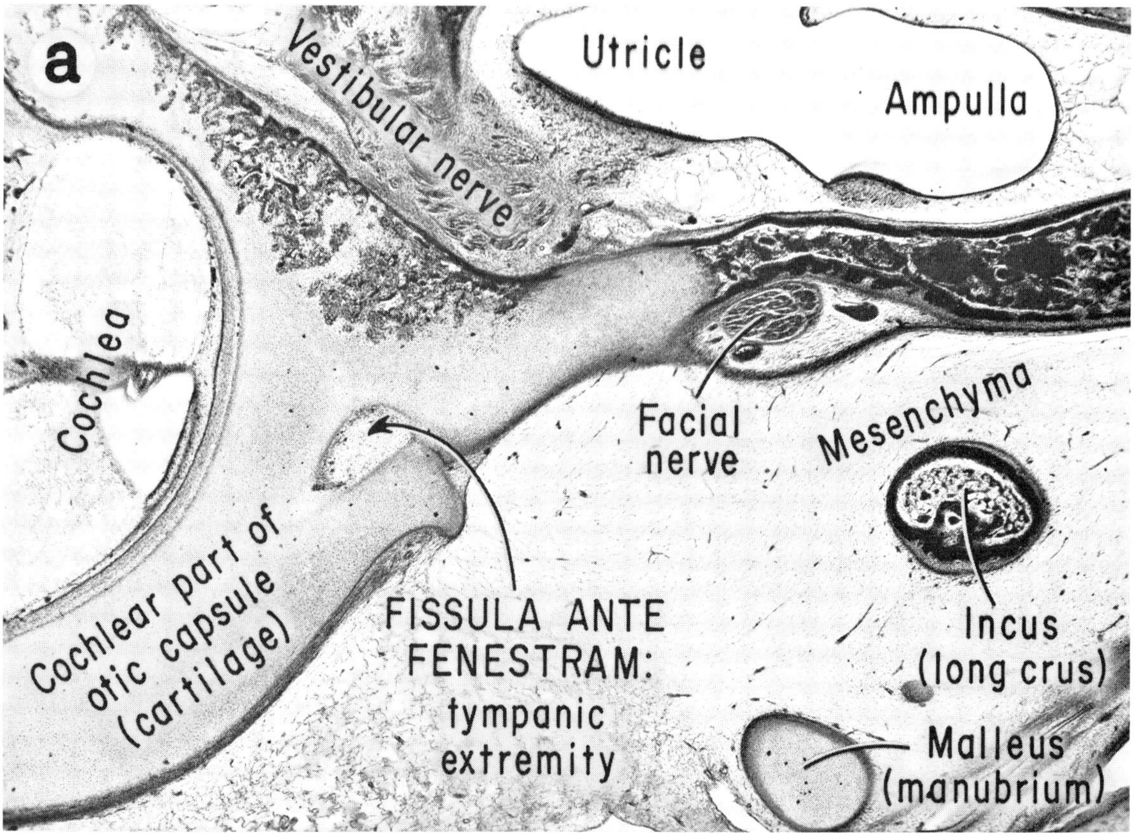

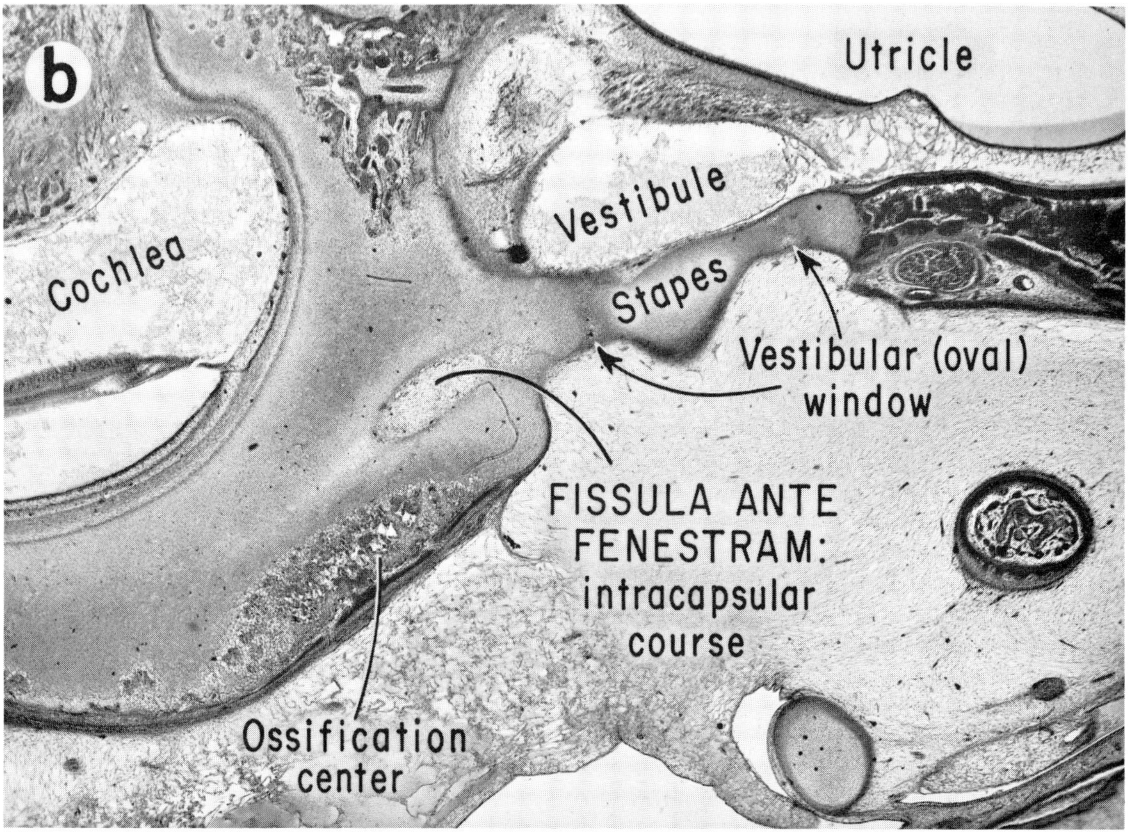

Figure II–41. See legend on the opposite page.

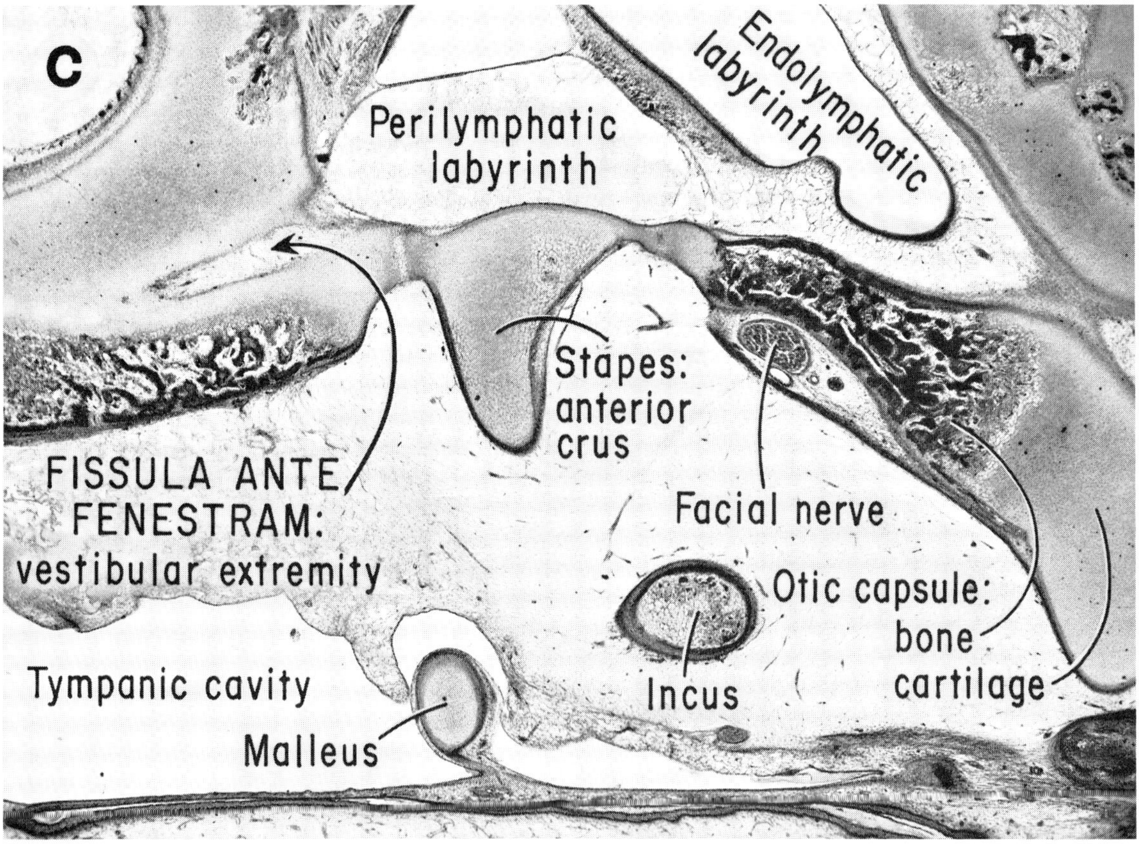

Figure II–41. FISSULA ANTE FENESTRAM: COURSE AND RELATIONS IN AN EARLY DEVELOPMENTAL STAGE. FETUS OF 19 WEEKS (161 MM.). *a*. TYMPANIC EXTREMITY. *b*. INTRAOSSEOUS COURSE. *c*. VESTIBULAR EXTREMITY (OR APERTURE).

The fissula ante fenestram develops as an anteriorly directed extension or outpouching of the layer of periotic tissue that lines the wall of the perilymphatic labyrinth. The tract extends from the labyrinthine wall (*a*), through the precartilaginous otic capsule (*b*), to a position just in front of the vestibular (oval) window (*c*).

The fissula makes its appearance between the 8-week and 10-week stage. In the fetus of approximately 5 months, as here pictured, it is a definite transcapsular tract.

The histological change is one in which the precartilage undergoes a retrogressive change, followed by differentiation of the primitive tissue into adult connective tissue. In the process of conversion of the cartilage into bone, the fissula persists as a fibrous stripe between periotic connective tissue and mucous membrane.

The fissula varies in size and form from one specimen to another. However, it is a constant structure and thus differs from the smaller channel, the fossula post fenestram which, when present, is a saclike outpouching from the vestibule just behind the vestibular window. The fissula is an anatomical feature of special interest in otology, since it is the predilected site for formation of otosclerotic bone.

Transverse sections, Wisconsin Collection, series 13, left ear. *a*, × 21; *b*, × 21; *c*, × 21.

ADULT STRUCTURE: Illustrated in Figures III–70 and III–123 to III–126.

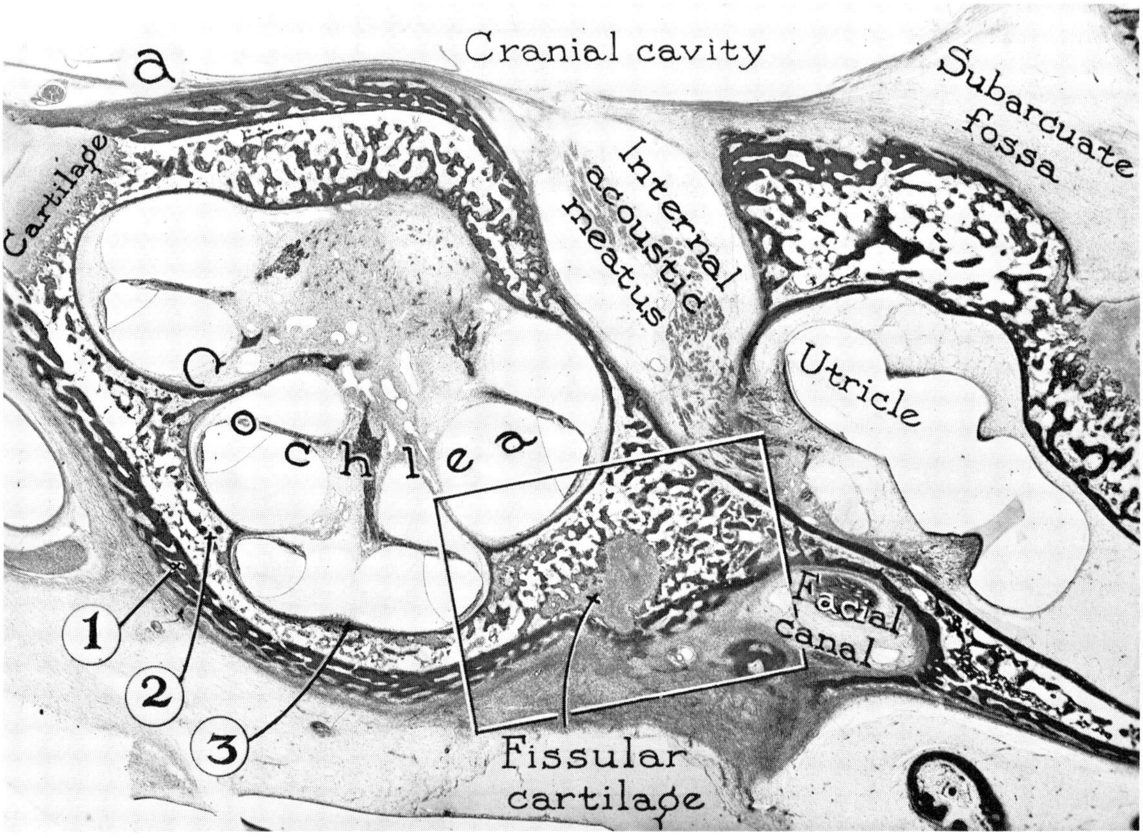

Figure II–42. FISSULA ANTE FENESTRAM: ABERRANT CONTENT. FETUS OF 21 WEEKS (183 MM.).

a. A chondral mass occupies the customary site of the trancapsular fissular tract of connective tissue. The blocked area is shown at higher magnification in *b.*

Figure II–42 continues on the opposite page.

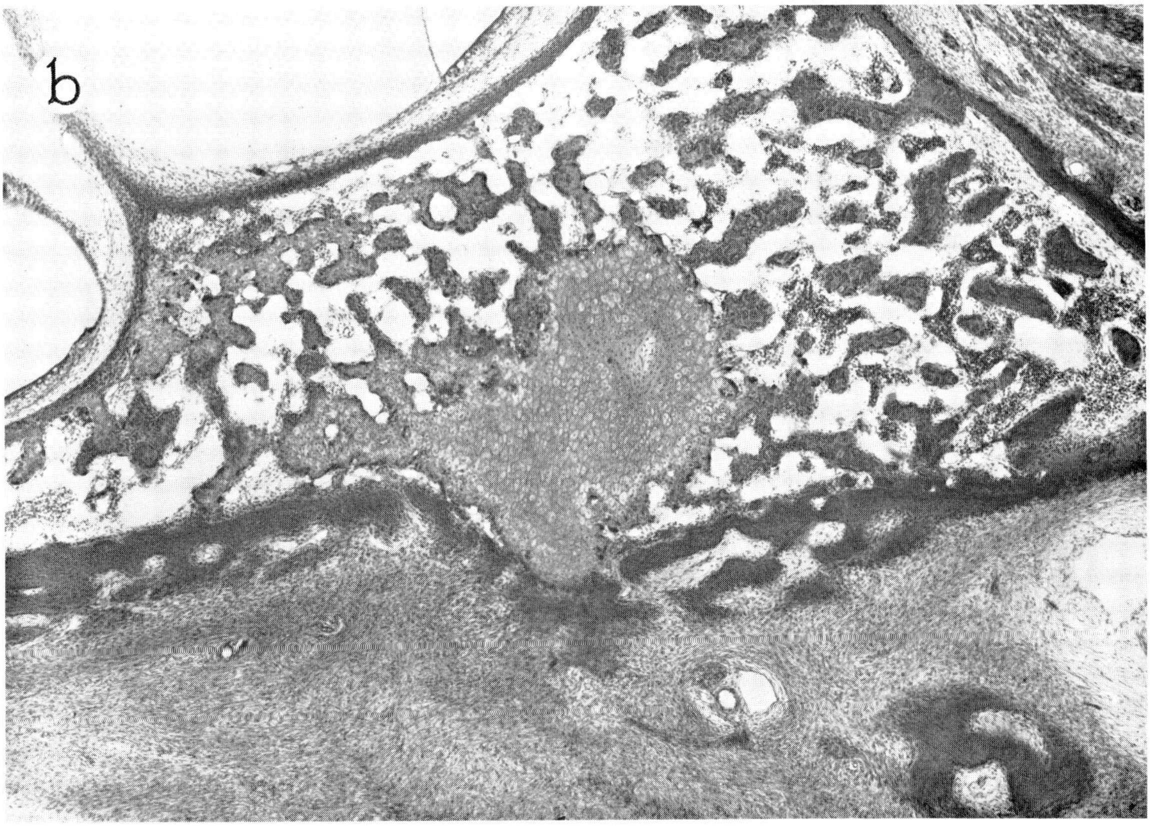

Figure II–42, Continued.

b. Demonstrating in detail the form of the cartilage mass and its histological gradation peripherally with the developing islands of intrachondral bone (see Figure II–35).

Transverse section, Wisconsin Collection, series 21. *a*, × 11; *b*, × 45.

ADULT STRUCTURE: Illustrated in Figures III–70 and III–123 to III–126.

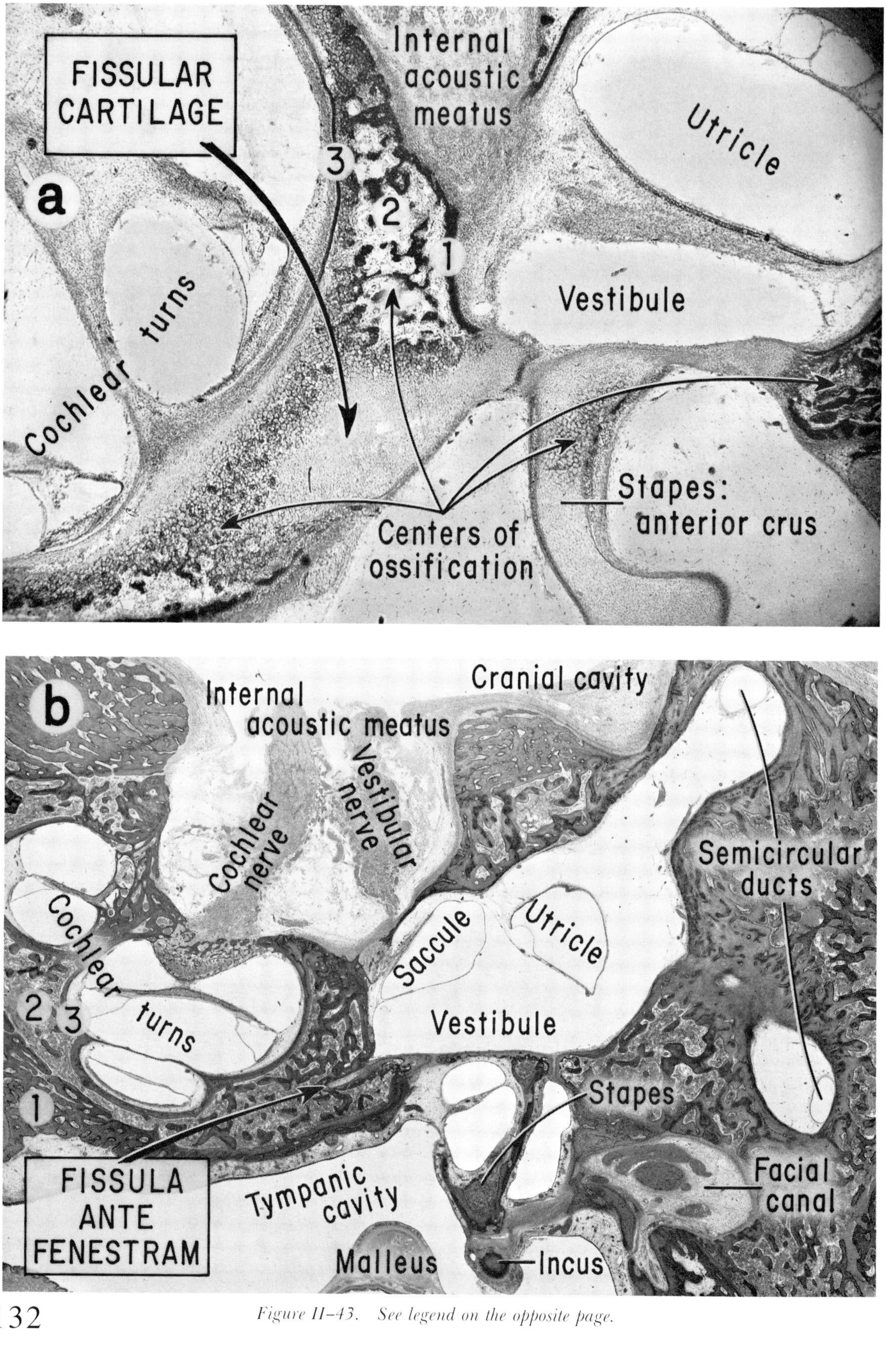

Figure II–43. See legend on the opposite page.

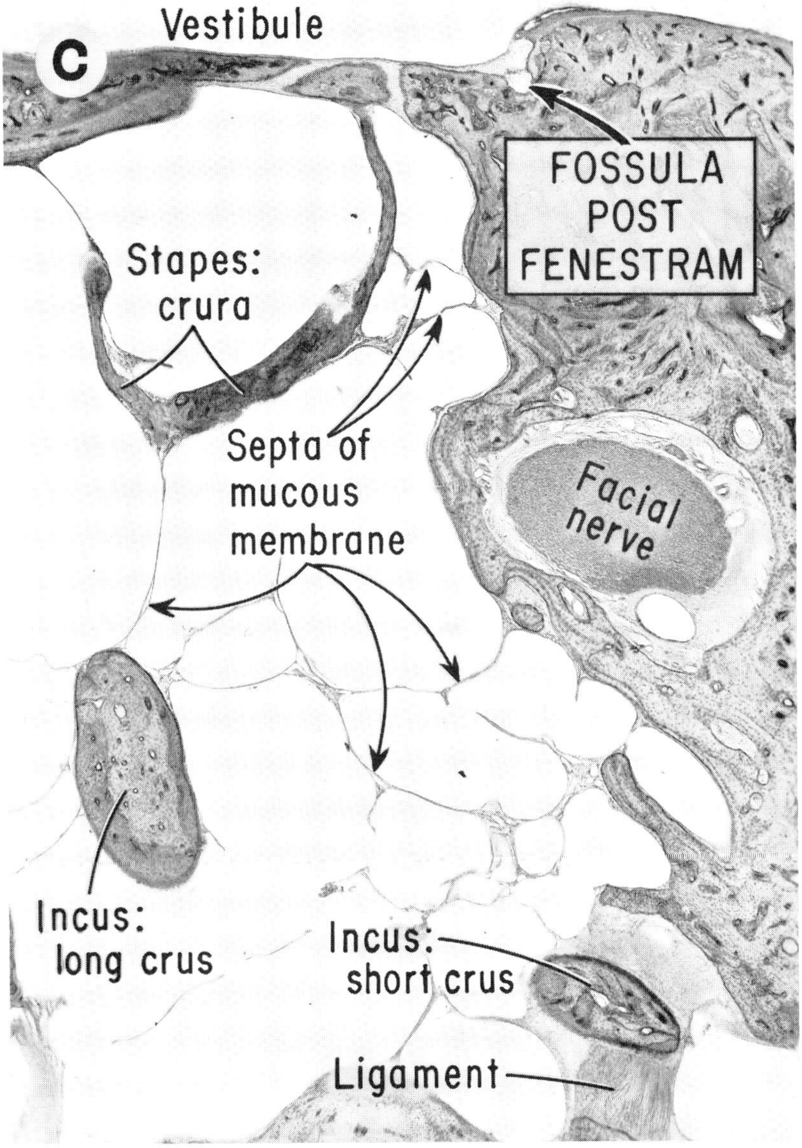

Figure II–43. Fissula ante fenestram and fossula post fenestram: developmental and adult anatomy. *a.* Fetus of 19½ weeks (160 mm.). *b.* Newborn (4-day premature). *c.* Adult, 19 years of age.

a. In the 5-month specimen, at the onset of ossification, cartilage persists in the fissular area of the otic capsule.

b. A fissula of typical form and position is here sectioned through the vestibular extremity.

c. The fossula is represented by a shallow cul-de-sac in the vestibule. Usually, as in this instance, it is not a complete transcapsular channel.

Transverse sections, Wisconsin Collection, series 41, 124, and 29, respectively. *a*, × 19; *b*, × 14; *c*, × 14.

Adult Structure: Illustrated in Figures III–70 and III–123 to III–126.

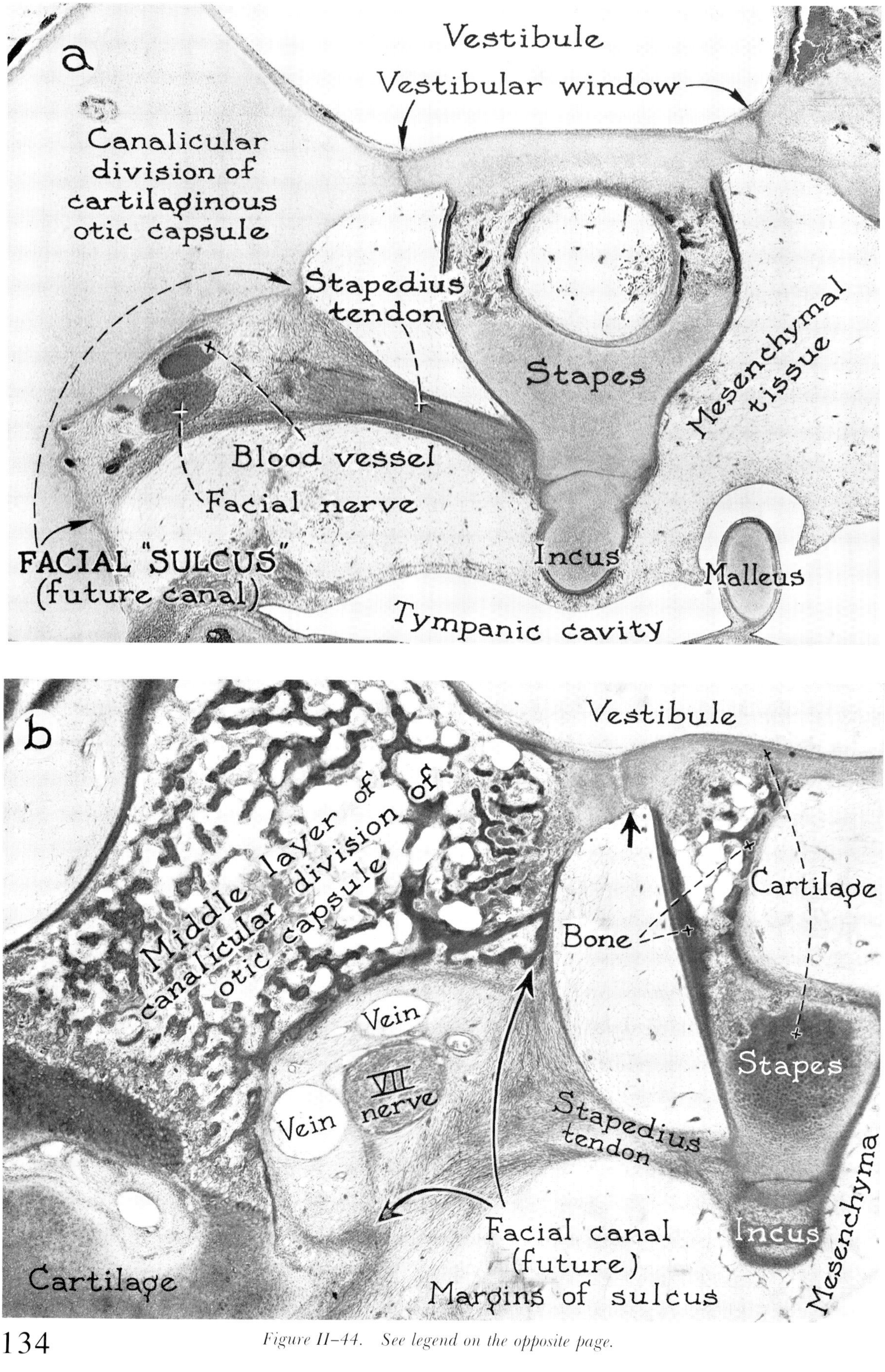

Figure II–44. See legend on the opposite page.

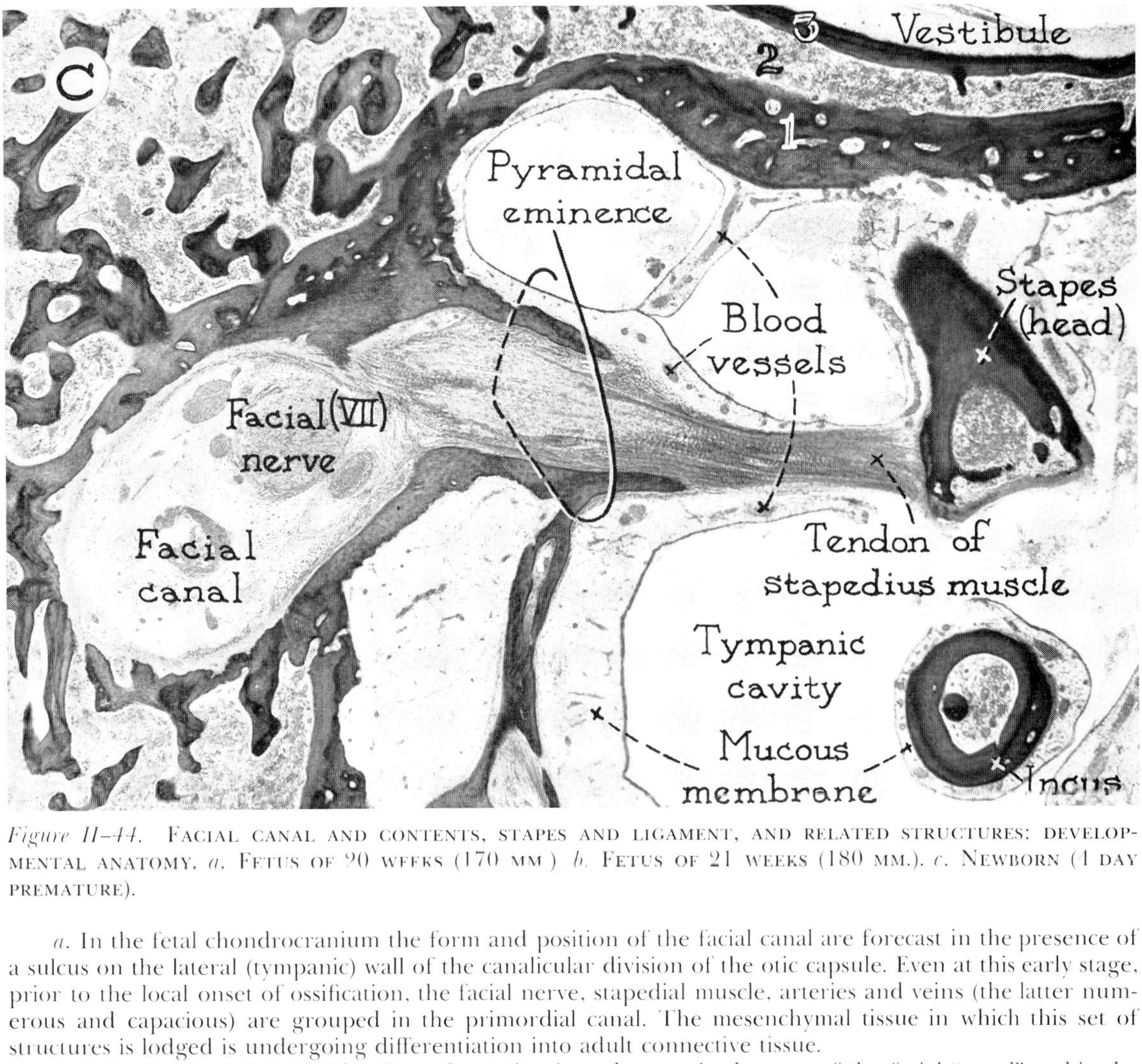

Figure II–44. FACIAL CANAL AND CONTENTS, STAPES AND LIGAMENT, AND RELATED STRUCTURES: DEVELOPMENTAL ANATOMY. *a.* FETUS OF 20 WEEKS (170 MM.). *b.* FETUS OF 21 WEEKS (180 MM.). *c.* NEWBORN (1 DAY PREMATURE).

a. In the fetal chondrocranium the form and position of the facial canal are forecast in the presence of a sulcus on the lateral (tympanic) wall of the canalicular division of the otic capsule. Even at this early stage, prior to the local onset of ossification, the facial nerve, stapedial muscle, arteries and veins (the latter numerous and capacious) are grouped in the primordial canal. The mesenchymal tissue in which this set of structures is lodged is undergoing differentiation into adult connective tissue.

b. In a specimen slightly older, bone formation is under way in the area of the facial "canal" and in the auditory ossicles. A nerve (VII), vessels, and the stapedius muscle (tendon at this level) are contained in the future canal. The unlabeled arrow points to the developing annular ligament. The mucous membrane of the expanding tympanic cavity is not yet draped over the stapes.

c. In the late fetus and in the newborn, the above-named structures are enclosed in a true canal. The stapedius tendon passes from the tip of the pyramidal eminence to insertion into the head of the stapes. The layers of the capsule are indicated by numerals: *1*, outer periosteal lamina; *2*, middle periosteal lamina; *3*, inner periosteal lamina (see Figure II–5). The mucous membrane now envelops the ossicles and covers the labyrinthine wall of the tympanic cavity.

Transverse sections, Wisconsin Collection, series 131, 29, and 124, respectively. *a*, × 24; *b*, × 24; *c*, × 26.

ADULT STRUCTURE: Illustrated in Figures III–64, III–65, III–69 to III–85, III–135, and III–136.

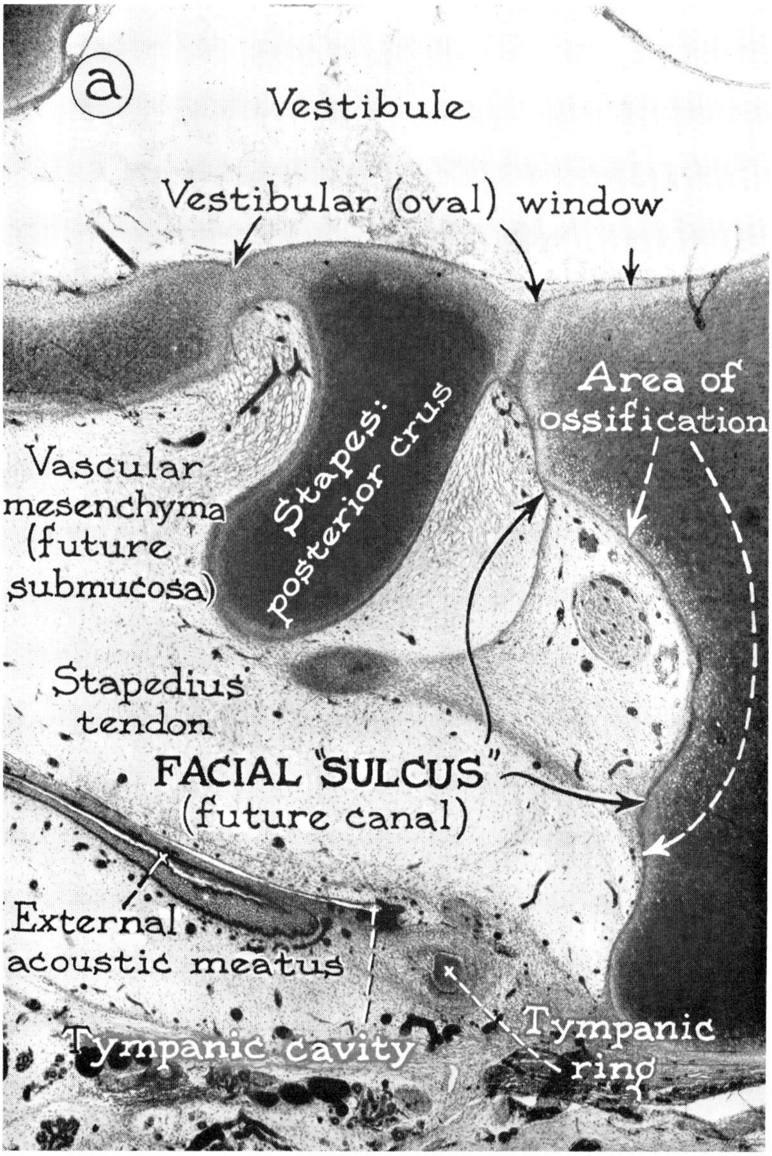

Figure II–45. STAPEDIUS MUSCLE, STAPES, FACIAL CANAL, AND RELATED STRUCTURES: DEVELOPMENT WITHIN APPROXIMATELY FIVE MONTHS. *a.* FETUS OF 16½ WEEKS (126 MM.). *b.* FETUS, 27 WEEKS (243 MM.). *c.* NEWBORN (4-DAY PREMATURE).

a. In the 4-month fetus, the otic capsule is still cartilaginous (periotic tissue indicated by unlabeled arrow). The stapedius muscle occupies a sulcus (the future canal) with the facial nerve and vascular mesenchymal tissue. At the level shown, the tendon is in midcourse to the stapedial insertion.

b. At approximately the 6-month stage, periosteal bone has begun to grow across the sulcus, to convert it into a canal. The result of growth is demonstrated in this 7-month specimen. At the level here shown, the stapedius tendon, having emerged from the pyramidal eminence, and invested by mucous membrane, crosses the tympanic cavity to the head of the stapes.

c. Showing, in the virtually adult condition, the manner in which the arteries and veins in the facial canal contribute to the blood supply of the auditory ossicles and the otic capsule (see also Figure III–67).

Transverse sections, Wisconsin Collection, series 11, 89, and 124, respectively. *a*, × 28; *b*, × 24; *c*, × 25.

ADULT STRUCTURE: Illustrated in Figures III–64, III–65, III–69 to III–85, III–135, and III–136.

Figure II–45 continues on the opposite page.

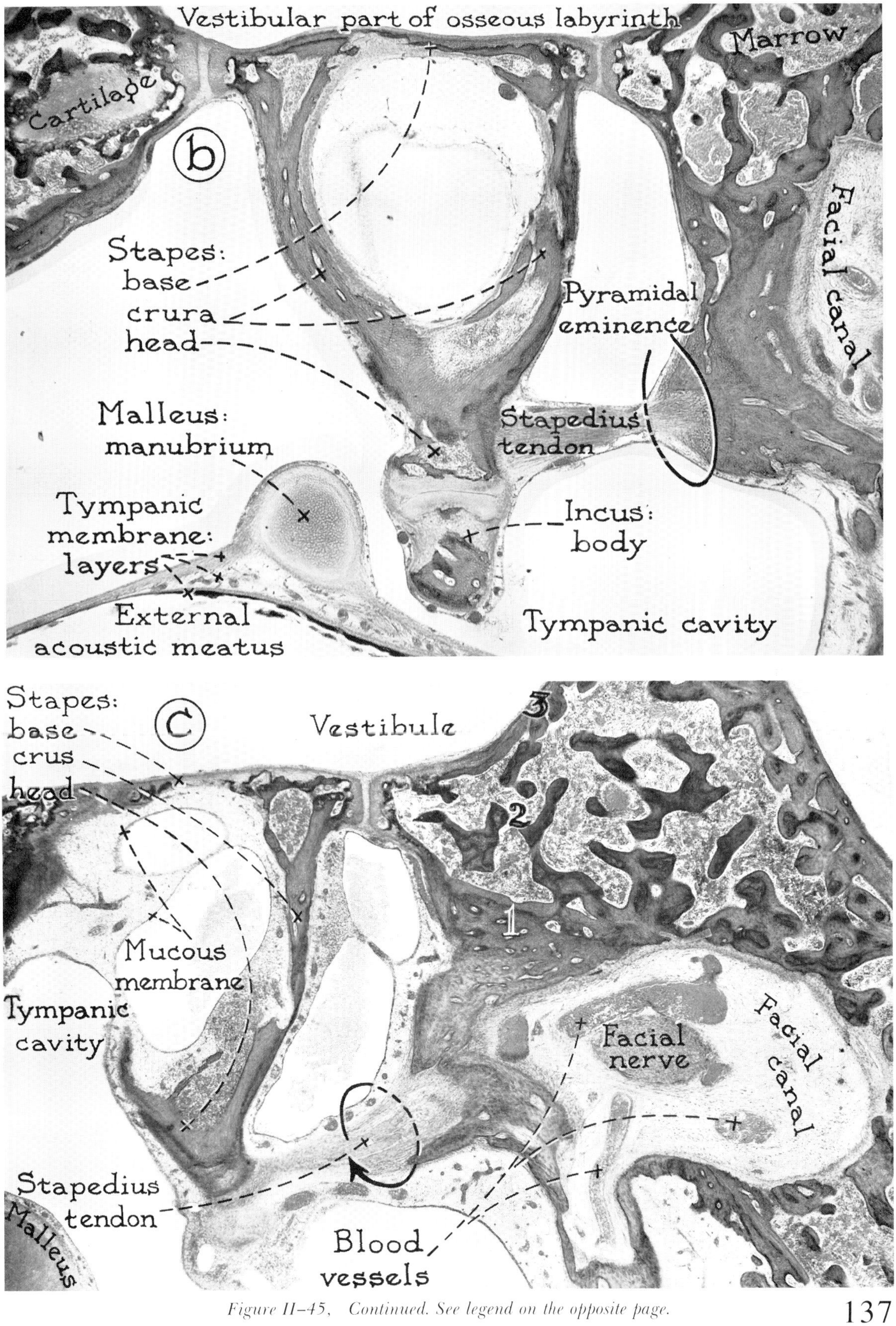

Figure II–45, Continued. See legend on the opposite page.

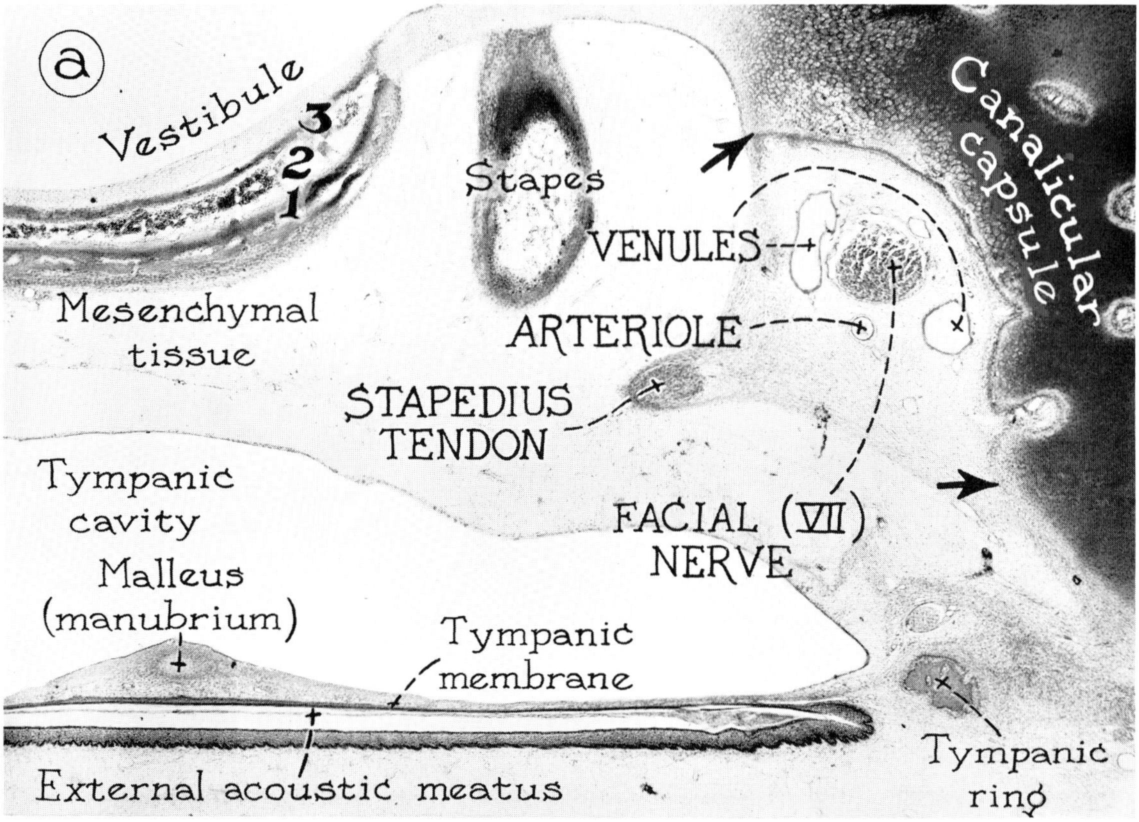

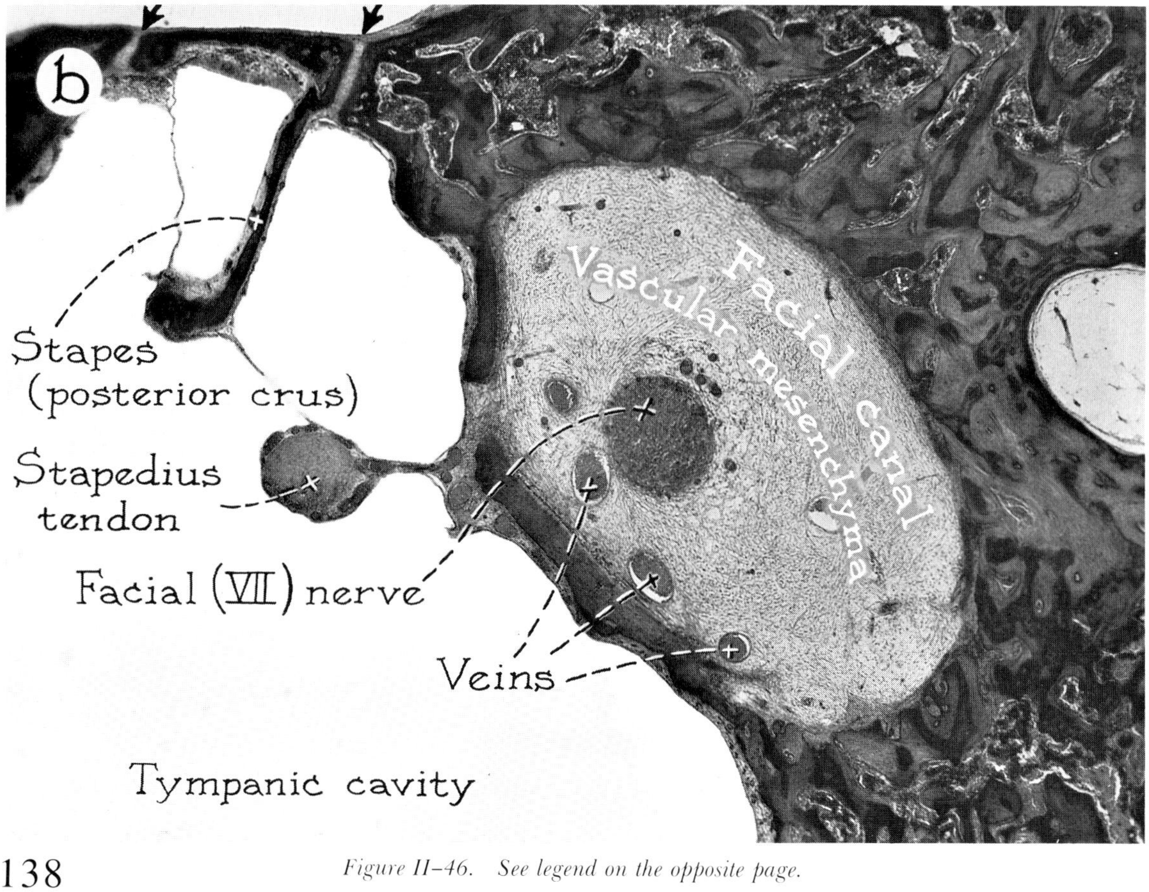

Figure II–46. See legend on the opposite page.

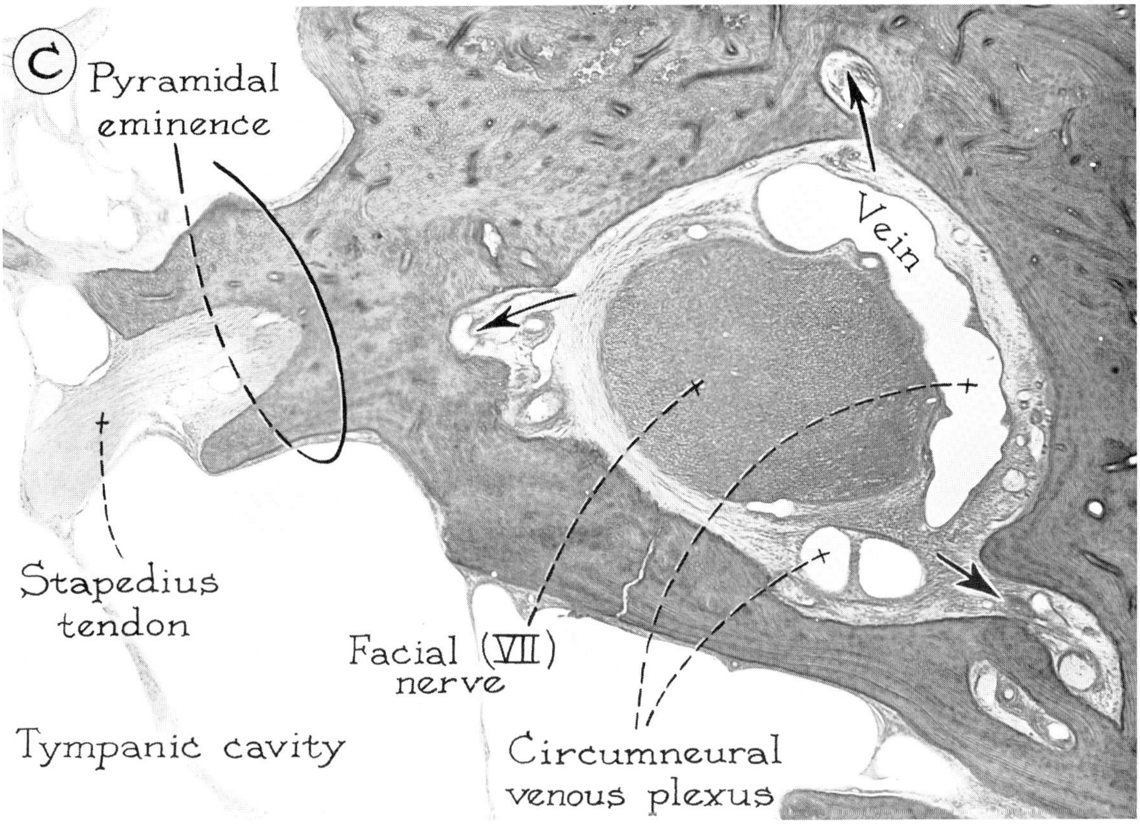

Figure II–46. FACIAL CANAL, ITS CONTENTS AND RELATED STRUCTURES: DEVELOPMENTAL AND ADULT ANATOMY. *a.* FETUS OF 21 WEEKS (183 MM). *b.* FETUS, 34 WEEKS (310 MM.). *c.* ADULT, 19 YEARS OF AGE.

a. The developing facial canal, although appearing as merely a shallow sulcus (at unlabeled arrows) on the canalicular part of the capsule, already houses the structures that are its contents in the adult. These include the facial nerve, the stapedius muscle (the tendon sectioned at the level shown), and vascular connective tissue. Even at this early stage, blood vessels are exchanged between the capsule and the "canal." Bone formation in the canalicular capsule is tardy, being represented by an area of calcified cartilage; in the cochlear capsule, the three typical layers of bone are present (numbered as in Figures II–5 and II–6).

b. In the 34-week specimen bone has spread from the margins of the sulcus to form a true canal. Unlabeled arrows point to the margins of the vestibular window.

c. The immediate wall of the facial canal in the adult is bone of periosteal origin; peripheral to this outer stratum, the bone of the middle layer remains identifiable through the presence of cartilage islands. In the highly vascular connective tissue around the nerve, veins are especially prominent, being large and plexiform. These blood vessels communicate with others which traverse vascular channels in the bone (at arrows) and with vessels in the submucosal tissue of the middle ear which contribute to the supply of the auditory ossicles. The latter vessels reach the ossicles in thin mesenterylike reflections of the mucous membrane (see Figure III–10*a*). At a level caudal to that of the pyramidal eminence, the stapedius muscle may either occupy the facial canal proper or an offset thereof, an independent "semicanal" (see Figure III–74*i*).

Transverse sections, Wisconsin Collection, series 21, 68, and 29, respectively. *a*, × 23; *b*, × 23; *c*, × 19.

ADULT STRUCTURE: Illustrated in Figures III–64, III–65, III–69 to III–85, III–135, and III–136.

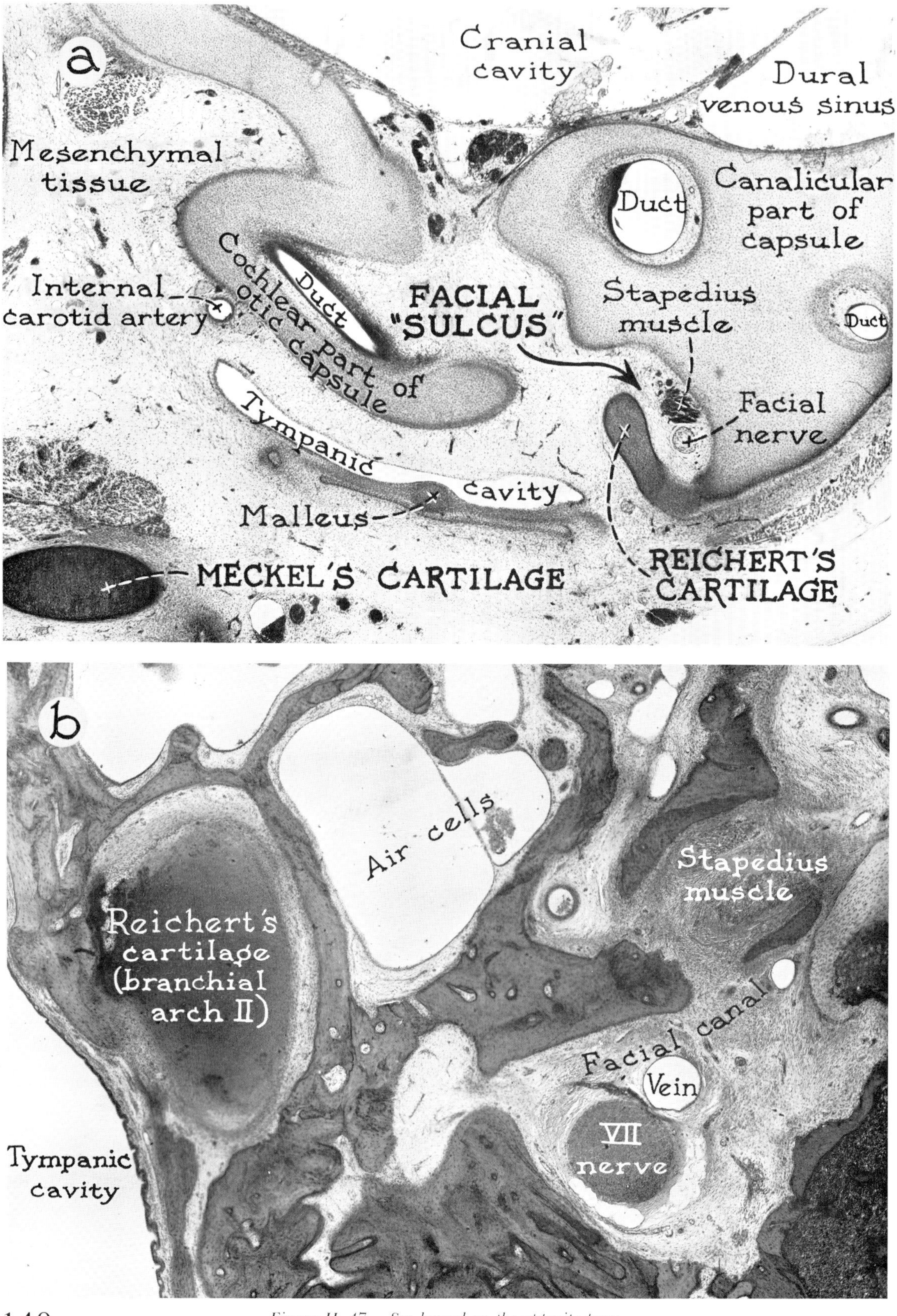

Figure II–47. See legend on the opposite page.

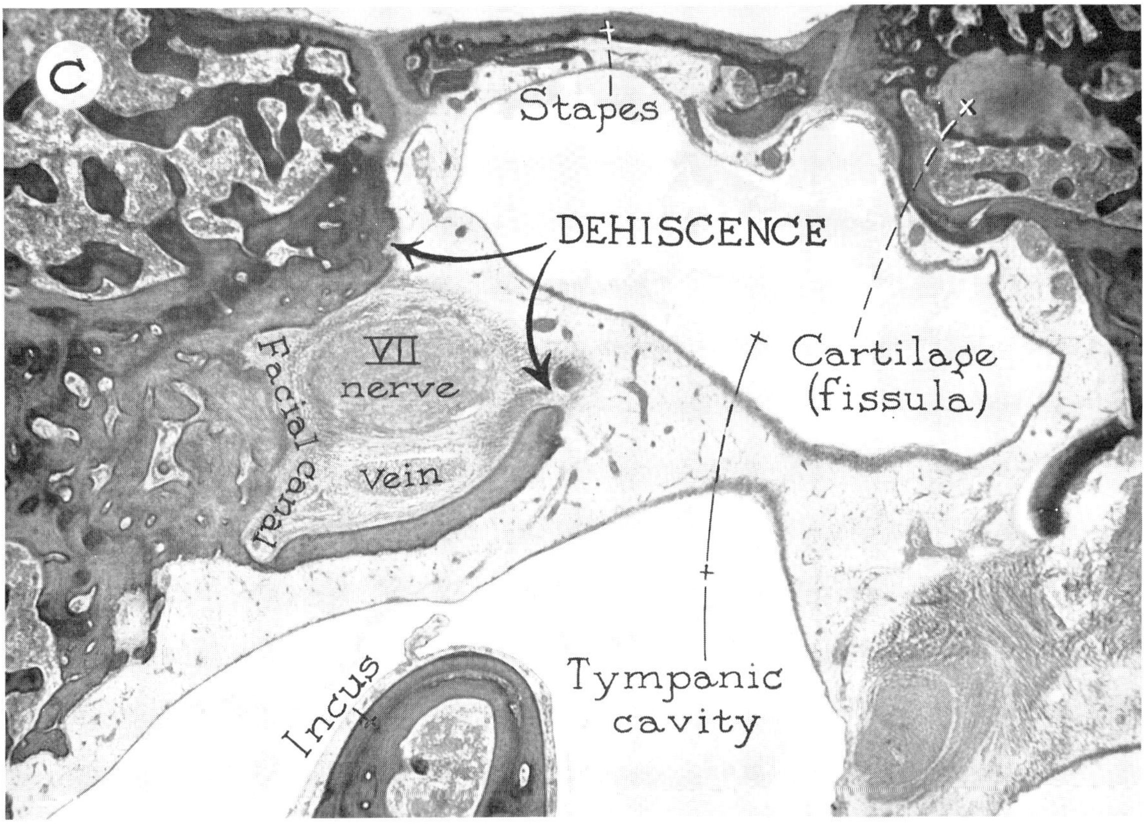

Figure II–47. FACIAL CANAL: EARLY FETAL, INFANTILE, AND ADULT ANATOMY. *a.* FETUS OF 10 WEEKS (48 MM.). *b.* INFANT OF 10 WEEKS. *c.* NEWBORN INFANT (4-DAY PREMATURE).

a. In the preosseous stage of the otic capsule, the future facial canal is a sulcus on the anterior part of the wall of the canalicular division of the cartilaginous capsule. The proximal extremity of the second visceral arch (Reichert's cartilage) contributes a transitory boundary for the "canal" (Figure II–7). On the opposite, or anterior, part of the otic capsule, the internal carotid artery is lodged in primitive mesenchymal tissue close to the wall of the developing cochlea. Just as the facial nerve will become enclosed by bone of the outer periosteal layer, so also will the artery be enveloped (See Figure II–35*b*).

b. Reichert's cartilage, here shown in a 10-week infant, persists as a readily identifiable chondral remnant through the first postnatal year. It becomes an element of the outer wall as a result of growth of periosteal bone between the nerve and the primitive cartilage. Far from being a smooth-walled conduit of circular outline, the lumen of the facial canal is strikingly irregular; communications with vascular channels in the surrounding bone are numerous and relatively capacious.

c. An example of failure in closure of the facial canal is demonstrated here. In this instance the dehiscence occurs on the anteromedial aspect of the canal, facing the vestibular window and the stapes.

Transverse sections, Wisconsin Collection, series 202, 83, and 124, respectively. *a*, × 27; *b*, × 27; *c*, × 26. (From Anson: Trans. Amer. Acad. Ophthal. Otolaryng., 73:17–38, 1969.)

ADULT STRUCTURE: Illustrated in Figures III–64, III–65, III–69 to III–85, III–135, and III–136.

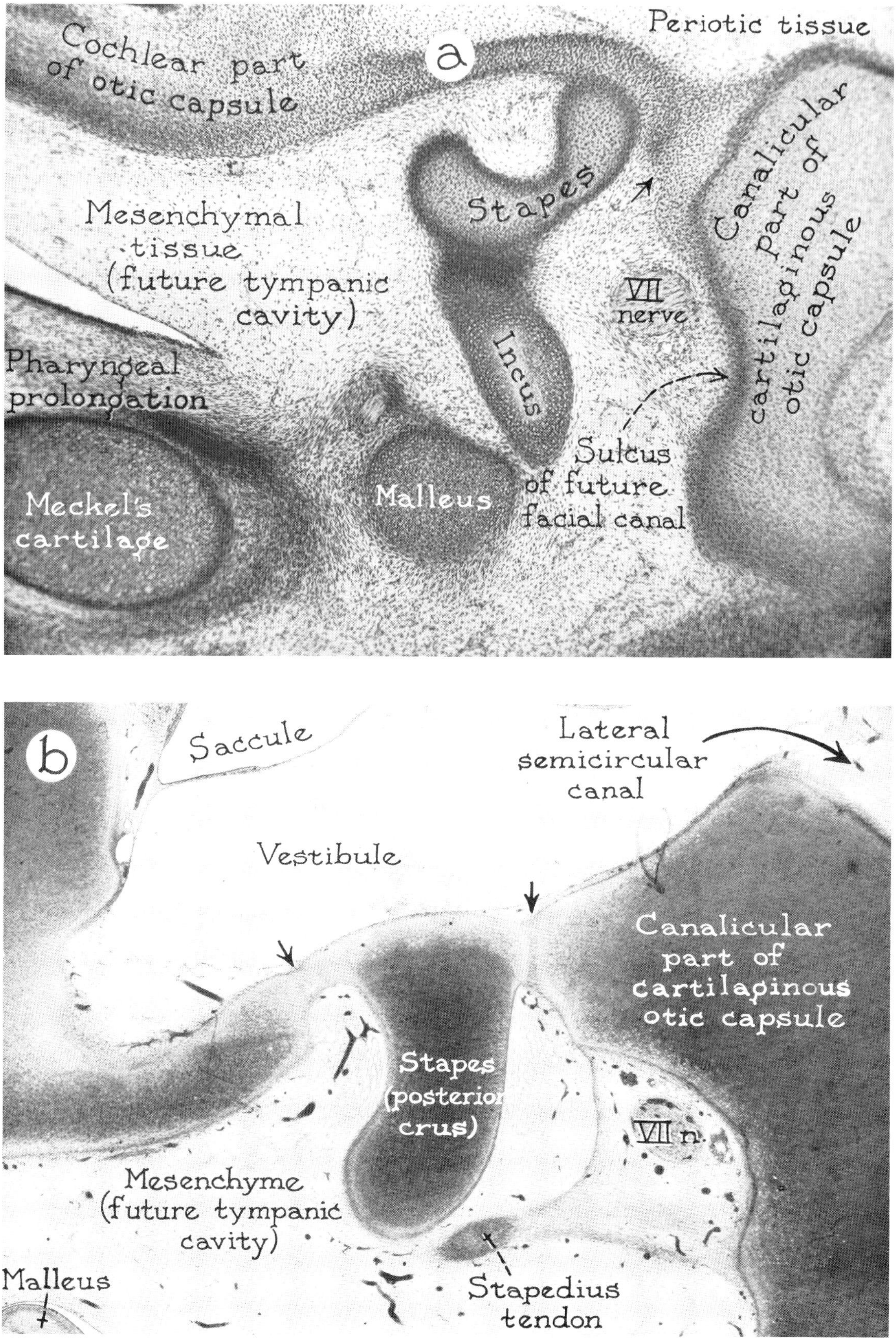

Figure II–48. See legend on the opposite page.

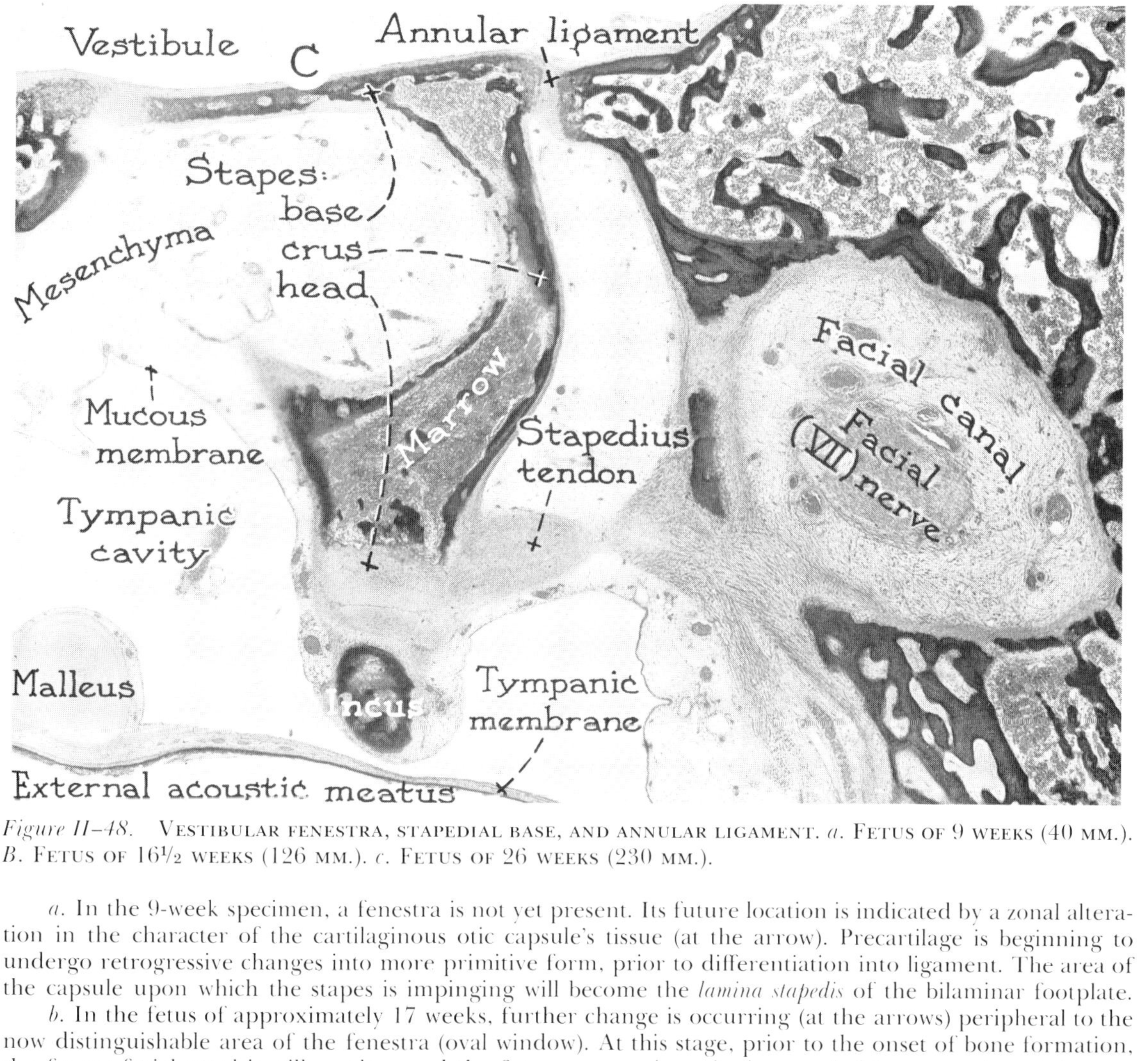

Figure II–48. VESTIBULAR FENESTRA, STAPEDIAL BASE, AND ANNULAR LIGAMENT. *a.* FETUS OF 9 WEEKS (40 MM.). *B.* FETUS OF 16½ WEEKS (126 MM.). *c.* FETUS OF 26 WEEKS (230 MM.).

a. In the 9-week specimen, a fenestra is not yet present. Its future location is indicated by a zonal alteration in the character of the cartilaginous otic capsule's tissue (at the arrow). Precartilage is beginning to undergo retrogressive changes into more primitive form, prior to differentiation into ligament. The area of the capsule upon which the stapes is impinging will become the *lamina stapedis* of the bilaminar footplate.

b. In the fetus of approximately 17 weeks, further change is occurring (at the arrows) peripheral to the now distinguishable area of the fenestra (oval window). At this stage, prior to the onset of bone formation, the future facial canal is still a sulcus and the future tympanic cavity is occupied by mesenchymal tissue.

c. In a specimen nine weeks older, a true window and annular ligament are present.

Transverse sections, Wisconsin Collection, series 168, 11, and 64, respectively. *a*, × 68; *b*, × 29; *c*, × 25.

(From Anson: Chapter 1 in Paparella and Shumrick (Eds.): Otolaryngology, Vol. I. Philadelphia, W. B. Saunders Co., 1973.)

ADULT STRUCTURES: Illustrated in Figures III–90 to III–92.

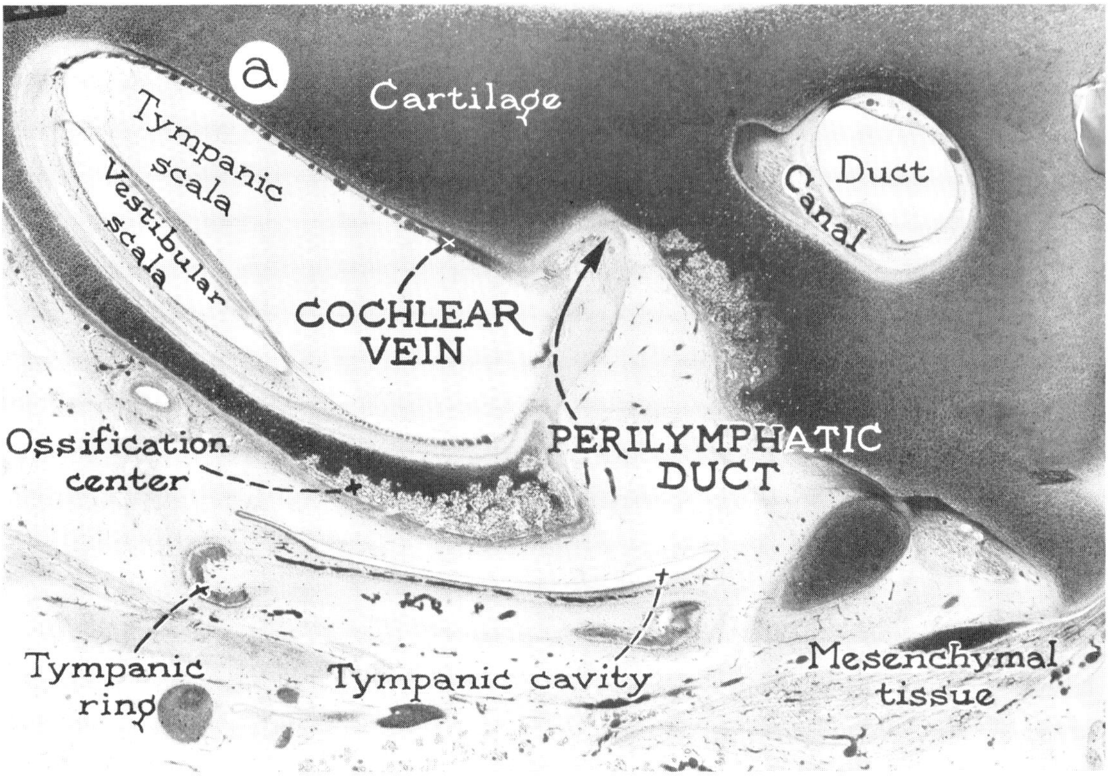

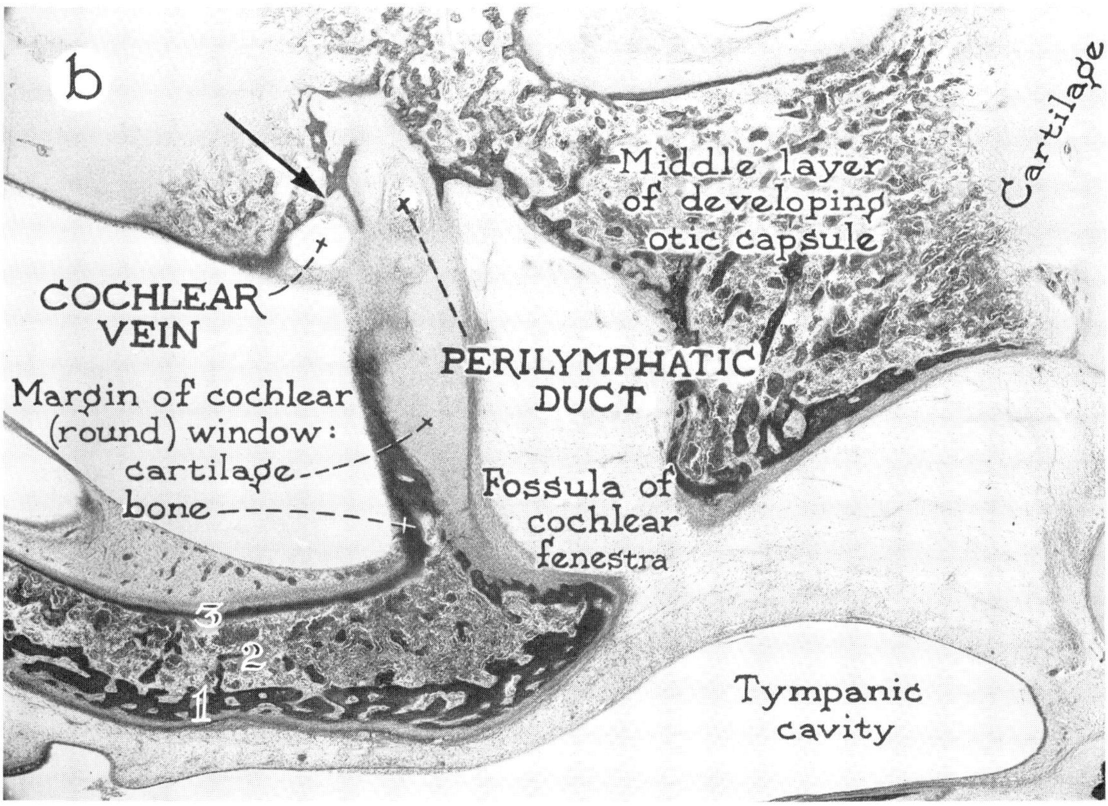

Figure II–49. See legend on the opposite page.

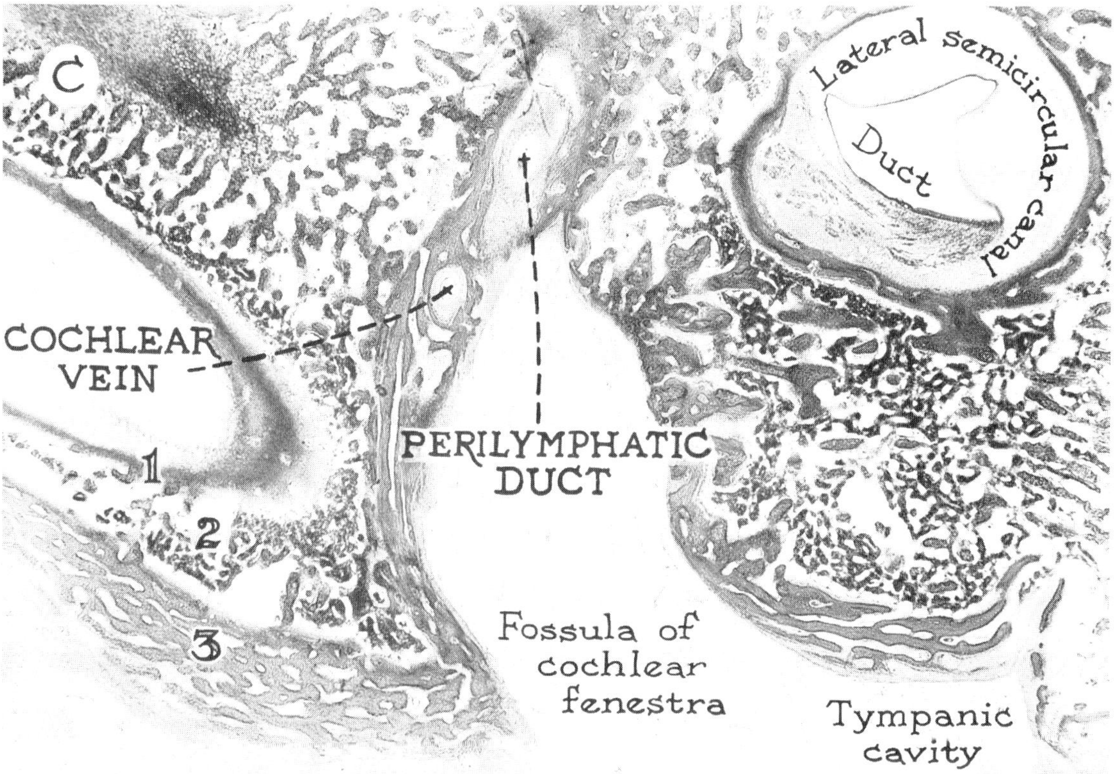

Figure II–49. COCHLEAR FENESTRA AND RELATED ANATOMY: DEVELOPMENT. *a.* FETUS OF 16½ WEEKS (126 MM.). *b.* FETUS OF 20 WEEKS (167 MM.). *c.* FETUS OF 21 WEEKS (183 MM.).

a. In the fetus at approximately the 4-month stage, the rim of the cochlear window is still formed in cartilage. The fundamental relations among the following are established: the tympanic scala (of the basal turn of the cochlea); the fossula of the cochlear fenestra (still occupied by primitive mesenchymal tissue); the cochlear aqueduct (or canaliculus), containing the tissue of the so-called perilymphatic duct and the cochlear vein.

b. In a specimen one month older, ossification of the capsule is in progress. At the level shown, the section passes through the wall of the fenestra where both cartilage and bone are present. Unlabeled arrow points to the area of developing bone which will intervene between the vein and the duct.

c. The capsule, now trilaminar, forms a complete osseous wall for the fenestra (see Figures III–93*b* and III–94*a* and *b*).

Transverse sections, Wisconsin Collection, series 11, 105, and 21, respectively. *a*, × 15; *b*, × 20; *c*, × 21.

(From Anson: Chapter 1 in Paparella and Shumrick (Eds.): Otolaryngology, Vol. I. Philadelphia, W. B. Saunders Co., 1973.)

ADULT STRUCTURE: Illustrated in Figures III–93 to III–97.

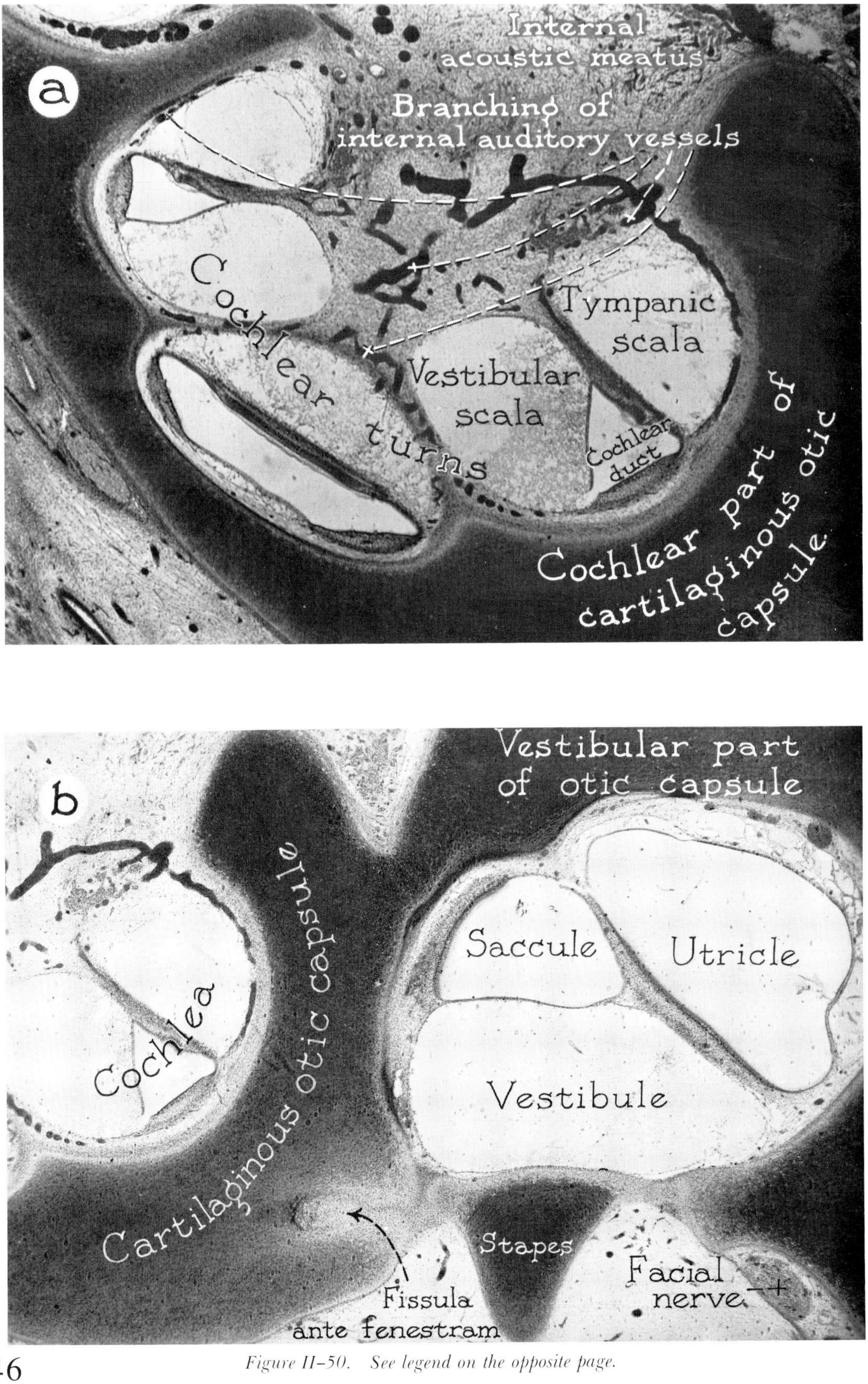

Figure II–50. See legend on the opposite page.

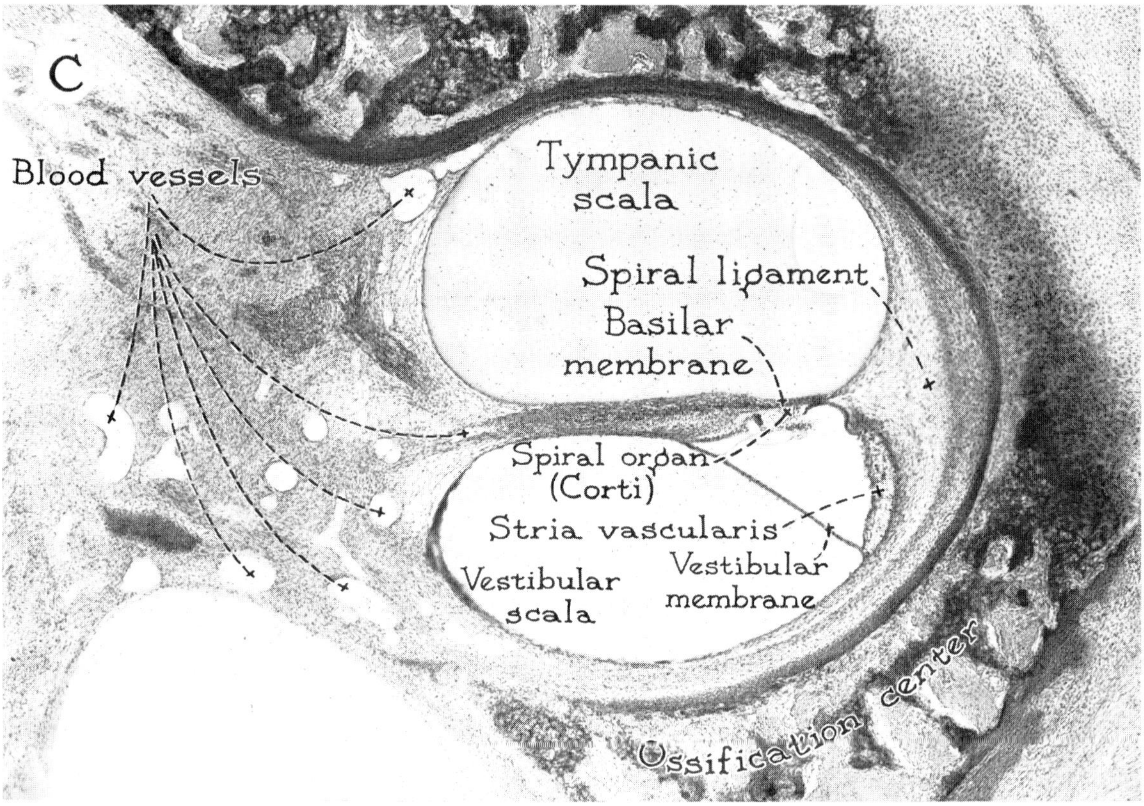

Figure 11–50. OTIC CAPSULE, BLOOD SUPPLY: DEVELOPMENTAL AND ADULT ANATOMY. *a* and *b*. FETUS OF 16 WEEKS (126 MM.). *c*. FETUS, 19+ WEEKS (160 MM.). *d*. FETUS OF 26 WEEKS (230 MM.). *e*. NEWBORN.

a. Demonstrating the early establishment of the internal auditory blood vessels in the internal acoustic meatus, and of their branches, as the latter course through the developing modiolus to the walls of the scalae, the osseous spiral lamina, and the partition between cochlear turns.

b. Showing the pattern of distribution of the blood vessels in the cochlear and vestibular division of the labyrinth. In the cochlea, the blood vessels course through the periotic tissue on the walls of the scalae and the cochlear duct. In the vestibule the main vessels are lodged in the periotic tissue on the attached surface of the saccule and utricle. This tissue is a remnant of the primordial reticulum (compare Figure 11–30, canalicular area). It will become the so-called "ligaments" for anchorage of the two vesicles.

The future facial canal is a sulcus on the wall of the canalicular division of the capsule; the fissula ante fenestram is an area of deorganizing precartilage in the wall of the cochlear division.

c. Detailing the blood vessels in the cochlea at the onset of ossification (in the 5-month fetus). They are traced from the internal acoustic meatus, through the modiolus to the attached extremity of the osseous spiral lamina, to the walls of the vestibular scala and the tympanic scala.

Figure 11–50 continues on the following page.

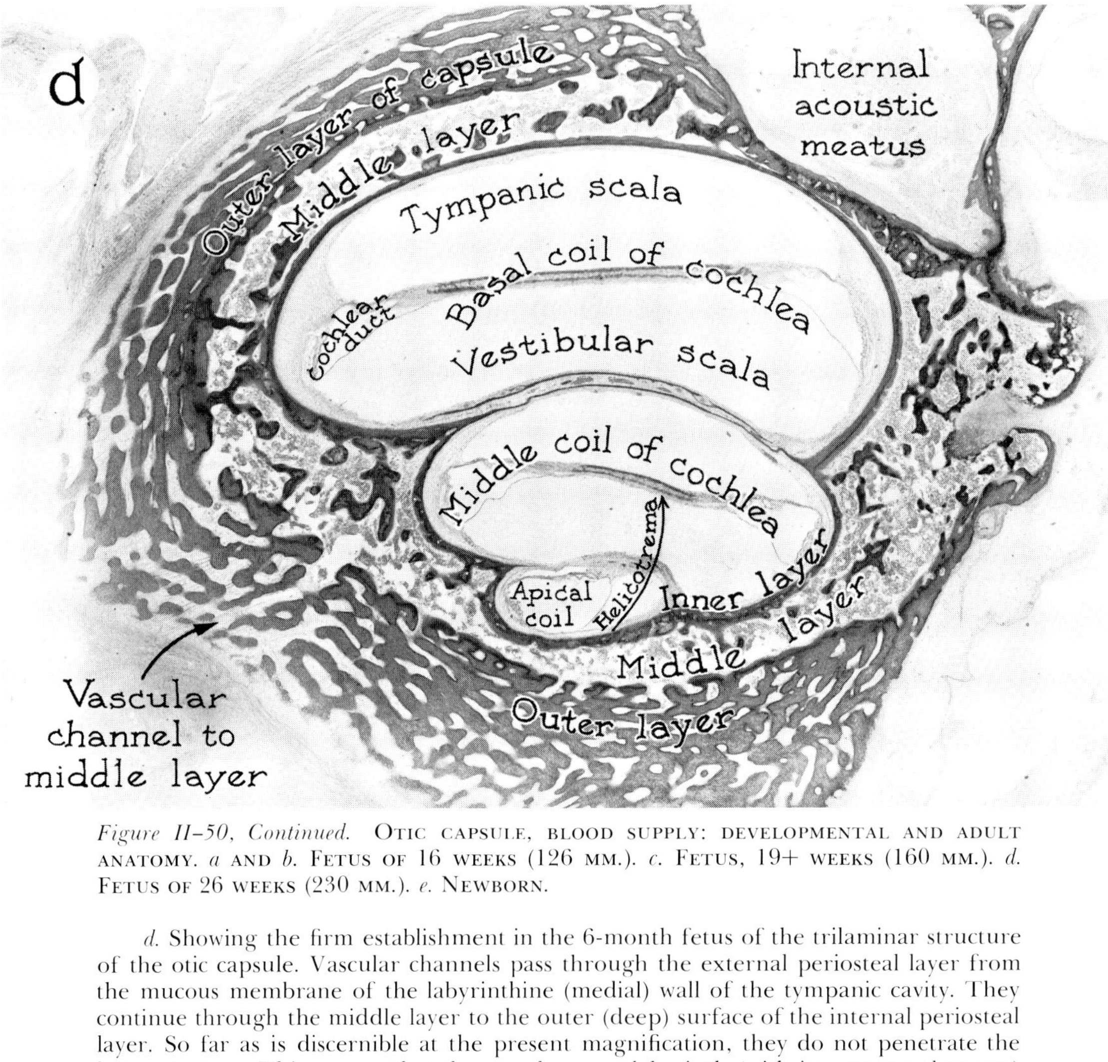

Figure II–50, Continued. OTIC CAPSULE, BLOOD SUPPLY: DEVELOPMENTAL AND ADULT ANATOMY. *a* AND *b*. FETUS OF 16 WEEKS (126 MM.). *c*. FETUS, 19+ WEEKS (160 MM.). *d*. FETUS OF 26 WEEKS (230 MM.). *e*. NEWBORN.

d. Showing the firm establishment in the 6-month fetus of the trilaminar structure of the otic capsule. Vascular channels pass through the external periosteal layer from the mucous membrane of the labyrinthine (medial) wall of the tympanic cavity. They continue through the middle layer to the outer (deep) surface of the internal periosteal layer. So far as is discernible at the present magnification, they do not penetrate the latter stratum. This means that the membranous labyrinth (with its sensory elements) and the periotic connective tissue must be supplied wholly or chiefly by the vessels that enter the capsule through the internal acoustic meatus.

Figure II–50 continues on the opposite page.

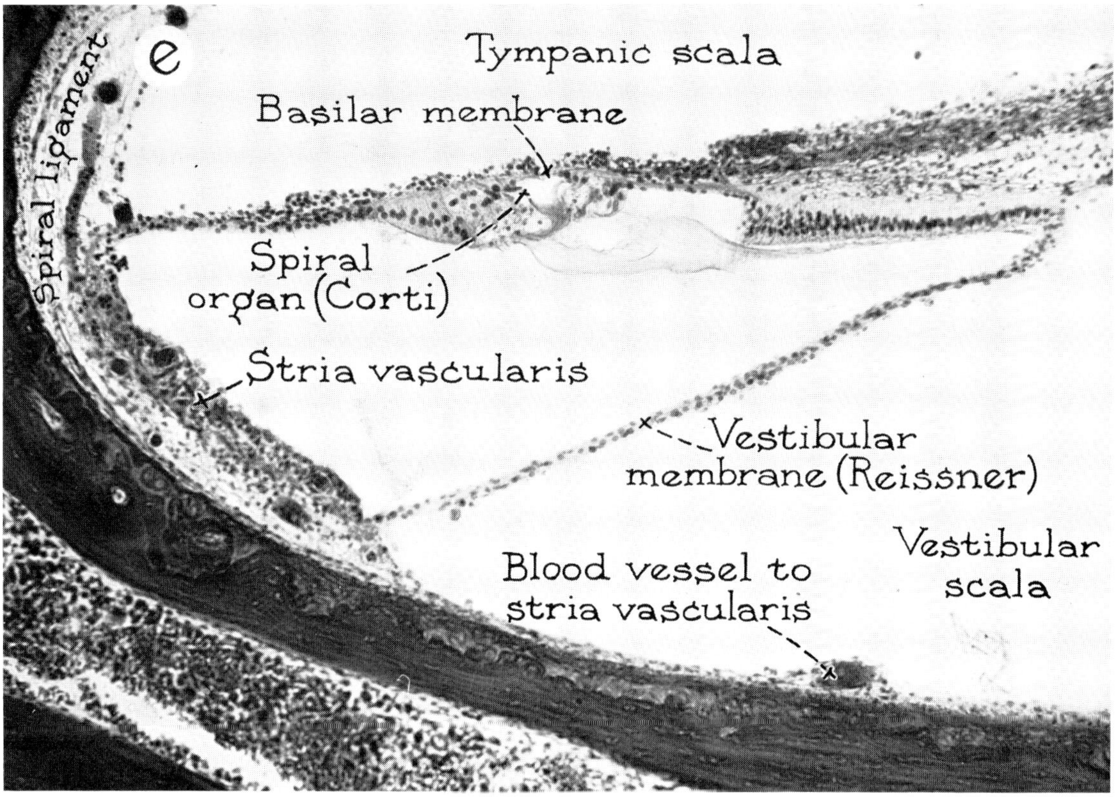

Figure II–50, Concluded.

e. Demonstrating the mature pattern of vascularization in a cochlear turn. Vessels coursing along the walls of the scalae (in the periotic tissue) and others transmitted by the osseous spiral lamina reach the *stria vascularis.*

Transverse sections, Wisconsin Collection, series as follows: *a* and *b*, 11; *c*, 207; *d*, 64; *e*, 124. *a*, × 20; *b*, × 18; *c*, × 44; *d*, × 15; *e*, × 138.

(*d* and *e* from Anson, Winch, Warpeha, and Donaldson: Ann. Otol., 75:921–944, 1966.)

ADULT STRUCTURE: Illustrated in Figures III–132 and III–137 to III–139.

TEMPORAL BONE WITH SITES OF CONTAINED STRUCTURES PORTRAYED IN PHANTOM VIEW.

In surgery of the temporal bone, familiarity with the interrelationship of the vital structures contained therein is as essential as knowledge of their individual morphology. The inherent problem posed by these features is further intensified by the fact that the pyramid is employed as a king's highway for the passage of neural, arterial, and venous elements that contribute little or nothing locally to the functional integrity of the labyrinthine systems.

The transverse venous sinus runs in a course curved lateralward in the transverse sulcus of the occipital bone and of the parietal bone in the attached margin of the *tentorium cerebelli.* Then it follows a tortuous course, medialward and downward in the sigmoid sulcus of the temporal bone and in the transverse sulcus of the lateral part of the occipital bone to the jugular foramen. There the sinus becomes continuous with the superior bulb of the internal jugular vein lodged in the jugular fossa on the inferior surface of the petrous part of the temporal bone.

The internal carotid artery ascends in the neck to the external carotid foramen on the inferior surface of the pyramid, this aperture being situated just anterior to the jugular fossa. In the carotid canal the artery follows a curving course, passing at first perpendicularly, then forward and medialward through the pyramid, to a point of emergence near the apex at the internal carotid foramen. There, at the *foramen lacerum*, the artery turns upward in the carotid sulcus on the body of the sphenoid bone.

The facial nerve is shown curving in a course through the facial canal, at first transversely above the vestibular (oval) window, then vertically in the mastoid wall of the tympanic cavity to the stylomastoid foramen.

The membranous duct system (in green) is shown as tubes contained in the osseous labyrinth (in buff tint). The long axis of the cone-shaped cochlea is placed horizontally, with the apex directed lateralward. The anterior wall adjoins the area of curvature of the carotid canal in the temporal bone. The basal turn ends at the cochlear (round) window (closed in the fresh state by the secondary tympanic membrane). The intermediate division, the vestibule, communicates with the middle ear through the vestibular (oval) window (closed in the fresh state by the stapes). In the vestibule, the cochlear duct is continuous with the saccule, the semicircular ducts with the utricle. The ducts appear as they lie in three planes nearly perpendicular to one another. They are contained in bony canals and correspond to them in both plane and course.

Part
III

THE EAR: Adult Anatomy

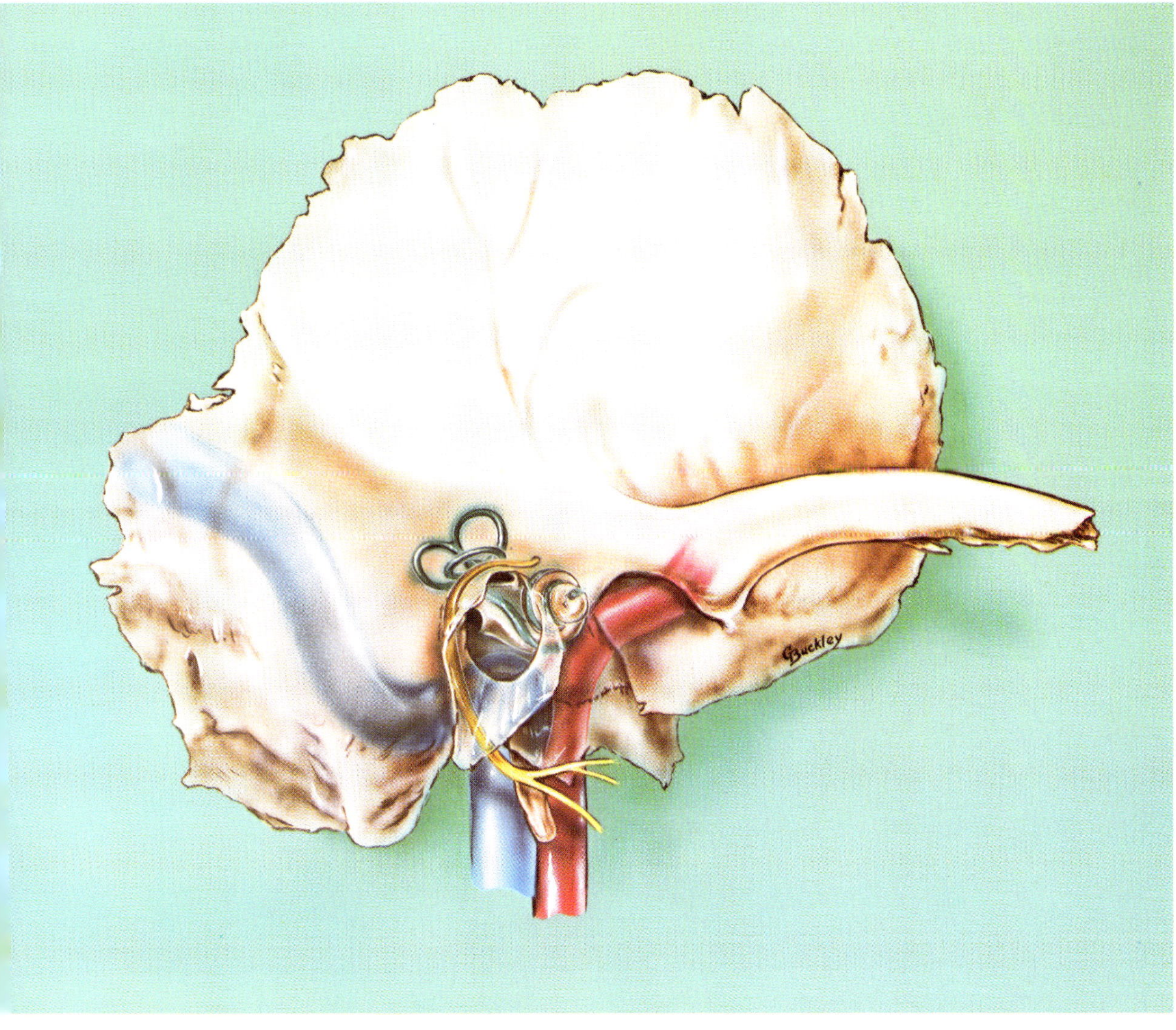

Parts of the Ear

Figure III–1[1]

The organ known as the *ear* (organum vestibulocochleare) is actually a compound organ that is sensitive to sound and to the effects of gravity and motion. The organ consists of three parts, each possessing distinctive structural and functional characters.

The first portion is known as the *external ear* (auris externa). It is subdivided into a sound-collecting part, the *auricle*, on the surface of the head; and a short conducting tube, the *external acoustic meatus*, that leads toward the interior and is closed at its deep end by the *tympanic membrane*.

The second component is termed the *middle ear* (auris media). It is represented chiefly by the *tympanic cavity*, a small, air-containing chamber in the petrous portion of the temporal bone. This cavity is not an isolated space; it communicates with the nasal part of the pharynx by a canal termed the *auditory* (eustachian) *tube*, and in the opposite direction, a recess passes from the tympanic chamber to the *tympanic antrum*. The antrum is continuous in turn with air spaces in the mastoid portion of the temporal bone. A chain of three small *ear bones* transmits, across the middle ear, the vibrational effects produced on the tympanic membrane by sound waves.

The third part, or *internal ear* (auris interna), contains the essential sensory apparatus and is extremely irregular in shape. It consists of membranous sacs and ducts, the *membranous labyrinth* (labyrinthus membranaceus); these lie within correspondingly intricate cavities in the interior of the petrous part of the temporal bone designated as the *osseous labyrinth* (labyrinthus osseus). The internal ear includes the *utricle* and *saccule*, two small, vesicular structures contained within the bony *vestibule* (vestibulum); three membranous *semicircular ducts* (ductus semicirculares), which are surrounded individually by corresponding bony *semicircular canals* (canales semicirculares ossei); and the membranous *cochlear duct* (ductus cochlearis) similar in general shape to the snail-like, bony *cochlea* (cochlea) encasing it. Of these several parts, the semicircular ducts are concerned with changes in the rate of movement, and the utricle and saccule are concerned with determination of static position; the cochlea is specialized for hearing.

[1]Unlike Part II, in which individual references to figures proved to be essential because of the progression in developmental steps, in Part III, the reader is referred to figures in sets which cover a general feature.

The External Ear

Figure III–1

The *external ear* consists of the auricle (auricula), attached to the side of the head, and the external acoustic meatus (meatus acusticus externus) leading from it to the middle ear.

AURICLE

Figure III–2

The *auricle* (auricula), or pinna, is a platelike structure that lies upon the side of the head. It presents a lateral and a medial surface. The lateral surface is irregularly concave and the medial surface correspondingly convex. The deepest part of its concavity, situated near the center, is termed the *concha auriculae;* this is partially divided by a prominent oblique ridge, the *crus of the helix* (crus helicis), into a superior part, the *cymba conchae,* and a larger, inferior part, the *cavum conchae.* The latter cavity leads into the external acoustic meatus.

The cavum conchae is bounded anteriorly by a prominent process, the *tragus,* which projects posteriorly over the entrance to the meatus. The tragus is separated from the crus of the helix by a well-marked depression, the *anterior incisure* (incisura anterior), and it sometimes bears a small *supratragic tubercle* (tuberculum supratragicum) superiorly. Bounding the cavum conchae posteriorly and inferiorly is a projection, the *antitragus,* lying opposite but somewhat inferior to the tragus, while between the two is a deep notch, the *intertragic incisure* (incisura intertragica). A prominent semicircular ridge, the *anthelix,* bounds the concha posteriorly and superiorly. Inferiorly it is separated from the antitragus by a slight depression, the *posterior auricular sulcus* (sulcus auriculae posterior). Superiorly the anthelix divides into two ridges, the *crura of the anthelix* (crura anthelicis), and between these is a shallow depression, the *triangular fossa* (fossa triangularis). The superior and posterior margin of the auricle is inverted and forms a prominent rim, the *helix,* which is continued anteriorly into the *crus of the helix* (crus helicis) and inferiorly into the *lobule* (lobulus auriculae). An elongated depression, partly overlapped by the helix and termed the *scapha*, separates the helix from the anthelix. Superiorly and posteriorly the free margin of the helix frequently presents a slight projection, the *auricular tubercle* (tuberculum auriculae), which is thought to correspond to the apex of the ear in lower mammals.

Upon the medial surface of the auricle the depressions of the lateral surface are represented by complementary elevations, *viz.*: the *eminence of the concha* (eminentia conchae), the *eminence of the scapha* (eminentia scaphae), and the *eminence of the triangular fossa* (eminentia fossae triangularis). Similarly, the lateral elevations become depressed areas on the medial surface, *viz.:* the *fossa of the anthelix* (fossa anthelicis), the *transverse sulcus of the anthelix* (sulcus anthelicis transversus), and the *sulcus of the crus of the helix* (sulcus cruris helicis). The attachment of approximately one-third of the medial surface to the head covers and hides the two latter depressions.

STRUCTURE

The features of the auricle, just described, are produced mainly by an internal plate of elastic cartilage, the *auricular cartilage* (cartilago auriculae). Besides the elevations and depressions already noted, it presents the following additional parts. Projecting anteriorly from the helix, near the crus, is a small tubercle, the *spine of the helix* (spina helicis). At the other end the posterior margin of the helix terminates in a pointed, taillike process, the *cauda helicis*, which is separated inferiorly from the antitragus by the deep *antitragohelicine fissure* (fissura antitragohelicina). Another deep notch, the *terminal incisure* (incisura terminalis auris), separates the cartilage of the auricle from that of the meatus, leaving only a narrow strip, the *isthmus* (isthmus cartilaginis auris), connecting the two. The cartilage of the tragus, the *lamina tragi*, is separated from that of the auricle proper and is attached to the lateral margin of the cartilage of the meatus.

The auricle is invested on both its medial and lateral aspects by integument that closely follows the irregularities of the underlying cartilage. Thus it is tightly bound to the perichondrium of the lateral surface by subcutaneous areolar tissue, but is much more loosely attached to the medial surface. In the subcutaneous tissue there is little fat except in the lobule, which is made up almost entirely of fat and tough fibrous tissue. *Hairs* are abundant, but for the most part rudimentary; however, in the region of the tragus and antitragus they may be large and long, particularly in males and in the aged. *Sebaceous glands* are found on both surfaces; they are especially well developed in the concha and triangular fossa, but *sudoriferous glands* are few and scattered.

LIGAMENTS AND MUSCLES

The auricle is attached to the side of the head by the skin, by the continuity of its cartilage with that of the acoustic meatus, and by certain extrinsic ligaments and muscles. Three extrinsic ligaments may be identified in the connective tissue: the *anterior ligament* (lig. auriculare anterius), stretching from the zygoma to the helix and tragus; the *superior ligament* (lig. auriculare superius), from the superior margin of the bony external acoustic meatus to the spine of the helix; and the *posterior ligament* (lig. auriculare posterius), from the mastoid process to the eminence of the concha.

There are also three extrinsic muscles—the *anterior, superior,* and *posterior auricular.* Six intrinsic muscles are distinguished, but in man they are poorly represented and vary greatly in degree of development. Upon the lateral surface the *helicis major* stretches from the spine of the helix to the anterosuperior margin; the *helicis minor* overlies the crus of the helix; the *tragicus* runs vertically upon the tragus; and the *antitragicus* stretches from the antitragus to the cauda helicis. Upon the medial surface the *transverse auricular muscle* stretches between the eminences of the concha and scapha, and the *oblique auricular muscle* passes between the eminences of the concha and the triangular fossa. Two additional small muscles occasionally present are the *pyramidalis auriculae* and the *incisurae helicis.*

EXTERNAL ACOUSTIC MEATUS

Figures III–3

The *external acoustic meatus* (meatus acusticus externus) is the auditory canal that extends from the concha to the tympanic membrane. It is approximately 25 mm. in length on the superoposterior wall; whereas, owing to the obliquity of the tympanic membrane, its anteroinferior wall is about 6 mm. longer. The canal consists of a more lateral *cartilaginous meatus* (meatus acusticus externus cartilagineus) and a more medial *osseous meatus* (meatus acusticus externus osseus). The acoustic meatus courses medially in a general anteroinferior direction in slightly tortuous S-fashion, but it is not confined to a single plane. Near the auricular end the meatus is convex anteriorly, whereas at the tympanic end the curve is reversed and is concave in the same direction. The lumen is irregularly elliptic in outline, the longer axis being vertical at the auricular end, but nearly horizontal at its tympanic extremity. The meatus is somewhat constricted about midway in its course, and also near the eardrum (tympanic membrane).

RELATIONS

The *anterior wall* of the meatus is related to the mandibular fossa medially and to the parotid gland laterally. The *inferior wall* is closely bound to the parotid gland. The *posterior wall* of the bony part is separated from the mastoid cells only by thin bone. The *superior wall* is separated at its medial end from the epitympanic recess by a thin plate of bone; laterally, thicker bone intervenes between meatus and cranial cavity.

STRUCTURE

The walls of the meatus are formed laterally of fibrocartilage and medially of bone, while both parts are lined with skin reflected inward from the auricle.

The *cartilage of the acoustic meatus* (cartilago meatus acustici) is trough-shaped; it is open superiorly and posteriorly, but the edges are united by dense fibrous tissue so that a tubular canal results. Medially the cartilage constitutes about one-third of the circumference; laterally, two-thirds. Two fissures, the *incisures of the cartilaginous meatus* (incisurae cartilaginis meatus acustici externi), usually occur in the anterior wall; these give mobility to the auricle. Laterally the cartilage of the meatus is directly continuous with that of the auricle, and medially it is connected firmly with the lateral lip of the bony meatus.

The osseous portion of the meatus, which comprises slightly more than half the length of the canal, is a tunnel through the temporal bone. The anterior wall, the floor, and the lower part of the posterior wall are formed by the tympanic part of the temporal bone; the remainder of the posterior wall and the roof are provided by the squama.

The *skin* of the meatus furnishes a continuous lining for the canal and an external covering for the tympanic membrane. It is relatively thick in the cartilaginous part of the meatus, but very thin in the bony portion, especially near the tympanic end where it is tightly bound to the periosteum. In the cartilaginous meatus the skin contains numerous fine hairs and sebaceous glands, whereas neither is found in the bony meatus. Tubular *ceruminous glands*, which represent modified sweat glands that secrete the *cerumen* (or ear wax), form a nearly continuous layer throughout the cartilaginous meatus, but occur on only small parts of the posterior and superior walls of the bony canal. The openings of their ducts appear as dark points to the unaided eye.

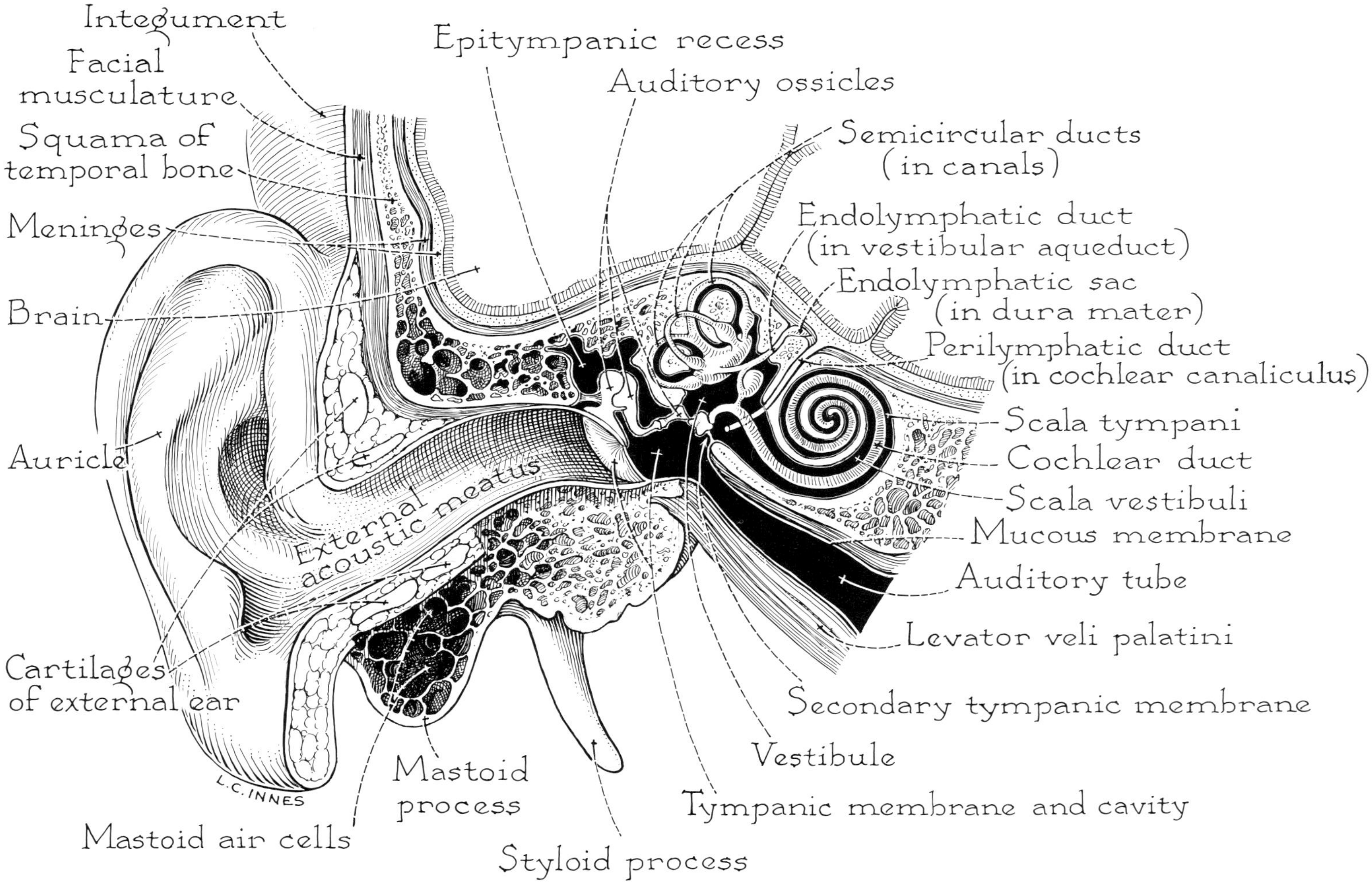

Figure III–1. Parts of the ear. A vertical section in the plane of the external acoustic meatus and the auditory tube. Semischematic.

The statoacoustic organ (*organum vestibulocochleare*) may be divided into three parts: the external, middle, and internal ears.

The external ear (*auris externa*) consists of the auricle (*auricula*) and the external acoustic meatus (*meatus acusticus externus*). The meatus, lined with skin, leads inward from the bottom of the concha of the auricle to the tympanic membrane.

The middle ear (*auris media*), or tympanic cavity, is a narrow chamber lined with mucous membrane and situated between the external acoustic meatus and the labyrinth. It communicates with the mastoid air cells and with the nasal pharynx. The

The internal ear (*auris interna*) contains the sensory organs of hearing and equilibrium in a labyrinthine system of cavities lodged within the petrous portion of the temporal bone. These cavities contain fluid, called perilymph, and a membranous counterpart of the bony chambers. The membranous labyrinth contains the endolymph.

The osseous labyrinth (*labyrinthus osseus*) consists of the cochlea (*cochlea*), three semicircular canals (*canales semicirculares ossei*), and an ovoid chamber, the vestibule (*vestibulum*). The vestibule lies between the medial wall of the tympanic cavity and the fundus of the internal acoustic meatus. Three semicircular canals open into its posterior part, while the *scala vestibuli* of the cochlea opens into the lower and anterior part. On the lateral wall is the oval, or vestibular, window (*fenestra vestibuli*), closed by the base of the stapes. From a small aperture on the medial wall, the vestibular aqueduct (*aqueductus vestibuli*) passes backward to the posterior surface of the petrous part of the temporal bone.

The three semicircular canals are posterior to the vestibule, turned at right angles to each other. They open into the vestibule through five round orifices, the adjoining extremities of the superior and posterior canals being fused into a common canal (*crus commune*). One extremity of each, where it joins the vestibule, expands into an ampulla (*ampulla ossea*).

The cochlea is a tapering tube coiled spirally for two and three-quarters turns around a central pillar, the *modiolus*. The cochlea lies anterior to the vestibule. Its base is directed toward the bottom of the internal acoustic meatus, the apex toward the middle ear. As the cochlea winds upward toward the apex, its diameter diminishes rapidly. The modiolus forms the inner wall of the cochlear tube; winding around it like the thread of a screw is a thin ledge of bone, the spiral lamina (*lamina spiralis ossea*), which partly subdivides the space of the osseous tube into two passages, the vestibular and cochlear staircases (*scala vestibuli, scala tympani*). The spiral lamina is tunneled by small canals that transmit filaments of the cochlear nerve to a larger canal within the central pillar of the cochlea.

The epithelial duct system of the membranous labyrinth is housed within the osseous labyrinth. Two components of the membranous labyrinth—namely the saccule (*sacculus*) and utricle (*utriculus*)—are contained in the vestibule. They communicate with the cochlear and canalicular parts of the system by the utricular duct (*ductus utriculosaccularis*) and with the endolymphatic duct (*ductus endolymphaticus*). The endolymphatic duct, prolonged through a channel in the osseous capsule—the latter also being known as the vestibular aqueduct—ends in a saclike enlargement in the cranial cavity on the posterior surface of the petrous part of the temporal bone.

Three membranous semicircular ducts (*ductus semicirculares*) open from the utricle. They are contained within the semicircular canals; although generally similar in form, they are smaller in diameter.

The saccule joins the membranous cochlear duct through a short, slender tube, the *ductus reuniens*. The cochlear duct occupies the osseous cochlea. Like the three ducts of the canalicular division, it is smaller than the osseous labyrinth in which it is housed. Each of the semicircular ducts lies within an undivided canal; but the cochlear duct, interposed between the free margin of the osseous spiral lamina and the opposite wall of the bony cochlea, divides the latter into two compartments: the tympanic scala and the vestibular scala. As its name indicates, the vestibular scala begins in the vestibule, where this portion of the internal ear is closed off from the middle ear (tympanic cavity) by the base of the stapes. At the apex of the cochlea, the scala vestibuli communicates with the scala tympani by means of an aperture termed the *helicotrema*. The tympanic scala matches the turns of the vestibular scala and ends at the base of the cochlea, where the secondary tympanic membrane (*membrana tympani secundaria*) in the round window (*fenestra cochleae*) separates the scala from the fossulate bay of the tympanic cavity.

Developmental Anatomy. A review of the contents of Part II may serve as a reminder of the degree to which a knowledge of embryonic and fetal anatomy is essential to an understanding of the adult structure of the temporal bone and ear.

This is true for the following reasons: the external ear is a derivative of an embryonic branchial groove; the space of the middle ear is an extension of the corresponding pharyngeal pouch; the auditory ossicles are, for the greater part, remodeled segments of the branchial skeleton; the labyrinthine spaces and their osseous walls reach adult dimensions in the fifth intrauterine month; the histologic fabric of the investing otic capsule and that of the ossicles remain identifiable—being, as it were, fetal skeletal elements in an otherwise adult skull.

Cross-references throughout Part II and Part III will aid in making the pictorial and textual material phases of a continuum.

(From Anson: Section X in Anson (Ed.): Morris' Human Anatomy, 12th ed. Copyright © 1966 by McGraw-Hill, Inc. Used by permission of McGraw-Hill Book Company.)

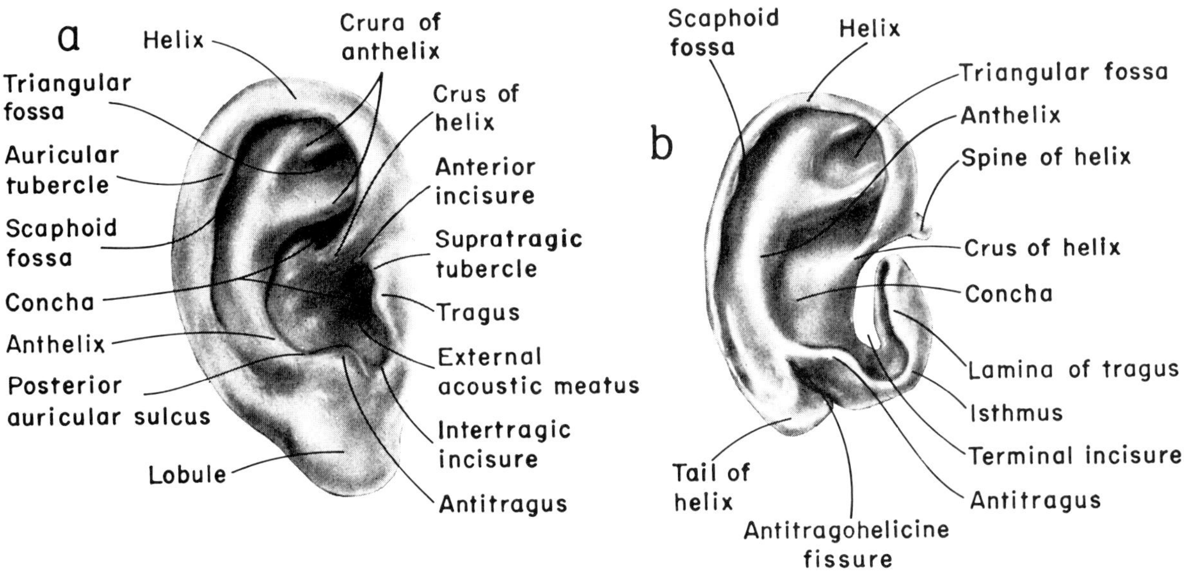

Figure III–2. EAR, AURICULAR CARTILAGE, AND MUSCLES: *a*, *b*, and *c* VIEWED FROM THE OUTSIDE; *d* VIEWED FROM THE INSIDE.

a and *b*. The auricle, or pinna, is completely invested by integument on the lateral surface. On the medial surface the skin covers only the upper and posterior part of the auricular cartilage (compare *d*), wherefrom it curves around into the skin of the head. Inferiorly the skin over the tail of the helix (see *b*) forms a flattened, rounded duplicature, the lobule of the ear. The fossae, sulci, crura, and other anatomical features are described on pages 154 and 155 of the text.

Figure III–2 continues on the opposite page.

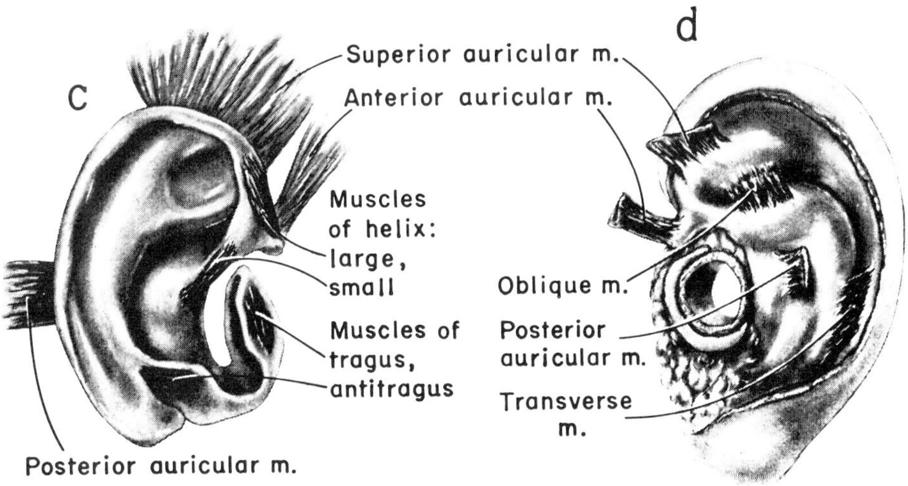

Figure III–2, Continued. EAR, AURICULAR CARTILAGE, AND MUSCLES: *a*, *b*, and *c* VIEWED FROM THE OUTSIDE; *d* VIEWED FROM THE INSIDE.

c and *d*. The extrinsic muscles are three in number; they converge from regions anterior, superior, and posterior to the auricle and are inserted into it. They arise from the galea aponeurotica of the epicranial musculature. Six intrinsic muscles are usually described; however, they are poorly represented in the human ear and, when present, vary greatly in degree of development. Details of origin and insertion are given in the text (pages 155 and 156).

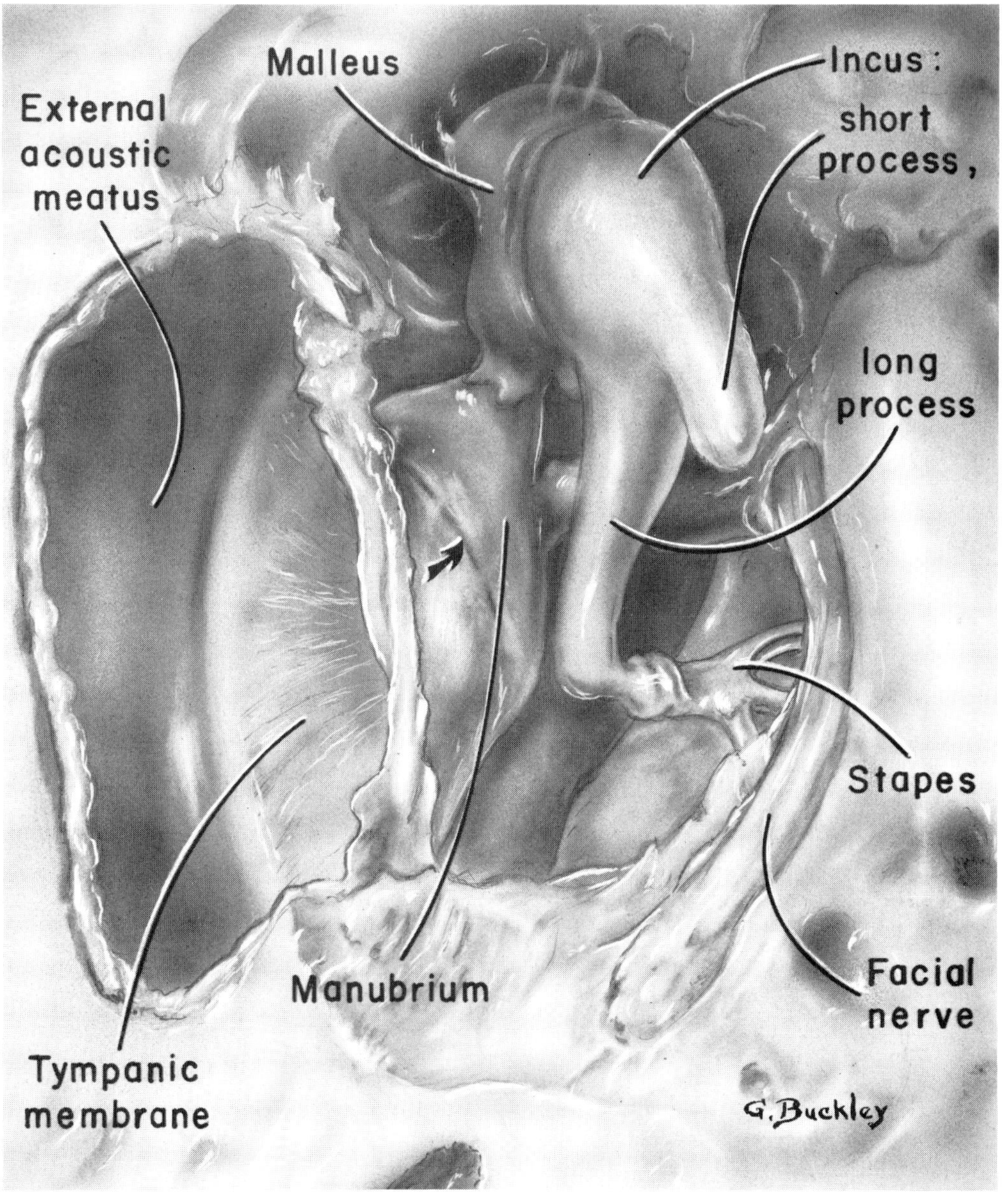

a

Figure III–3. EXTERNAL ACOUSTIC MEATUS OF THE OUTER EAR, TYMPANIC MEMBRANE, AND TYMPANIC CAVITY OF THE MIDDLE EAR WITH THE CONTAINED AUDITORY OSSICLES. THE TYMPANIC RING IS INTACT (FREED MARGIN TOWARD THE READER). *a.* FIRST STAGE IN THE DISSECTION OF AN UNEMBALMED SPECIMEN.

a. The external skin lining the meatus contributes the cutaneous stratum of the tympanic membrane. The membrane is stretched out in the tympanic sulcus and incisure (*incisura Rivini*) of the *pars tympanica* of the temporal bone. It is drawn inward, funnel-shaped, by the tip of the manubrium of the malleus. Internally, the lining of the middle ear forms the mucosal stratum of the tympanic membrane. This epithelial layer is carried over the manubrium from the inner aspect of the drum membrane (at arrow). The head of the malleus and part of the incus occupy the epitympanic recess. The long process of the incus descends almost parallel to the manubrium. On its medial side a small eminence is offset as a lenticular process for articulation with the foveate head of the stapes. The stapedius tendon (unlabeled) attaches to the head of the stapes.

Figure III–3 continues on the opposite page.

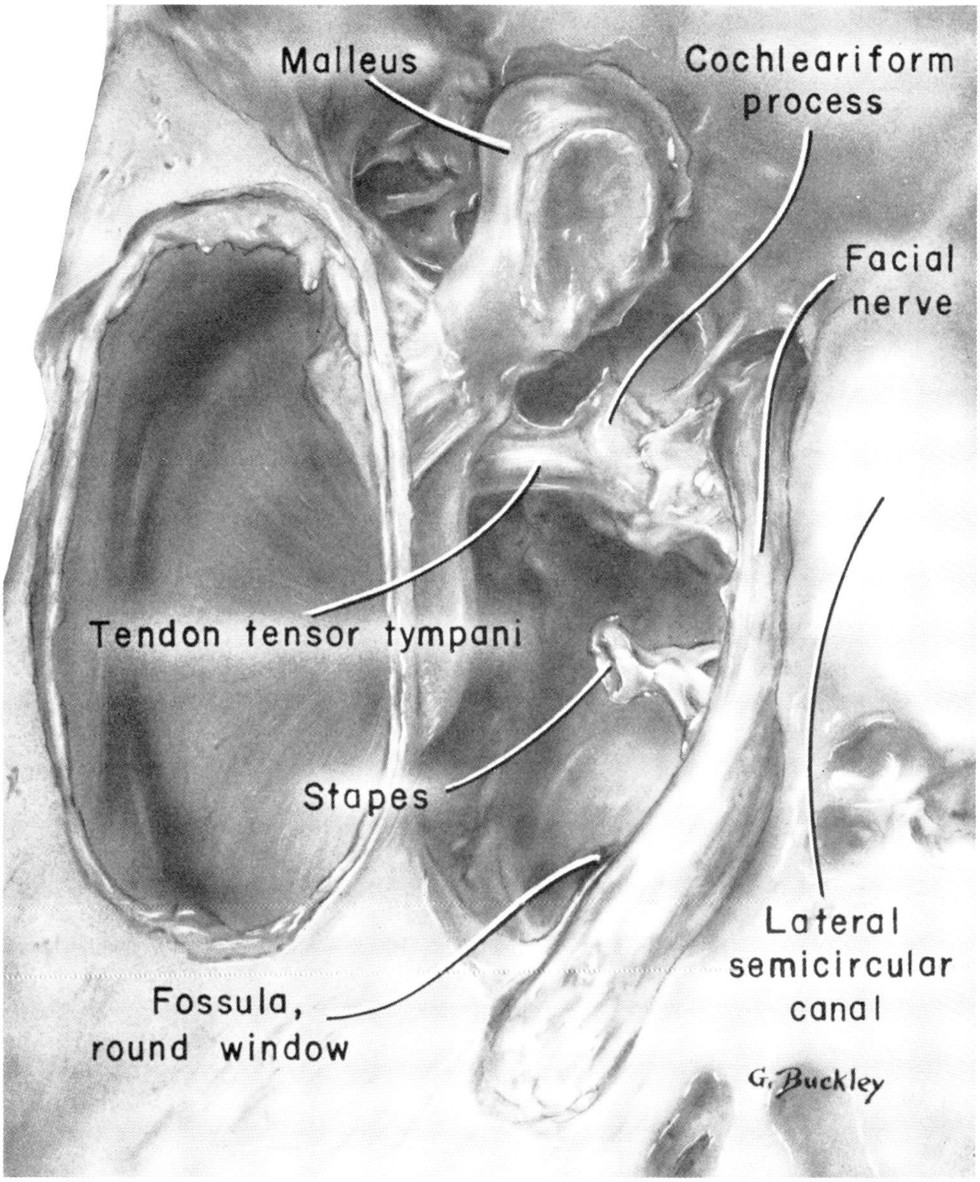

b

Figure III–3, Continued. *b.* SECOND STAGE IN DISSECTION.

b. The incus has been removed in order to demonstrate the articular surfaces of the malleus and the stapes and the tympanic part of the tensor tympani tendon. The mucous membrane has been dissected from the body of the malleus and reflected from the reader's side of the tendon of the tympanic tensor. The facial nerve is exposed from the *geniculum* to a point, inferiorly, near its emergence at the stylomastoid foramen.

The club-shaped head of the malleus presents on its posteromedial aspect a somewhat elongate, saddle-shaped articular surface for the body of the incus (see preceding illustration). The head of the stapes is foveate for reception of the lenticular process of the incus. The tendon of the tensor tympani is seen as it crosses the middle ear from the semicanal to the neck of the malleus.

The Middle Ear

Figure III–1

The *middle ear* includes the *tympanic cavity* (cavum tympani), the *tympanic antrum* (antrum mastoideum), and the *auditory tube* (tuba auditiva). These constitute a continuous, irregular, pneumatic chamber and passage, located through the greater part of its extent in the temporal bone. The centrally located tympanic cavity is shut off from the external ear by the *tympanic membrane* (membrana tympani), and from the chamber that forms the internal ear by the structures that occupy the cochlear and vestibular windows. It communicates with the pharynx by means of the auditory tube and connects backward through the antrum with the mastoid cells.

The parts to be considered are, in order: the tympanic membrane, the tympanic ring, the tympanic cavity and its contents (including the tympanic antrum and mastoid cells), and the auditory tube.

TYMPANIC MEMBRANE

Figures III–3, III–4, and III–64

The *tympanic membrane* (membrana tympani), or eardrum, serves as a common membranous partition between the external acoustic meatus and the tympanic cavity; in this way it furnishes a medial wall for the one and a lateral wall for the other. The membrane is a thin, semitransparent disk, elliptic in shape. Its long axis is nearly vertical, measuring 9 to 10 mm.; the least diameter is 8 to 9 mm. Set obliquely, the membrane slopes medially from the posterosuperior to the antero-inferior wall of the auditory meatus. The angle formed with the superior wall is usually 140 degrees, but the membrane varies greatly in form, size, and obliquity. It is slightly concave on its external aspect because of traction from the manubrium of the malleus (the outermost of the three small ear bones), which is firmly attached to the inner (medial or tympanic) surface.

The most depressed point, the *umbo membranae tympani,* is slightly inferior and posterior to the center of the membrane and corresponds to the tip of the manubrium. From here a whitish streak, the *mallear stria* (stria mallearis), caused by the manubrium shining through, is seen in an external view passing toward the superior margin. At the superior end of the stria is a slight projection, the *mallear prominence* (prominentia mallearis), formed by the lateral process of the malleus. Therefrom the *anterior* and the *posterior mallear folds* (plicae mallearis anterior et posterior) stretch to the respective extremities of the tympanic sulcus of the temporal bone. The small, triangular area of the membrane bounded by the plicae is termed the *flaccid portion* (pars flaccida), or Shrapnell's membrane. It is thin and lax, and is attached directly to the petrous bone at the *tympanic notch* (incisura tympanica). The larger part of the tympanic membrane, the *tense portion* (pars tensa), is inferior to the plicae and is tightly stretched. Its thickened *border* (limbus membranae tympani) is attached by a *fibrocartilaginous ring* (anulus fibrocartilagineus) to the tympanic sulcus of the temporal bone; at the terminal spines of the sulcus-bearing tympanic ring the limbus is continuous with the plicae.

STRUCTURE

The tympanic membrane is about 0.1 mm. thick and consists of four sheetlike lamellae: The lateral surface is covered by a *cutaneous layer* (stratum cutaneum), which is merely a thin continuation of the skin lining the external auditory meatus. On the next deeper level is a *radiate fibrous layer* (stratum radiatum), composed of connective tissue; its fibers are attached to the manubrium of the malleus and radiate outward, finally passing directly into the peripheral fibrocartilaginous ring. Still deeper is the *circular fibrous layer* (stratum circulare), which has its fibers arranged concentrically and is best developed near the circumference. These two closely united, fibrous layers are not represented in the pars flaccida. The *mucous layer* (stratum mucosum), which is a portion of the mucous membrane of the middle ear cavity, covers the medial surface of the tympanic membrane smoothly except where the embedded manubrium of the malleus causes an elevation.

VESSELS AND NERVES

The *arteries* occur in two sets, one on each surface of the tympanic membrane, and the two connect through anastomoses. The cutaneous vessels originate from the deep auricular branch of the internal maxillary artery; the supply to the mucous surface is from the anterior tympanic branch of the internal maxillary and from the stylomastoid branch of the posterior auricular. The *veins* communicate with those of the external meatus and tympanic cavity. *Lymphatics*, like the blood vessels, are arranged in two communicating sets; they probably drain into lymph nodes in the region of the mastoid process, tragus, and auditory tube.

The *nerves* accompany the vessels; they are derived chiefly from the auriculotemporal branch of the mandibular nerve, supplemented by twigs from the auricular branch of the vagus, and the tympanic branch of the glossopharyngeus.

TYMPANIC RING

Figures III–3 to III–7

The tympanic ring, or annulus, is an incomplete circle, in the concavity of which is a groove, the tympanic sulcus, for attachment of the circumference of the tympanic membrane.

The sulcus is situated on the posterior surface of the tympanic part of the temporal bone. Superiorly, the sulcus runs out into small pointed extremities, the greater and lesser tympanic spines. The space between the spines is not entirely filled up by attachment to the subjacent bone (to which it fused as a "ring" in the course of fetal development); on the contrary, there remains an indentation called the tympanic incisure (notch of Rivinus). Growth of the original ring results in movement inward of the sulcus—which then occupies a position deep within the external acoustic meatus.

TYMPANIC CAVITY AND CONTENTS

Figures III–8 to III–13, III–16, III–17, III–20, III–23, and III–64

The *tympanic cavity* (cavum tympani), or *tympanum* (drum), is an irregular space within the temporal bone, situated between the external and internal ear. It is lined with mucous membrane and not only contains air, entering from the auditory tube, but also is traversed by a chain of small bones that transmit vibrations from the tympanic membrane across the cavity to the labyrinth. The tympanum is a flattened cleft which extends in an oblique, anteroposterior plane. The longer vertical and anteroposterior diameters measure about 15 mm. each; the transverse dimension varies between 2 mm. at the narrowest region midway to 6 mm. superiorly and 4 mm. inferiorly. Frequently the jugular fossa is deep, a circumstance that results in corresponding reduction of the capacity of the tympanic cavity.

Considered as a chamber lined with mucous membrane (i.e., in the fresh state), the cavity may be divided into two regions: a lower part, corresponding in vertical extent to the tympanic membrane, constitutes the tympanic cavity proper; the upper region, extending above the upper border of the membrane, is known as the *epitympanic recess* (recessus epitympanicus). It is on the posterior part of this latter chamber that a communication into the *tympanic antrum* (antrum mastoideum) is found.

The tympanic cavity proper has the shape of a very short cylinder with concave ends, the outer end being formed by the tympanic membrane and the inner end by the lateral wall of the labyrinth. The epitympanic recess is a definite chamber whose height is about one-third that of the entire tympanic cavity; it overlies somewhat the external acoustic meatus and contains the head of the malleus and the body and short limb of the incus.

BOUNDARIES OF THE TYMPANIC CAVITY

Considered as a whole, the tympanic cavity may be said to be bounded by six not too clearly demarcated walls, facing one another in pairs.

The roof, or *tegmental wall* (paries tegmentalis), is furnished by a portion of the tegmen tympani, a thin plate of bone which separates the space from the cranial cavity.

The floor, or *jugular wall* (paries jugularis), is very narrow transversely and is related intimately with the fossa for the internal jugular vein. The surface is rendered irregular by the *tympanic cells* (cellulae tympanicae), or air cells, while near the back there is occasionally a marked *styloid prominence* (prominentia styloidea) corresponding to the root of the styloid process.

The posterior boundary, or *mastoid wall* (paries mastoideus), is wider above than at its lower part, where there are many additional tympanic air cells. Above these occurs an elevation, the *pyramidal eminence* (eminentia pyramidalis), on whose apex is an aperture transmitting the tendon of the stapedius muscle. The fleshy belly of that muscle is contained in a cavity within the center of the pyramid itself and is frequently continuous with the facial canal. Lateral to this is a foramen, the *apertura tympanica canaliculi chordae tympani*, through which the chorda tympani nerve enters the tympanic cavity, covered by a reflection of the mucous membrane. Between this opening and the pyramidal eminence is a fossa termed the *posterior sinus* (sinus posterior), frequently referred to by clinicians as the "facial sinus" or "facial recess." Above this again is a recess, known as the *fossa of the incus* (fossa incudis), where the posterior ligament of the incus is attached. The epitympanic recess occupies the upper part of the posterior wall; from the recess opens the tympanic antrum.

The anterior boundary, or *carotid wall* (paries caroticus), is also wider above than below. It presents superiorly the *tensor tympani muscle* in its semicanal; at a lower level is the tympanic orifice of the *auditory tube*, by means of which a direct communication is established into the nasopharynx. Inferiorly a thin, bony wall, covered with tympanic air cells and pierced by the caroticotympanic nerves, separates the tympanic cavity from the carotid canal.

The medial boundary, or *labyrinthine wall* (paries labyrinthicus), presents various features, most of which are related, interiorly, to the labyrinthic systems of the internal ear. Inferiorly there is the *promontory* (promontorium), produced by the bulging basal turn of the cochlea, with the nervous *tympanic plexus* (plexus tympanicus) lodged in grooves upon its surface. Inferior and posterior to the promontory is a depression, the *fossula fenestrae cochleae*, at the bottom of which is the *cochlear window* (fenestra cochleae), or round window of older usage; its orifice is closed by the fibrous, mucosa-covered *secondary tympanic membrane* (membrana tympani secundaria). Posterior to the promontory is a smooth projection, the *support of the promontory* (subiculum promontorii), which forms the inferior border of a rather deep depression known as the *tympanic sinus* (sinus tympani). Superiorly and posteriorly are three landmarks: a depression (the *fossula fenestrae vestibuli*) leading to the *vestibular window* (fenestra vestibuli), formerly called the oval window, which is closed by the base of the stapes and the annular ligament; the *prominence of the facial canal* (prominentia canalis facialis), which indicates the position of the canal containing the facial nerve as it crosses the medial wall and turns downward along the mastoid wall; and the broadly bulging *prominence of the lateral semicircular canal* (prominentia canalis semicircularis lateralis). Anterosuperior is the curved end of the bony semicanal in which the tensor tympani muscle runs; this is the *cochleariform process* (processus cochleariformis).

The lateral boundary, or *membranous wall* (paries membranaceus), is formed mainly by the tympanic membrane (already considered) together with the small rim of temporal bone to which it is attached. This osseous *tympanic ring* (anulus tympanicus), deficient superiorly at the *tympanic notch* (incisura tympanica), bears the *tympanic groove* (sulcus tympanicus) where the tympanic membrane is attached. Superiorly the lateral wall of the epitympanic recess is represented by the *scutum*, a plate of bone belonging to the squama.

BOUNDARIES OF THE EPITYMPANIC RECESS

With the foregoing descriptions of the middle-ear landmarks in mind, the walls of that subdivision of the tympanic cavity called the *epitympanic recess* (recessus epitympanicus) can now be stated. Superiorly, it is bounded by the rooflike tegmen tympani; medially, by the prominence of the lateral semicircular canal and the prominence of the facial canal; laterally, by the scutum; and posteriorly, by the fossa of the incus and the irregular bony surface just behind it. The boundary line between the tympanic cavity proper and the epitympanic recess is marked by the prominence of the facial canal medially and the fossa of the incus posteriorly.

Tympanic Mucous Membrane

Figures III–10a, III–11, III–18, and III–22

The tympanic cavity is supplied with a *mucous membrane* (tunica mucosa cavi tympani) which lines its wall completely and also invests its exposed contents. The lining is continuous anteriorly with the mucosa of the auditory tube and posteriorly with that of the tympanic antrum and mastoid cells. Structurally it is a thin, transparent, vascular membrane, intimately united to the periosteum; the epithelium is simple and mostly of the low, nonciliated type. Passing from the walls to the contents of the tympanic cavity, the mucosa not only covers the ligaments of the malleus and the incus, the tendons of the tensor tympani and stapedius muscles, but also forms a number of special folds and pouches.

The *anterior mallear fold* (plica mallearis anterior) is reflected from the tympanic membrane over the anterior process and ligament of the malleus and over the adjacent part of the chorda tympani. The *posterior mallear fold* (plica mallearis posterior), stretching between the manubrium of the malleus and the posterior tympanic wall, surrounds the lateral ligament of the malleus and the posterior part of the chorda tympani. Each of these folds presents inferiorly a concave, free border; and between them and the tympanic membrane are two blind pouches, the *anterior* and the *posterior recess of the tympanic membrane* (recessus membranae tympani anterior et posterior), or pouches of von Tröltsch. Connected with the posterior recess is a third cul-de-sac, the *superior recess of the tympanic membrane* (recessus membranae tympani superior), or Prussak's space, situated between the pars flaccida of the tympanic membrane and the neck of the malleus. The floor of this recess is formed by the lateral process of the malleus. A somewhat variable fold of mucosa, the *incudal fold* (plica incudis), passes from the roof of the tympanic cavity to the body and short limb of the incus. The body and short limb of the incus, the head of the malleus, and the incudal fold incompletely separate off a lateral *cupular portion* (pars cupularis) of the epitympanic recess. A *stapedial fold* (plica stapedis) stretches from the posterior wall of the tympanic cavity and surrounds the stapes, including the obturator membrane that stretches between its two limbs. Other inconstant folds have been described.

Associated Air Chambers and Cells

Figures III–18 to III–20, III–22, and III–32 to III–39

An aperture (aditus ad antrum) in the upper part of the posterior wall of the epitympanic recess leads into the chamber known as the *tympanic antrum* (antrum mastoideum). This is a relatively large cavity, about the size of a small bean and irregular in form. It lies mainly behind the tympanic cavity, but is also somewhat above and lateral to it.

The antrum is lined with thin mucous membrane, continuous with that of the tympanic cavity and epitympanic recess; into it open the abundant *mastoid cells* (cellulae mastoideae). These cells are small, irregular cavities mostly located behind and below the antrum within the substance of the mastoid process of the temporal bone. They communicate with one another freely and vary exceedingly in size and arrangement.

Auditory Ossicles

Figures III–3, III–4, III–7, III–27, and III–67

The tympanic cavity contains three small, movable bones: the *malleus*, or hammer; the *incus*, or anvil; and the *stapes*, or stirrup.

The auditory ossicles extend like a chain across the tympanic cavity to connect functionally the tympanic membrane with the vestibular (oval) window. The outermost ossicle is the malleus, firmly attached to the tympanic membrane; the innermost, the stapes, is fixed in the vestibular window and is in direct contact with the fluid perilymph of the internal ear; intermediate between the other two lies the incus. The three bones are bound together by articulations, and they also effect ligamentous connections with the walls of the containing cavity. This compound osseous system acts like a bent lever to convert the vibrations of the tympanic membrane into intensified thrusts of the stapes against the perilymph.

MALLEUS

Figure III–26b to d

The *malleus*, or hammer, is the largest of the auditory ossicles. It lies farthest laterally and forward. Its upper part, the *head* (capitulum mallei), occupies the recessus epitympanicus. This part of the malleus is thick and club-shaped and presents on its posterior and medial surfaces an elongated saddle-shaped articular surface for the body of the incus, which encroaches below upon a toothlike process, *tooth* or *cog of the hammer*. The head is separated by a constriction, the *neck* (collum mallei), from the *handle of the hammer* (manubrium mallei). The latter is a thin, bony rod, oval in cross section, which tapers off toward the tip, where it terminates in the form of a spatula. On the lateral margin it is covered by cartilage; the lateral surface gives rise to the *stria mallearis* and is covered medially by the mucous membrane of the tympanic cavity. The handle forms an angle of about 130 degrees with the head of the hammer. Its angle with the horizontal plane varies also, and amounts on the average on the right to about 50 degrees, on the left to 45 degrees. Above and to the lateral side, the handle of the hammer is continued into the small, tapered *lateral process* (processus lateralis), which produces a bulging of the tympanic membrane. From the anterior surface of the neck a thin *anterior process* (processus anterior) passes forward.

INCUS

Figure III–26b, c

The *incus*, or anvil, has approximately the configuration of a tooth with two roots. To the crown of the tooth corresponds the flattened *body* (corpus incudis). On its free basis the incus presents a saddle-shaped articular surface which encroaches somewhat upon a ridge on the lateral surface, the *tooth* or *cog of the anvil*, that serves for the reception of the head of the hammer. The *short leg* (crus breve) and *long leg* (crus longum) correspond to the roots of a tooth. The short leg is the thicker of the two; both taper toward their tips and diverge from one another, forming an angle of about 100 degrees. The short leg is directed horizontally backward; its tip is covered with cartilage and lies in the fossa incudis. The long one runs parallel to the manubrium of the malleus and lies somewhat medially and dorsally from it. On the medial side of the tip of the long leg is a *small process* (processus lenticularis).

STAPES

Figures III–24, III–25, and III–26a

The *stapes*, or stirrup, lies farthest medially. It possesses a *footplate* (basis stapedis), two *legs* (crus anterius and crus posterius), and a small *head* (capitulum stapedis). The footplate fills the vestibular fenestra (or oval window) almost completely. It is flat and possesses an upper convex and a lower straight or slightly concave margin. The two legs are hollowed on their concave side in groovelike fashion and are of approximately equal length; the anterior crus is finer than the posterior crus and less markedly curved (hence, the terms curvilineum and rectilineum, respectively). The posterior crus possesses near the head a small rough area for the insertion of the stapedius tendon. A thin connective tissue membrane (membrana obturatoria stapedis) is occasionally stretched out between the crura and the base. The head of the ossicle is variable in form and size. The lateral free end presents a small convex surface, covered with cartilage, for articulation with the lenticular process of the incus. The plane of the stirrup is approximately horizontal.

Ossicular Ligaments and Muscles

Figures III–27 to III–29

The manubrium and lateral process of the malleus are embedded in the tympanic membrane. The head of the malleus bears an elliptic articular surface on its posterior side; the margin of this is bound to the body of the incus by a thin capsular ligament, forming a diarthrodial joint known as the *incudomallear articulation* (articulatio incudomallearis). From the inner surface of the capsular ligament a wedge-shaped circular rim projects into the joint cavity and incompletely divides it. The long limb of the incus lies parallel to the superior and medial aspect of the manubrium of the malleus and ends in the lenticular process. The convex extremity of this process fits into the concavity on the head of the stapes, thereby creating a diarthrodial joint, the *incudostapedial articulation* (articulatio incudostapedia). From this connection with the incus the stapes passes across the tympanic cavity to its junction with the wall of the labyrinth. The cartilage-covered edge of the stapedial base is bound to the cartilage-covered rim of the vestibular window by the annular ligament of the base of the stapes, thus constituting the *tympanostapedial syndesmosis* (syndesmosis tympanostapedia).

In addition to the attachment of the manubrium of the malleus and the base of the stapes to the walls of the tympanic cavity, the bones have additional ligamentous attachments. The *superior malleal ligament* (lig. mallei superius) descends almost vertically from the roof of the epitympanic recess to the head of the malleus. The *anterior malleal ligament* (lig. mallei anterius) extends from the angular spine of the sphenoid bone through the petrotympanic (Glaserian) fissure to the anterior, or long, process of the malleus which it surrounds; the actual insertion is into the neck of the malleus. The *lateral malleal ligament* (lig. mallei laterale) is short and thick, connecting the margins of the tympanic notch with the neck of the malleus. The *posterior incudal ligament* (lig. incudis posterius) is little more than a fold of mucous membrane that descends from the tympanic roof to the body of the incus. The *annular ligament of the stapedial base* (lig. anulare stapedis) is a ring of elastic fibers encircling the base of the stapes and uniting it to the rim of the vestibular window.

Each of the two muscles of the ossicles is contained within a bony canal. The *tensor tympani muscle* is a penniform muscle about 2 cm. long. It arises from the cartilaginous part of the auditory tube, from the adjacent part of the great wing of the sphenoid bone, and from the bony walls of the *semicanal* (semicanalis m. tensoris tympani) that encloses it. It ends in a round tendon that turns almost at right angles over the cochleariform process and passes laterally across the tympanic cavity to be attached to the manubrium of the malleus near its neck. This muscle serves to draw the manubrium medially and thus tighten the tympanic membrane; it is supplied by the trigeminal nerve through the tensor tympani branch from the otic ganglion. The *stapedius muscle,* smallest of all skeletal muscles, arises in the interior of the hollow pyramidal eminence and from a sulcus in the wall of the facial canal. Its tendon escapes through the opening at the apex and then turns anteriorly to insert on the posterior surface of the neck and posterior crus of the stapes. The muscle draws laterally the anterior border of the base of the stapes; it is innervated by the stapedial branch of the facial nerve.

AUDITORY TUBE

Figures III–7, III–11, III–18, III–64a, and III–65d

The *auditory tube* (tuba auditiva), or eustachian tube, extends from the *tympanic ostium* (ostium tympanicum tubae auditivae) on the carotid (anterior) wall of the tympanic cavity inferiorly to reach the pharynx. In the course of this descent it also inclines medially and anteriorly. The entire tube is about 37 mm. long. In the lateral (or tympanic) one-third of its length it has a bony wall that constitutes a *semicanal* (semicanalis tubae auditivae); in the medial (or pharyngeal) two-thirds the wall is cartilaginous.

The *osseous portion* (pars ossea tubae auditivae) begins at the tympanic ostium on the anterior wall of the tympanic cavity. Superiorly a thin *septum* (septum canalis musculotubarii) alone separates the lumen from the tensor tympani muscle; the medial wall is in relation with the carotid canal. The irregularly triangular lumen gradually contracts toward the jagged anteromedial extremity of the bony tube; this is the narrowest point in the entire auditory tube and is named the *isthmus* (isthmus tubae auditivae).

The *cartilaginous portion* (pars cartilaginae tubae auditivae) is firmly attached to the osseous segment and lies in a sulcus at the base of the angular spine of the sphenoid bone. It expands gradually in its passage toward the lateral wall of the pharynx, where its opening, the *pharyngeal orifice* (ostium pharyngeum tubae auditivae), is situated just posterior to the inferior nasal concha and in front of the lateral pharyngeal recess (Rosenmüller). The walls of the cartilaginous portion are supported chiefly by the *tubal cartilage* (cartilago tubae auditivae) in the form of a plate that is folded so as to make a troughlike structure; this consists of a broad *medial lamina* (lamina medialis) and a narrower *lateral lamina* (lamina lateralis), completed laterally and inferiorly by a *membranous lamina* (lamina membranacea) of connective tissue.

The lining of the auditory tube is a *mucous membrane* (tunica mucosa) continuous with that of the tympanic cavity at one end, and with that of the nasopharynx at the other extremity. The epithelium is ciliated, varying in type from simple columnar at the tympanic end to pseudostratified as the pharynx is approached. The mucosal lining of the osseous portion is thin and firmly attached to the bony supporting wall. In the cartilaginous portion the mucosa becomes thicker, looser, and folded; here it contains *mucous glands* (gl. mucosae). They are especially abundant near the pharynx, where there is also lymphoid tissue aggregated into *lymph nodules* (noduli lymphatici tubarii). The walls are in contact except during swallowing, yawning, and sneezing, when they are opened by the tensor veli palatini muscle.

The Internal Ear

Figure III–1

The *internal ear* (auris interna), located within the petrous part of the temporal bone, receives the terminations of the cochlear and vestibular divisions of the acoustic nerve and is the essential part of the organs of hearing and equilibrium. It consists of three main parts: the endolymphatic (membranous) labyrinth; the perilymphatic (osseous) labyrinth; and the surrounding otic capsule.

MEMBRANOUS LABYRINTH

Figures III–14, III–15, III–40 to III–46a, III–47, and III–48

The *membranous labyrinth* (labyrinthus membranaceus) is a system of epithelial spaces and tubes filled with a clear fluid, the endolymph (Scarpa's fluid). It is for the most part surrounded by the *perilymphatic labyrinth* (spatium perilymphaticum) and its supporting connective tissue. Both labyrinths lie within the so-called *bony labyrinth* (labyrinthus osseus) of the otic capsule.

The main parts of the membranous labyrinth are the cochlear duct, the utricle, three semicircular ducts and their ampullae, the saccule, and the endolymphatic duct and sac. Smaller connecting channels are the utricular duct, the saccular duct, and the ductus reuniens.

These lesser channels, like the endolymphatic duct (with which they communicate directly or indirectly), possess special features of configuration that require modification of the familiar conventionalized descriptions and stylized illustrations: the proximal segment of the endolymphatic duct, enlarged to sinus-like form, is continued as the less capacious duct into the saccule; the excessively fine ductus reuniens, in passing from the saccule into the cochlear part of the labyrinth, joins the cul-de-sac (or cecal chamber) of the cochlear duct where the wall is closely related to a corresponding bay of the perilymphatic scala; the endolymphatic duct, in communicating with the utricle, does so through a slitlike orifice guarded by a fold of the utricular wall.

The *cochlear duct* (ductus cochlearis) and the *semicircular ducts* (ductus semicirculares) follow quite closely the configuration of the similarly named bony canals. On the other hand, the membranous components of the vestibule do not preserve so faithfully the form of the containing cavity; instead, they are fashioned into two sacs, the *utricle* (utriculus) and *saccule* (sacculus). These latter connect indirectly with each other and also with the cochlear and semicircular ducts. The membranous labyrinth is filled with a fluid, the *endolymph* (endolympha), wholly separate from the perilymph; the arborizations of the acoustic nerve terminate in the internal lining of this epithelial duct system.

UTRICLE

Figures III–50 to III–53b, c, and III–58

The *utricle* is an ovoid, slightly flattened sac whose rounded end occupies the elliptical recess in the superoposterior region of the vestibule. Here it is attached firmly by connective tissue and by entering filaments from the utricular branch of the vestibular division of the acoustic nerve. Anteriorly and laterally an oval, thickened area, the *macula acustica utriculi*, marks the region of the utricular sense organ. On the posterior wall are the openings of the semicircular ducts, and on the anterior wall is a slender tube, the *utriculosaccular duct* (ductus utriculosaccularis), which communicates with the saccule.

SACCULE

Figures III–50 to III–53c

The *saccule* is also ovoid, but is smaller than the utricle. It lies in the anterior and inferior part of the vestibule, bound to the spherical recess by fibrous tissue and by the saccular branch of the vestibular division of the acoustic nerve. An oval thickening occurs anteriorly where the saccular nerve filaments end in the *macula sacculi.*

At its inferior surface the saccule passes into the short, extremely slender tube, the *ductus reuniens*, which connects with the cochlear duct. Posteriorly the saccule gives off the utriculosaccular duct already mentioned. At an angle along this canal the slender *endolymphatic duct* (ductus endolymphaticus) arises to extend through the vestibular aqueduct and reach the posterior surface of the petrous part of the temporal bone; here it ends in a dilated, relatively capacious pouch, the *endolymphatic sac* (saccus endolymphaticus), situated within the cranial meningeal tissue.

ENDOLYMPHATIC DUCT AND SAC

Figures III–41, III–44, III–60 to III–62, III–104, III–105, III–107, and III–108

The *endolymphatic duct* (ductus endolymphaticus) lies within a bony canal, the *vestibular aqueduct* (aqueductus vestibuli), and is immediately surrounded, through the greater part of its length, by a loosely textured connective tissue that is continuous with the periosteum; however, at its proximal (utricular) extremity, the duct is within the perilymphatic labyrinth, where the internal aperture of the aqueduct arises from the vestibule. The distal end of the duct is continuous with the *endolymphatic sac* (saccus endolymphaticus), part of which lies in a fovea on the posterior surface of the petrous part of the temporal bone between the layers of the cranial dura mater. At the inner end of the vestibular aqueduct the endolymphatic duct enters the vestibule, where it unites with two ducts that meet it like the arms of the letter Y. One of these, the utricular duct, opens into the utricle; the other, the saccular duct, opens into the saccule. In earlier literature the term *utriculosaccular* was applied to these two connecting ducts.

The expanded part of the duct which lies chiefly within the vestibule may be termed the *sinus*. The next, or intermediate, segment of the duct which passes through the narrow part of the vestibular aqueduct is correspondingly constricted and could appropriately be named the isthmus. The duct system widens again to become the sac.

The type of lining epithelium of the ducts varies regionally from cuboidal to flattened. In the sinus and occasionally in the isthmus, the epithelium is generally columnar.

The *endolymphatic sac* (saccus endolymphaticus) is the terminal enlargement of the duct. Two regions of the sac are now recognized; *viz.*, the proximal or rugose portion, and a distal or smooth portion. The proximal part is characterized by an irregular lumen, owing to the presence of numerous folds of the lining epithelium. The sac lies for the most part in the funnel-shaped cranial portion of the aqueduct, but a part of the rugose portion and the remainder of the sac extend between the periosteal part of the dura and the dura proper. The connective tissue in which the rugose segment of the sac is lodged is more loosely textured and more vascular than that which surrounds the smooth portion.

The histologic structure of the endolymphatic sac varies with the individual and also with age. The lining is mostly a cuboidal epithelium. The cells are usually somewhat taller in the rugose portions. The greatest variation occurs in the form of the lumen; in some cases it is completely open, in others the epithelial walls are locally contiguous or even adherent. In sections this feature causes the lumen to have the appearance of discontinuous vacuolated spaces.

The sac is a gross structure, not a miniature expansion of a duct. It may be quite readily inflated or injected by a syringe inserted into the cranial dura mater, most advantageously where the dural layer is carried over the osseous crest of the external aperture of the vestibular aqueduct. Distended in this way, the sac may have a width of 1 cm. or more.

SEMICIRCULAR DUCTS

Figures III–53a; III–54a, b, c, e, f; III–58; and III–59

Three membranous tubes open into the utricle by five orifices. They run within the bony semicircular canals and resemble them in name, number, shape, and position. However, each *semicircular duct* (ductus semicircularis) is less than one-third the diameter of the containing bony canal, from which it is separated by a large perilymphatic space, except at a line of attachment along the greater curvature. Each *membranous ampulla* (ampulla membranacea) bears on its attached surface an external transverse groove, the *ampullary groove* (sulcus ampullaris), for the entrance of the ampullary branch of the vestibular division of the acoustic nerve; corresponding to the sulcus internally there is a ridge, the *ampullary crest* (crista ampullaris), which projects into the lumen and receives the nerve endings.

COCHLEAR DUCT

Figures III–52, III–54d, III–55, and III–56

This spirally coiled tube lies within the bony cochlea and is attached to its outer wall. The *cochlear duct* (ductus cochlearis) begins as a blind pouch, cul-de-sac, or the *vestibular cecum* (caecum vestibulare), which occupies the cochlear recess of the vestibule. The epithelial duct, following the spiral canal of the bony cochlea, makes a basal, middle, and incomplete apical turn, then ends blindly just beyond the hamulus of the spiral lamina in a second blind pouch named the *cupular cecum* (caecum cupulare). This projection helps to form the *helicotrema.* Close to the vestibular cecum the cochlear duct is continuous with the saccule through the *ductus reuniens* as a small-calibered intermediary.

The cochlear duct is an epithelium-lined tube, somewhat triangular in transverse section. Its floor is formed partly by thickened periosteum, overlying the peripheral part of the bony lamina spiralis; this tissue continues as a fibrous *basilar membrane* (lamina basilaris), reaching from the free border of the spiral lamina to the periosteum that lines the peripheral wall of the osseous cochlear canal. The epithelium of the cochlear floor is greatly elevated and specialized, constituting the complicated *spiral organ* (organum spirale) *of Corti* in which the fibers of the cochlear nerve terminate and constitute the peripheral sense organ of hearing. The peripheral supporting wall of the cochlear duct is supplied by the thickened periosteum of the outer wall of the bony cochlear canal; this is designated as the *spiral ligament of the cochlea* (lig. spirale cochleae). The third wall, or roof, is a thin *vestibular membrane* (paries vestibularis ductus cochlearis) that passes unsupported from the spiral ligament to the osseous spiral lamina near its free margin, forming with the latter an angle of 45 degrees.[1]

The cochlear duct and the bony spiral lamina divide the entire cochlear canal into an upper perilymphatic passage, the *scala vestibuli*, and a lower passage, the *scala tympani*. The two scalae unite apically at the *helicotrema* where the cochlear duct comes to an end.

The cul-de-sac of the cochlear duct is closely related to the corresponding prolongation of the scala tympani, the two being separated by the thin basilar membrane; they lie in intermediate position between the fossula of the cochlear fenestra and the vestibule of the inner ear. In progression from without inward, from the fossular bay of the general tympanic cavity to the vestibular part of the perilymphatic labyrinth, a series of four spaces is produced by the successive interposition of three membranes.

Structure of the Utricle, Saccule, Semicircular Ducts, and Cochlear Duct

Figures III–54a, b and III–55 to III–59

The walls of the utricle, saccule, and semicircular ducts consist of three layers. Externally there is loose connective tissue containing blood vessels and pigment cells and bordering upon the perilymphatic spaces. The intermediate layer is an ordinary basement membrane; the internal lining is mostly a simple, low epithelium. At the maculae and cristae all three layers are thickened to produce the elevations characteristic of these regions. Here the epithelium elongates to the columnar type in which slender *supporting cells* and flask-shaped, sensory *hair cells* intermingle. Between and upon the projecting hairs is a gelatinous membrane, which in the utricle and saccule contains superficially a mass of minute calcareous granules, the *otoconia*. Branches consisting of naked axis cylinders of the vestibular division of the acoustic nerve form basketlike terminations about the hair cells.

The *vestibular membrane* (membrana vestibularis) is only 0.003 mm. thick. It consists of a middle layer of connective tissue, bordered on each free surface by thin epithelium. The lateral wall of the cochlear duct is supported by thickened and altered periosteum. This so-called *spiral ligament* (lig. spirale cochleae) contains many blood vessels in its upper portion (i.e., nearer the junction with the vestibular membrane), and these extend even into the irregular pseudostratified epithelium that clothes it. Accordingly, this highly vascular region is designated as the *vascular stripe* (stria vascularis).

---

[1] It should be noted that the concept of a cochlear chamber possessing roof and floor represents an artistic liberty growing out of the convenience of placing illustrations of the elongate spiral organ in a horizontal position on a page. In the standing position the modiolus lies in the horizontal plane, whereupon the "floor" becomes a medial wall.

The floor of the cochlear duct is the most highly specialized of all. On the side of the scala tympani the periosteum of the osseous spiral lamina is continued past the lamina itself and, as the fibrous *basilar membrane* (lamina basilaris), stretches to the spiral ligament of the lateral wall. On the side next to the lumen of the duct the periosteum is thicker, forming the *border of the osseous spiral lamina* (limbus laminae spiralis osseae) which serves for the attachment of the *tectorial membrane* (membrane tectoria). The latter is a delicate, flexible, gelatinous membrane overlying the rest of the sensory receptive mechanism; it is an epithelial derivative, cuticular in nature. The *spiral organ of Corti* (organum spirale) is the highly specialized epithelial apparatus that is affected by sound. It is an elevated epithelial band, placed upon the basilar membrane and extending the full length of the cochlear duct. The organization of the spiral organ is complex; it consists of inert *supporting cells* and shorter *hair cells*. The supporting cells are all tall, slender elements, extending from the basilar membrane to the free surface. Conspicuous are the pillar cells which bound the central *tunnel*, an axial canal throughout the whole length of the organ. The two groups of hair cells, inner and outer according to their relation to the tunnel, are short cylinders with rounded bases reaching scarcely halfway to the basilar membrane; their free ends bear numerous stiff cilia. Nerve fibers from the cochlear division of the acoustic nerve take a complex course, but their terminal branches finally embrace the bodies of hair cells. These specialized, neuroepithelial cells are the receptor elements of sound waves.

Vestibulocochlear (VIII) Nerve

Figures III–45a, III–47b, III–51, III–53, III–69a, and III–70

The *nerve* of the membranous labyrinth, the vestibulocochlear, divides into two parts. The vestibular nerve arises from cells of the vestibular ganglion situated at the bottom of the internal acoustic meatus; its fibers are distributed in two rami to the maculae of the utricle and saccule and to the ampullae of the semicircular ducts. Contained in the spiral canal of the modiolus is the spiral ganglion of the cochlear nerve; its peripheral fibers pass from the modiolus through the spiral lamina to reach the hair cells in the organ of Corti about which the fibers arborize.

Areas of Fundus of Internal Acoustic Meatus

Figures III–106, III–133, and III–134

The floor of the acoustic canal is closed by a plate of bone which serves, on its opposite side, as the medial wall of the vestibule and the cochlea.

The *fundus of the internal acoustic meatus* (fundus meatus acustici interni) is divided into upper and lower portions by a sharp horizontal ridge, the *transverse crest.*

In an anterior depression in the upper, smaller area of the fundus is situated the internal opening of the facial canal; and a posterior, funnel-shaped depression, the *superior vestibular area,* contains several small openings of canals that conduct branches of the upper terminal ramus of the vestibular nerve to the *superior cribrose macula* (macula cribrosa superior) of the vestibule.

Anteriorly the lower, larger area presents a rounded depression, the *cochlear area;* here begins a spiral band of small openings, the *spiral tract of foramina.* Its curve matches that of the cochlea. The orifices transmit the bundles of the cochlear nerve directly to the basal turn or through the *longitudinal modiolar canals* to the middle and apical turns. In the posterior part of the same area, closely adjacent to the transverse crest, lies a zone with small openings, the *inferior vestibular area,* for transmission of fibers to the *middle cribrose macula* (macula cribrosa media) of the vestibule. Medialward from this area is situated a single larger opening, the *singular foramen* (foramen singulare) by which the posterior ampullary nerve passes to the *inferior cribrose macula* (macula cribrosa inferior).

Within the vestibule the utricle lies in the *elliptical recess*; its *acoustic macula* (macula acustica utriculi) is supplied by the utricular nerve, which emerges from the *superior cribrose macula* (macula cribrosa superior). The saccule is lodged in the *spherical recess* of the vestibule; fibers of the saccular nerve reach its *acoustic macula* (macula acustica sacculi) from the macula cribrosa media.

On the anterior wall of the *posterior osseous ampulla* (ampulla ossea posterior) is a small perforated area, the *inferior cribrose macula* (macula cribrosa inferior); it contains openings of small canals that begin in the *singular foramen* (foramen singulare) and through which the *posterior ampullary nerve* reaches the vestibule on the way to the ampulla of the semicircular duct.

Facial (VII) Nerve and Canal

Figures III–63, III–67 to III–85, III–132, III–135, and III–136

At the fundus of the internal acoustic meatus the facial nerve separates from the acoustic, thereupon entering its own *facial canal* (aqueductus fallopii) in the petrous portion of the temporal bone. Within the substance of the bone it first courses lateralward in the region between the cochlea and the semicircular canals. As the nerve approaches the tympanic cavity, it makes an abrupt bend posteriorly, running in the medial wall of the cavity immediately above the vestibular (oval) window. Then the nerve dips downward, adjacent to the mastoid air cells, to emerge at the stylomastoid foramen. Where the nerve changes its course abruptly, there occurs an exaggeration of the bend in a **U**-shaped structure, the *knee* (geniculum n. facialis). The swelling is the *geniculate* *ganglion* (ganglion geniculi). Not infrequently the facial canal is incomplete. In such cases of dehiscence the nerve is exposed.

Chorda Tympani and Canaliculus

Figures III–64 and III–65

The chorda tympani takes origin from the facial nerve either within the facial canal or before the nerve enters the stylomastoid foramen. Upon emergence from the *iter chordae posterius*, the nerve crosses to the opposite side of the tympanic cavity at the *iter chordae anterius*. In this course it is invested by mucous membrane, either in the malleal folds or in the tympanic membrane.

Variations occur, especially in the nature of the canaliculus through which the chorda tympani ascends through the bone to reach the posterior iter. The canaliculus may be totally independent of the facial canal. But whether the proximal division of the course be typical or atypical, emergence of the chorda from its canaliculus occurs at the posterior iter.

Invested by mucous membrane, the chorda tympani crosses between the long crus of the incus and the manubrium of the malleus. It passes along the anterior process of the malleus toward the aperture of the petrotympanic (Glaserian) fissure through the anterior and posterior malleal ligaments.

The chorda tympani leaves the tympanic cavity through the *iter chordae anterius* (canal of Huguier), thereupon entering the petrotympanic fissure. Through this fissure it descends to the mandibular fossa (the latter being divided by the fissure). The sensory fibers supply the anterior two-thirds of the tongue.

OSSEOUS LABYRINTH[1]

Figures III–45, III–46b, III–86, and III–87

The *bony labyrinth* (labyrinthus osseus) is about 2 cm. long. The osseous matrix bordering the cavities is harder than the rest of the petrous bone; this difference in texture makes it possible, in the fetus

[1] The terminology employed in describing the internal ear is both inadequate and misleading. The term *osseous labyrinth* is inappropriate, since its use fallaciously implies that a bony wall may be shelled away, as an independent investment for the system of continuous labyrinthic spaces which contain the perilymph. This is not possible in the temporal bone after it has assumed adult consistency—which it actually does in the fetus. Thereupon the bone of the primordial bony capsule fuses with the compact periosteal bone surrounding it.

Now, were the term *otic labyrinth* used for the ectodermal epithelial tube system (as a substitute for membranous), the space between the otic labyrinth and the otic capsule would become *periotic labyrinth*.

The name otic labyrinth would have logical appeal, on the basis of its derivation from the otic vesicle, the latter in turn differentiated from the otocyst. The names *otic fluid*, *periotic fluid*, and *periotic tissue* would be equally logical, as would *otic duct* and *otic sac* (replacing endolymphatic duct and endolymphatic sac, respectively). The term endolymphatic would then become an inclusive name, applied to the whole system of epithelium-lined labyrinthic channels.

This revision has been suggested by the senior author to the International Anatomical Nomenclature Committee.

and in the young infant, to separate away this most internal part of the labyrinth as a bony shell. The entire shell is the primitive otic capsule. There are three incompletely divided, component regions: the *vestibule* (vestibulum), the *semicircular canals* (canales semicirculares ossei), and the *cochlea*. The entire bony labyrinth is lined with thin periosteum which, in turn, is surfaced internally with a delicate epithelioid layer; it contains a fluid—*perilymph*—that surrounds the smaller, membranous labyrinth.

The perilymphatic labyrinth lies within the petrous part of the temporal bone. The labyrinthic wall is the medial boundary of the tympanic cavity. On the medial side is the fundus of the internal acoustic meatus. The labyrinth is surrounded by a very hard layer of bone 2 to 3 mm. thick, the bony labyrinthine capsule. In the fetus and in the newborn the capsular bone reaches the surface of the pars petrosa in some places; in other places it is separated by spongy bone substance from the remainder of the bony mass of the pyramid of the temporal bone. In the adult temporal bone the capsular bone is in large part fused with the compact bony substance of the neighborhood. The labyrinth is approximately 20 mm. in length; it lies approximately parallel to the posterior surface of the pyramid of the temporal bone. The base of the cochlea, adjoining the internal acoustic meatus, is directed parallel to the plane of the posterior semicircular canal. This canal and the meatus form an angle of 45 degrees with the median plane; so also does the plane of the superior semicircular canal, which stands perpendicular to both. The internal acoustic meatus is directed horizontally and frontally.

VESTIBULE

Figures III–13 to III–15, III–45, III–52, III–57, III–69a, III–91a, III–93a, and III–122

The bony *vestibule* (vestibulum) is an ovoid, central chamber about 4 mm. in diameter. It is the most capacious part of the labyrinth. Anteroinferiorly the vestibule leads into the cochlea; posterosuperiorly it receives the ends of the semicircular canals. Although for the most part free of remnants of the primordial reticulum, some strands of connective tissue cross the perilymphatic space to the outer wall of the utricle and saccule. These periotic bands support small blood vessels.

The interior of the vestibular wall shows depressions and ridges that correspond to definite parts of the contained membranous labyrinth. Superiorly and posteriorly on the medial wall is the *elliptical recess* (recessus ellipticus) for the utricle; inferiorly and anteriorly occurs the *spherical recess* (recessus sphericus) which accommodates the saccule. Between these two hollows is an oblique ridge, the *vestibular crest* (crista vestibuli) that divides posteriorly into two limbs bounding a small depression; this concavity is the *cochlear recess* (recessus cochlearis), which lodges the blind beginning of the cochlear duct or scala media of the older terminology.

There are also definite openings in the bony wall. Tiny grouped foramina, the *cribrose maculae* (sieve areas), accommodate the nerves entering to supply the several sensory fields of this central labyrinthine region. A larger aperture opens into the *vestibular aqueduct* (aqueductus vestibuli), which transmits the endolymphatic duct. Still larger apertures serve as openings of the semicircular canals and as a communication with the cochlea. On the lateral wall, next to the tympanic cavity occurs the *vestibular window* (fenestra vestibuli or oval window) which is closed by the base of the stapes.

SEMICIRCULAR CANALS

Figures III–53a; III–54a, b, c, e, f; III–58; III–59a; III–104; III–106; and III–109

There are three *osseous semicircular canals* (canales semicirculares ossei) superoposterior to the vestibule. Each describes about two-thirds of a circle and lies at right angles to the other two; this makes the relation of their planes like the three adjoining sides about the corner of a cube. The bony canals measure about 1 mm. in diameter, but at one end each becomes dilated into an *osseous ampulla* (ampullae osseae) twice as large. The canals open into the vestibule by five (instead of six) apertures, since in one instance a single orifice serves for two fused canals.

The *superior* and *posterior semicircular canals* (canales semicirculares superior et posterior) lie in nearly vertical planes, the right angle included between them opening laterally. The anterolateral end of the superior canal and the inferior end of the posterior canal are ampullated. The other extremities of these two canals join to form the *common limb* (crus commune) which opens into the vestibule by a single orifice. The *lateral semicircular canal* (canalis semicircularis lateralis) bows in the horizontal plane and is the shortest of the three; its ampulla lies close to that of the superior canal. The lateral canal occupies the same plane as its mate of the other ear, whereas the superior canal of one ear is parallel to the posterior canal of the other.

COCHLEA

Figures III–52; III–53c; III–54c, d; III–55; III–69a; III–70; III–86; and III–87a

The bony cochlea resembles a snail shell, from which the name is taken. In form the cochlea is conical, its *base* (basis cochleae) lying upon the internal acoustic meatus and its apex, or *cupula*, directly anteriorly and laterally. The base measures 9 mm., while the axial height is 5 mm. Most of the cochlea consists of the *spiral cochlear canal* (canalis spiralis cochleae). This is a spiral tube over 30 mm. long, coursing through nearly two and three-quarters turns about a central bony axis, or *modiolus*. Projecting outward from the modiolus is a thin, bony plate, the *osseous spiral lamina* (lamina spiralis ossea); it winds about the modiolus like the flanged thread of a screw and ends apically in the hooklike *hamulus*. In this manner the cochlear canal is partially subdivided into an upper passage, the *vestibular staircase* (scala vestibuli), and a lower passage, the *tympanic staircase* (scala tympani). The two scalae join apically at the *helicotrema*, where the partitioning spiral lamina ends freely at the *hook* (hamulus laminae spiralis).

The base of the cochlea corresponds to the *cochlear area* (area cochleae) at the bottom of the internal acoustic meatus. This area lies on the medial wall of the vestibule and contains the *spiral tract of foramina* (tractus tegmentalis centralis) for the passage of nerves to the cochlea. Nearby, other cribriform areas transmit nerves to the rest of the membranous labyrinth. The modiolus is a short, tapering column, which is tunneled by *longitudinal modiolar canals* (canales longitudinales modioli) and a *spiral modiolar canal* (canalis spiralis modioli); these serve for the conduction of both blood vessels and nerves.

The beginning of the bony cochlear canal presents three chief openings. One effects a connection with the vestibule; another, the *cochlear window* (fenestra cochleae or round window), leads to the tympanic cavity but is closed by the *secondary tympanic membrane*; the third is the orifice of the *cochlear canaliculus* (canaliculus cochleae) which, through its contained *perilymphatic duct*, establishes a communication between the scala tympani and the subarachnoid cavity. In addition, five appendages of the perilymphatic labyrinth call for consideration: the space around the proximal portion of the endolymphatic duct, the fissular tracts situated anterior and posterior to the vestibular fenestra, and the cul-de-sac of the scala tympani. These "Transcapsular Channels" are discussed individually, beginning page 186.

SCALA VESTIBULI

Figures III–45; III–52; III–54d; III–55; III–94b; and III–122a to c

The scala vestibuli is an extension of the vestibule along the anterior surface of the cochlear duct, or scala media. This space, like that of the vestibule, is largely free of trabeculae of the periotic connective tissue. The outer wall of the scala vestibuli consists of a mesenchymal epithelium whose delicate basement membrane is partly fused to the basement membrane of the epithelium on the anterior wall of the cochlear duct. This partition between the cavities of the two scalae is the *vestibular membrane* (Reissner). The remainder of this wall lines the anterior surface of the osseous spiral lamina. At the tip, or *blind end* (caecum cupulare), of the cochlear duct the scala vestibuli communicates with the scala tympani, the point of union being the helicotrema.

SCALA TYMPANI

Figures III–45; III–52; III–54d; III–55; III–94b; and III–122 a to c

The scala tympani, like the scala vestibuli, is a fluid-filled space from which trabeculae of the periotic tissue are virtually absent. The scala lies along the posterior side of the cochlear duct and the spiral lamina, and extends from the helicotrema to the cochlear (round) window. The only point of communication with other portions of the perilymphatic labyrinth occurs at the helicotrema. The anterior wall of the scala tympani is partly fused to form the basilar membrane. Central to the cochlear duct the osseous spiral lamina separates the scala vestibuli and scala tympani.

OTIC CAPSULE

Figure III–88

The otic capsule, surrounding the labyrinths, belongs in a special category for the following reasons: it ossifies from numerous (fourteen or more) centers, thus differing from the other bones of the skull; its originally independent centers of ossification fuse to form a protective shell for the organs of special sense—and do so with complete obliteration of suture lines; although the capsule is derived from cartilage, there remain no peripheral areas of chondral growth which would correspond to the epiphyseal and diaphyseal zones of a typical long bone (e.g., a femur); the osseous tissue of the constituent centers remains fetal in character, never being replaced by bone of familiar haversian pattern and texture; maximum dimensions are reached during the fifth month of intrauterine life. Despite the fact that morphogenesis proceeds with surprising speed, histogenesis lags, the capsular fabric changing slowly from the sixth fetal month to the first postnatal year. Some of the bone of the capsule is destined to be removed to make way for air spaces, the formation of which may be initiated in the late fetus.

STRUCTURE

In the ears of late fetuses and of all postnatal specimens, it is possible to distinguish, histologically, a line which separates the bone of the original otic capsule from the innermost of the incremental layers of periosteal bone. The addition of such periosteal layers, accompanied by concurrent fusion with adjacent squamous and occipital elements of the developing cranium, results in the incorporation of the otic capsule into the greater bulk of the so-called petrous part of the temporal bone. Actually, only the primordial capsule retains a relatively petrous fabric; the surrounding bone (and, in some instances, part of the capsule itself) is highly cancellous, through the presence of marrow spaces, or even more porous because of the widespread distribution of air cells.

These features of capsular architecture are readily distinguishable both in the formative and in the mature condition of the cochlea. Primitively, within each center of ossification, the middle layer consists of sparsely distributed trabeculae in a circumferential area where space outbulks bone. This relationship persists in later fetal stages. Even in the adult, the three layers remain identifiable.

Almost without exception, the adult temporal bone retains an opening on its posterior surface that is reminiscent of a crucial stage in the development of the otic capsule. This is the *subarcuate fossa* (fossa subarcuata). It is the route of invasion by vascular buds of connective tissue from the meninges.

As a result of their resorptive action, the cartilage of the canalicular division of the otic capsule becomes spongy, and expansion of the arcs of the semicircular canals is thereby permitted. The activity reaches its maximum in the 21-week fetus. The residual aperture in the adult assumes any one of a variety of forms. It transmits small branches from the internal auditory artery and the accompanying vein. Within the bone it is represented by the petromastoid canal.

Transcapsular Channels, Sulci, and Fenestrae

The otic capsule and the *pars petrosa* of which it is, so to speak, the labyrinthic core, is fundamentally a protective osseous box whose contributory centers of ossification fuse without sutural demarcation. However, it differs from a simple encasement in two very diverse ways: first, it opens to the exterior at two windows, oval and round, whose service is acoustic; second, it is crossed by channels or indented by sulci whose contained structures, in several instances, are of little or no service to the sense of hearing or balance. This means that the pyramid behaves as an anatomic king's highway for blood vessels and nerves whose destinations are in territories beyond the ear.

VESTIBULAR (OVAL) FENESTRA

Figures III–89, III–90, III–92, and III–93a

Anterolaterally, as seen in a macerated specimen, the vestibule opens into the tympanic cavity through the *vestibular (oval) window* (fenestra vestibuli), to the margin of which, in the fresh state, the base of the stapes is fastened by the annular ligament.

COCHLEAR (ROUND) FENESTRA

Figures III–89, III–92, III–93b to III–97, and III–109

The space situated anterior to the osseous spiral lamina, *i.e.*, the scala vestibuli, opens into the vestibule; that situated posterior to the lamina, *i.e.*, the scala tympani, ends blindly. In the macerated specimen the scala tympani opens into the tympanic cavity by means of the *cochlear (round) window* (fenestra cochleae), which, in the fresh state, is closed by the *secondary tympanic membrane* (membrana tympani secundaria) situated within the depths of the fossula of the cochlear window.

The membrane arises from the *crest of the cochlear window* (crista fenestrae cochleae). It is usually bulged slightly inward, into the tympanic scala. The lateral surface is covered by a continuation of the mucous membrane of the tympanic cavity. The medial surface is invested by the excessively thin periotic connective tissue.

VESTIBULAR AQUEDUCT

Figures III–98; III–100 c, d to III–106; and III–109 to III–118

In the area of the elliptical recess (for reception of the utricle) is found the internal aperture of the *vestibular aqueduct* (aqueductus vestibuli). This channel transmits the endolymphatic duct, which is surrounded only at its vestibular extremity by a short extension of the perilymphatic labyrinth.

COCHLEAR CANALICULUS

Figures III–98; III–100 a, b; III–101; III–109; and III–119 to III–122

The periotic, or perilymphatic, duct is not a true duct but a potential space containing an arachnoid type of connective tissue and fluid. It begins in the scala tympani, near the cochlear window, and terminates in a funnel-shaped aperture situated medial to the jugular fossa. This periotic channel lies within the cochlear canaliculus, where it is surrounded by the periosteum of the latter.

FISSULA ANTE FENESTRAM

Figures III–123a and III–124 to III–126

Considered as an appendage of the perilymphatic labyrinth, the fissula ante fenestram is a strip of periotic connective tissue extending from the vestibule just anterior to the vestibular window through an irregular, slitlike space in the bony otic capsule to the periosteum of the tympanic cavity near the pulley of the tensor tympani muscle. Interest is centered around the fissula because it is the predilective site for the formation of chondromatous nodules and otosclerotic bone.

FOSSULA POST FENESTRAM

Figure III–123b

The fossula post fenestram is an evagination of the periotic tissue into the otic capsule just posterior to the vestibular window at a point about one-third of the way between the window and nonampullated end of the lateral semicircular canal. Differing from the fissula, it occurs inconstantly and, when present, is likely to open only into the vestibule.

CUL-DE-SAC OF THE SCALA TYMPANI

Figures III–42, III–44a, and III–46

The vestibular cecum of the cochlear duct is a blind sac which projects for a short distance beyond the opening of the ductus reuniens into the vestibule, there to be lodged in the cochlear recess. Even more striking than this cecal prolongation, or cul-de-sac, is the larger and adjacent cul-de-sac of the scala tympani. This perilymphatic sacculation lies external to the osseous spiral lamina, between whose facing free margins it is separated from the cochlear duct (of the endolymphatic system of channels) by the basilar membrane.

SUBARCUATE FOSSA

Figures III–102, III–103b, III–111a, III–113a, III–115, III–127, and III–128

The subarcuate fossa is typically a small opening into the bone on the posterior surface of the pyramid, situated above and behind the opening of the internal acoustic meatus. It lies just below the superior angle of the petrous part of the temporal bone. It is relatively capacious in fetal stage and in the newborn, small in the adult. The fossa transmits offsets of the internal auditory artery and vein. It is highly variable in form, position and dimensions. It is sometimes continuous with elongate vascular sulci which reach the sigmoid sulcus or the superior petrosal sulcus.

The arteries that enter the fossa are sometimes large enough to be consequential features in surgery at the cerebellopontine angle.

CAROTID CANAL

Figures III–129 and III–132

The carotid canal traverses the petrous part of the temporal bone. It transmits the internal carotid artery and accompanying venous and neural plexuses. The canal begins at an external foramen on the inferior surface of the bone, just in front of the jugular foramen. The canal follows a curving course, passing upward and forward to an internal foramen situated near the apex of the bone.

In this course, the canal forms the anterior (or carotid) boundary of the tympanic cavity. It is regularly related to air cells which may reach relatively great size and appear in a variety of patterns.

JUGULAR FOSSA

Figures III–108c and III–130 to III–132

The jugular fossa, situated on the inferior surface of the pyramid posteromedial to the external carotid foramen, sometimes is separated from the posterior cranial fossa by a thin plate of bone. In some specimens the fossa is broadly continuous with the sigmoid sulcus. When the fossa is deep, the space of the tympanic cavity is correspondingly reduced When the "roof" of the fossa is dehiscent, nothing more substantial than mucous membrane would intervene between the bulbous vein and the tympanic cavity.

Blood and Nerve Supply

ARTERIES AND VEINS

Figures III–137 to III–141

The arteries to the middle and the internal ear are derived from branches of the subclavian and the external and internal carotid. As the branches approach the areas or structures that they or their rami will ultimately supply, there is a definite division between those destined chiefly for the tympanic cavity and its contents and the vessels to the neural elements of the membranous labyrinth and the bone of the enveloping wall. These may be discussed conveniently under headings of the arteries that ascend in the neck, there giving off branches that enter the following foramina, canals, or fissures: *foramen magnum*, stylomastoid foramen, petrosquamous fissure, petrotympanic fissure, jugular foramen, vestibular aqueduct, caroticotympanic canaliculi (in the carotid canal), tympanic canaliculus (in the *fossula petrosa*), hiatus of the facial canal, and the small openings that make up the subarcuate fossa.

In addition to these, the minute channel for transmission of the cochlear vein must be added (as it follows the general course of the cochlear canaliculus, but remains separate therefrom). Otherwise, the veins accompany arteries of the same name.

ANTERIOR AND MEDIAL SURFACES

The vertebral branch of the subclavian artery, upon leaving the transverse foramen in the atlas, enters the cranial cavity through the foramen magnum. It unites with the vessel of the opposite side to form the unpaired basilar artery. The internal auditory artery is a branch of either the basilar artery or the anterior inferior cerebellar artery. The internal auditory artery goes lateralward with the facial and vestibulocochlear nerves to course through the internal acoustic meatus to the cochlea. At the *porus* of the meatus a very small branch is sent to the subarcuate fossa for supply of the canalicular part of the petrous pyramid.

The external aperture of the vestibular aqueduct, situated posterior to the opening of the meatus, receives small vessels from the meningeal branch of the occipital artery. The latter is a branch of the external carotid; it ascends through the jugular foramen (with the vein) in dura mater of the posterior cranial fossa.

In a medial view of the temporal bone is also seen the petrosquamous fissure through which the superior tympanic branch of the middle meningeal artery reaches the bone. The middle meningeal, a branch of the maxillary (the latter from the external carotid), reaches the cranial cavity by passing through the foramen spinosum.

On the anterior surface of the petrous pyramid, near the apex, is seen the hiatus of the facial canal. In addition to the nerve, it transmits the superficial petrosal ramus of the middle meningeal artery. This vessel anastomoses with the stylomastoid branch of the posterior auricular.

Veins, additional to those accompanying the arteries of the same name, are received from the bone by the superior and inferior sulci and the sigmoid sulcus.

LATERAL SURFACE

The petrotympanic fissure transmits the anterior tympanic branch of the maxillary from the external division of the common carotid; upon reaching the middle ear, it ramifies in the mucous membrane and anastomoses with tympanic vessels of other sources.

INFERIOR SURFACE

In the wall of the carotid canal a small foramen (or foramina) of the caroticotympanic canaliculus transmits a similarly named artery into the middle ear. The branches anastomose on the promontory with those from the maxillary and middle meningeal artery.

The stylomastoid branch of the posterior auricular (from the external carotid) ascends through the facial canal to the canaliculus of the chorda tympani, through which it reaches the middle ear as the posterior tympanic artery. It anastomoses with the superficial petrosal branch of the middle meningeal.

The inferior tympanic branch of the ascending pharyngeal (the latter from the external carotid) passes the petrosal fossula and tympanic canaliculus into the middle ear, where its twigs contribute to the plexus on the promontory.

Those vessels are accompanied by corresponding veins. In addition, a separate vein from the cochlea, following the general course of the cochlear canaliculus, reaches the inferior surface of the pyramid between the jugular fossa and the carotid canal.

Most of the vessels are tympanic; they contribute to a plexus that is richest in the mucous membrane of the promontory. Some of these vessels give off branches to the auditory ossicles and to the tympanic membrane. Additionally, the outer and middle layers of bone on the labyrinthine wall of the tympanic cavity receive lesser supply.

External Ear

The arteries of supply to the auricle are branches of the posterior auricular and the superficial temporal vessels—both subdivisions of the external carotid artery. The veins are the anterior auricular tributaries of the temporal vein and the auricular branches of the posterior auricular vein. The latter vessels sometimes reach meningeal territory by joining the transverse sinus through the mastoid emissary vein.

The external acoustic meatus is supplied by the external carotid artery through branches from the posterior auricular, superficial temporal and deep auricular vessels. The veins connect with those of the auricle and drain similarly.

The arteries to the tympanic membrane occur in two sets, one on each surface. The two sets communicate through anastomoses. The cutaneous vessels arise from the deep auricular branch of the internal maxillary. The supply to the mucosal surface is from the anterior tympanic branch of the internal maxillary and from the styloid branch of the posterior auricular. The veins communicate with those of the external acoustic meatus and the tympanic cavity.

Middle Ear

The blood supply of the middle ear is relatively rich, numerous vessels course through the submucosal tissue, not only in the part which covers the walls of the tympanum, but also in that which invests the ossicles, the stapedial tendon, and the tensor tympani muscle. There is a paucity of vessels in the bone of the primordial otic capsule. However in the outer, periosteal layers of the *pars petrosa*, there are numerous vascular channels. The sparse periotic tissue in the vestibule forms several attenuate bridges which cross the space intervening between the osseous wall of the labyrinth and epithelium of the saccule and utricle. These serve as supports for small blood vessels. Similar tissue occurs in the semicircular canals. Special forms of vascular supply are found in the cochlea and in the vestibular aqueduct. In the former, the *stria vascularis* is richly provided with vessels; in the latter, the vessels occupy the areolar tissue of the rugae. The abundant blood vessels in the submucosal tissue of the wall of the labyrinth provide branches to the ossicles. Many of these pass first to the stapes by following the tendon of the stapedius muscle; then they send rami medialward toward the stapedial base, lateralward toward the head of the ossicle and to the incus and malleus. The supply is augmented by vessels which, after coursing through the facial canal, emerge therefrom through channels near the pyramidal eminence.

Most of the vessels for the stapes pass along the crura; few pass through a crus, by way of foramina, from one surface to the other. Upon reaching the base, they occupy channels in the thickened bone at the crurobasal junction, spreading therefrom circumferentially.

In the incus and malleus the pattern of vascularization differs from that in the stapes: because their structure is less profoundly altered in the course of prenatal development, they retain a more nearly typical scheme of internal blood supply than does the stapes. Some of the vascular spaces are located along the line of contact of the periosteal and endosteal layers of bone. From these channels, others pass to prominent intercommunicating channels inward, ultimately to a small, centrally located marrow cavity. The blood vessels that are carried to the incus and malleus by the mucosal septa enter each ossicle at openings in the periosteal layer at the site of attachment of these mesenterylike reflections of the mucous membrane.

Internal Ear

The *internal auditory artery*, a branch of the basilar artery, supplies the entire membranous labyrinth. This artery passes through the internal auditory meatus and then divides into three branches. The first of these branches, the *vestibular artery*, supplies the vestibular nerve and parts of the saccule, utricle, and semicircular ducts. The second branch, the *vestibulocochlear artery*, supplies the basal turn of the cochlea, the greater part of the saccule, the body of the utricle, the posterior semicircular duct, and parts of the lateral and superior semicircular ducts. The third, or terminal, branch is the *cochlear artery*. After entering the modiolus, it gives rise to the spiral arteries. The branches of the internal auditory artery, in addition to supplying the otic labyrinth, also vascularize the framework of the surrounding periotic labyrinth.

The venous drainage of the labyrinth is accomplished by three main veins and their tributaries. The first, the *internal auditory vein*, which drains the apical and middle turns of the cochlea, leaves the temporal bone by way of the internal acoustic meatus. The second, the so-called *vein of the cochlear aqueduct*, arises from capillaries at the basal turn of the cochlea, the saccule, and part of the utricle. It leaves the labyrinth near the internal aperture of the cochlear canaliculus, not occupying the connective tissue in the perilymphatic "duct." The vein is transmitted by a separate bony canal in the otic capsule; paralleling the cochlear aqueduct, it terminates in the inferior petrosal sinus. The third, the *vein of the vestibular aqueduct*, drains blood from the semicircular ducts and part of the utricle. This vein, accompanying the endolymphatic duct in its course through the bony vestibular aqueduct, reaches the dura mater where, together with the numerous small veins of the rich venous plexus which surrounds the endolymphatic sac, it opens into the lateral sinus.

NERVES

External Ear

The sensory nerves of the auricle are branches of the great auricular and small occipital nerves from the cervical plexus and auricular branch of the vagus. The muscles are supplied by the temporal and posterior auricular branches of the facial nerve.

The nerves to the external acoustic meatus are sensory branches from the auriculotemporal ramus of the mandibular nerve and from the auricular ramus of the vagus.

Middle Ear

The nerves of the middle ear accompany the vessels of supply (see above). They are derived chiefly from the auriculotemporal branch of the mandibular nerve; these fibers are supplemented by twigs from the auricular branch of the vagus and the tympanic branch of the glossopharyngeal.

Internal Ear

The nerve of the membranous labyrinth is the acoustic[1] (VIII cranial nerve). It divides into two parts, vestibular and cochlear. The vestibular nerve arises from cells of the vestibular ganglion situated at the bottom of the internal acoustic meatus. Its fibers are distributed in two rami to the maculae of the utricle and saccule and to the ampullae of the semicircular ducts. The spiral ganglion of the cochlear nerve is contained in the spiral canal of the modiolus. The peripheral fibers pass from the modiolus through the spiral lamina to reach the hair cells in the organ of Corti, about which they arborize.

---

[1] Modern term in the *Nomina Anatomica* is vestibulocochlear.

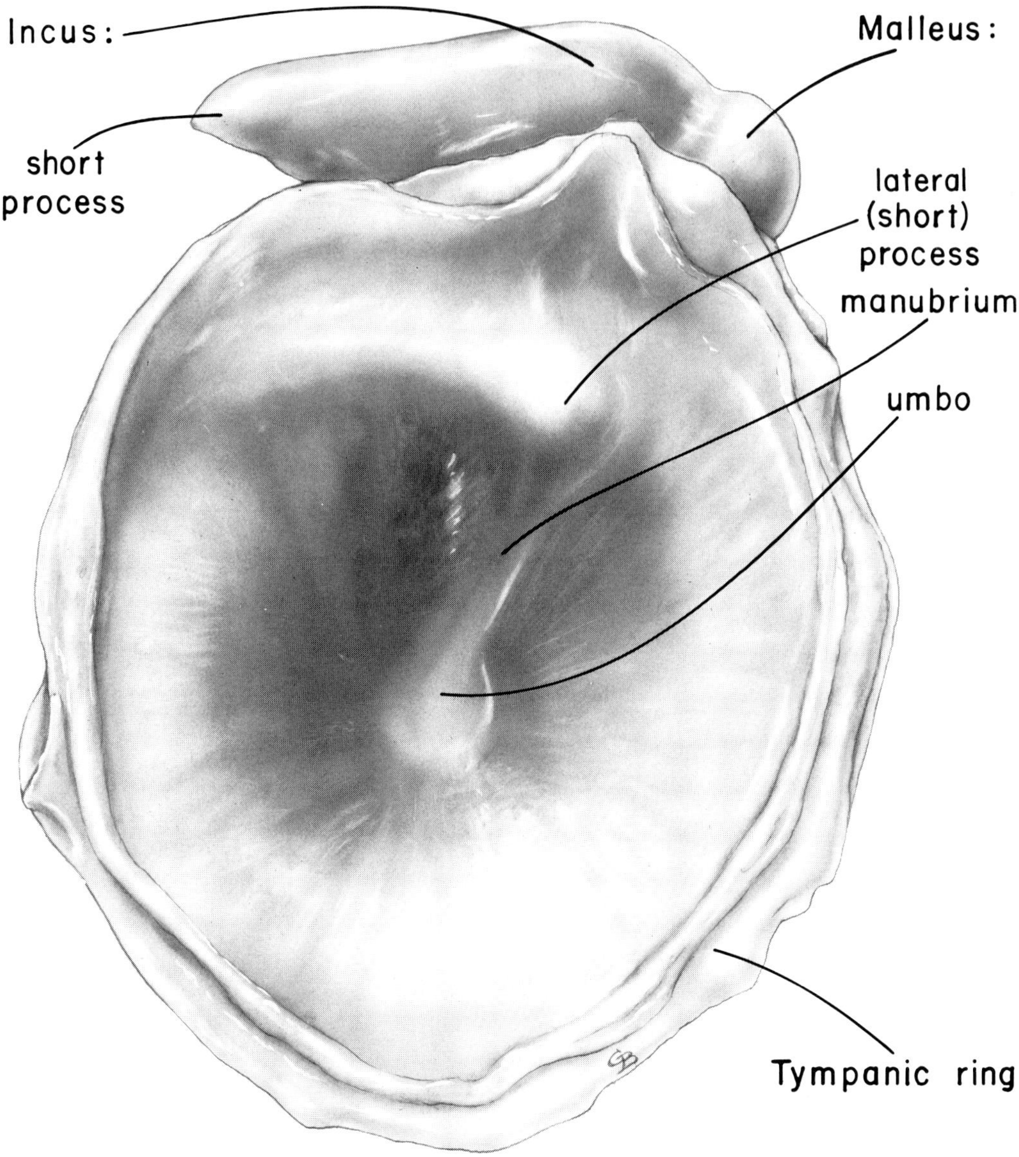

Figure III–4. TYMPANIC RING AND MEMBRANE, EXCISED IN ONE PIECE WITH THE AUDITORY OSSICLES FROM AN UNEMBALMED SPECIMEN. *a.* LATERAL ASPECT, AS IF VIEWED FROM THE EXTERNAL ACOUSTIC MEATUS.

a. The tympanic membrane, or eardrum, is thin, smooth, and either oval or elliptical in form. It is stretched out in the tympanic sulcus and tympanic incisure of the *anulus tympanicus*, thus separating the external acoustic meatus from the tympanic cavity. It is clothed on the outside by a continuation of the external skin, and on the inside by mucous membrane. The upper flaccid portion is pushed forward by a buttonlike mallear prominence, produced by the lateral (or short) process of the malleus. In the larger inferior, tense part it is drawn inward by the tip of the manubrium, so as to be funnel-shaped medianward. The depression thus produced is called the umbo. The opposite surface is pictured in the following illustration.

Figure III–4 continues on the opposite page.

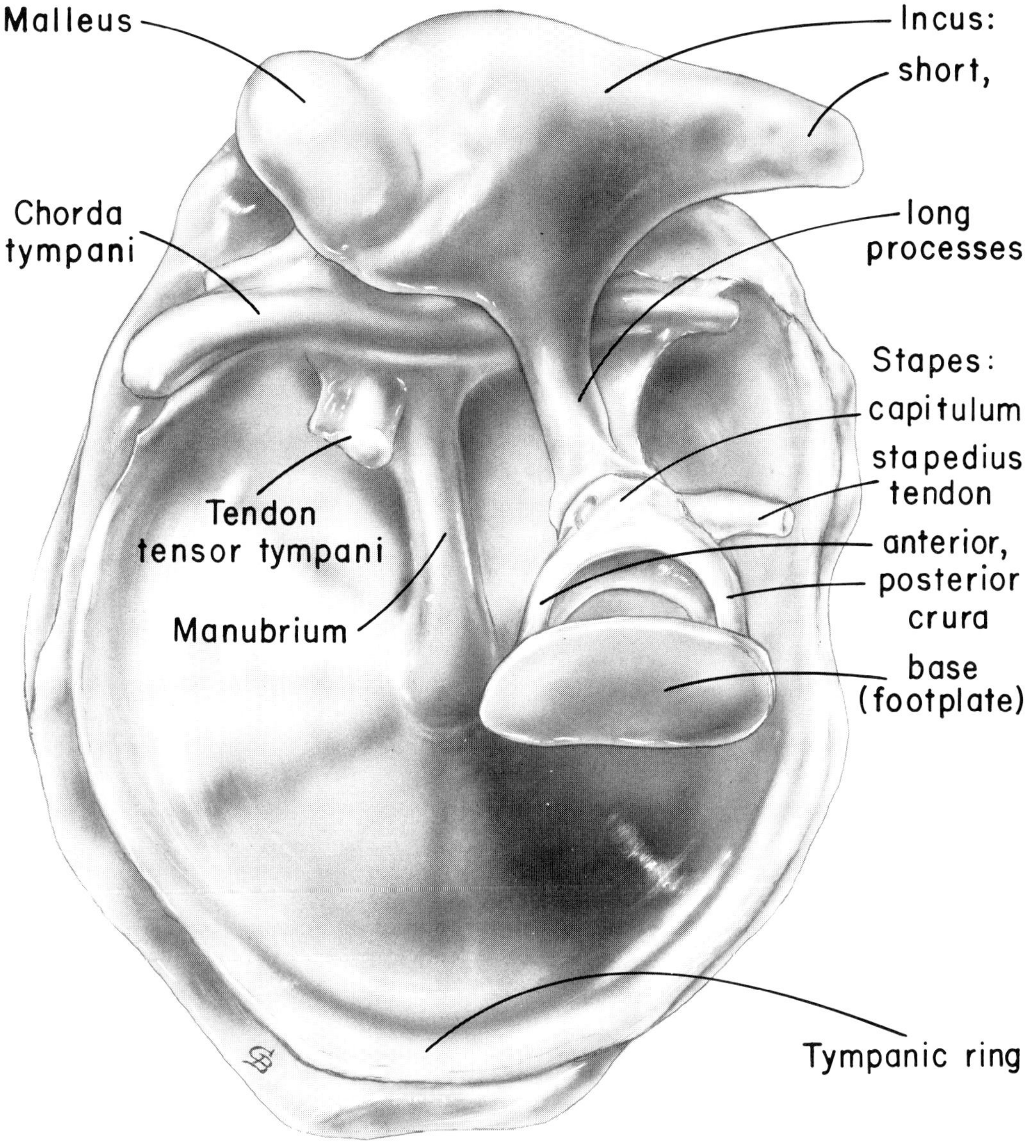

b

Figure III–4, Continued. TYMPANIC RING AND MEMBRANE WITH AUDITORY OSSICLES. *b.* MEDIAL ASPECT OF THE SPECIMEN SHOWN IN *a*.

b. The chorda tympani and the tendons of the two ossicular muscles have been transected near their attachments. The head *(capitulum)* and handle *(manubrium)* of the malleus, or hammer, are in view. All parts of the incus, or anvil, are seen in relation to this middle ear aspect of the tympanic membrane. These subdivisions are the body *(corpus)* and the legs or processes *(crus breve, crus longum)*. Similarly, all parts of the stapes, or stirrup, are in this view: footplate *(basis)*, legs *(crura)*, and head *(capitulum)*. The tympanic tensor is shown at its mallear attachment, the stapedial tendon at the point of implantation into the head of the stapes. The important ossicular relations of the chorda tympani are demonstrated; this branch of the facial nerve courses through the posterior and anterior folds of the mucous membrane, between the long crus of the incus and the manubrium of the malleus.

Figure III–5. TYMPANIC RING AND RELATED ANATOMICAL STRUCTURES. MACERATED SPECIMEN IN LATERAL VIEW.

The dissection shows in greater detail the following structures on the medial (labyrinthine) wall of the tympanic cavity as they are seen through the tympanic ring: the facial canal, the tympanic cavity, and the several groups of air cells.

The vestibular window is situated in approximately the middle of the labyrinthine wall. It appears (in the macerated bone) as a transversely oval opening that leads into the vestibular part of the osseous labyrinth. It is placed at the bottom of a fossa *(fossula fenestrae vestibuli)*, plainly in view from the lateral side. Below the window, the wall projects into the cavity as the promontory, the latter produced by the basal turn of the cochlea.

A sharp declivity on the posterior aspect of the promontory leads into a second fossa *(fossula fenestrae cochleae)*. The fossula is bounded above by a smooth projection of bone, the subiculum of the promontory (not in view). In passing dorsalward from the promontory, the subiculum forms the inferior boundary of the tympanic sinus. This deep fossa is continuous above with the fossula of the vestibular fenestra; it is bounded laterally by the pyramidal eminence and the promontory of the facial canal, medial to which it passes to a variable extent. The fossula continues forward and somewhat upward and medialward into the cochlear fenestra (round window), the latter out of view as the observer sees the tympanic cavity through the ring. The fenestra opens into the basal cochlear turn. The aperture is bordered by a narrow bony ridge, or *crista*, for attachment of the secondary tympanic membrane (see Figures III–93, III–94, and III–95).

The facial canal is shown throughout its length (the osseous shell opened) from the geniculum to the stylomastoid foramen. The geniculum begins on the roof of the internal acoustic meatus. After a short course lateralward, it bends at a right angle (hence the term "knee"). From this point the canal passes backward in a horizontal plane. Then it turns downward in the mastoid wall of the tympanic cavity to the stylomastoid foramen.

The bone is extensively pneumatized; air cells are abundant posteriorly (in the mastoid process), anteriorly (to the petrous apex), inferiorly (in the jugular wall of the tympanic cavity), and medially (on the labyrinthine wall of the tympanic cavity). In the latter situation they are continuous with the space of the epitympanic recess and tympanic antrum.

Dissection by Dr. Bruce B. Shilling.

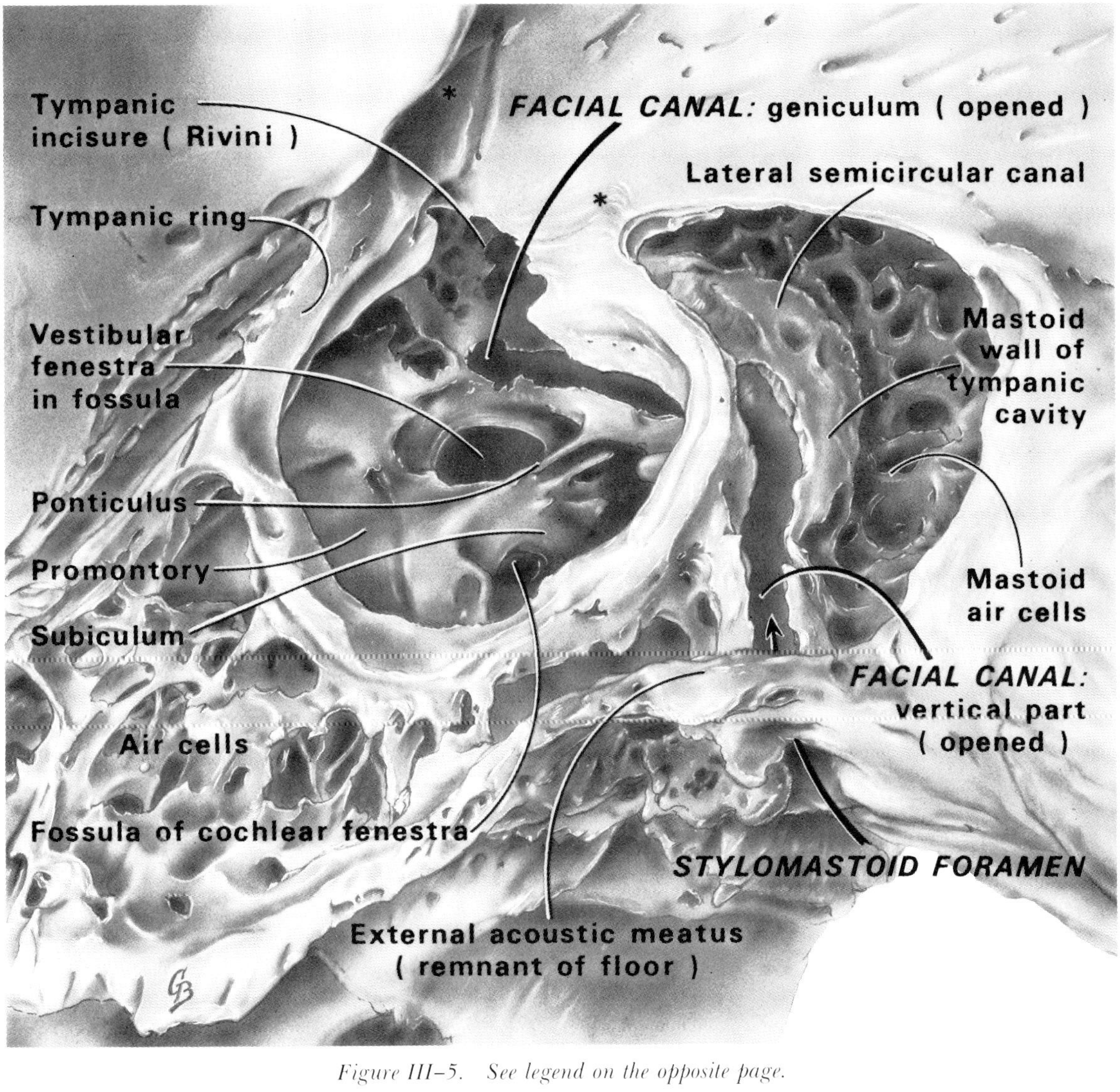

Figure III–5. See legend on the opposite page.

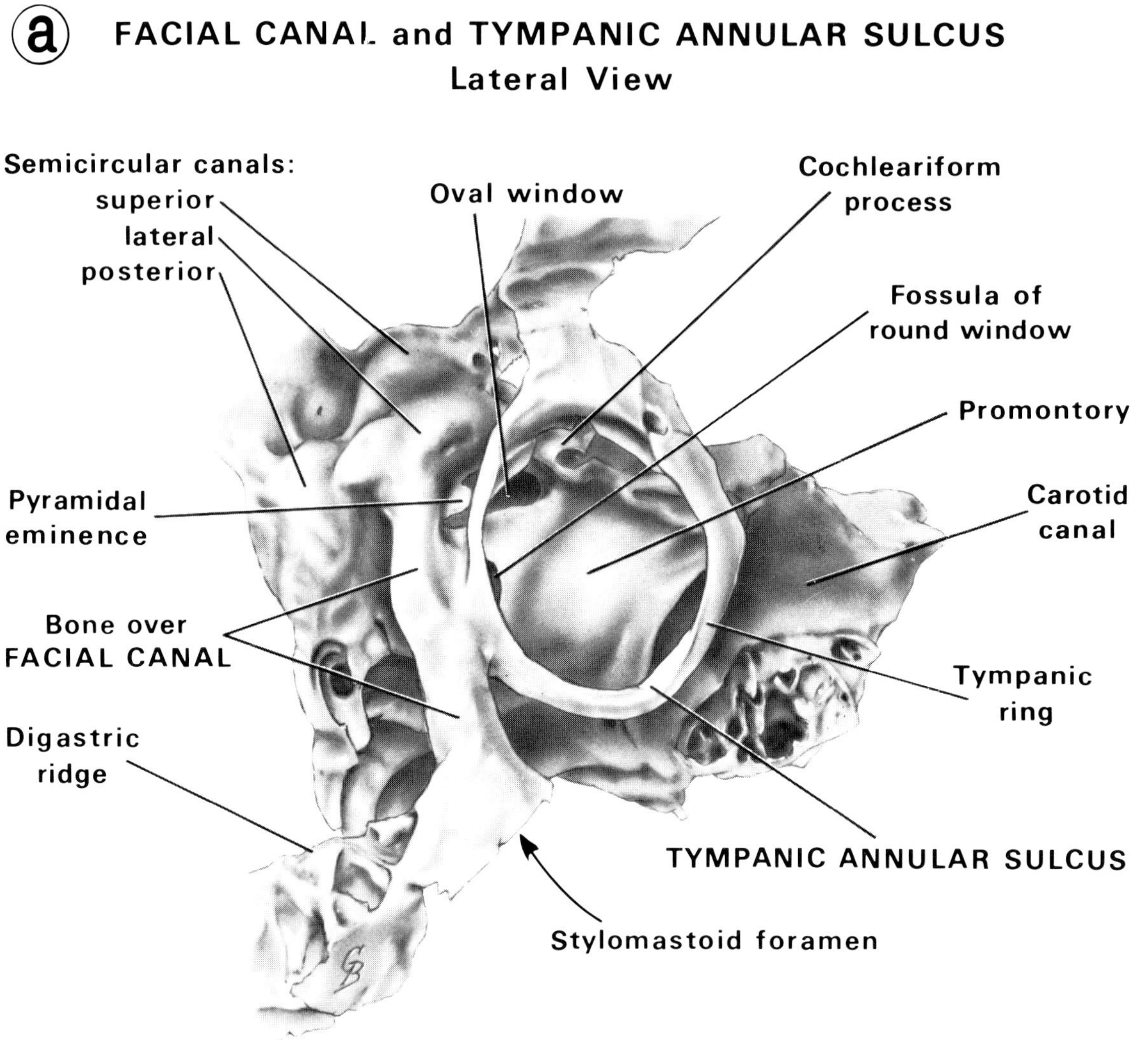

Figure III–6. TYMPANIC RING AND FACIAL CANAL. *a.* DISSECTION OF A SKELETAL PREPARATION. THE BONE HAS BEEN REMOVED TO THE LEVEL OF THE WALL OF THE FACIAL CANAL AND TO THE RIM OF THE VESTIBULAR (OVAL) WINDOW.

a. Demonstrating in lateral view the most frequent relationship between the horizontal segment of the facial canal and the tympanic ring; namely, one in which the anterior part is more medial to the ring than the posterior part (this segment coming lateralward from a position deep to the ring). The following features are also demonstrated: the curvature of the facial canal as it changes direction from horizontal to vertical; proximity of the curving segment to the semicircular canals; proximity of the stylomastoid foramen to the digastric fossa or notch (mastoid incisure) which gives origin to the posterior belly of the digastric muscle.

(From Litton, Krause, Anson, and Cohen: Laryngoscope, 79:1584–1604, 1969.)

Figure III–6 continues on the opposite page.

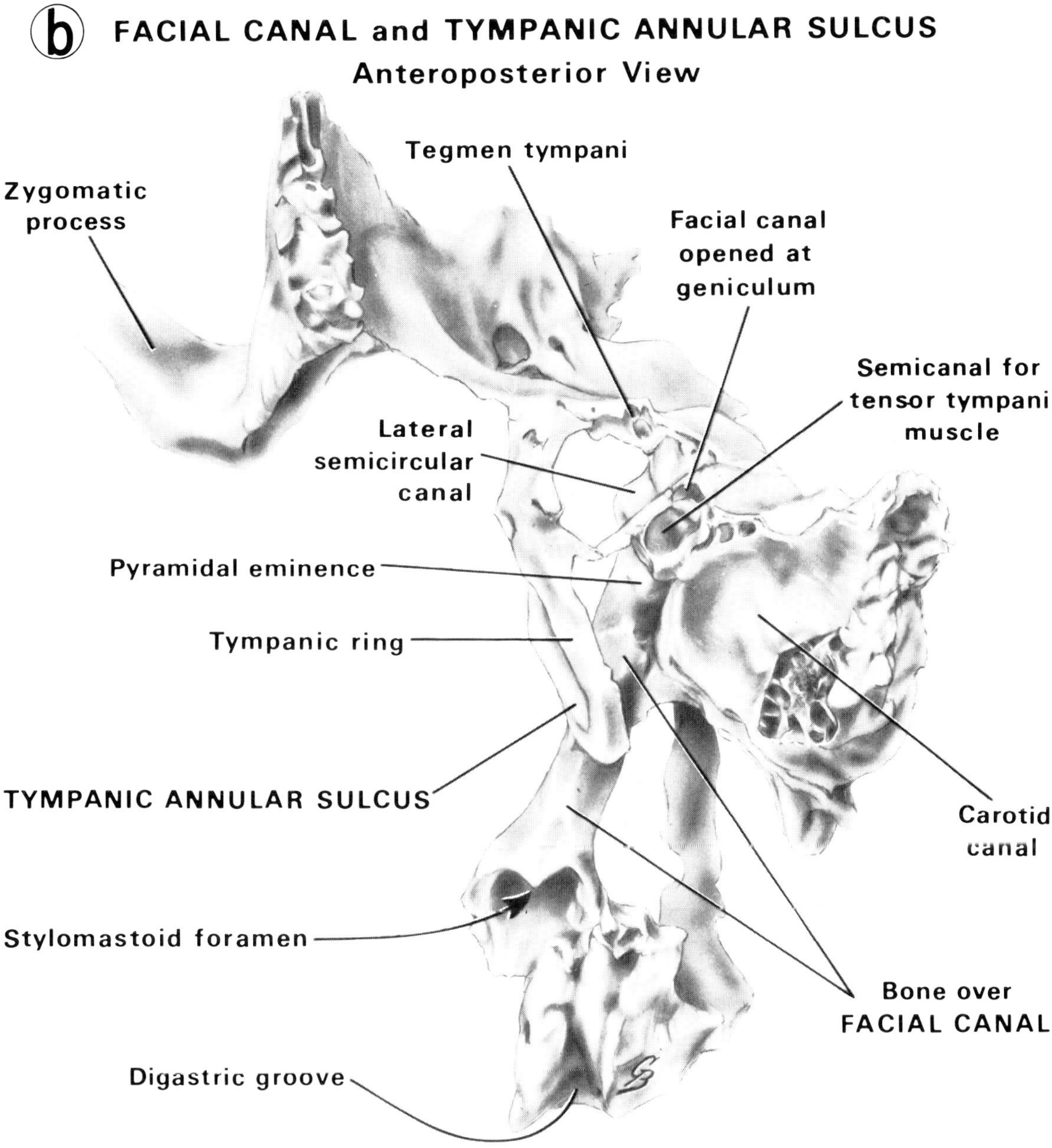

Figure III–6, Continued. TYMPANIC RING AND FACIAL CANAL. *b.* TOPOGRAPHIC RELATIONSHIP.

b. Showing the angular relation of the plane of the tympanic ring to the long axes of the facial canal. Viewed from in front (anteriorly) and slightly below (inferiorly). This is the anteroposterior plane of roentgenology.

Here the tympanic annulus crosses the facial canal to intersect at an angle of 40 degrees; the point of crossing is at the approximate midpoint in the length of the vertical (descending) segment. However, the medial-to-lateral slant is subject to great variation, a fact established by a study of 50 specimens: in one specimen the vertical segment lay completely lateral to the plane of the annulus; in 16, the crossing occurred in the upper (cranial) half of the plane; in 16, in the lower half; and in 17, the canal was entirely medial to the ring.

(From Litton, Krause, Anson, and Cohen: Laryngoscope, 79:1584–1604, 1969.)

Figure III–7. CONTENTS OF THE TYMPANIC CAVITY EMPHASIZING OSSICULAR AND NEURAL ANATOMY.

Dissection of an unembalmed specimen of temporal bone (with tunica mucosa of the tympanic cavity intact), showing the lateral wall of the middle ear as seen in medial view.

The following structures are demonstrated: the chorda tympani (of the facial nerve) throughout its course in the middle ear, the malleus and incus (medial aspect), and the orifice of the auditory (eustachian) tube. It would be difficult to displace the chorda tympani downward. Even with minimal displacement, it would be crushed between the instrument used and the tensor tendon.

In this specimen the long crus of the incus is slightly more anterior in position and nearer the long process of the malleus than is usually the case.

The nerve enters the tympanic cavity through a posterior canaliculus, passes across the manubrium (handle) of the malleus, and leaves the cavity by an anterior canaliculus to reach the infratemporal fossa through the petrotympanic fissure (see Figure III–65 *a* to *h*).

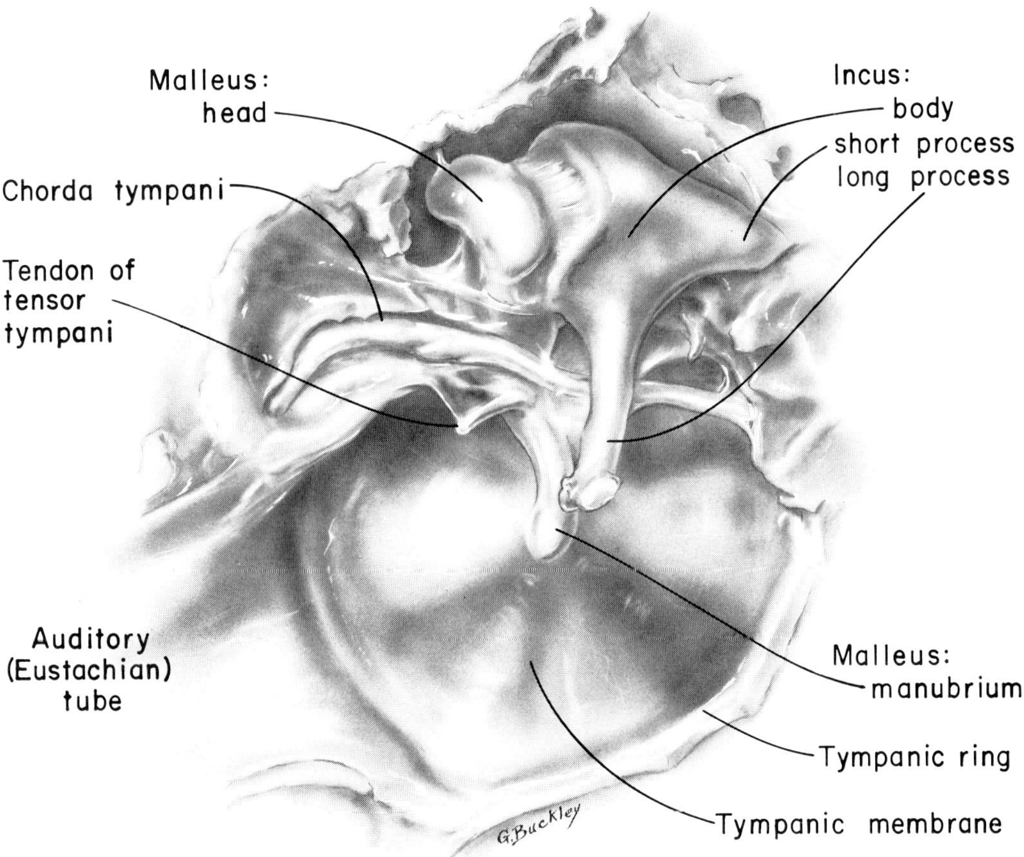

Figure III–7. See legend on the opposite page.

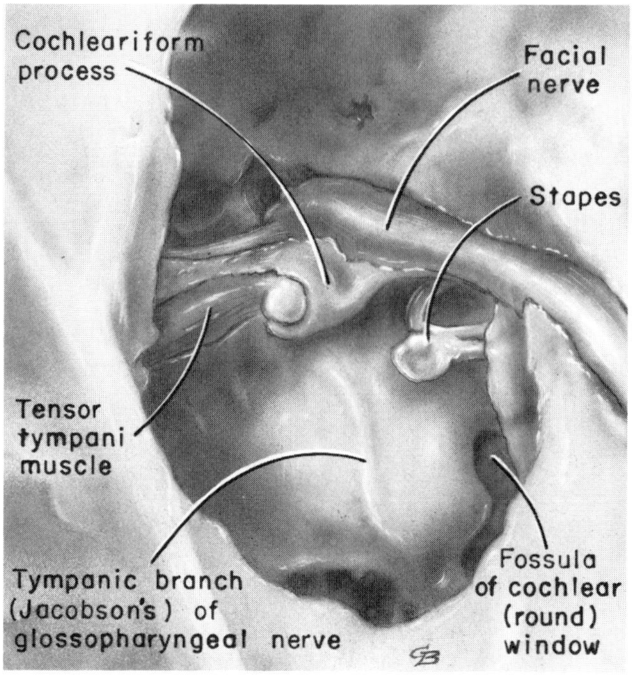

a

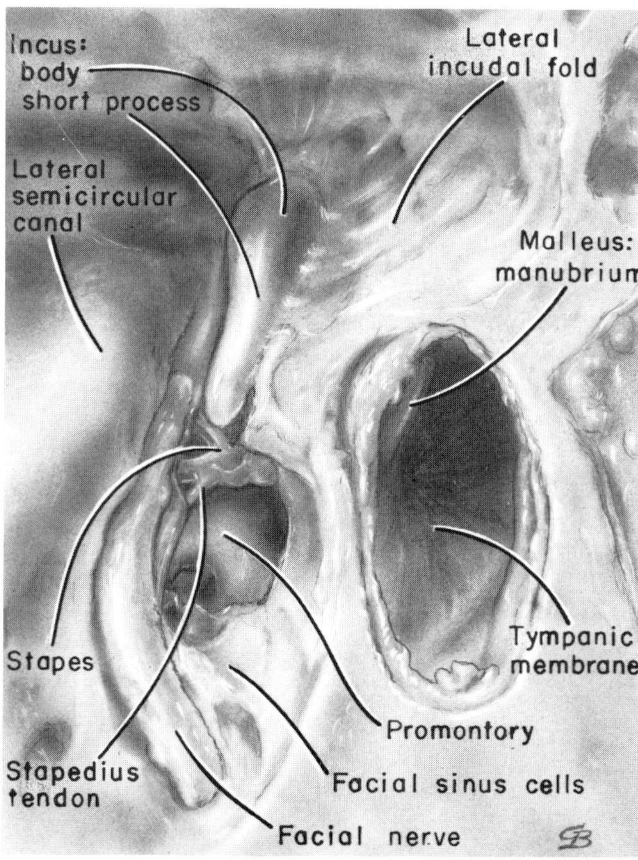

b

Figure III–8. See legend on the opposite page.

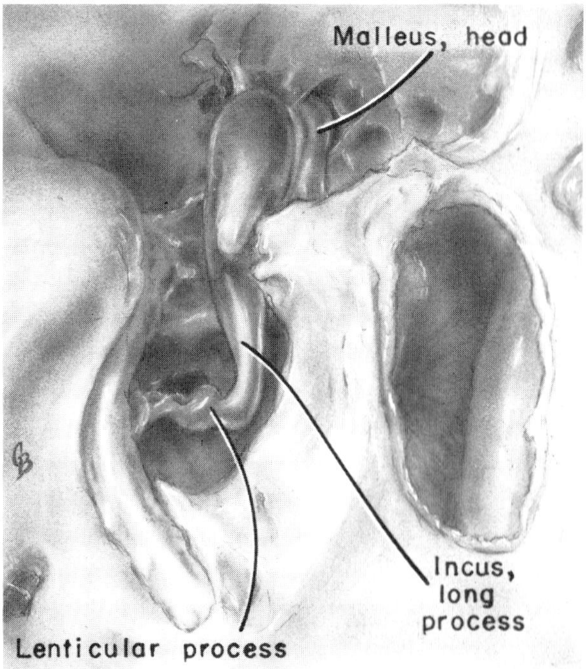

C

Figure III–8. ANATOMY OF THE MEDIAL, OR LABYRINTHINE, WALL OF THE TYMPANIC CAVITY. DISSECTION OF AN UNEMBALMED SPECIMEN.

a. The facial canal and the semicanal have been opened, the incus and malleus removed and the tendon of the tensor tympani transected. Here the facial nerve leaves the bottom of the internal acoustic meatus to enter the facial canal and run lateralward to the facial knee, or *geniculum.* Next, turning backward and lateralward, the nerve arches over the vestibular, or oval, window (this segment exposed in the dissection). Then, in the third segment, the course of the nerve changes from horizontal to vertical. The stapes occupies the fossula of the vestibular fenestra. Below the vestibular window a sharp declivity marks the edge of the fossula of the cochlear fenestra. The fossula leads upward and medianward to the cochlear, or round, window; the latter is closed in the natural state by the secondary tympanic membrane. The depth and plane of the fossula are such that the membrane is out of view when the surgeon looks into the tympanic cavity from the external acoustic meatus. Just beneath the cochleariform process a bulging, termed *promontorium,* is produced by the basal turn of the cochlea. The tympanic branch of the glossopharyngeal nerve descends beneath its mucous membrane. If the cochleariform process is to be removed, care must be taken not to pry it with a motion that could rotate bone fragments into the facial nerve.

b. External acoustic meatus of the outer ear; ossicles and related structures of the middle ear (seen through the mastoid); and the tympanic membrane interposed between the two spaces. First stage in the dissection of an unembalmed specimen.

The impression of the handle of the malleus is seen in the upper part of the lateral surface of the tympanic membrane. The mucous membrane that lines the surface of the whole tympanic cavity is draped over the auditory ossicles in the form of folds, or *plicae* (for example, the lateral incudal fold here shown). It is also carried into irregularities in the walls of the tympanic cavity and auditory tube as well as the spaces in the mastoid part of the temporal bone.

c. Ossicles and related structures of the middle ear. Second stage in dissection. The incudal fold has been removed in order to reveal the incudomallear joint; the cells of the facial sinus have been dissected away.

The head of the malleus is situated in the epitympanic recess where it articulates with the body of the incus. The short process of the incus is directed horizontally backward (here, toward the reader). The long one runs parallel to the manubrium, lying posteromedial to it. On the medial side of the tip of the long process, a small process articulates with the head of the stapes.

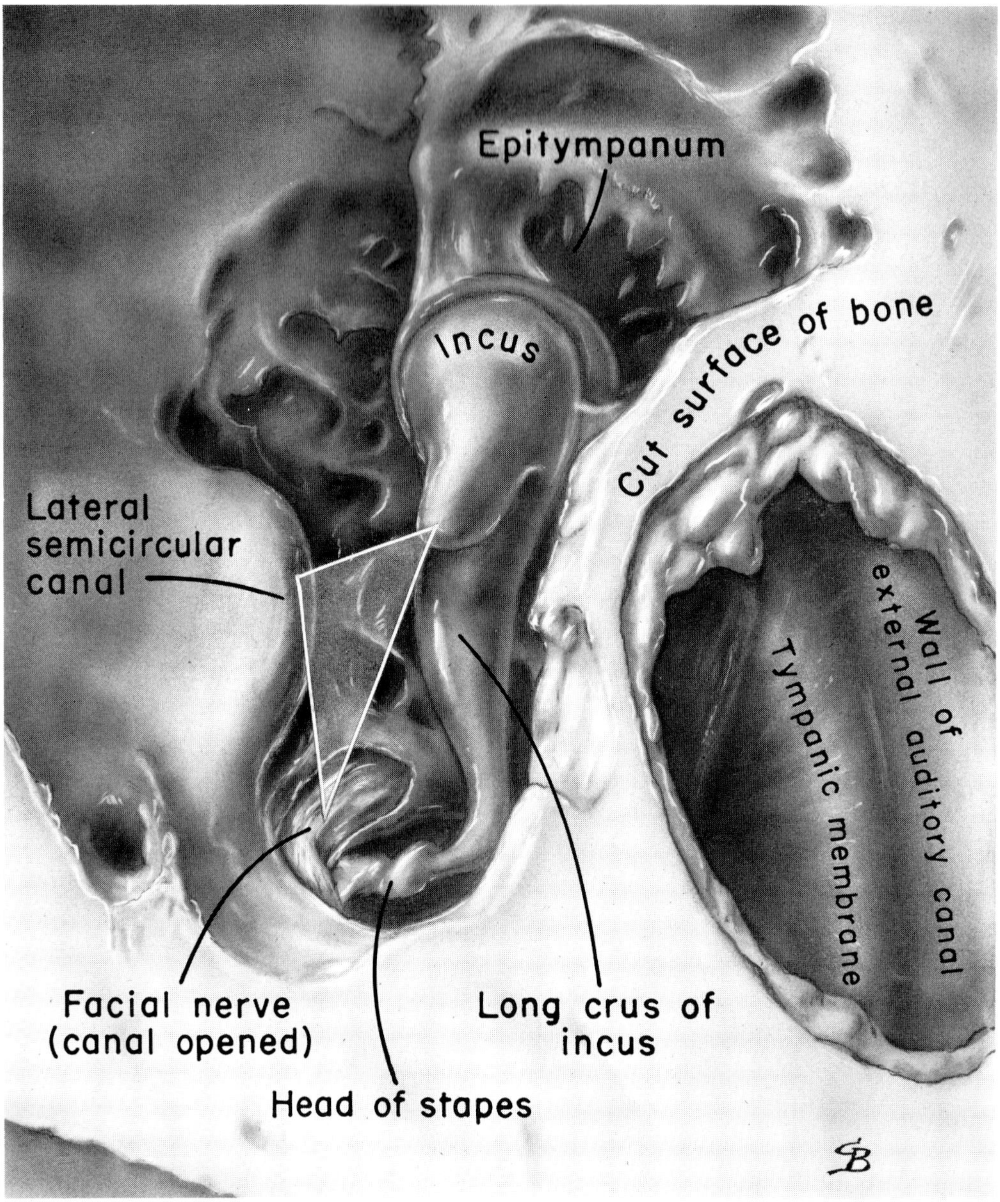

a

Figure III–9. RELATIONSHIP OF THE FACIAL NERVE (AT THE TURN IN ITS COURSE), TO ADJACENT STRUCTURES.

The triangle, here superimposed on a drawing of a dissection, connects the short process of the incus, the bulge of the semicircular canal, and the facial nerve.

a. At the downward-directed apex of the triangle, the facial canal has been opened to expose the nerve. Here the nerve, after crossing horizontally above the stapes, changes direction to descend vertically toward the stylomastoid foramen. At the lower right the tympanic membrane is seen in the depths of the external acoustic meatus.

Figure III–9 continues on the opposite page.

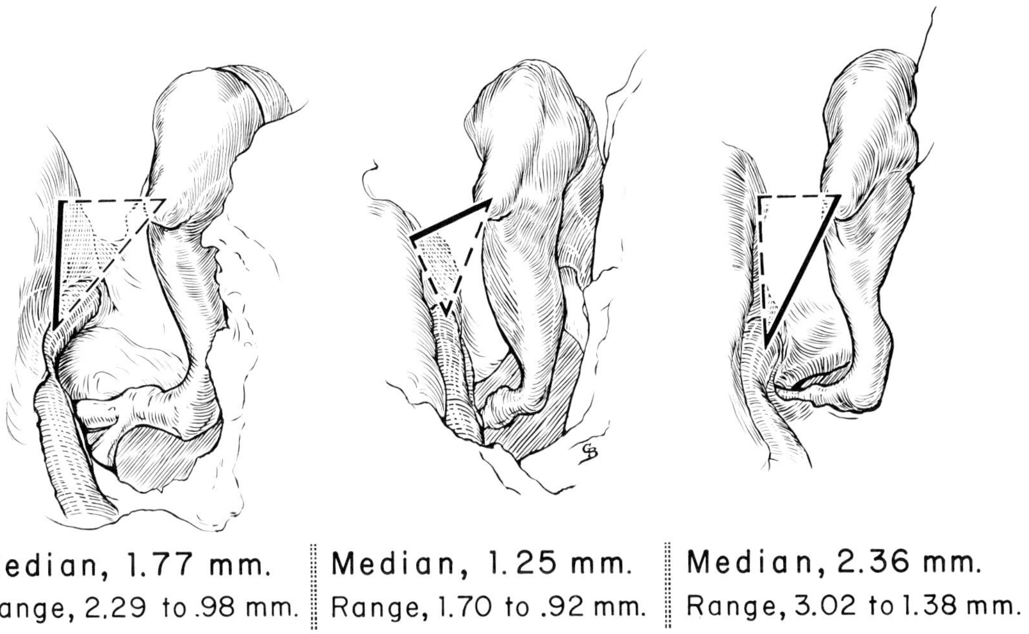

Figure III–9, Continued. RELATIONSHIP OF THE FACIAL NERVE (AT THE TURN IN ITS COURSE), TO ADJACENT STRUCTURES.

b. The accompanying diagrams record measurement of length for each of the three distances in 25 specimens.

The key structure in the surgical anatomy of the temporal bone is the facial nerve. The identification and preservation of this source of motor innervation for the facial musculature are of first importance in the removal of pathology which may resemble, abut upon, or even surround the nerve.

When pathology in the temporal bone is approached through the mastoid cortex, the mastoid antrum is located, the lateral semicircular canal is identified, and the short process of the incus is uncovered. Further surgery may entail decompression of the facial nerve for Bell's palsy or removal of facial sinus cells (located lateral to the vertical portion of the nerve and caudal to the short process of the incus). In either case, the relationship of the nerve to the short process of the incus and to the horizontal semicircular canal is evident.

The surgically important relationships in this area may be considered as forming the angles of a triangle, with the operator viewing the short process of the incus on end. The short process of the incus, the lateral semicircular canal, and the facial nerve make up the landmarks. A triangle is then constructed by drawing three lines as follows: from the tip of the short process of the incus to the nearest portion of the lateral semicircular canal; from the canal to the nearest part of the facial nerve; and a third line connecting the ends of the first two. The interdistances for the 25 bones were as follows: the median distance from the tip of the short process of the incus to the nearest portion of the horizontal semicircular canal was 1.25 mm., with a range of 1.70 to 0.92 mm.; that from the horizontal canal to the facial nerve was 1.77 mm., with a range of 2.29 to 0.98 mm.; and that from the short process of the incus to the facial nerve 2.36 mm., with a range of 3.02 to 1.38 mm.

(From Donaldson and Anson: Ann. Otol., 74:59–62, 1965.)

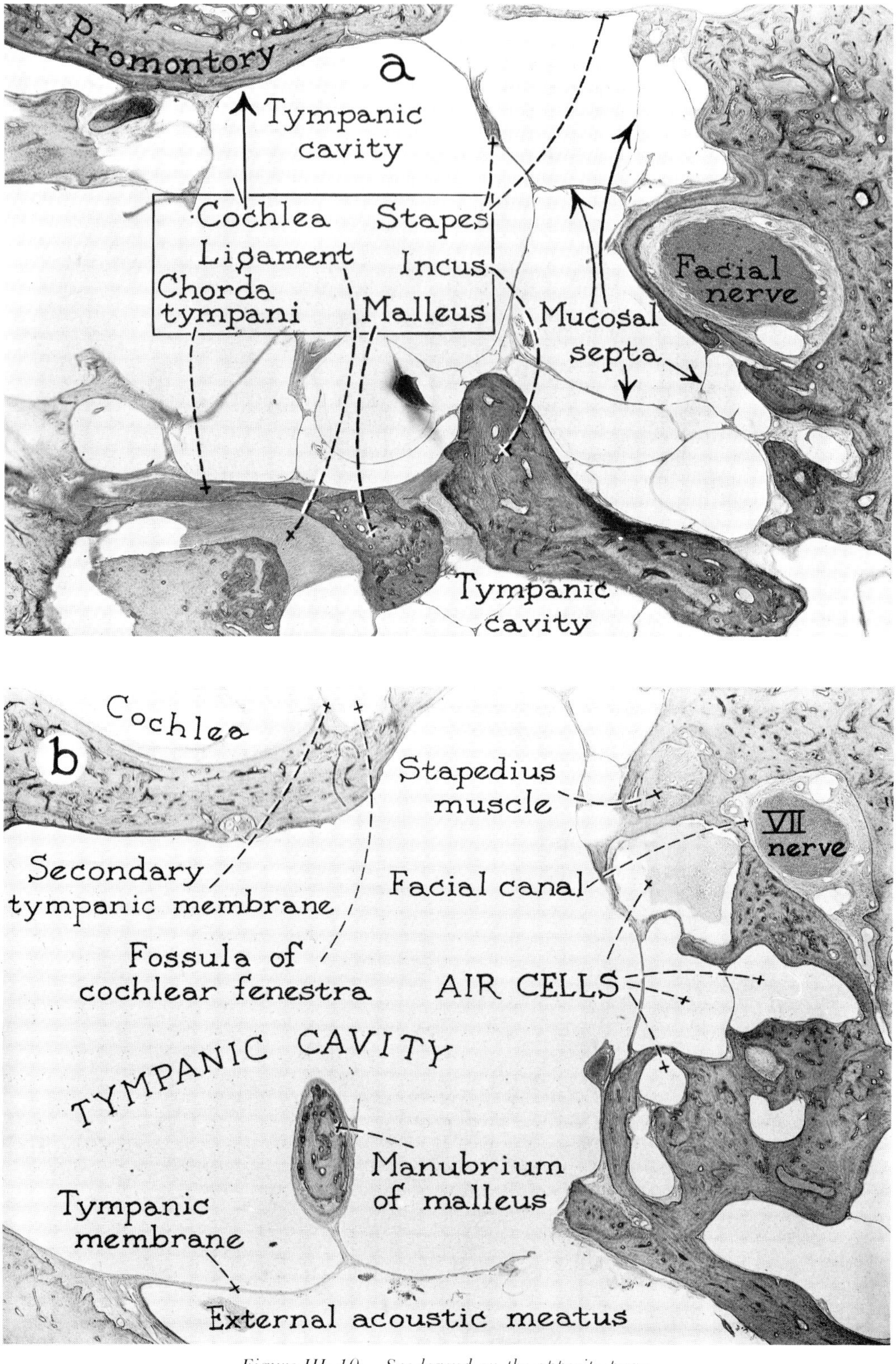

Figure III–10. See legend on the opposite page.

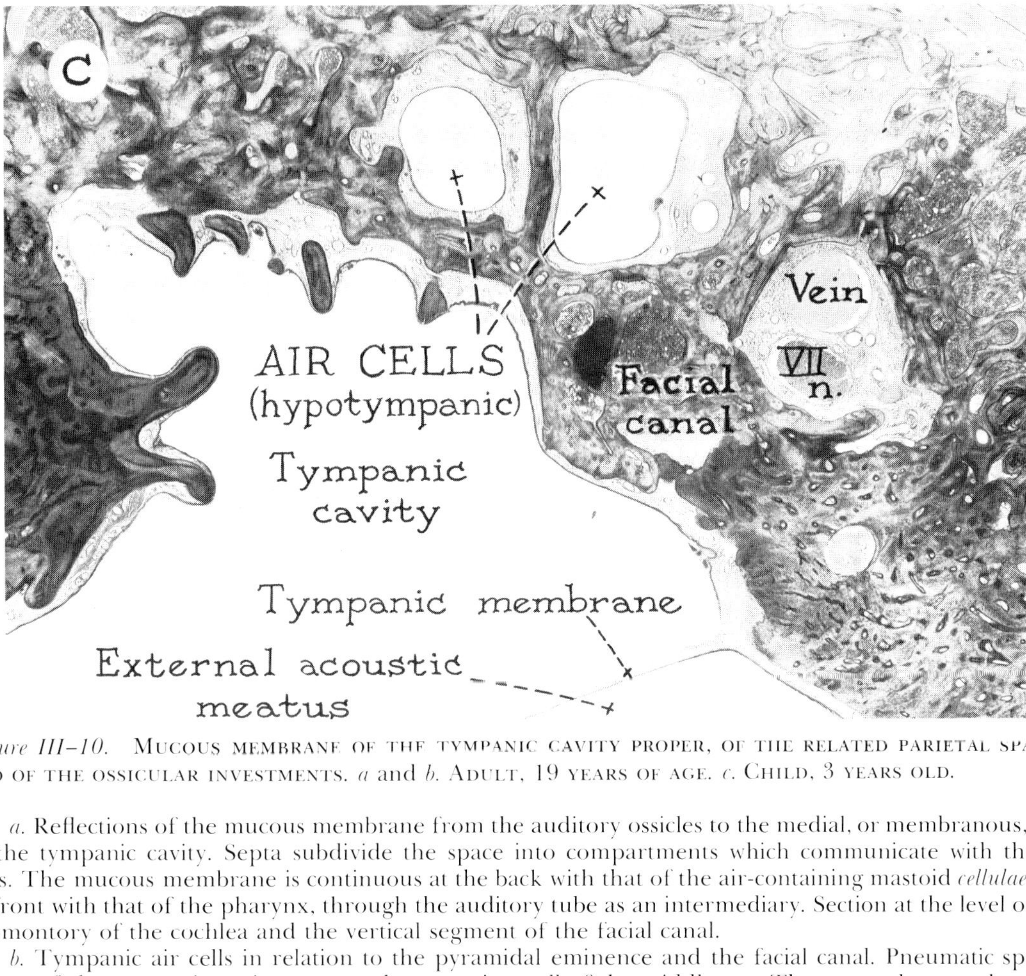

Figure III-10. MUCOUS MEMBRANE OF THE TYMPANIC CAVITY PROPER, OF THE RELATED PARIETAL SPACES, AND OF THE OSSICULAR INVESTMENTS. *a* and *b*. ADULT, 19 YEARS OF AGE. *c*. CHILD, 3 YEARS OLD.

a. Reflections of the mucous membrane from the auditory ossicles to the medial, or membranous, wall of the tympanic cavity. Septa subdivide the space into compartments which communicate with the air cells. The mucous membrane is continuous at the back with that of the air-containing mastoid *cellulae* and in front with that of the pharynx, through the auditory tube as an intermediary. Section at the level of the promontory of the cochlea and the vertical segment of the facial canal.

b. Tympanic air cells in relation to the pyramidal eminence and the facial canal. Pneumatic spaces, offsets of the tympanic cavity, occupy the posterior wall of the middle ear. The mucosal septa, shown in *a*, bound these air cells.

c. Hypotympanic air cells, in relation to the facial canal. These cells, situated on the floor of the tympanic cavity, lie anteromedial to the facial canal.

Transverse sections, Wisconsin Collection, series as follows: *a* and *b*, 29; *c*, 96. *a*, ×13; *b*, ×7; *c*, ×12.

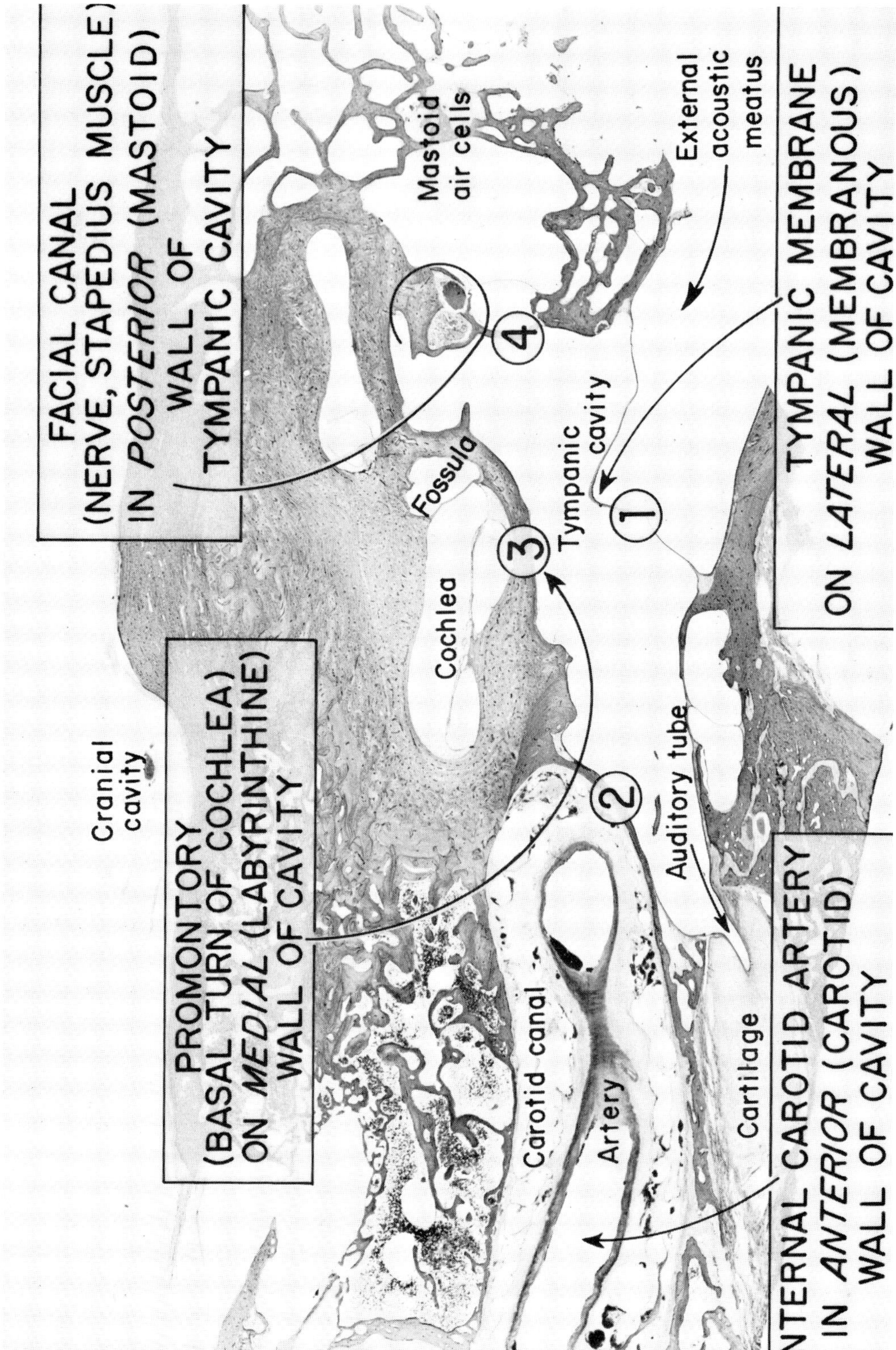
FACIAL CANAL (NERVE, STAPEDIUS MUSCLE) IN POSTERIOR (MASTOID) WALL OF TYMPANIC CAVITY
Mastoid air cells
External acoustic meatus
4
Fossula
Tympanic cavity
1
3
Tympanic
TYMPANIC MEMBRANE ON LATERAL (MEMBRANOUS) WALL OF CAVITY
Cochlea
Cranial cavity
PROMONTORY (BASAL TURN OF COCHLEA) ON MEDIAL (LABYRINTHINE) WALL OF CAVITY
2
Auditory tube
Carotid canal
Artery
Cartilage
INTERNAL CAROTID ARTERY IN ANTERIOR (CAROTID) WALL OF CAVITY

Figure III–11. TYMPANIC CAVITY: WALLS AND RELATED ANATOMY. FEMALE, 55 YEARS OF AGE.

The tympanic, or eardrum, cavity is continuous behind and lateralward with the air cells in the mastoid part of the temporal bone, and in front and medialward with the pharynx through the auditory (eustachian) tube.

The lateral wall (at *1*) of the cavity is in large part occupied by the tympanic membrane and is termed the *paries membranaceus.* The anterior wall (*2*) is formed by the carotid canal; hence it is designated *paries caroticus.* The medial wall (*3*) adjoins the labyrinth and is therefore called the *paries labyrinthicus.* At the level here shown, the basal turn of the cochlea bulges into the space as the promotory, and the tympanic scala is separated at the cochlear fenestra (round window) from the fossula of the fenestra by the secondary tympanic membrane. At a more superior level are situated the vestibular fenestra and stapes and the semicanal for the tensor tympani muscle. The posterior wall (*paries mastoideus*, at *4*) is studded with numerous tympanic air cells. This wall contains the facial canal which transmits the facial nerve and stapedius muscle.

The inferior wall (not shown) is termed the *paries jugularis* since it is, in large measure, the "roof" of the fossa for the superior bulb of the jugular vein. The superior wall (not shown) is termed the *paries tegmentalis* since it is formed by the tympanic tegmen (part of the floor of the middle cranial fossa).

Transverse section, Iowa Collection, series 67–500 2R, ×4.

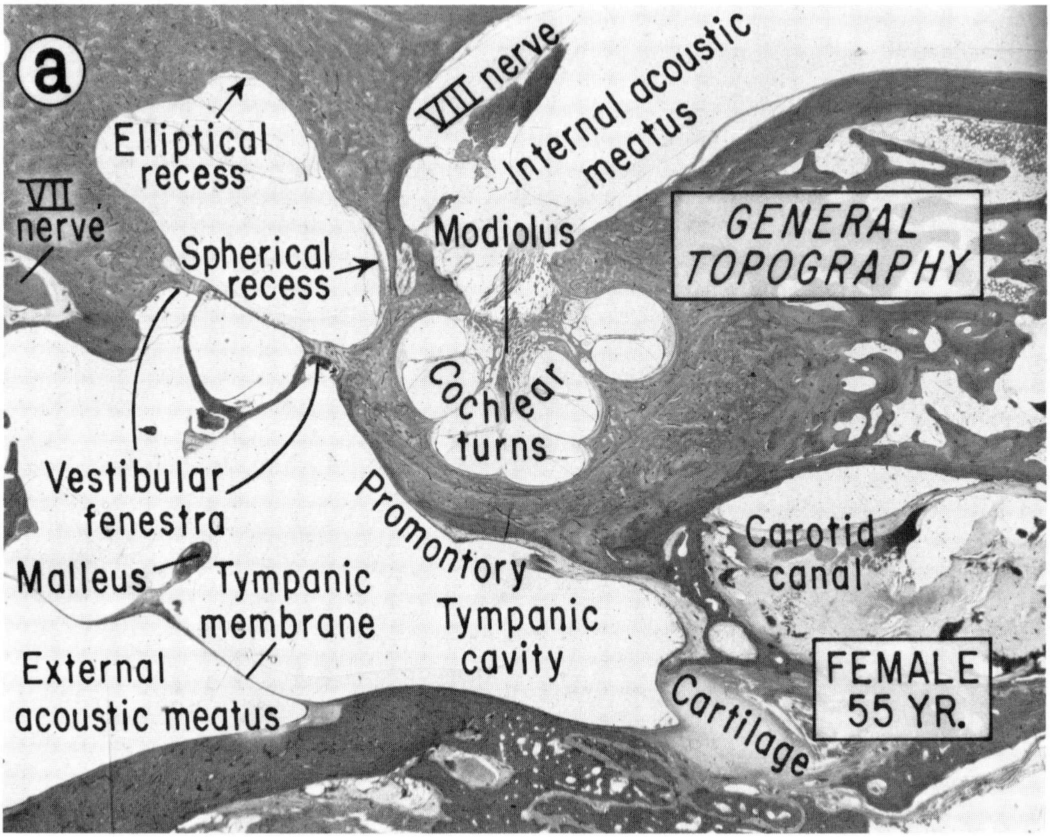

Figure III–12. CRITICAL DISTANCES IN THE MIDDLE AND THE INNER EAR. *a* and *b*. FEMALE, 55 YEARS OF AGE.

a. General topography for the following figure *(b)*, in which measurements are recorded for interdistances in the middle and inner ear and for the depth of the internal acoustic meatus.

Figure III–12 continues on the opposite page.

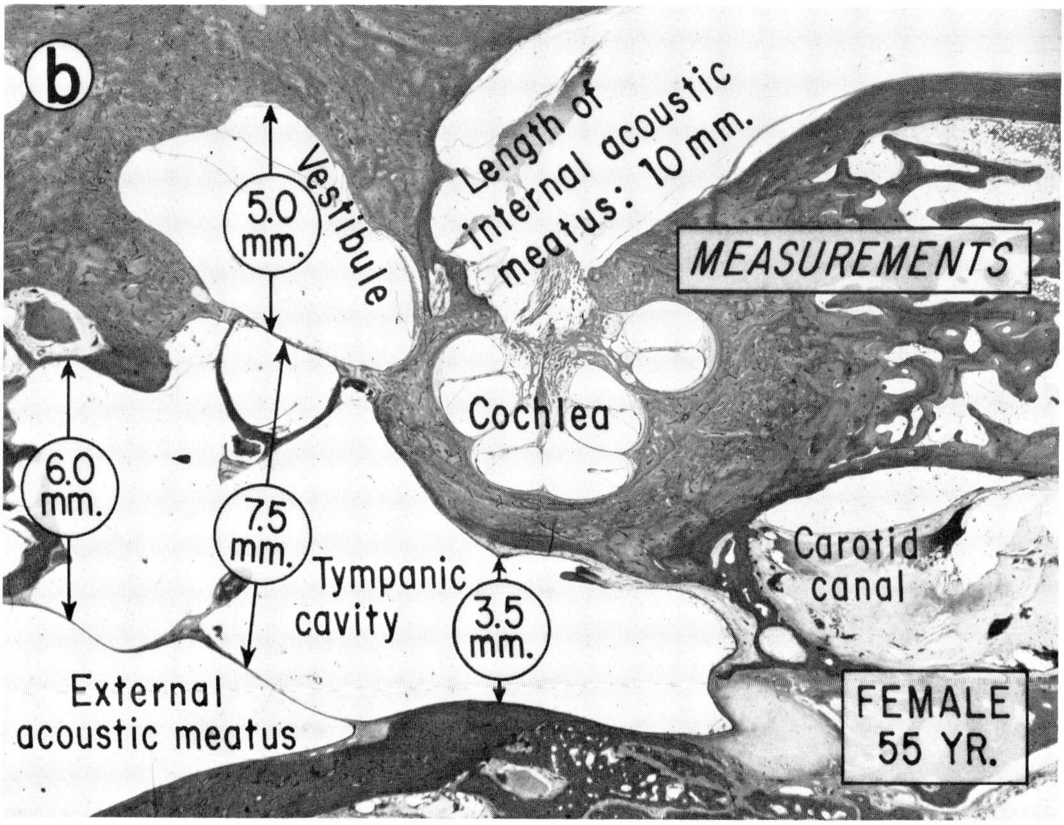

Figure III–12, Continued. CRITICAL DISTANCES IN THE MIDDLE AND THE INNER EAR. *a* and *b*. FEMALE, 55 YEARS OF AGE.

b. At this horizontal level through the entire stapes and the modiolus of the cochlea, the following measurements are recorded for the middle ear: tympanic membrane to the facial canal and to the stapedial footplate; from the lateral wall to the promontory. For the inner ear, the measurement is given for the distance from the footplate of the stapes to the wall of the elliptical recess of the utricle.

Figure III–12 continues on the following page.

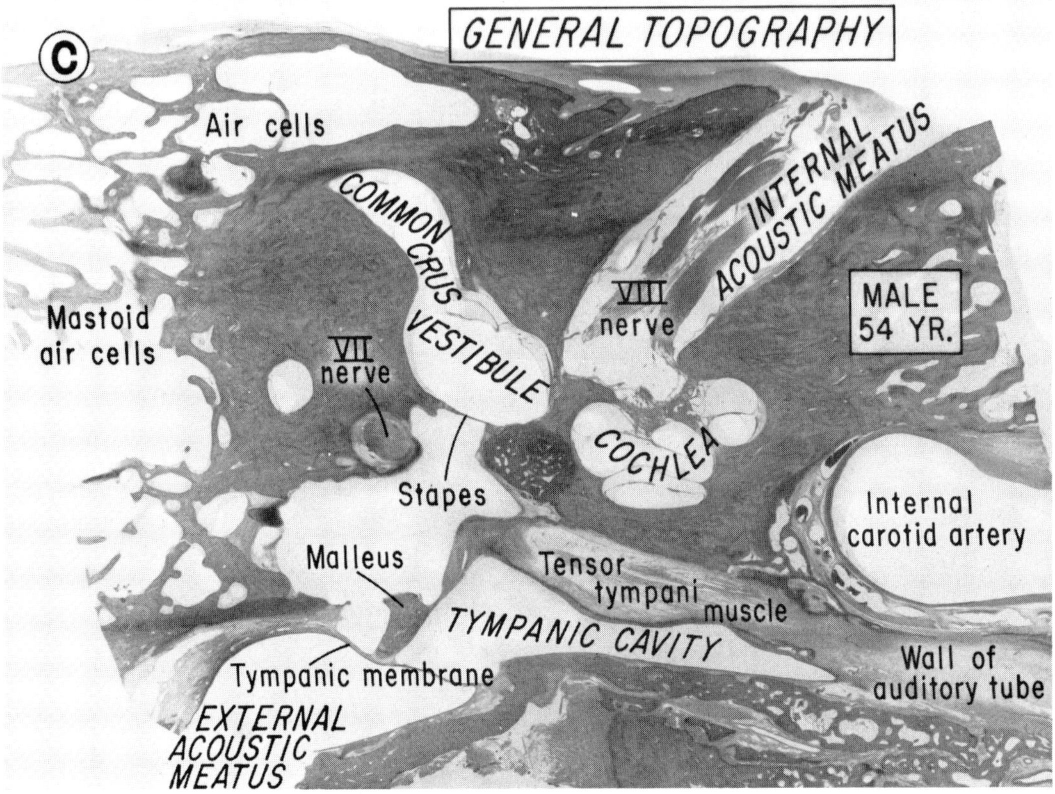

Figure III–12, Continued. CRITICAL DISTANCES IN THE MIDDLE AND THE INNER EAR. *c.* MALE, 54 YEARS OF AGE.

c. Showing the structures in the tympanic cavity and in its labyrinthine (medial) and membranous (lateral) walls: the manubrium of the malleus in the tympanic membrane; the tensor tympani muscle in the semicanal on the cochlear division of the labyrinthine wall; the facial nerve (in a dehiscent canal); an area of otosclerotic bone (in antefenestral position); the stapes (closing the vestibular window). The facial canal and the promontory of the cochlea form the posterior and anterior boundaries, respectively, of the fossula which houses the stapes.

Figure III–12 continues on the opposite page.

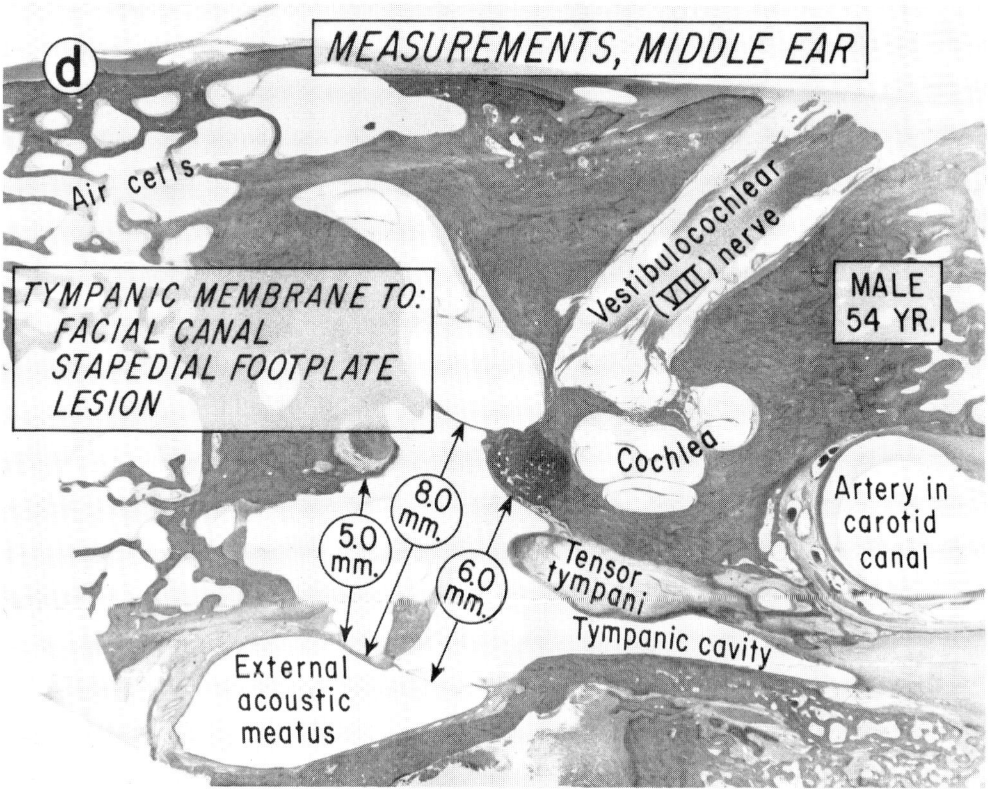

Figure III–12, Concluded. CRITICAL DISTANCES IN THE MIDDLE AND THE INNER EAR. *d.* MALE, 54 YEARS OF AGE.

d. Recording the distances across the tympanic cavity to the following: the facial canal; the stapedial base (footplate); and the otosclerotic area of the cochlear wall.

Transverse sections, Iowa Collection, series as follows: *a* and *b*, 67–500 2 R; *c* and *d*, 583; right temporal bones. *a* ×6; *b*, ×6; *c*, ×4; *d*, ×4.

(*d* from Anson: Trans. Amer. Acad. Ophthal. Otolaryng., 76:108–129, 1972.)

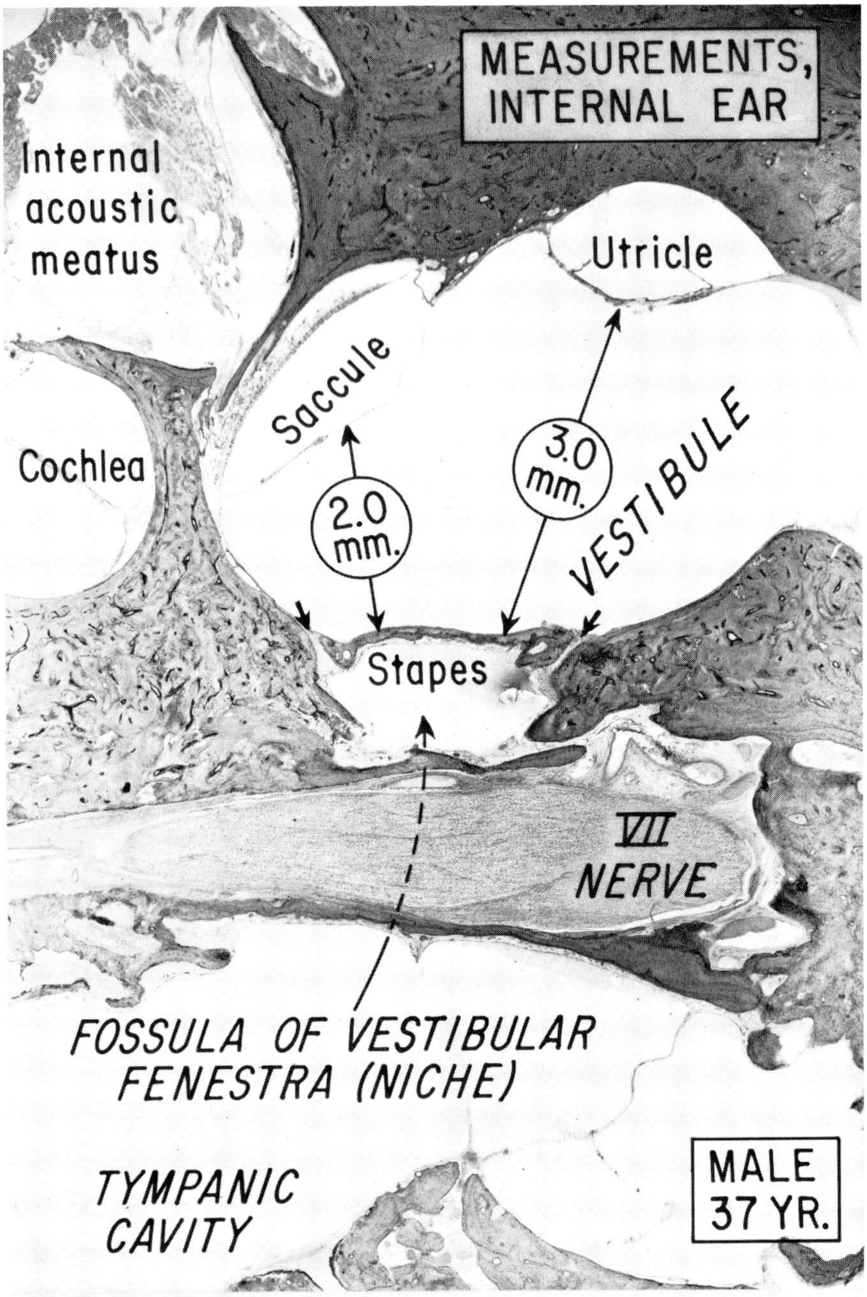

Figure III–13. RELATIONSHIPS IN THE MIDDLE AND INTERNAL EAR AND CRITICAL MEASUREMENTS IN THE LATTER. MALE, 37 YEARS OF AGE.

At the level of the stapedial footplate, the general space of the tympanic cavity is divided by the transversely coursing facial canal. The locally sequestered part of the cavity is the fossula of the vestibular fenestra, or stapes "niche" of otological surgery.

The distances are recorded from the base (footplate) of the stapes, across the vestibule, to the saccule and to the utricle.

The following important features are also shown: the fossular space between the stapes and the facial canal in horizontal course; and the conformation of the rim of the stapedial footplate (at arrows) in the vestibular (oval) window.

Transverse section, Wisconsin Collection, series, 21. ×15.

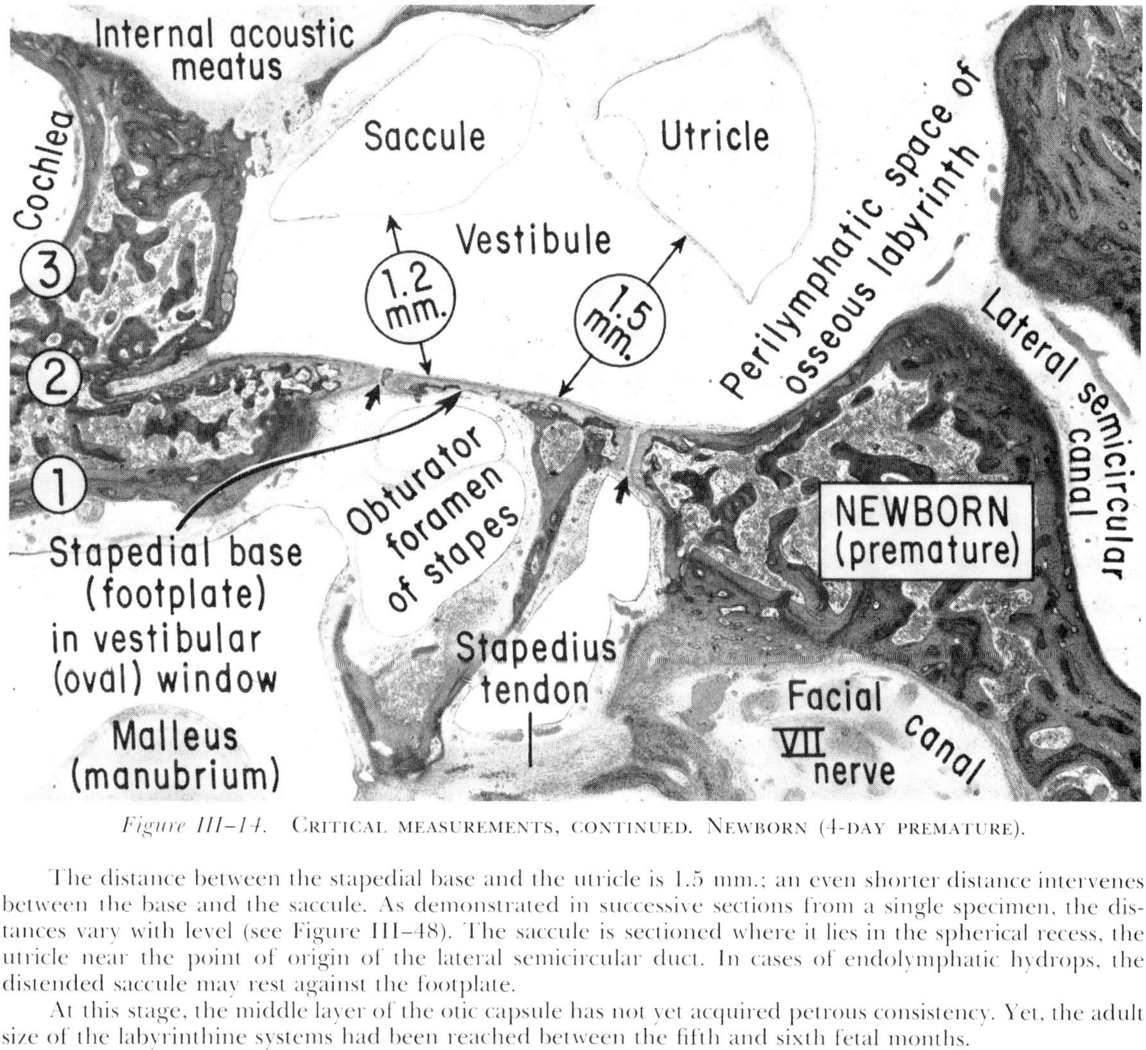

Figure III–14. CRITICAL MEASUREMENTS, CONTINUED. NEWBORN (4-DAY PREMATURE).

The distance between the stapedial base and the utricle is 1.5 mm.; an even shorter distance intervenes between the base and the saccule. As demonstrated in successive sections from a single specimen, the distances vary with level (see Figure III–48). The saccule is sectioned where it lies in the spherical recess, the utricle near the point of origin of the lateral semicircular duct. In cases of endolymphatic hydrops, the distended saccule may rest against the footplate.

At this stage, the middle layer of the otic capsule has not yet acquired petrous consistency. Yet, the adult size of the labyrinthine systems had been reached between the fifth and sixth fetal months.

Transverse section, Wisconsin Collection, series 124. ×18.

Figure III–15. CRITICAL MEASUREMENTS, CONCLUDED. FETUS OF 6 MONTHS.

Demonstrating the early establishment of the "adult" relationship between the stapes and the vestibular elements (saccule and utricle) of the membranous labyrinthine system. Maturity in size of the vestibule and of the utricle and saccule is attained just as soon as the inner periosteal layer of the otic capsule is completely formed. At this stage the middle layer of the capsule is partly cartilaginous; the fissula ante fenestram (at asterisk) still contains cartilage. Abbreviations: *S.S.C.*, superior semicircular canal; *L.S.C.*, lateral semicircular canal.

Transverse section, Wisconsin Collection, series 70. ×13.

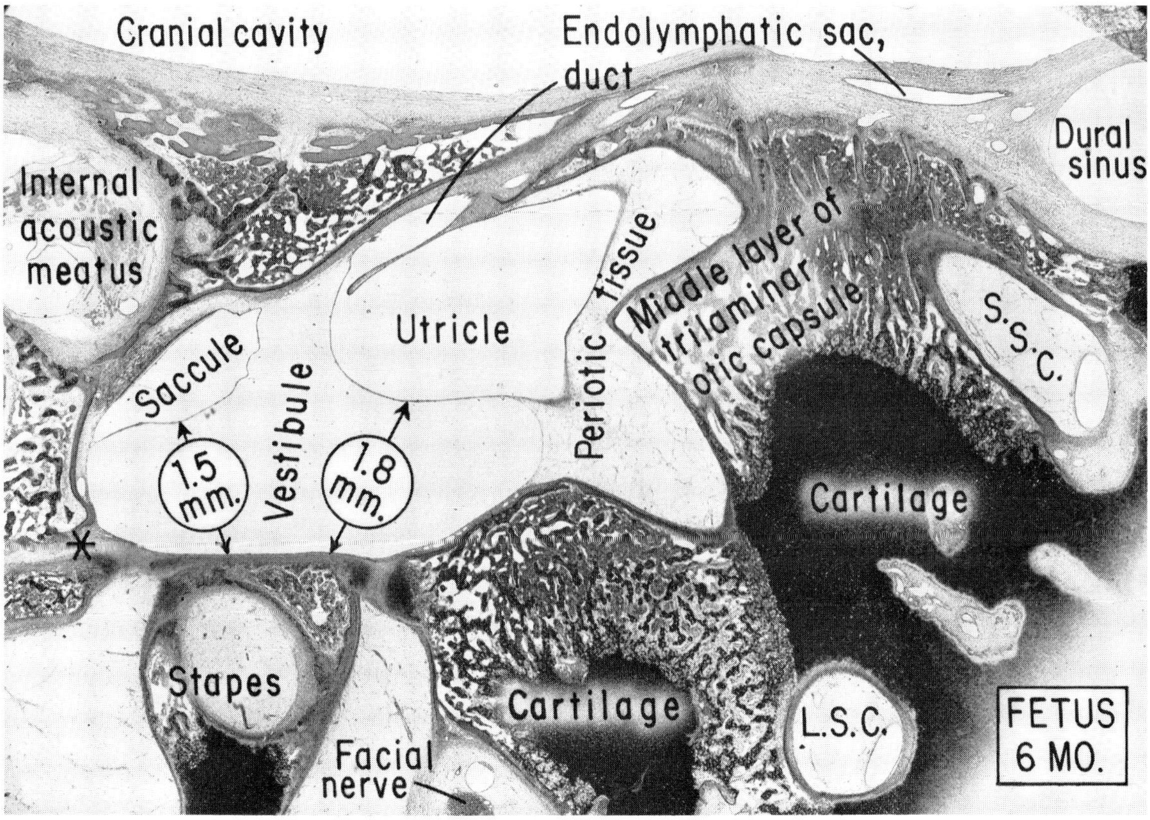

Figure III–15. See legend on the opposite page.

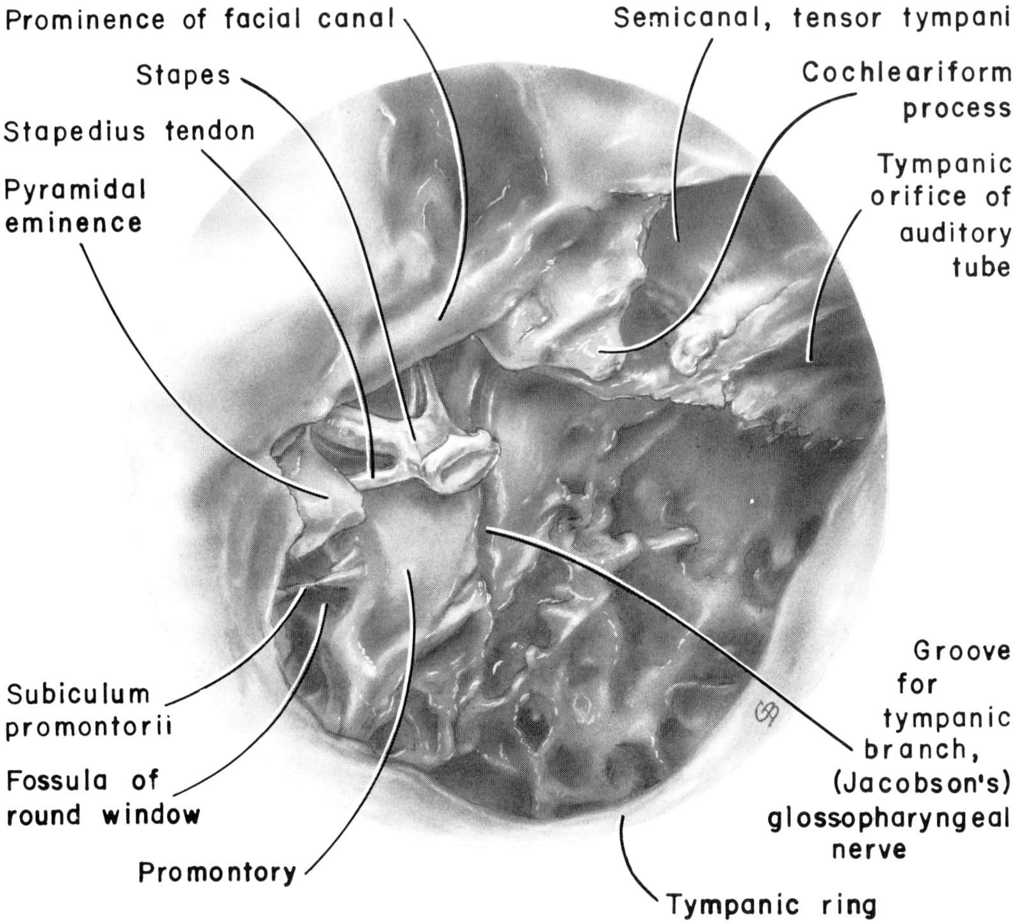

a

Figure III–16. Anatomy of the medial, or labyrinthine, wall of the tympanic cavity; demonstrating especially the tympanic air cells. Dissections of unembalmed specimens.

a. The malleus and incus have been excised; the tensor tympani has been removed from the semicanal and Jacobson's nerve from its sulcus. The stapes and the tendon of its muscle remain *in situ.*

The tympanic cells, numerous in this case, may extend as tracts into the tympanic sinus and medial to the vertical segment of the facial canal. They are frequently continuous with pneumatized areas in the bone of the inner ear, sometimes extending to the apex of the petrous pyramid to form an unbroken succession with air cells in the auditory tube. In the specimen illustrated the cells are abundant in the area bounded by the opening of the auditory tube anteriorly and the fossula of the cochlear (round) window posteriorly.

Figure III–16 continues on the opposite page.

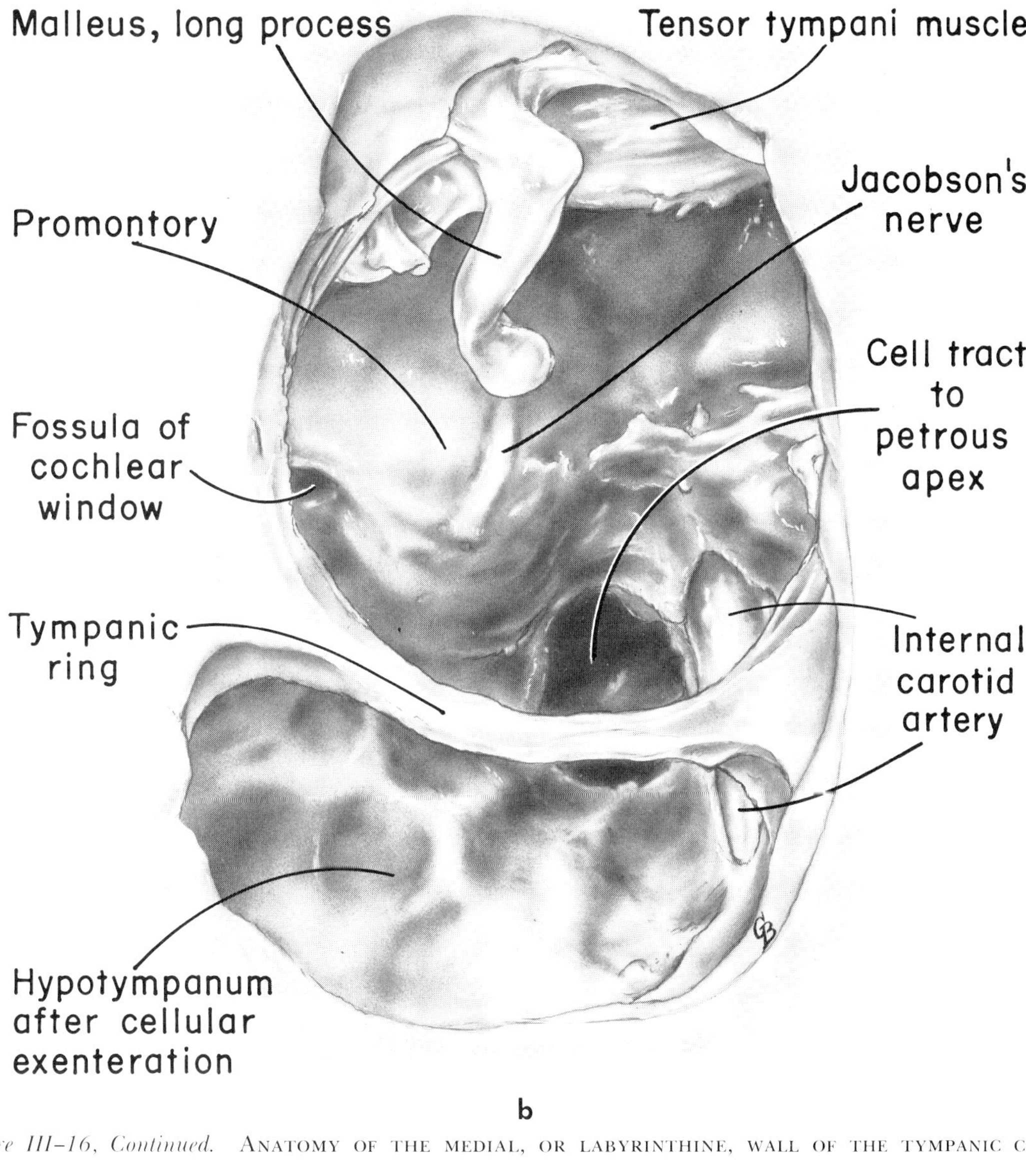

Figure III–16, Continued. ANATOMY OF THE MEDIAL, OR LABYRINTHINE, WALL OF THE TYMPANIC CAVITY; DEMONSTRATING ESPECIALLY THE TYMPANIC AIR CELLS. DISSECTIONS OF UNEMBALMED SPECIMENS.

The cells invade mainly the bone of the promontory formed by the basal turn of the cochlea, as far as the sulcus for the nerves contributory to the tympanic plexus (*Jacobsoni*).

b. The tympanic membrane has been excised, the inferior segment of the tympanic ring retained in order to demonstrate its topographical relation to the air cell tracts.

The dissection demonstrates the extent of hypotympanic pneumatization, the presence of cells below the level of the tympanic ring, their broad communication with similar cells of the petrous apex, and the nearness of this aperture to the internal carotid artery.

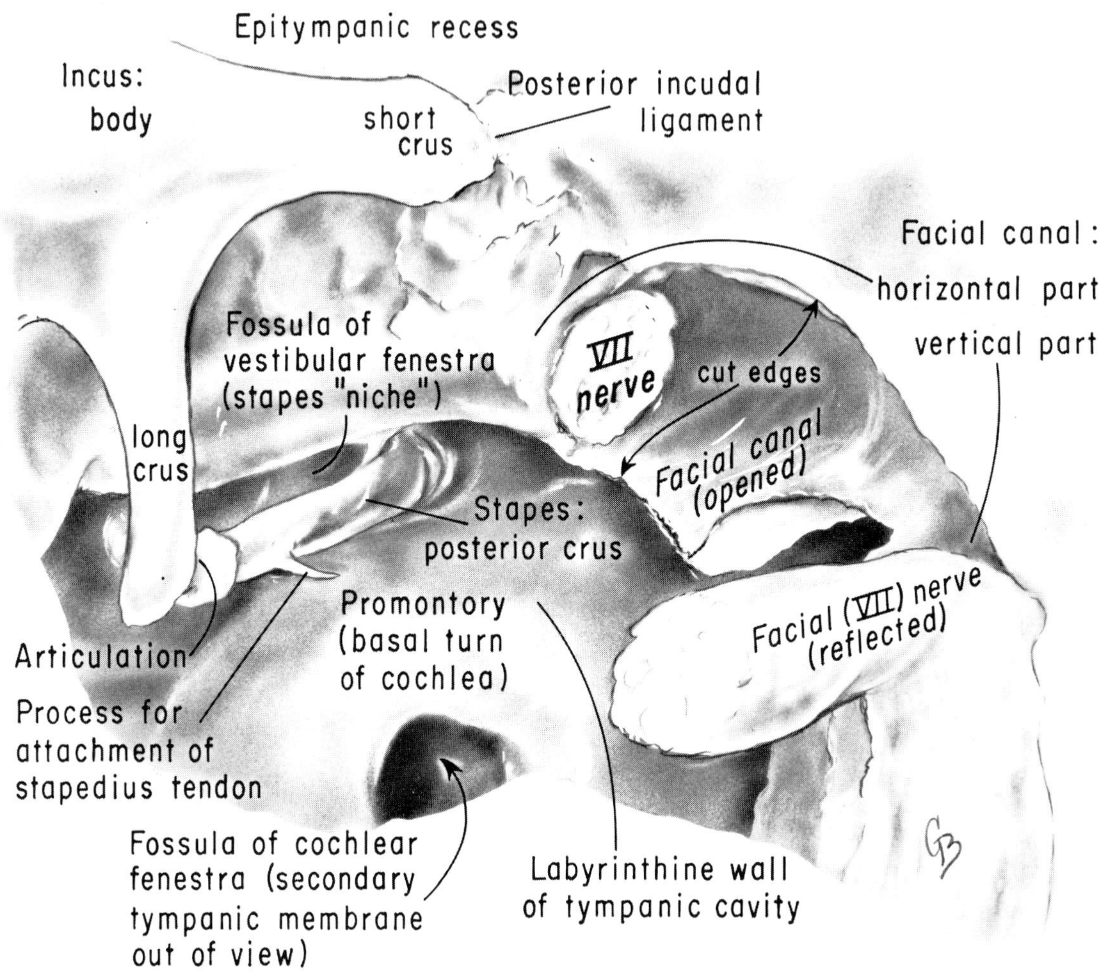

Figure III–17. Tympanic cavity: structures on the medial (tympanic) wall. *a.* Dissection of an unembalmed specimen, left temporal bone.

a. The facial canal has been opened in the curving segment between the horizontal and vertical portions; the nerve has been transected, the distal part reflected. The canal is intact in the area of the geniculum. The canal overarches the fossula of the vestibular (oval) window (the stapes "niche"). The prominence formed by the basal turn of the cochlea forms a "roof" for a comparable space that leads into the cochlear (round) window. The window and the secondary tympanic membrane that closes the fenestra are seen in lateral view. In this specimen the stapedius muscle was absent; the normal site of attachment of its tendon on the posterior crus is marked by the presence of an osseous spur.

Figure III–17 continues on the opposite page.

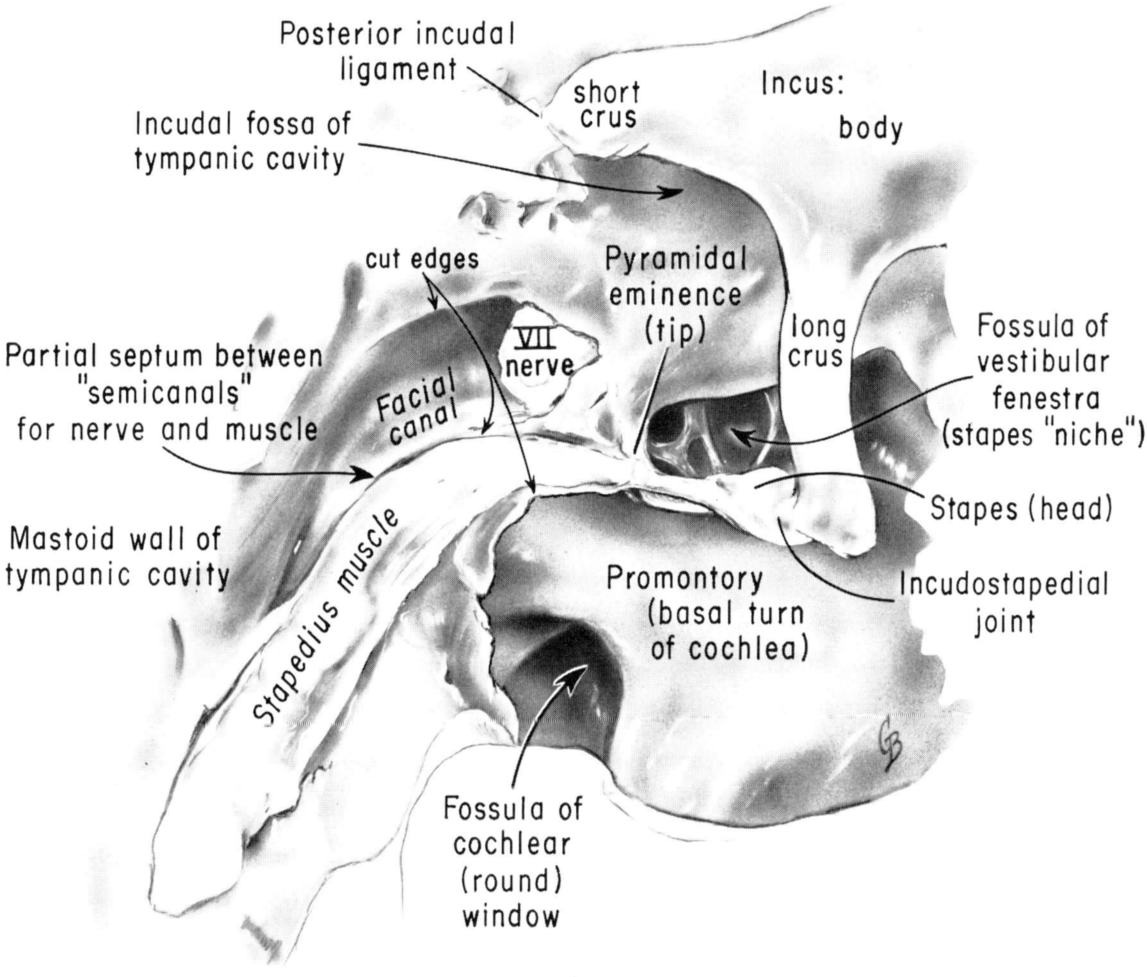

Figure III–17, Continued. TYMPANIC CAVITY: STRUCTURES ON THE MEDIAL (TYMPANIC) WALL. *b.* DISSECTION OF AN UNEMBALMED SPECIMEN, RIGHT TEMPORAL BONE.

b. The compartments of the facial canal have been opened. The facial nerve has been transected and removed in order to demonstrate its depth and the way in which it is divided by an osseous septum into channels (each a "semicanal") for the facial nerve and the stapedius muscle. The latter is shown in its entirety, from the lower extremity to the tendon of attachment on the head of the stapes. The horizontal segment of the facial canal is intact as it overarches the fossula of the vestibular fenestra.

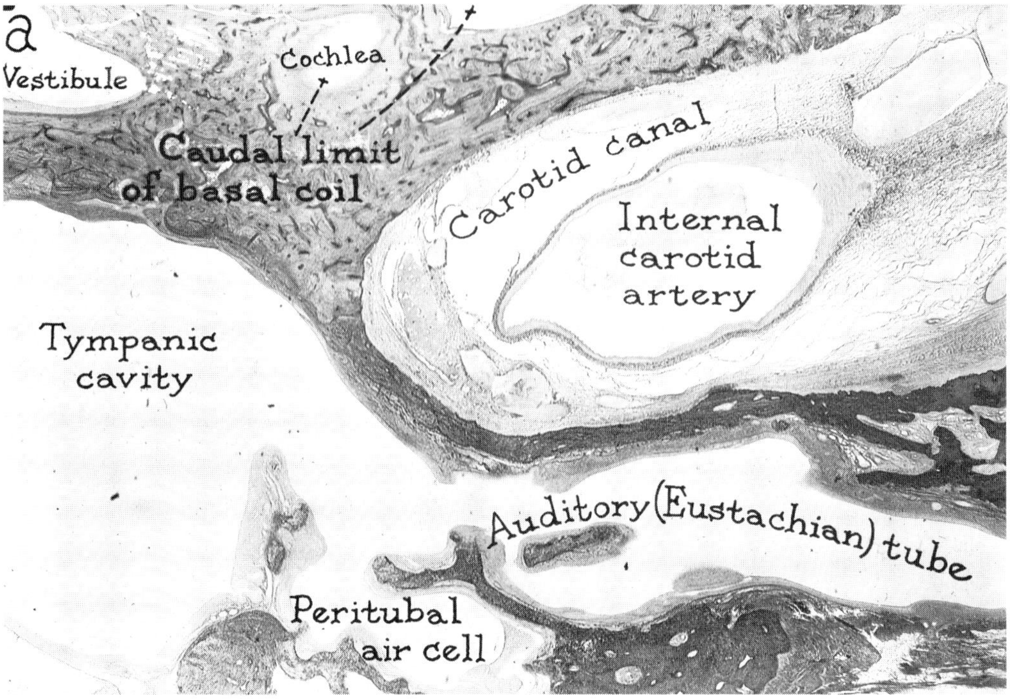

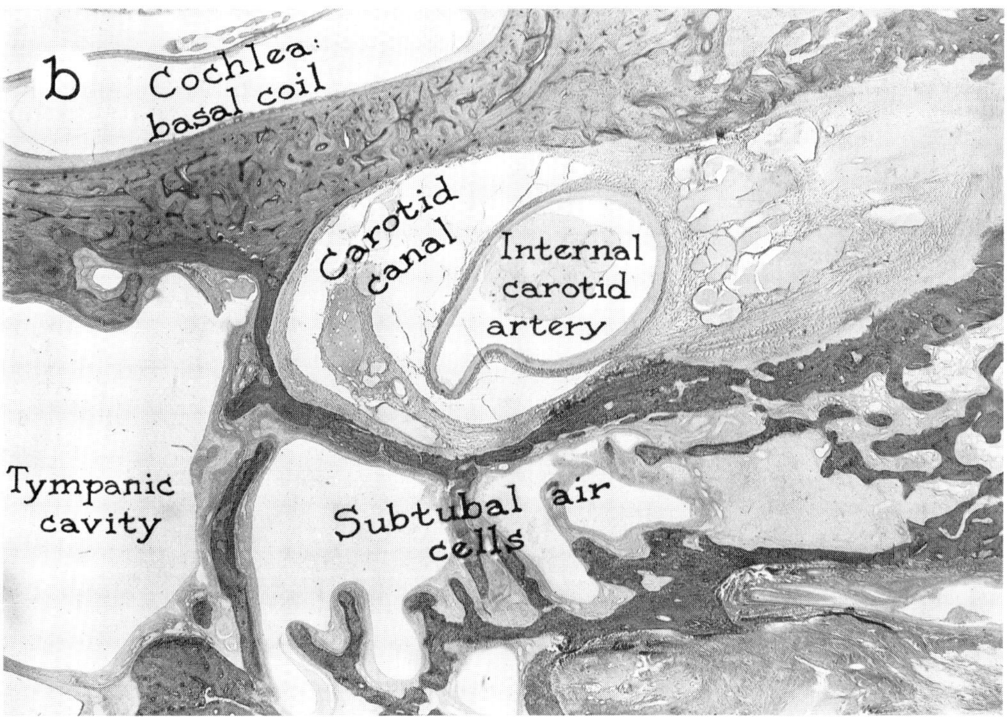

Figure III–18. See legend on the opposite page.

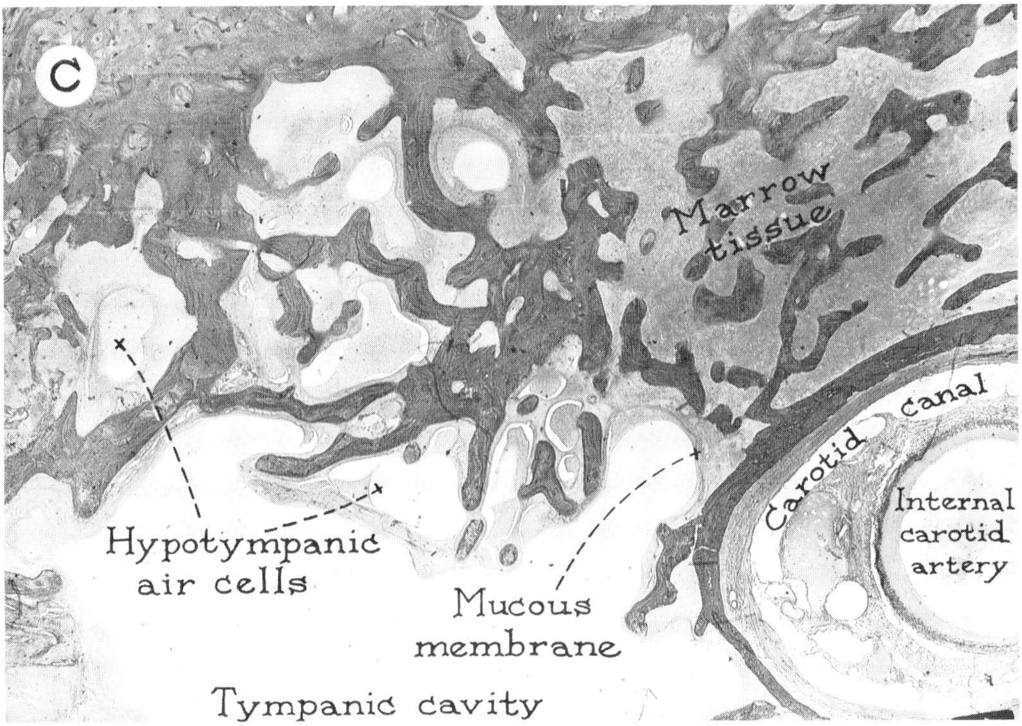

Figure III–18. AIR CELLS RELATED TO THE AUDITORY (EUSTACHIAN) TUBE AND THE TYMPANIC CAVITY. INFANT, 10 MONTHS OLD.

a. Here the cells are situated on the lateral wall of the auditory tube at the entrance of the latter into the tympanic cavity. Section at the lower limit of the cochlea.

b. This group of cells opens into the auditory tube from below. Section passing through the basal coil of the cochlea.

c. These pneumatic spaces occupy the "floor" and medial wall of the tympanic cavity.

In addition to the air cells in the mastoid process, pneumatic spaces in the petrous part of the temporal bone develop as outpocketings of the antrum, the tympanic cavity proper, and the auditory tube. Next to the mastoid and antral cells, carotid air cells are the most common. They arise as an epithelial inbudding into the developing bone as early as the twenty-seventh week of fetal life. They have been observed (in specimens from the Wisconsin Collection) in the following five regions: (1) anterior to the carotid canal and below the auditory (eustachian) tube, hence the term subtubal (or peritubal) air cells; (2) posterior to the carotid canal, as extensions of the subtubal cells; (3) between the auditory tube and carotid canal, again as extensions; (4) lateral to the carotid canal, between the canal and the mouth of the auditory tube, as precochlear cells; and (5) rarely, in the form of extensions of the precochlear set, above the carotid canal, just medial to the top of the cochlea (supracarotid cells).

Transverse sections, Wisconsin Collection, series 97. ×12.

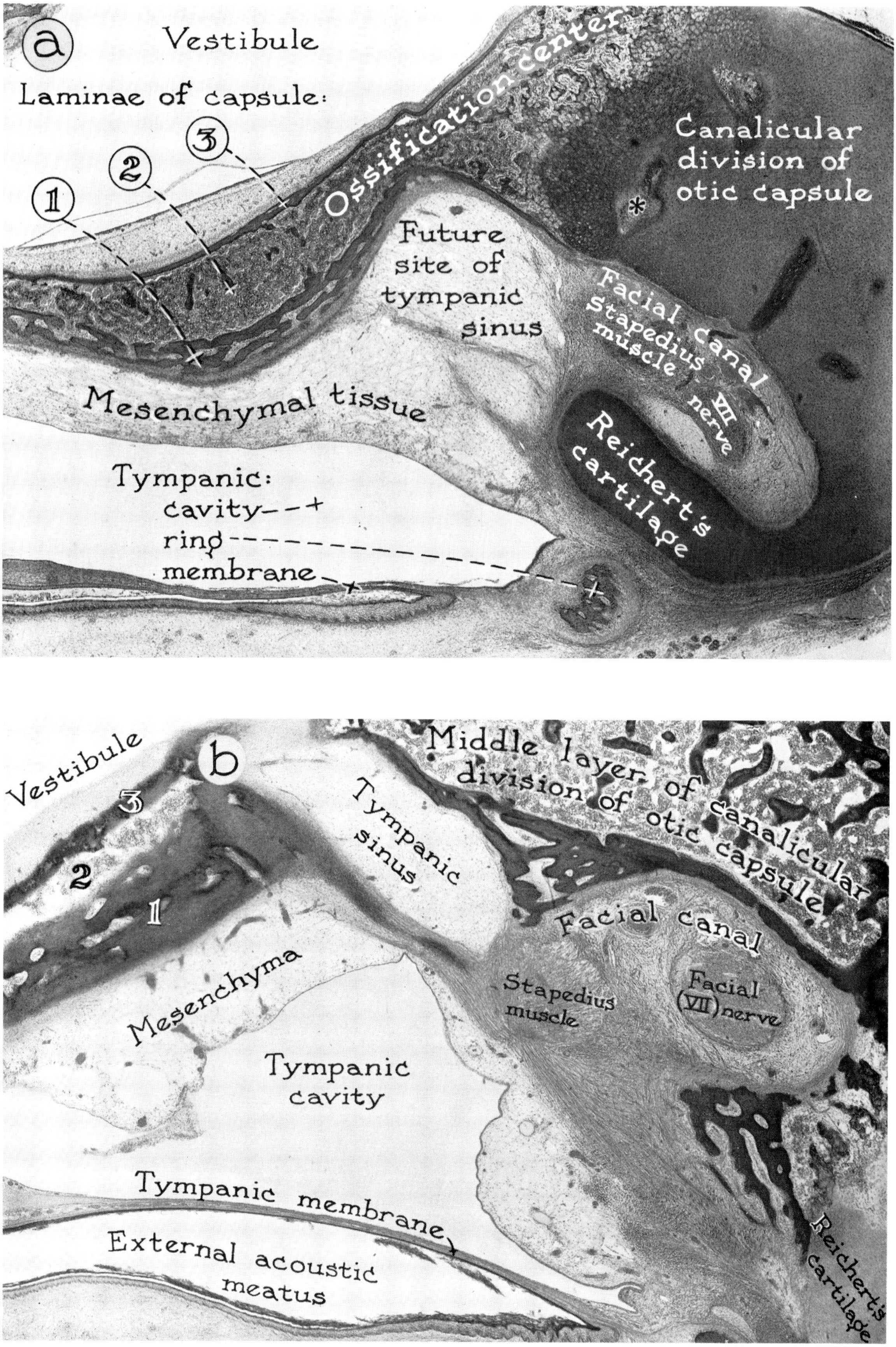

Figure III–19. See legend on the opposite page.

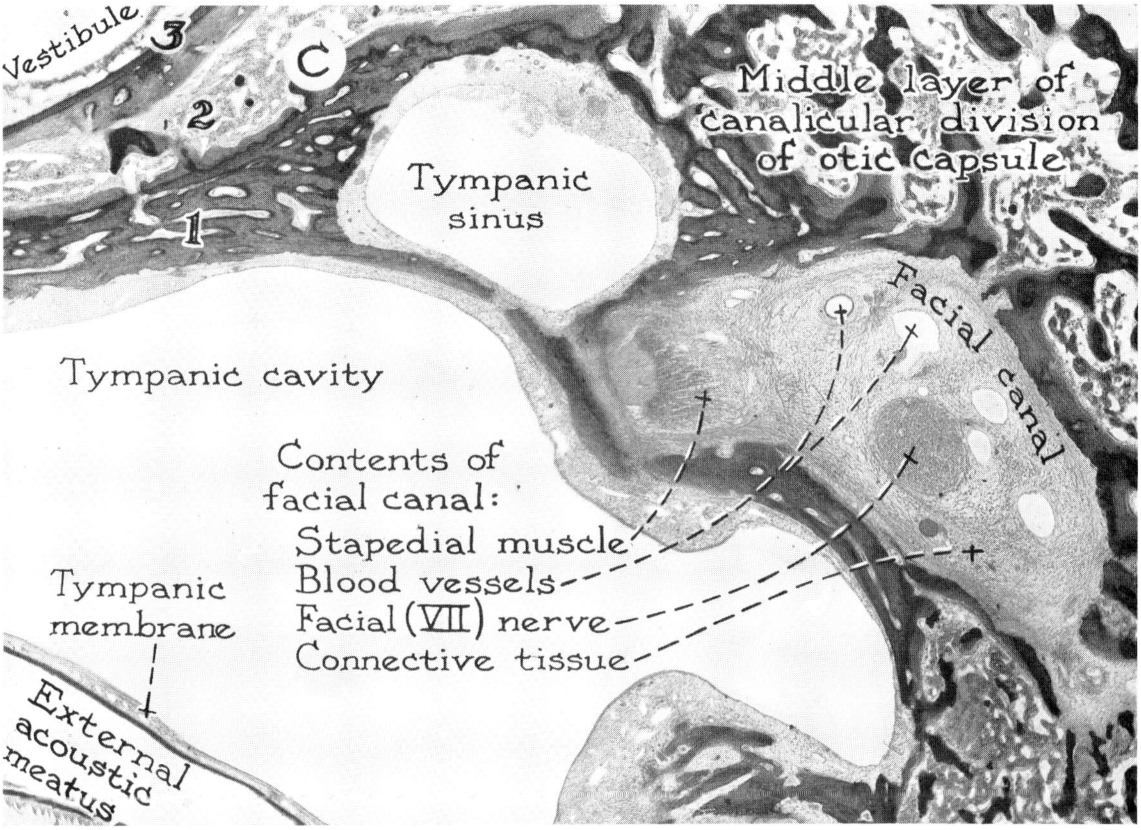

Figure III–19. TYMPANIC SINUS: DEVELOPMENTAL AND ADULT ANATOMY. *a.* FETUS OF 20 WEEKS (170 MM.). *b.* FETUS OF 26 WEEKS (230 MM.). *c.* FETUS OF 29 WEEKS (260 MM.).

a. In the 5-month fetus, part of the medial wall of the future tympanic sinus is still cartilaginous. Where ossification is occurring, the typical layers of bone are formed: *1*, outer periosteal layer; *2*, middle layer (mainly cartilage islands); *3*, inner periosteal layer. The facial canal is in a similarly primitive stage of morphogenesis, its lateral wall being formed by Reichert's cartilage (second branchial arch). The mucous membrane of the expanding cavity has not yet reached the labyrinthine wall of the tympanum and, therefore, has not yet formed a tympanic sinus. On the opposite (lateral) wall, the mucous membrane is the innermost layer of the trilaminar tympanic membrane.

b. Spread of the tympanic mucous membrane is a relatively slow process, the sinus still being occupied by primitive mesenchymal tissue. The sulcus that will become the facial canal contains the typical structures: namely, facial nerve, stapedius muscle, and blood vessels (veins being both numerous and capacious).

c. In a fetal stage of approximately seven months, bone formation in the canalicular division of the otic capsule has resulted in separation, superiorly, of the tympanic sinus from the space of the general tympanic cavity and in formation of the true (closed) facial canal. At this level, below the pyramidal eminence, the sinus occupies a surgically significant position between the vestibule and the facial canal.

Figure III–19 continues on the following page.

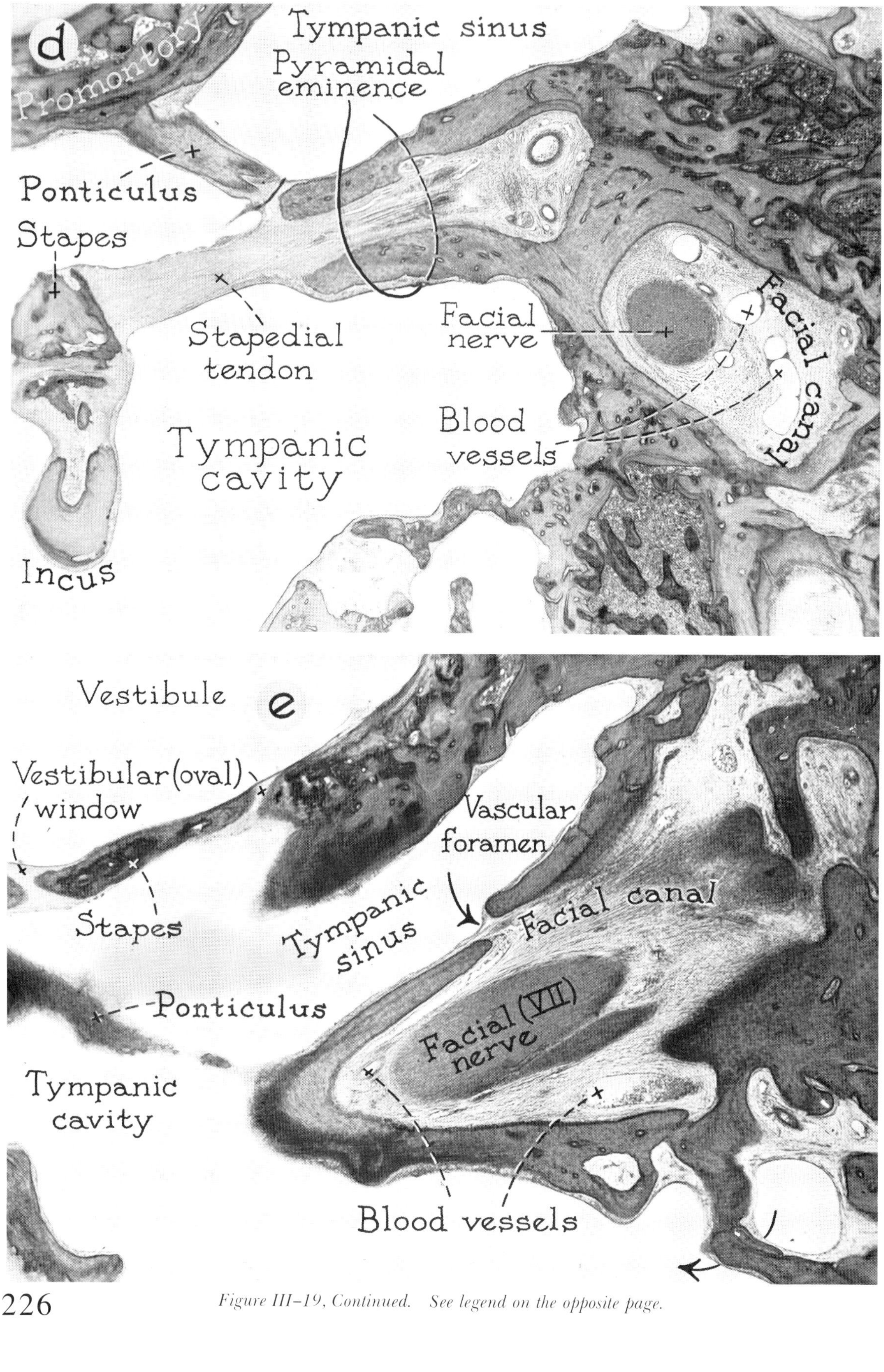

Figure III–19, Continued. See legend on the opposite page.

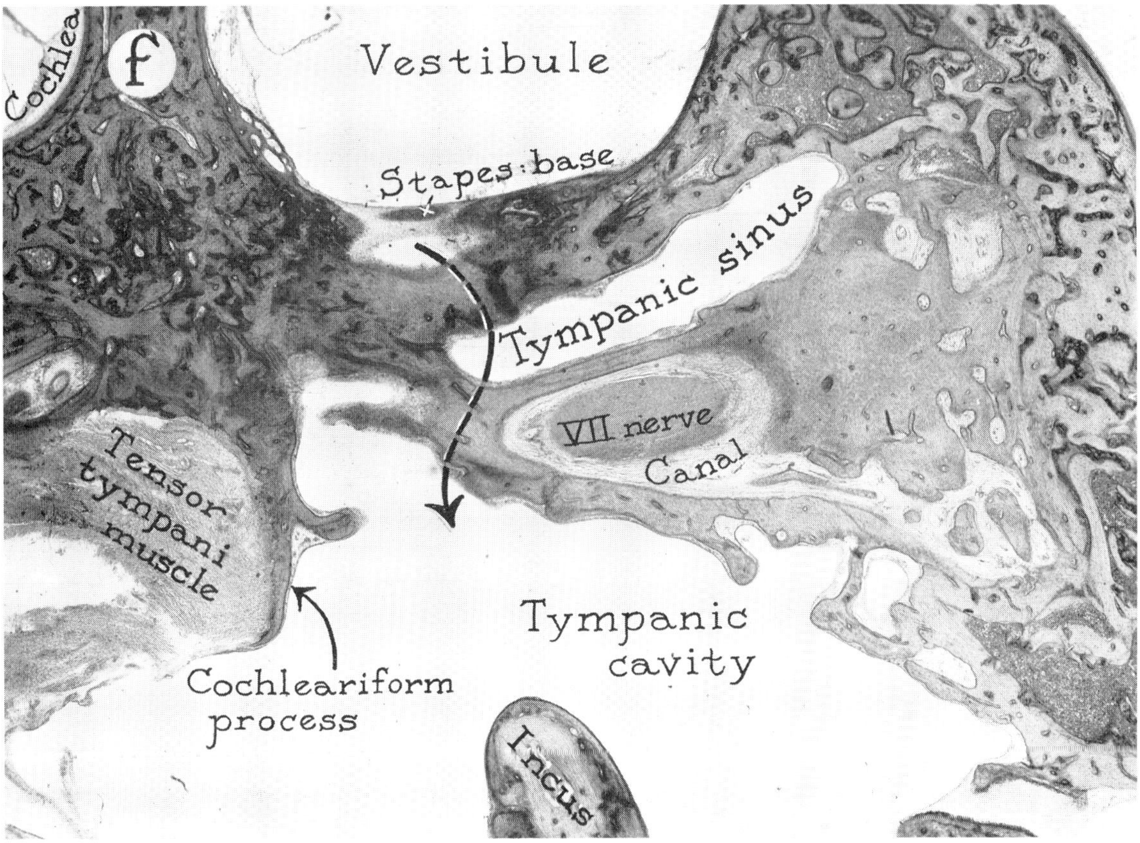

Figure III–19, Continued. TYMPANIC SINUS: DEVELOPMENTAL AND ADULT ANATOMY. *d* to *f*. INFANT, 10 WEEKS OLD.

d. In the infant, the form and relationships of the tympanic sinus are established. At the horizontal level of the stapedius tendon, the tympanic sinus is closed in by bone: medially by the promontory, laterally by the pyramidal eminence, and anteriorly by the ponticulus. It communicates with the general space of the tympanic cavity below but not above—becoming less capacious as it is traced cranialward (compare *f*).

e. Just above the level of the stapedius tendon, the tympanic sinus is closely related to the vestibular window. The sinus is bounded posterolaterally by the wall of the facial canal, as the latter changes from a horizontal to a vertical course.

f. Farther cranialward, at the upper limit of the vestibular window, the tympanic sinus is a small chink. In this specimen, the level marks the summit of the fossula of the vestibular fenestra, or stapes "niche" (from which the unlabeled arrow is directed into the tympanic cavity). Here the facial canal, in prefenestral position, is approximately in midcourse between the geniculum and the junction of the transverse and vertical segments.

Transverse sections, Wisconsin Collection, series as follows: *a*, 131; *b*, 64; *c*, 45 A; *d* to *f*, 83. *a*, ×23; *b*, ×24; *c*, ×29; *d*, ×19; *e*, ×29; *f*, ×19.

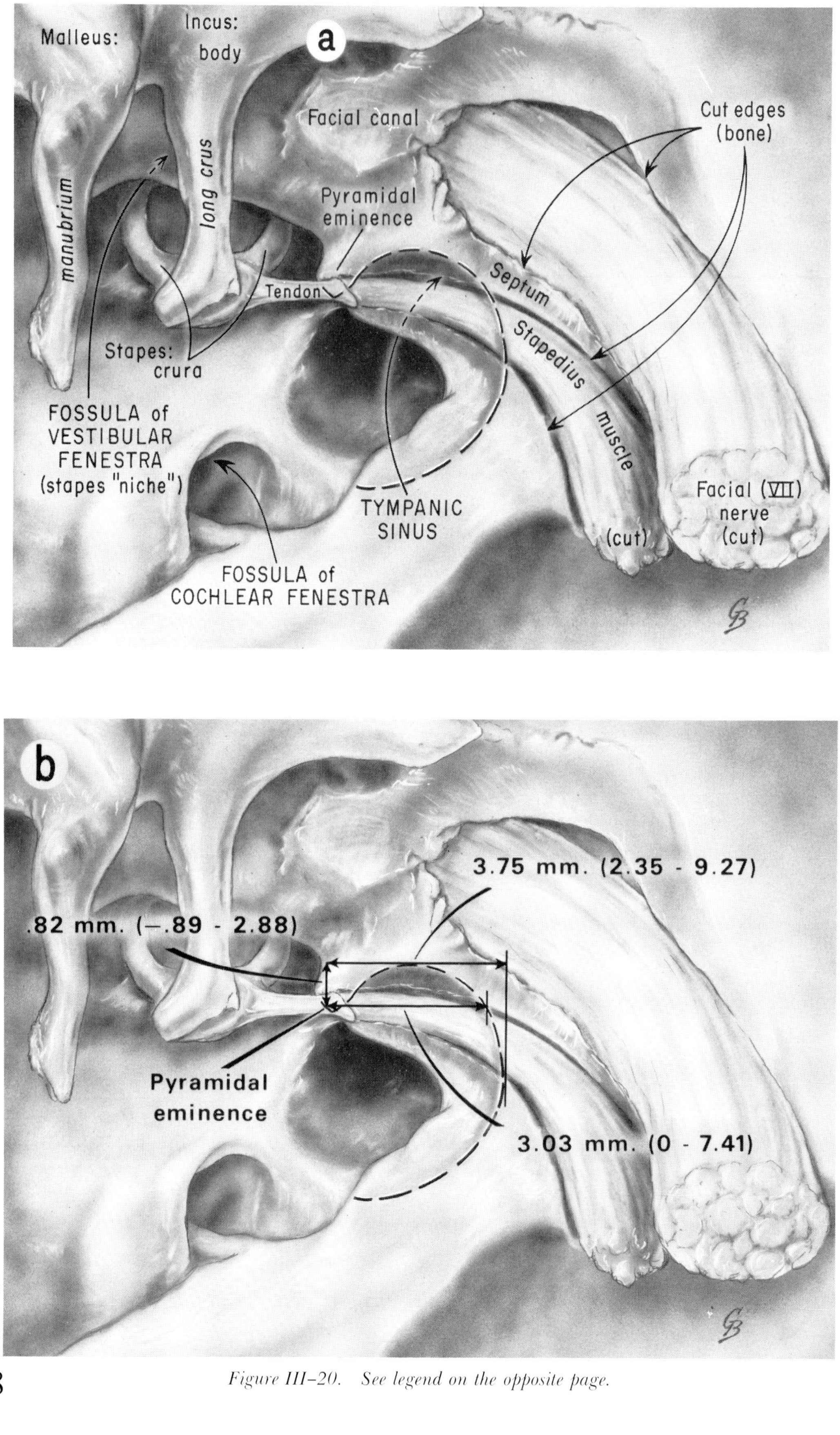

Figure III–20. See legend on the opposite page.

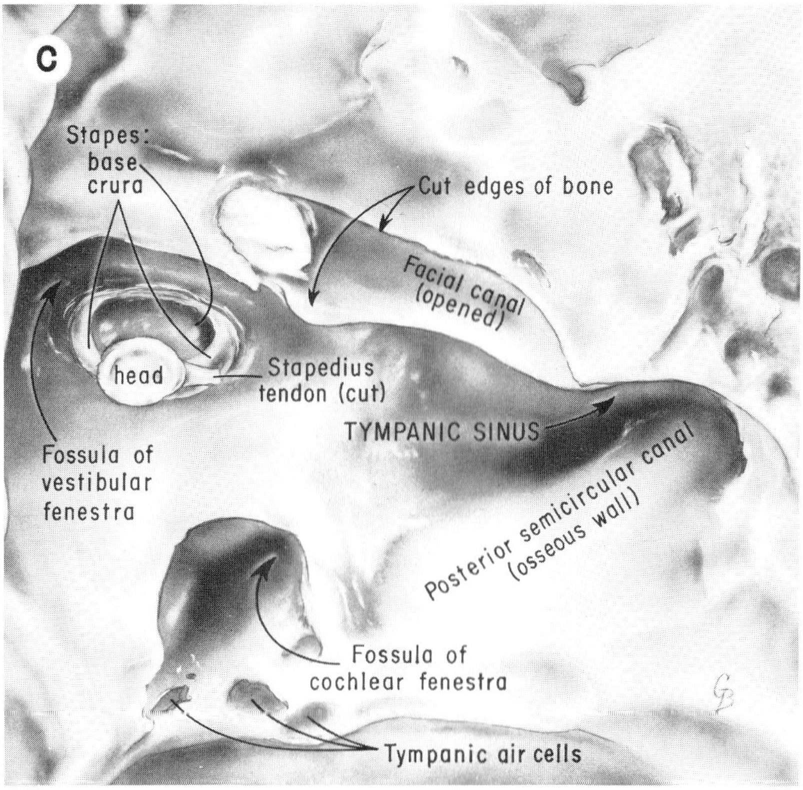

Figure III–20. TYMPANIC CAVITY AND SINUS: VARIATIONAL ANATOMY SHOWN IN FIVE UNEMBALMED SPECIMENS.

a. The facial canal has been opened in order to expose the facial nerve and the stapedius muscle. It is shown that these structures are housed in separate compartments for part of their course. The size and relations of the tympanic sinus are demonstrated. The sinus extends posteriorly (along the broken line) deep to the compartment for the muscle.

b. The same section as shown in *a*, with measurements

c. The stapedius muscle has been excised, and the facial nerve has been transected in its horizontal course and removed. The lateral wall of this exceptionally large tympanic sinus has been dissected away to expose the space in its entirety, as it reaches the posterior margin of the posterior semicircular canal.

Figure III–20 continues on the following page.

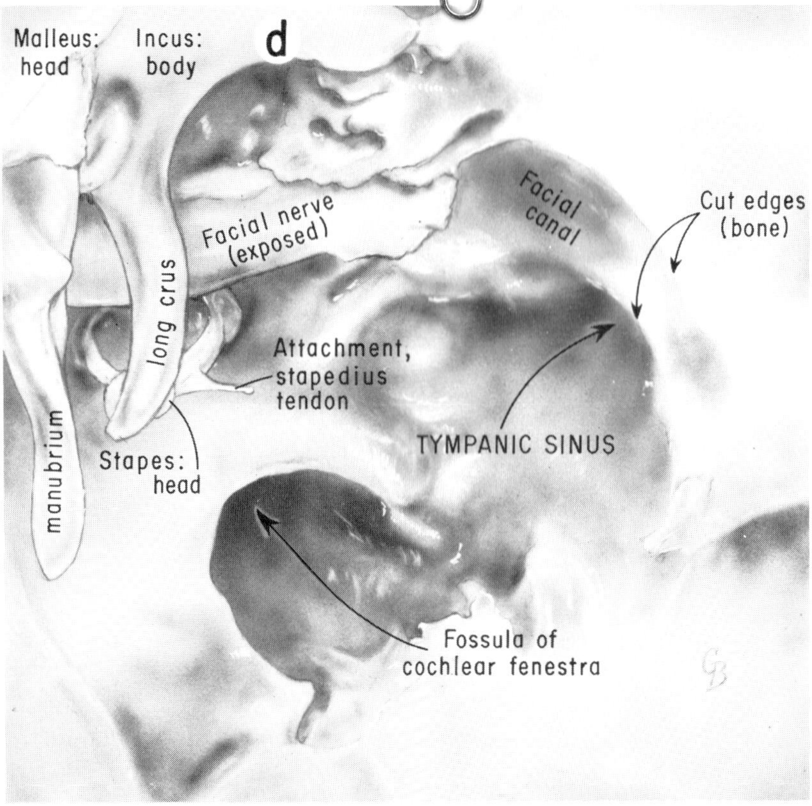

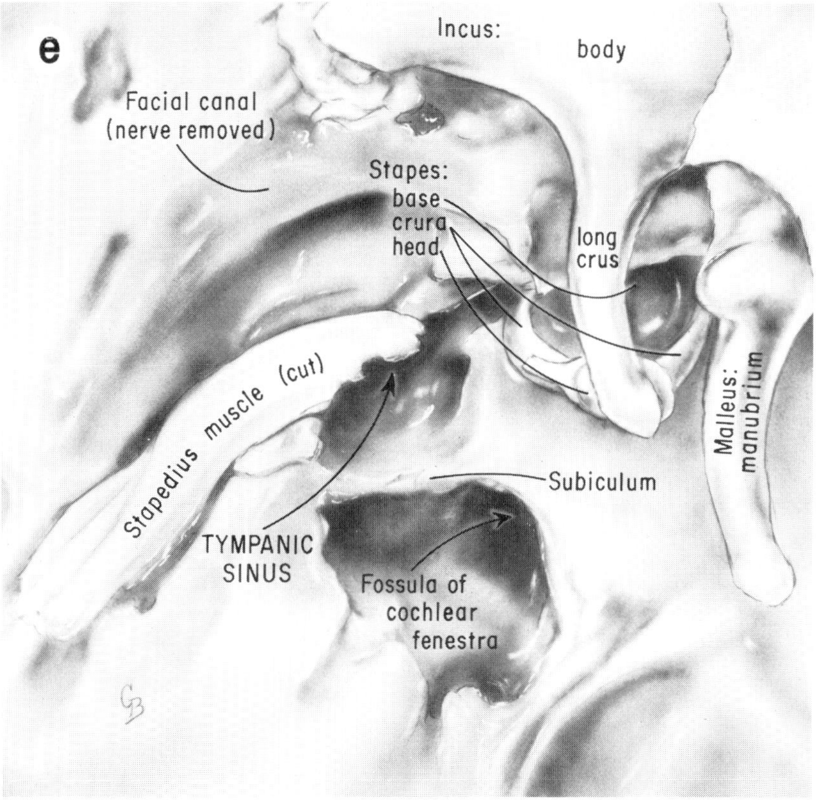

Figure III–20, Continued. *See legend on the opposite page.*

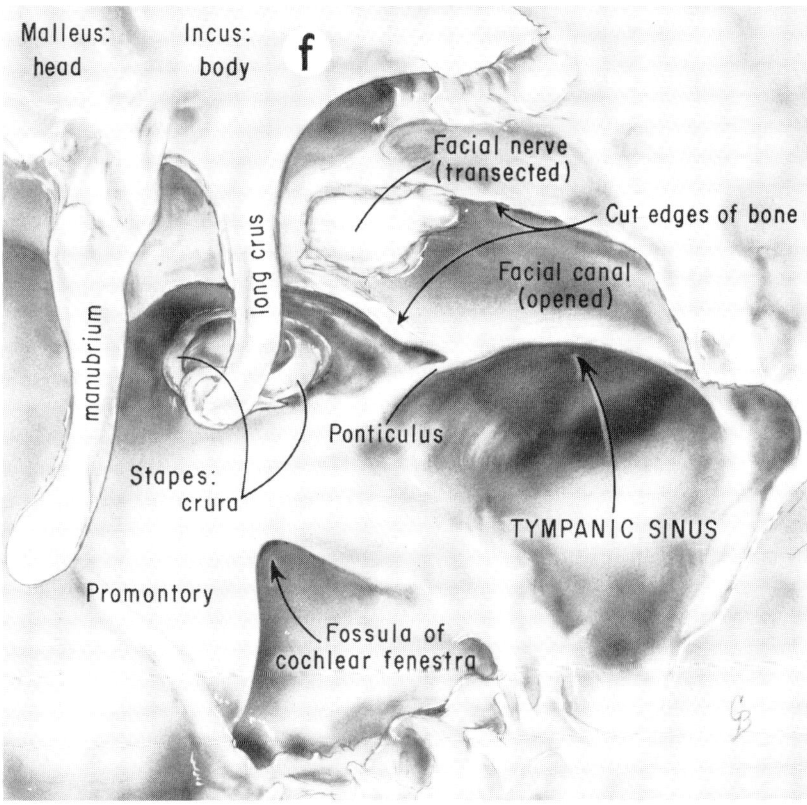

Figure III–20, Continued. TYMPANIC CAVITY AND SINUS.

d. The sinus tympani has been exposed as in the preceding figure. Although the sinus does not extend as far posteriorly, it almost reaches the posterior margin of the vertical portion of the facial nerve.

e. The sinus has been exposed as in the preceding instance. It is quite small and could have been adequately exposed and cleaned without damaging the facial nerve. The subiculum bounds the sinus inferiorly.

f. The sinus has been exposed by removing its lateral wall, demonstrating the relation of the ponticulus to the sinus.

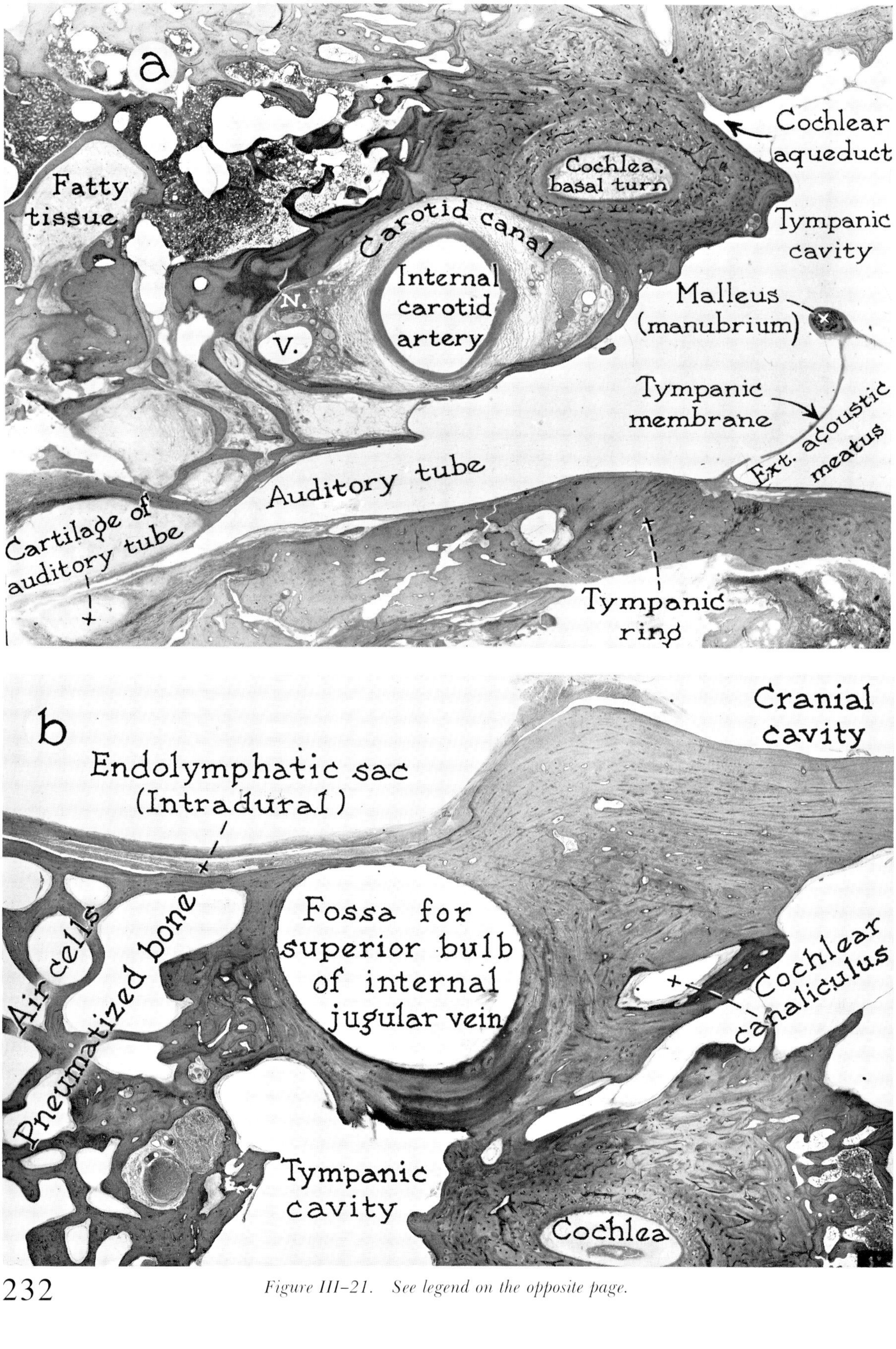

Figure III–21. See legend on the opposite page.

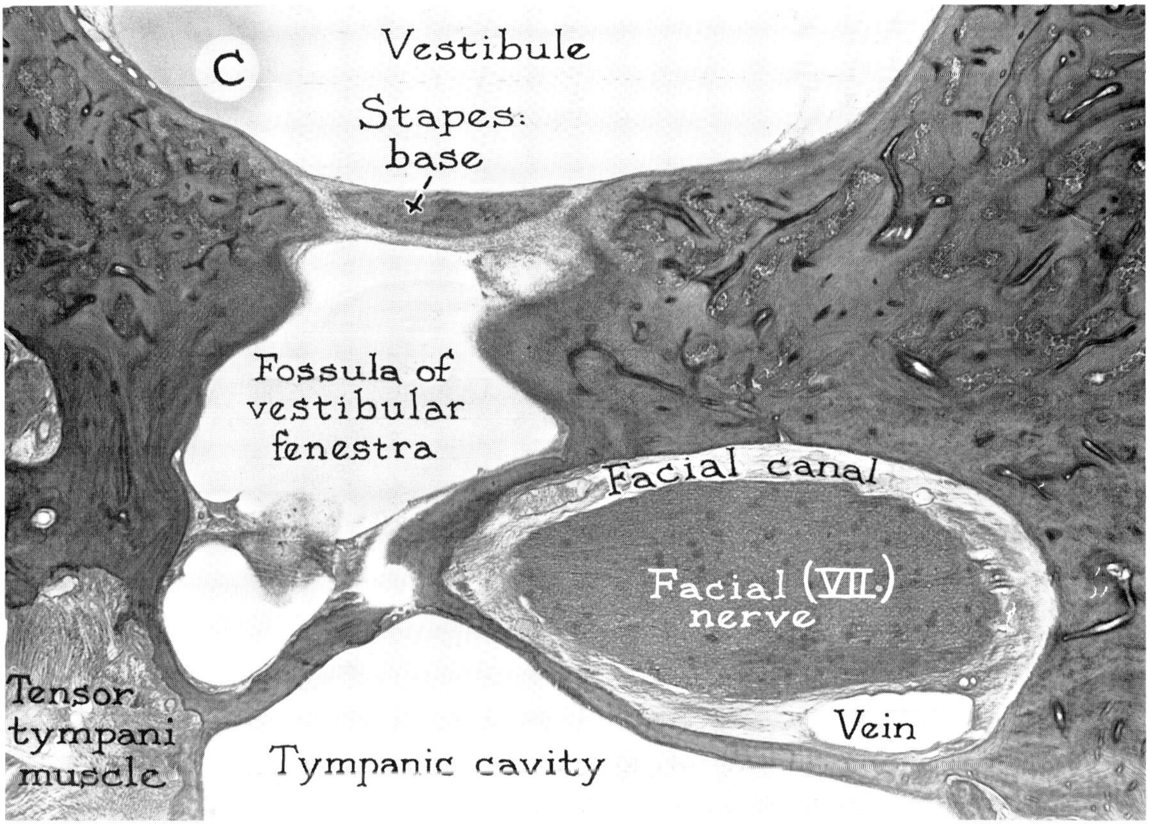

Figure III–21. TYMPANIC CAVITY, MAJOR VASCULAR AND NEURAL RELATIONS: TOPOGRAPHY OF THE CAROTID CANAL, JUGULAR FOSSA, AND FACIAL CANAL. *a* and *c*. ADULT, 19 YEARS OF AGE. *b*. ADULT, 38 YEARS OLD.

a. The carotid canal, in following a curving course through the petrous part of the temporal bone, is closely related to the promontory formed by the basal turn of the cochlea. It projects into the tympanic cavity at the junction of the promontory with the auditory tube.

b. The fossa that houses the superior bulb of the jugular vein frequently invades the space of the tympanic cavity. In some instances the "roof" of a deep fossa is dehiscent, mucous membrane alone intervening between the jugular bulb and the surgeon's exploring instrument. A high dehiscent jugular bulb may be mistaken for a glomus tumor (see Figure III–101).

c. The facial canal transmits numerous arteries and capacious veins in addition to the facial nerve (see reconstruction, Figure III–69*c*). The vessels are branches of the stylomastoid and greater petrosal. Leaving the canal through the pyramidal eminence and vascular foramina in the wall, they contribute importantly to the blood supply of the tympanic mucous membrane, auditory ossicles and tympanic membrane (see Figure III–67).

Transverse sections, Wisconsin Collection, series as follows: *a* and *c*, 29; *b*, 24. *a*, ×8; *b*, ×7; *c*, ×28.

(*a* and *b* from Anson: Trans. Amer. Acad. Ophthal. Otolaryng., 73:17–38, 1969.)

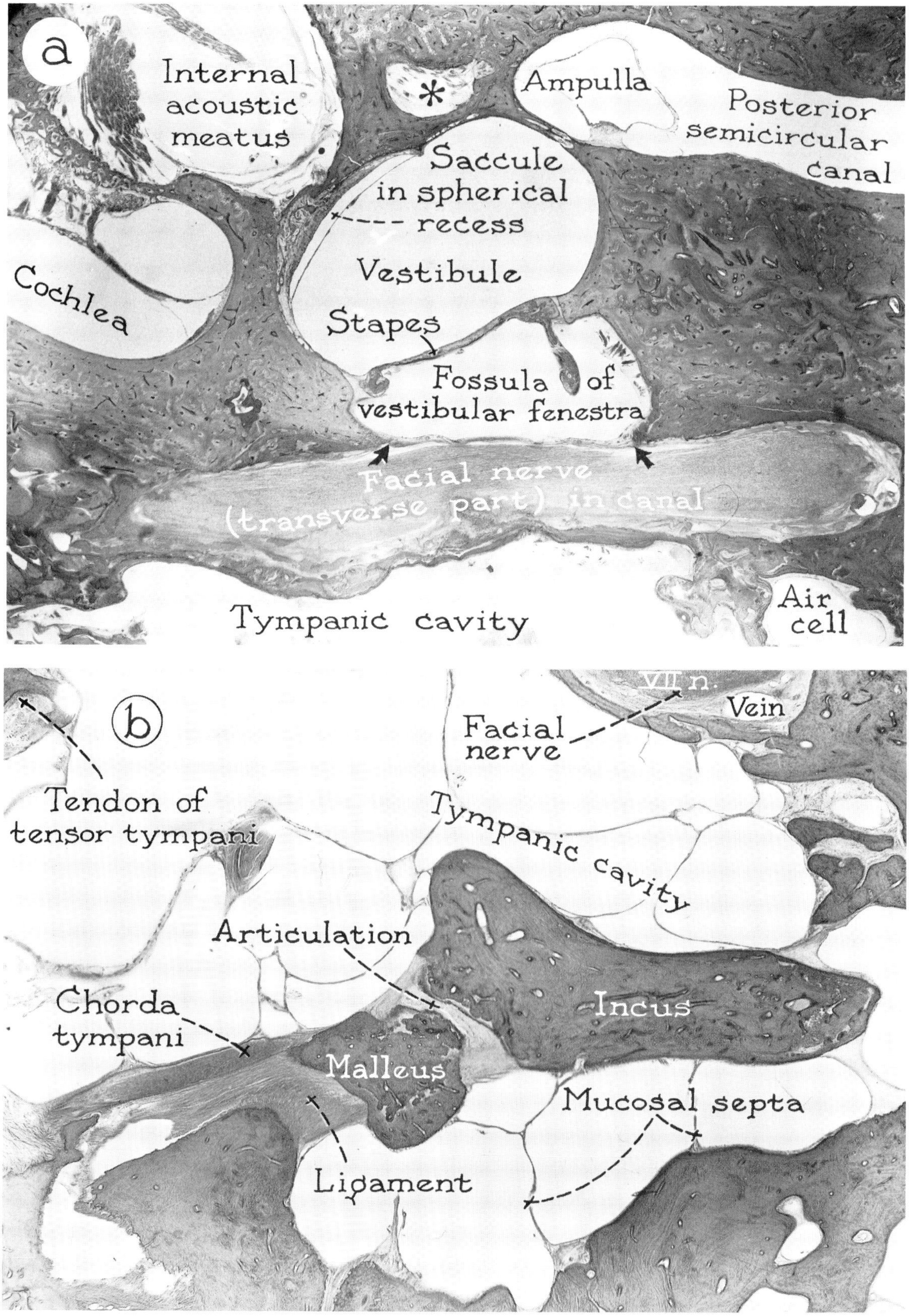

 Figure III–22. See legend on the opposite page.

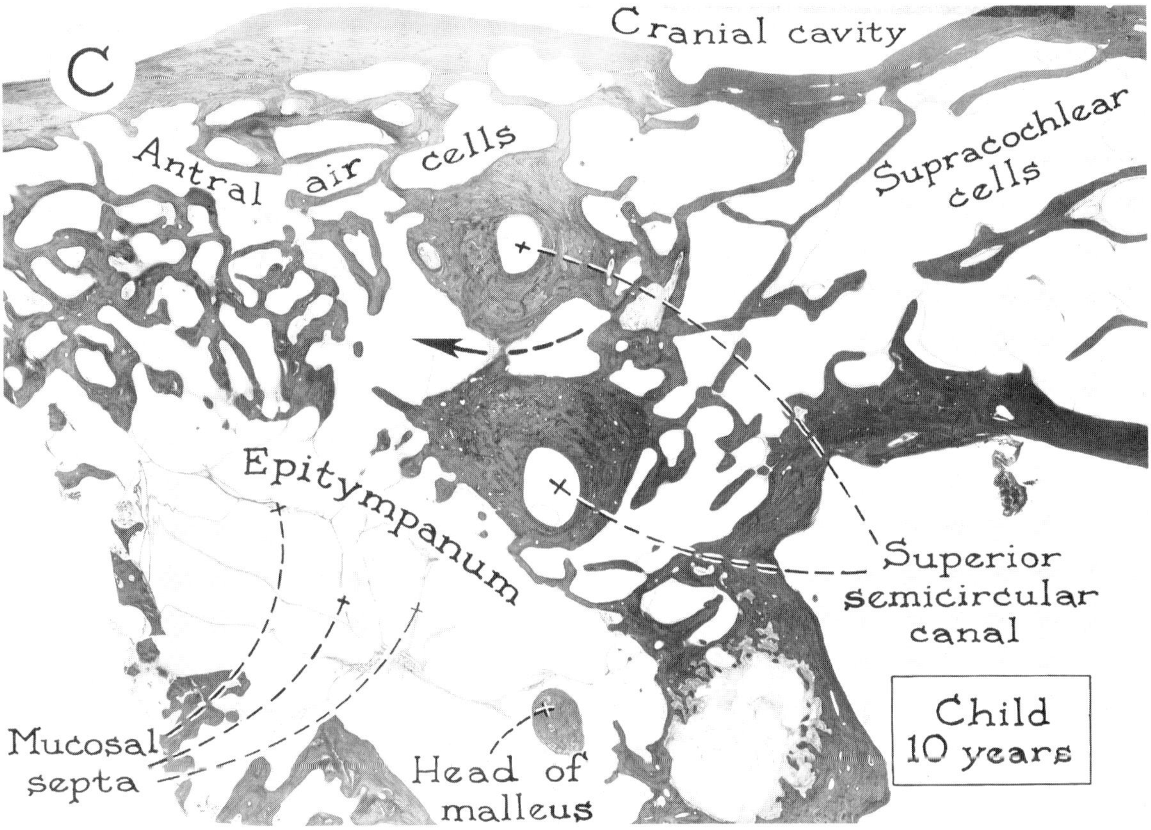

Figure III–22. TYMPANIC CAVITY AND RELATED AIR SPACES: ADULT ANATOMY. *a.* ADULT, 40 YEARS OLD. *b.* ADULT, 19 YEARS OF AGE. *c.* CHILD, 10 YEARS OLD.

a. Showing one of the numerous tympanic air cells and the fossula of the vestibular fenestra. The fossula is situated above the ponticulus. In its superior part, the fossula is bounded by the stapedial base (footplate) medially and the facial canal laterally. In this specimen, where the canal is dehiscent (between arrows), the nerve is exposed on the wall of the fossula. The asterisk indicates the nerves of supply to the ampulla of the posterior semicircular duct.

b. Demonstrating the manner in which the tympanic cavity is subdivided into lesser spaces by septa of the mucous membrane (see also Figures III–91*c* and III–141). Blood vessels, coursing in the connective tissue between the apposed layers of membrane, carry smaller vessels to the auditory ossicles.

c. Showing the degree to which the *pars petrosa* may be pneumatized: in this instance, leaving the osseous wall of the superior semicircular canal supported only by thin trabeculae. The cells intercommunicate freely (see arrow). The larger spaces (the epitympanum, for example) are crossed by numerous mucosal septa (compare preceding figure). The cells at the reader's right overlie the cochlea.

Transverse sections, Wisconsin Collection, series 18, 29, and 57, respectively. *a*, ×13; *b*, ×16; *c*, ×6.

Figure III–23. CHOLESTEATOMA: THE SAC OF A PRIMARY ACQUIRED CHOLESTEATOMA.

The sac has been opened to demonstrate its relation to the epitympanum and to the auditory ossicles. The arrow points to the attic tract into the sac, the medial wall of which is approximated to the head of the malleus and the body of the incus. An incision has been made superiorly into the skin of the canal extending into the sac. The dissection simulates the way in which the procedure would be carried out in a modified radical mastoidectomy.

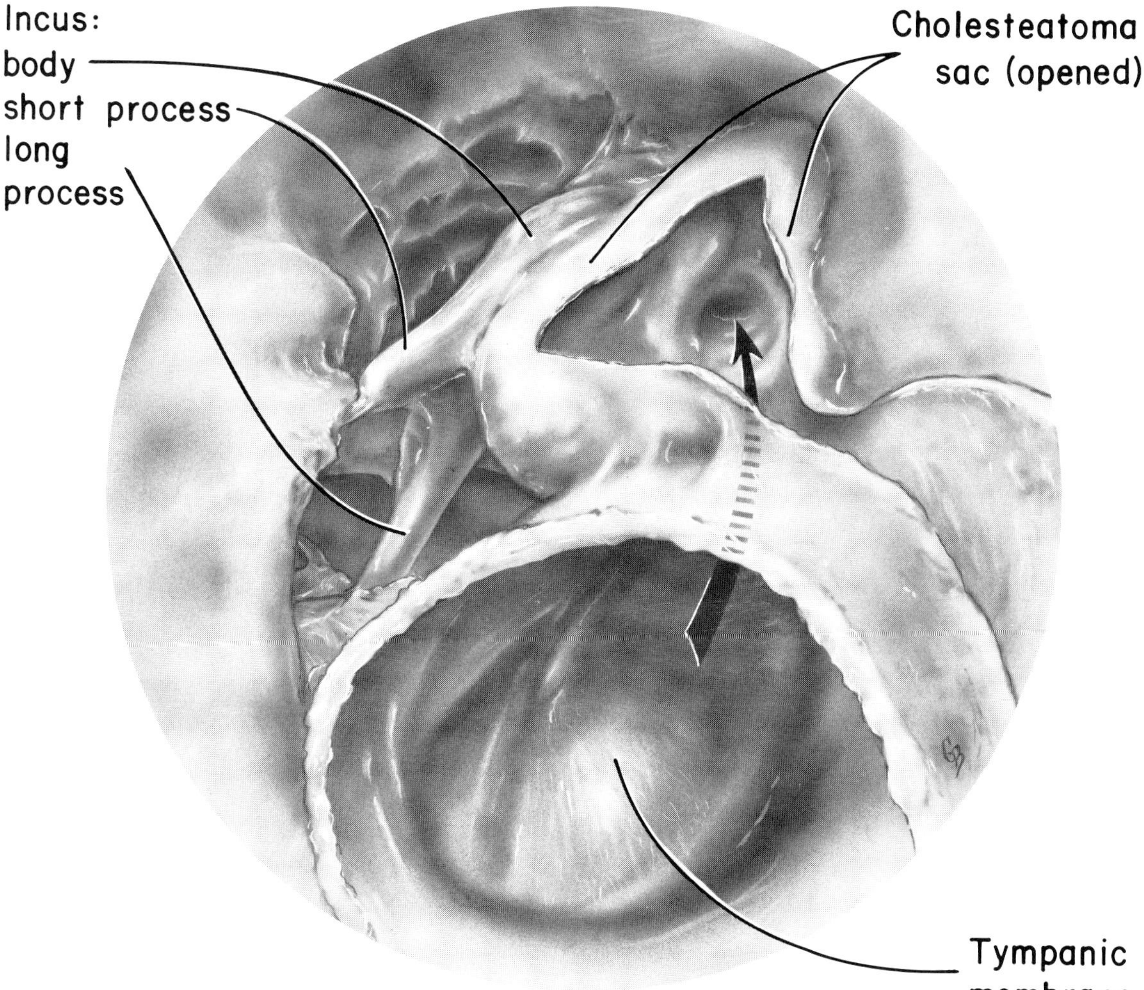

Figure III–23. See legend on the opposite page.

Figure III–24. Auditory ossicles, normal form. Drawings prepared with the use of a dissection microscope.

Upper left. The stapes, or stirrup, possesses a footplate (base), two legs (crura), and a small head (capitulum). A neck (collum) is also sometimes described. The footplate occupies the vestibular (oval) window, almost completely filling it. The vestibular surface is flat; on the tympanic aspect, the margin is lipped circumferentially, an excavation being thus produced. The legs, or columns, are hollowed out in groovelike fashion on their facing surfaces, these excavations being continuous with the concavity on the footplate and with a space in the head (hereinbelow). The upper margin of the footplate is convex, the lower margin straight or concave. The posterior leg is usually more sharply curved than the anterior and, therefore, the slightly longer of the two; it possesses near the head a small roughened area or a projection for insertion of the stapedial muscle. The anterior crus is the finer of the two. The head is highly variable in form. The lateral surface is usually foveate, for reception of the lenticular process of the incus. Like the medial surface of the footplate, the lateral surface of the head is covered with cartilage. In the natural state the intercrural space is closed by a reflection of the mucosal lining of the middle ear, termed the obturator membrane of the stapes.

The form of the incus, or anvil, suggests that of a tooth with two roots. To the crown of the "tooth" corresponds the flattened body. The free surface of the latter presents a saddle-shaped articular surface for reception of the head of the malleus. To the roots correspond the crura, long and short; the latter is the thicker of the two. The long leg ends in a lenticular process.

The malleus, or hammer, is the largest of the three ossicles. The upper part, or head, is thick and club-shaped, and presents on the posteromedial aspect an elongate saddle-shaped articular surface for the body of the incus. The head is separated by a constriction, the neck, or *collum*, from the handle, or *manubrium*. The latter tapers toward a spatulate tip. The manubrium is continued, in superolateral direction, into a small lateral process, which, in the natural state, produces a bulging in the tympanic membrane. A thin anterior process (*Folii*) is directed forward from the neck of the ossicle.

Lower line. Stapes, with records of variation in size obtained from measurement of 75 consecutive specimens.

Upper right. Specimens of stapes selected to demonstrate variation in form. Viewed from above. The specimen in the lower figure possesses crura of markedly different form. As regularly described, the posterior crus is curved, the anterior crus relatively straight. The superior crural arch is more expansive than the inferior one. In the specimen shown in the upper figure the posterior crus, although the longer of the two, is less curved than that of the following case. The superior crural arch is opened more widely than the inferior arch. The neck of the ossicle is foraminous; the articular surface of the head is flattened (in contrast to the form assumed by the capital portion in the following specimen).

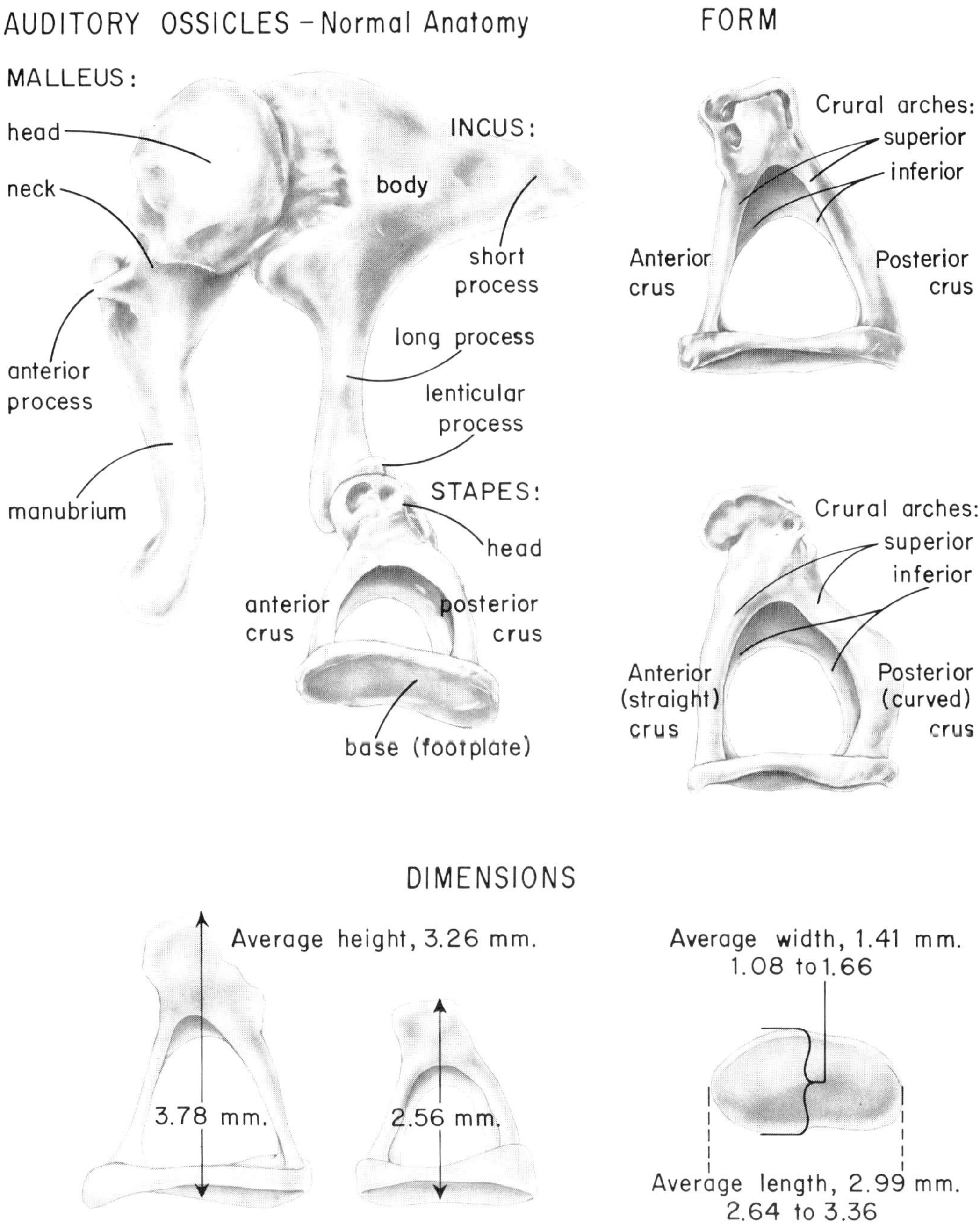

Figure III–24. See legend on the opposite page.

Figure III–25. Stapes, vestibular fenestra, and periotic appendages. Selected levels from the same otological series. Adult, 19 years of age.

The unlabeled arrows in *b* and *c* point to the vestibular apertures of, respectively, the fissular and fossular tracts in the area of the vestibular fenestra (oval window).

a and *b*. Demonstrating the mature form and histological structure of the base (footplate) and crura of the stapes, together with such related structures as the fissula ante fenestram on the vestibular aspect and mucosal septa on the tympanic side.

Between the fifth and sixth fetal month the footplate and the head of the stapes acquire a layer of endosteal bone, applied to the layer of primordial cartilage. This bilaminar structure is retained throughout life. The cartilage lamina is carried around the margin of the footplate, thus facing similar tissue that lines the window. The jutting edge of the window underlies the footplate (see *b* and *c*). Centrally, the osseous layer is excessively thin, sometimes locally absent. It is thick circumferentially, where it contains intercommunicating vascular channels.

The fissula ante fenestram crosses the bone on the cochlear side of the fenestra. Its contained tissue is continuous with that which lines the osseous labyrinth; its wall, at the vestibular extremity, is lined by cartilage continuous with that of the fenestra.

Septa, derived from the mucosal lining of the tympanic cavity, are carried across the latter space to the auditory ossicles. Having form and location that suggest miniature mesenteries, they transmit small blood vessels of ossicular supply from arteries and veins in the submucosal tissue and the bone (see Figures III–22*b* and III–26*b*).

c. Illustrating the anatomical structures described above, and additionally the vestibular extremity of the fossula post fenestram (at unlabeled arrow). Unlike the fissula ante fenestram, the fossula is an inconstant structure, and, when present, is usually represented only by a medial portion. Also, differing from the fissula, it is rarely the primary site of otosclerotic bone formation. Both of these transcapsular channels, like the cochlear and vestibular aqueducts, may be regarded as appendages of the perilymphatic space.

Transverse sections, Wisconsin Collection, series 29.

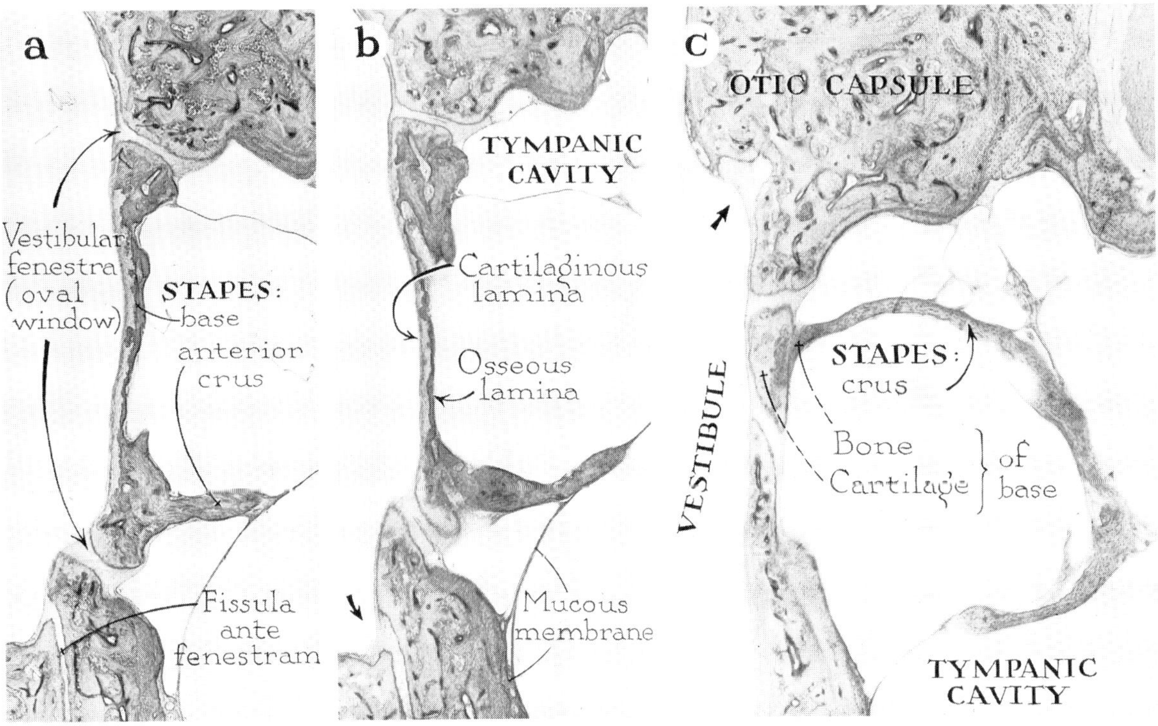

Figure III–25. See legend on the opposite page.

Figure III–26. BLOOD SUPPLY OF THE AUDITORY OSSICLES. *a.* NEWBORN INFANT (4-DAY PREMATURE). *b* to *d.* ADULT, 19 YEARS OLD.

a. Stapes, with tendon and contents of the facial canal; *b* and *c*, malleus and incus at the level of their articulation; *d*, malleus, near its area of attachment of the manubrium to the tympanic membrane.

The auditory ossicles do not receive their chief intraosseous supply through nutrient foramina situated near their extremities; rather, differing from the pattern common for typical long bones, openings are distributed throughout the length of each ossicle. The closest approximation to a familiar schema is encountered in the stapes, where vessels are concentrated at the crurobasal junctions. Three other features affecting structure and relationships place the ossicles in a special category, separating them from classification with the bones of leg and arm: they are nonhaversian (hence, fetal) in histological architecture; they lack true marrow cavities; they are invested by the mucosal lining of the tympanic cavity.

a. The blood supply of the stapes is intimately associated with vessels which find their chief source and termination in the facial canal. In young individuals, at least, the veins form an intricate plexus in a canal which is far more capacious than would be required by the actual contents. The arteries are fewer and smaller than the veins—a proportion common to other parts of the human body from sole to scalp. In passing to and from the ossicle, some vessels accompany the stapedius tendon through the orifice of the pyramidal eminence; others (in fact, most of them) join their less numerous companions by employing foramina situated near the eminence. The veins form an anastomotic network around the tendon; the arteries, on the contrary, follow a more direct course. Upon reaching the head of the ossicle, the vessels pass in both directions.

b and *c.* Throughout much of its body and crura, the incus, when seen in section, seems virtually riddled by these vascular canals. The marrow cavity, early reduced to minimal caliber, remains in the adult as an inconsiderable channel, bearing little resemblance to that of a typical bone. The vessels transmitted by the canals communicate at frequent points with those of submucosal position and without regional concentration. Some then continue through mucosal septa (at arrow in *b*), or pass into the tissue of the articulation. This relation between foramina and septa is also strikingly displayed in the malleus. The blood supply to the lenticular process is decreased by removal of the stapes with its associated vessels. Care must be taken when crimping a prosthesis to the long process of the incus in order to avoid crushing the cortex in which the numerous vascular channels are circumferentially arranged at a superficial level. This could further interfere with blood supply to the lenticular process.

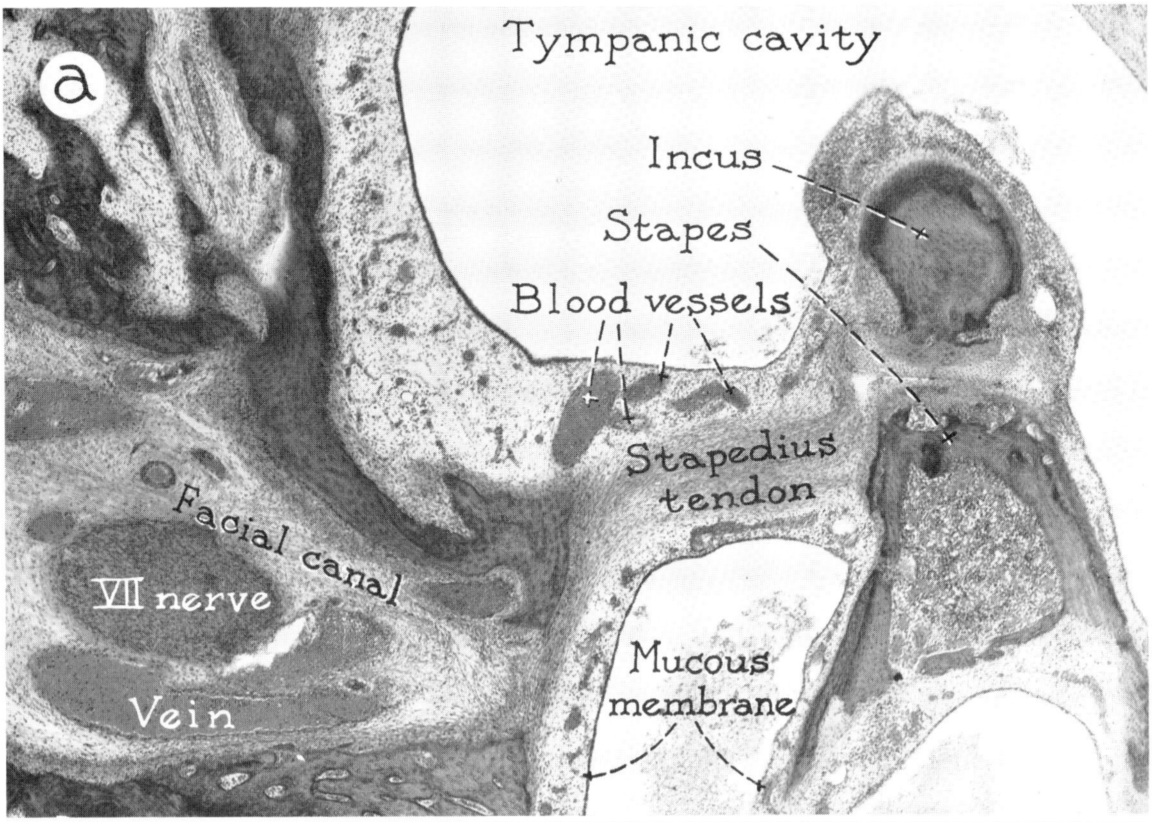

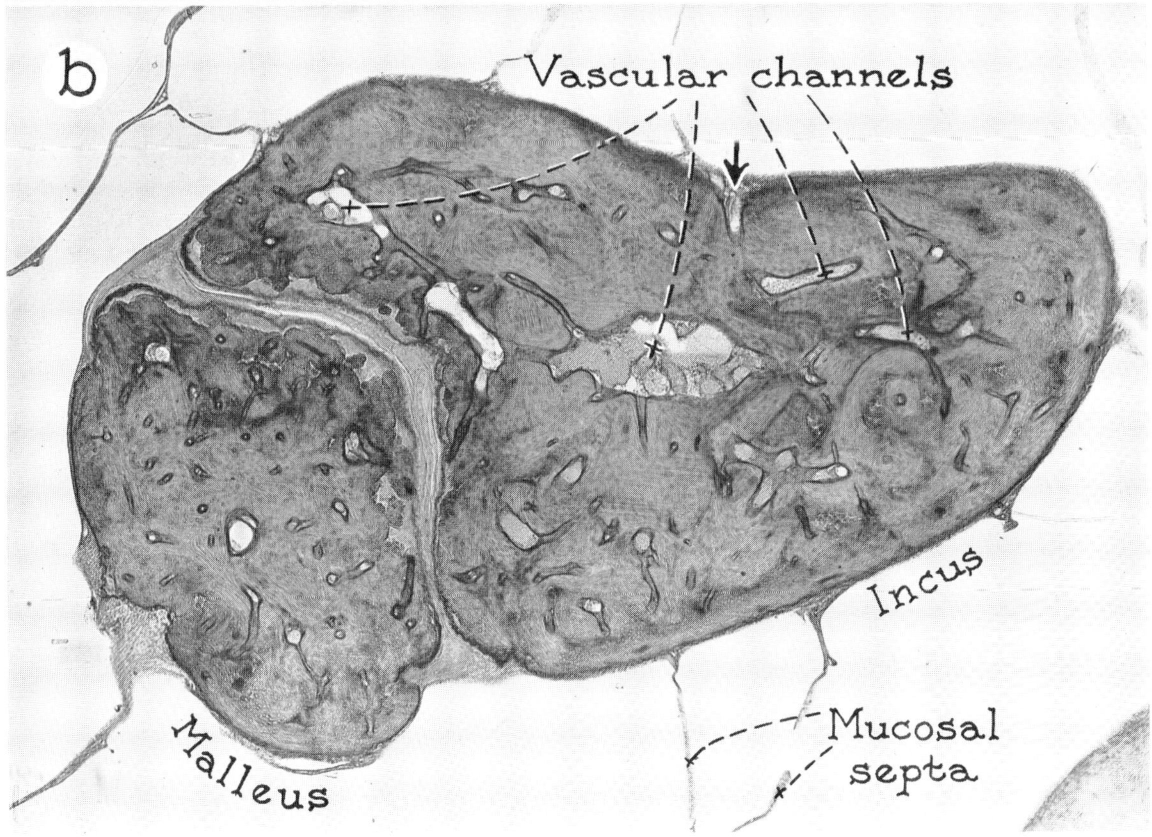

Figure III–26. See legend on the opposite page.

Figure III–26 continues on the following page.

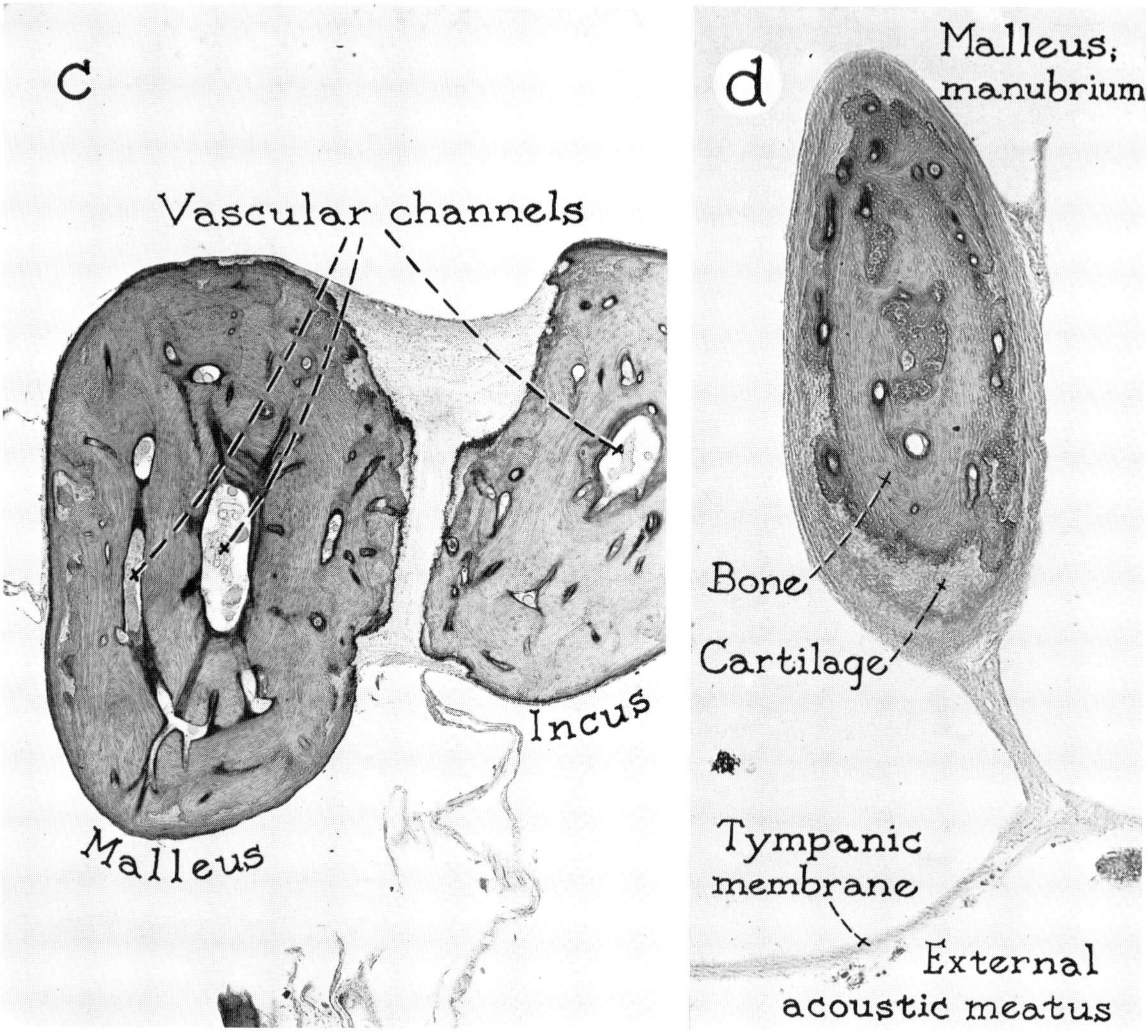

Figure III–26, Continued. BLOOD SUPPLY OF THE AUDITORY OSSICLES. *a*. NEWBORN INFANT (4-DAY PREMATURE). *b* to *d*. ADULT, 19 YEARS OLD.

d. In the manubrium of the malleus, toward the area of contact with the tympanic membrane, vessels of lesser caliber are numerous near the surface. Here, where cartilage covers the bone as a submucosal investment, the vessels near the surface are invested, each by an osseous shell which presses into the external, chondral pellicle. At this level, the mucous membrane is reflected from the inner aspect of the tympanic membrane to the manubrium of the malleus in the form of a lesser "ligament" (see Figure III–3*a*).

Transverse sections. Wisconsin Collection, series as follows: *a*, 124; *b* to *d*, 29. *a*, ×32; *b*, ×25; *c*, ×31; *d*, ×38.

(From Anson, Harper, and Winch: Ann. Otol., 73:645–658, 1964.)

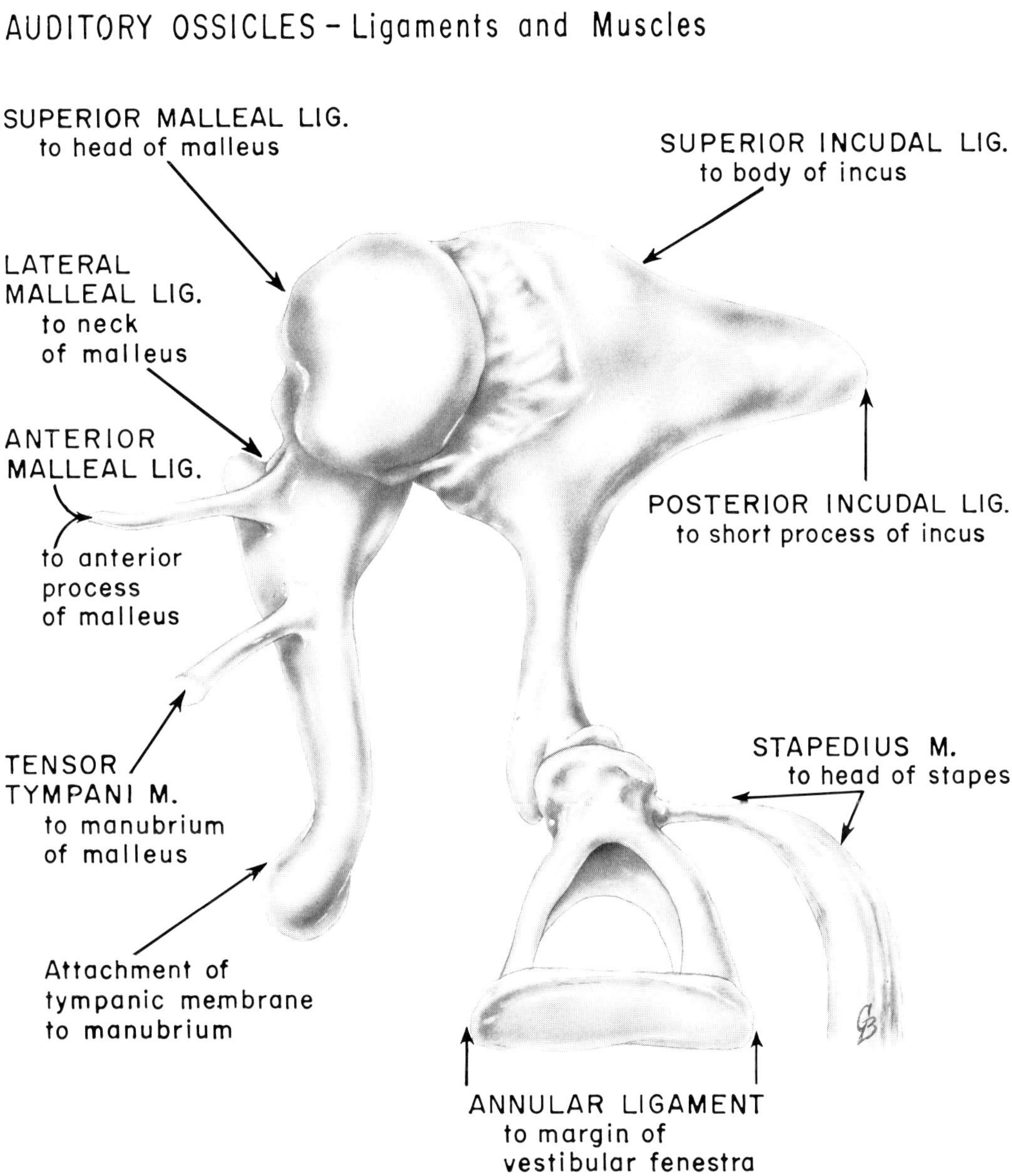

Figure III–27. Auditory ossicles, their ligaments and muscles. Viewed from the medial aspect.

The areas of attachment of the tensor tympani muscle and of the several ossicular ligaments are indicated. A portion of the stapedius muscle is shown, removed from the facial canal and the pyramidal eminence.

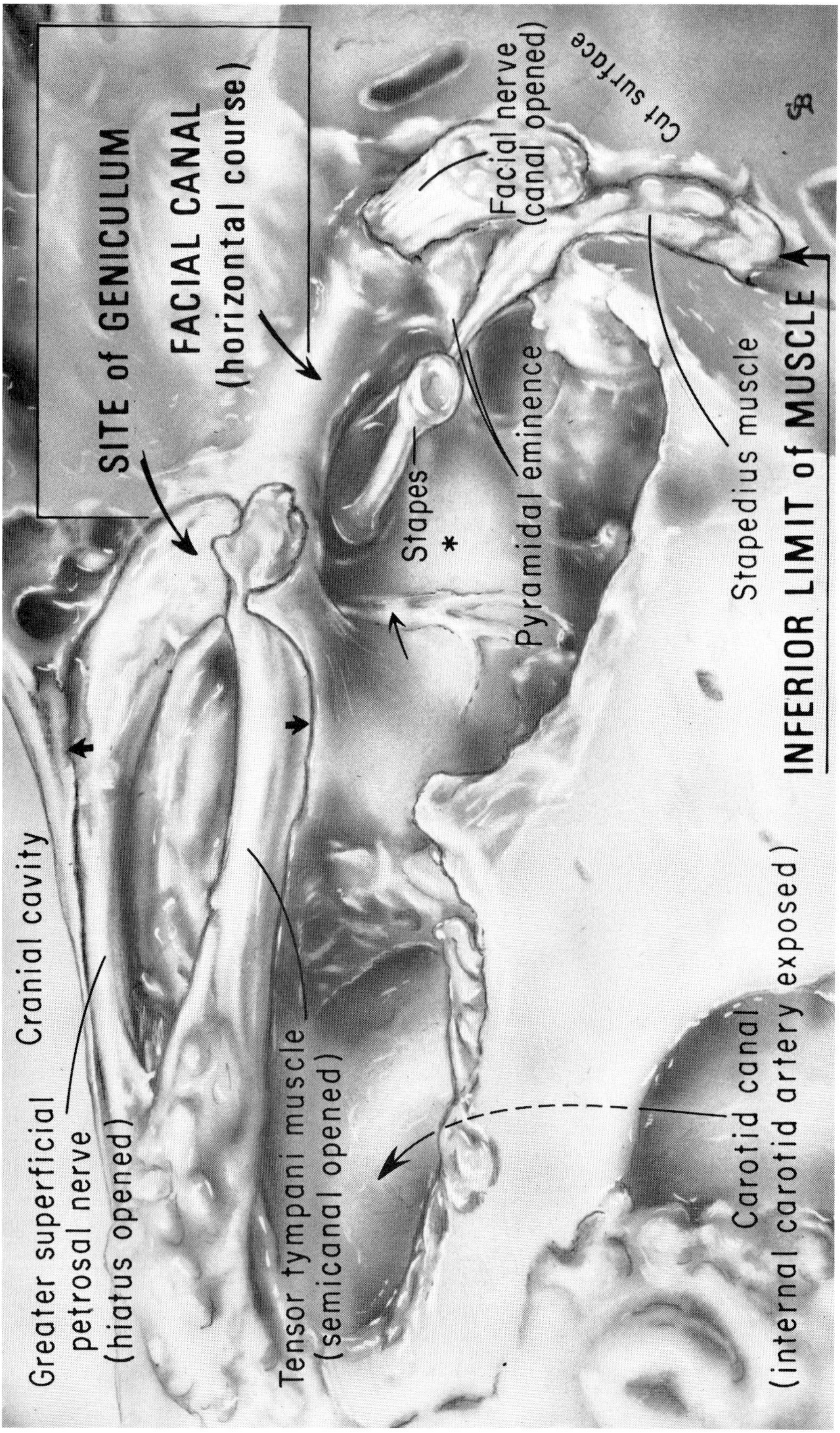

SITE of GENICULUM
FACIAL CANAL
(horizontal course)
Facial nerve
(canal opened)
Cut surface
Stapes
Pyramidal eminence
Stapedius muscle
INFERIOR LIMIT of MUSCLE
Cranial cavity
Greater superficial
petrosal nerve
(hiatus opened)
Tensor tympani muscle
(semicanal opened)
Carotid canal
(internal carotid artery exposed)

Figure III–28. Ossicular muscles: tensor tympani and stapedius. Dissection of an unembalmed specimen.

The tensor tympani, arising in part from the bony walls of the semicanal, ends in a round tendon that turns almost at a right angle (at which point it is cut). It would continue across the tympanic cavity, to be attached to the manubrium of the malleus (see Figure III–3*b*).

The stapedius muscle occupies a portion of the facial canal, separated from the nerve by an incomplete septum. The tendon fills the space of the pyramidal eminence. There, bending somewhat downward at an obtuse angle and invested by mucous membrane, it courses forward and medialward to an attachment on the posterior margin of the head of the stapes (see Figures III–27, III–78*d*, and III–20*a*).

The tympanic nerve of Jacobson, upon emerging from the tympanic canaliculus, ascends on the medial wall of the tympanic cavity. The internal carotid artery, here partly exposed in its petrosal portion, first ascends in front of the cochlea of the internal ear. Then, turning forward and medialward, it lies just behind the auditory (eustachian) tube. Asterisk indicates the promontory.

(From Anson, Donaldson, Warpeha, and Rensink: Ann. Otol., 79:710–727, 1970.)

Figure III–29. Ossicular muscles. Tympanic cavity, medial or labyrinthine wall. Dissection of an unembalmed specimen.

a. The stapedius muscle has been exposed through its full extent. The stapes is *in situ*; the incus and malleus have been removed. The wall of the facial canal has been removed, where the horizontal segment becomes continuous with the vertical portion, and the contained nerve has been transected.

The origin of the stapedius muscle arises from walls of a troughlike "semicanal" in the superior part of the facial canal. It narrows to a tendon that appears at the tip of the eminence. Here, inclining upward, at an angle, and invested by mucous membrane, it courses medialward and forward to an attachment on the posterior surface of the head of the stapes. The facial canal is shown as it overarches the stapes; the nerve, partially exposed, here begins the downward course toward the stylomastoid foramen. The tympanic sinus appears as a deep *cul-de-sac* extending medialward and posteriorly from the general tympanic cavity. A bony projection, the *subiculum promontorii*, intervenes between the sinus and the fossula of the cochlear window.

b. Anatomy of the medial or labyrinthine wall of the tympanic cavity with details of structure shown in the preceding figure. Arrows point to the cut edges of the osseous channels.

The greater superficial petrosal nerve is seen as it comes off the facial nerve at the geniculate ganglion and begins its course through the hiatus of the facial canal. The rostrum of the cochleariform process overlaps the facial nerve, slightly along a superoinferior axis, considerably from an anteroposterior axis. The tympanic branch of the glossopharyngeal nerve (of Jacobson), in contributing to the tympanic plexus, passes medial to the cochleariform process. Here, as the facial canal passes horizontally lateralward, it forms the *prominentia* just below the more evident prominence of the lateral semicircular canal. In this segment of its course, the canal is situated between the latter eminence and the stapes; it forms the superior boundary of the fossula of the vestibular fenestra, or stapes "niche."

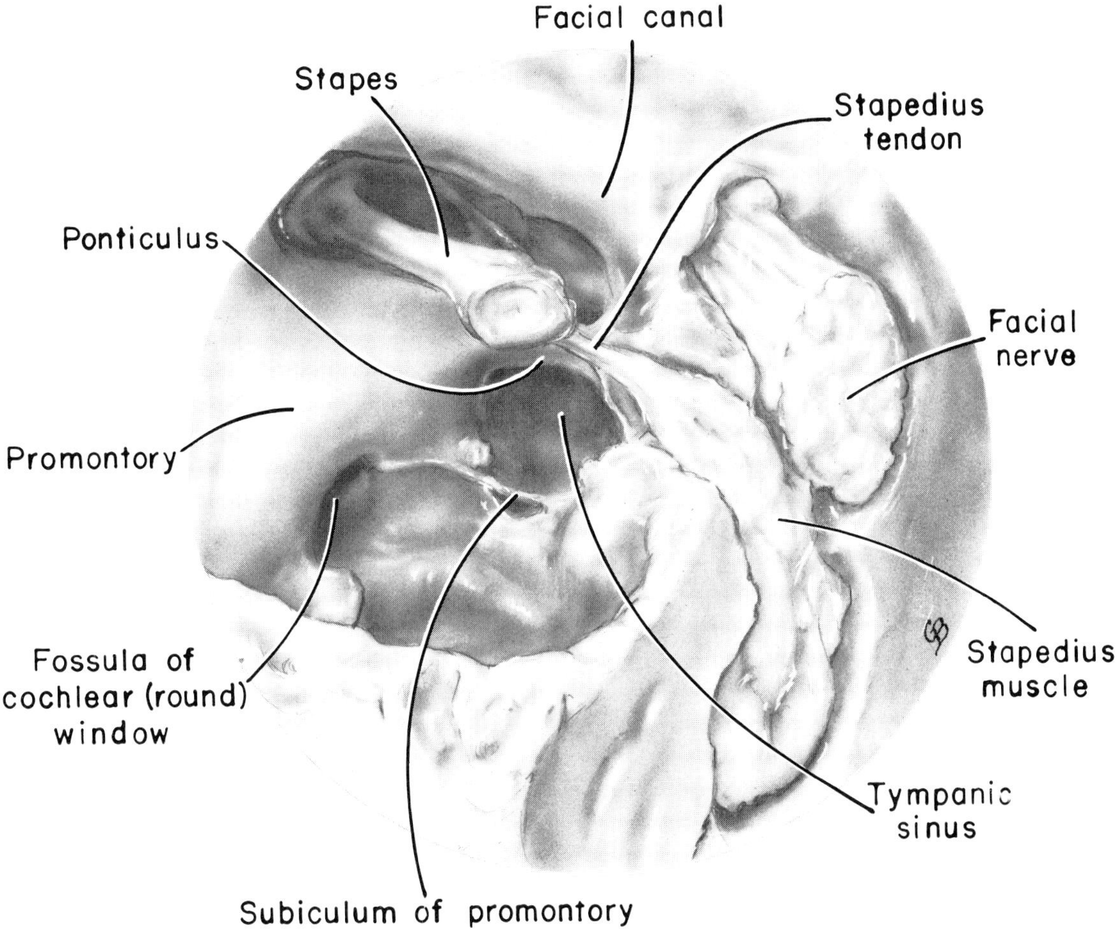

a

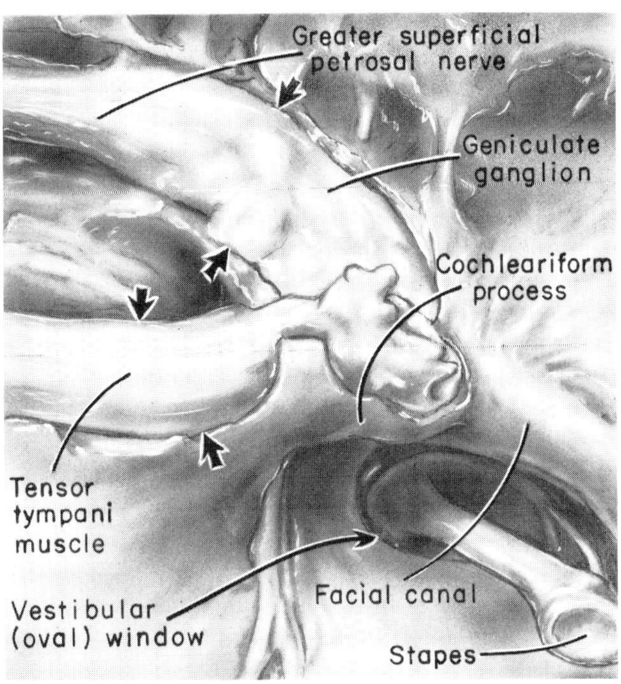

b

Figure III–29. See legend on the opposite page.

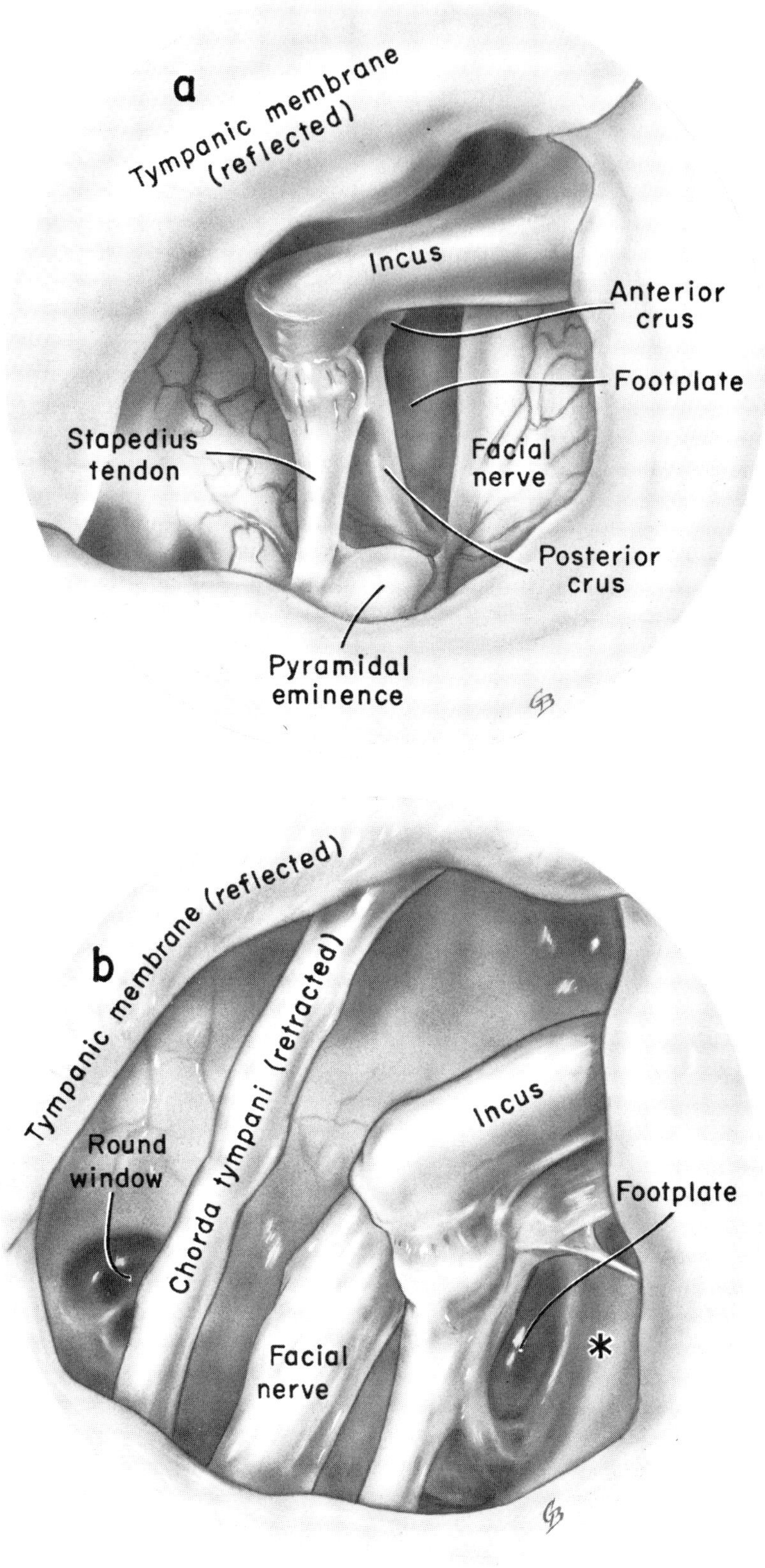

Figure III–30. See legend on the opposite page.

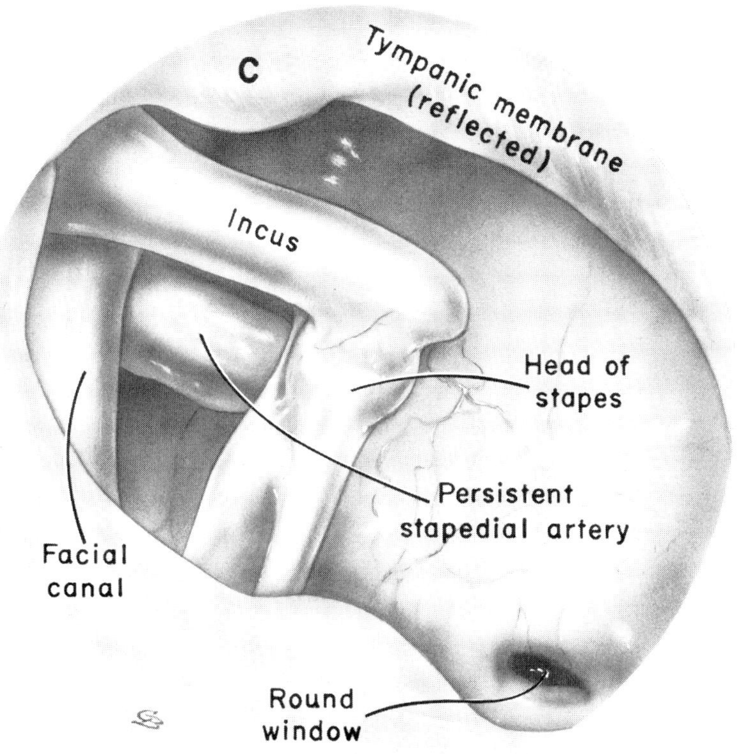

Figure III–30. ANOMALIES OF THE FACIAL NERVE AND THE STAPEDIAL ARTERY AS RELATED TO THE AUDITORY OSSICLES.

The view in each instance is from the external acoustic meatus, the tympanic membrane having been reflected as in a conventional tympanotomy.

a. Complete absence of a bony covering for the facial nerve throughout the extent of the surgical field. The ossicles and the stapedius tendon were normal.

b. Similar dehiscence of the facial canal, with malposition of the facial nerve. In the absence of an osseous canal, the facial nerve lay exposed in an abnormal position, inferior to the stapes and upon the promontory. The normal location is indicated by the asterisk. The chorda tympani, of unusually large size, has been retracted in the customary manner.

c. Persistence of the stapedial artery. The large artery paralleled the course of the long crus of the incus, lying deep to the latter and to the head of the stapes. Superiorly it was situated beneath the ridge formed by the facial canal. It passed from surgical view under the stapedial head.

Selected cases generously provided by Dr. J. V. D. Hough.

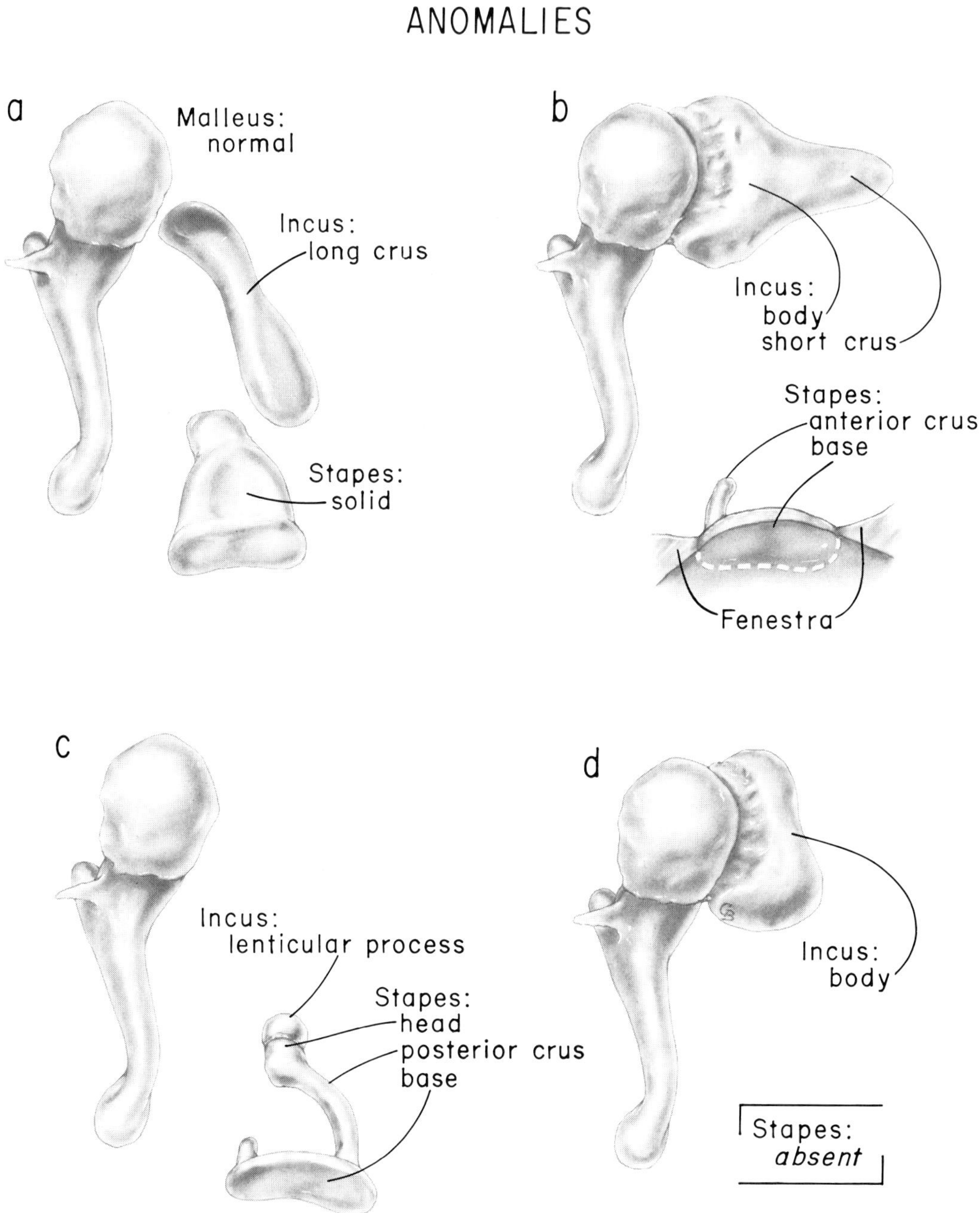

Figure III–31. AUDITORY OSSICLES OF ABERRANT, OR "ANOMALOUS," FORM.

a. Incus represented only by a long crus; stapes solid. *b.* Incus lacking a long crus; stapes aberrant in being fixed to the oval window and having only a remnant of the "crural arch." *c.* Incus represented by a lenticular process; stapes having a partial anterior crus. *d.* Incus lacking crura; stapes absent.

Drawings prepared from semischematic sketches provided by Dr. Victor Goodhill.

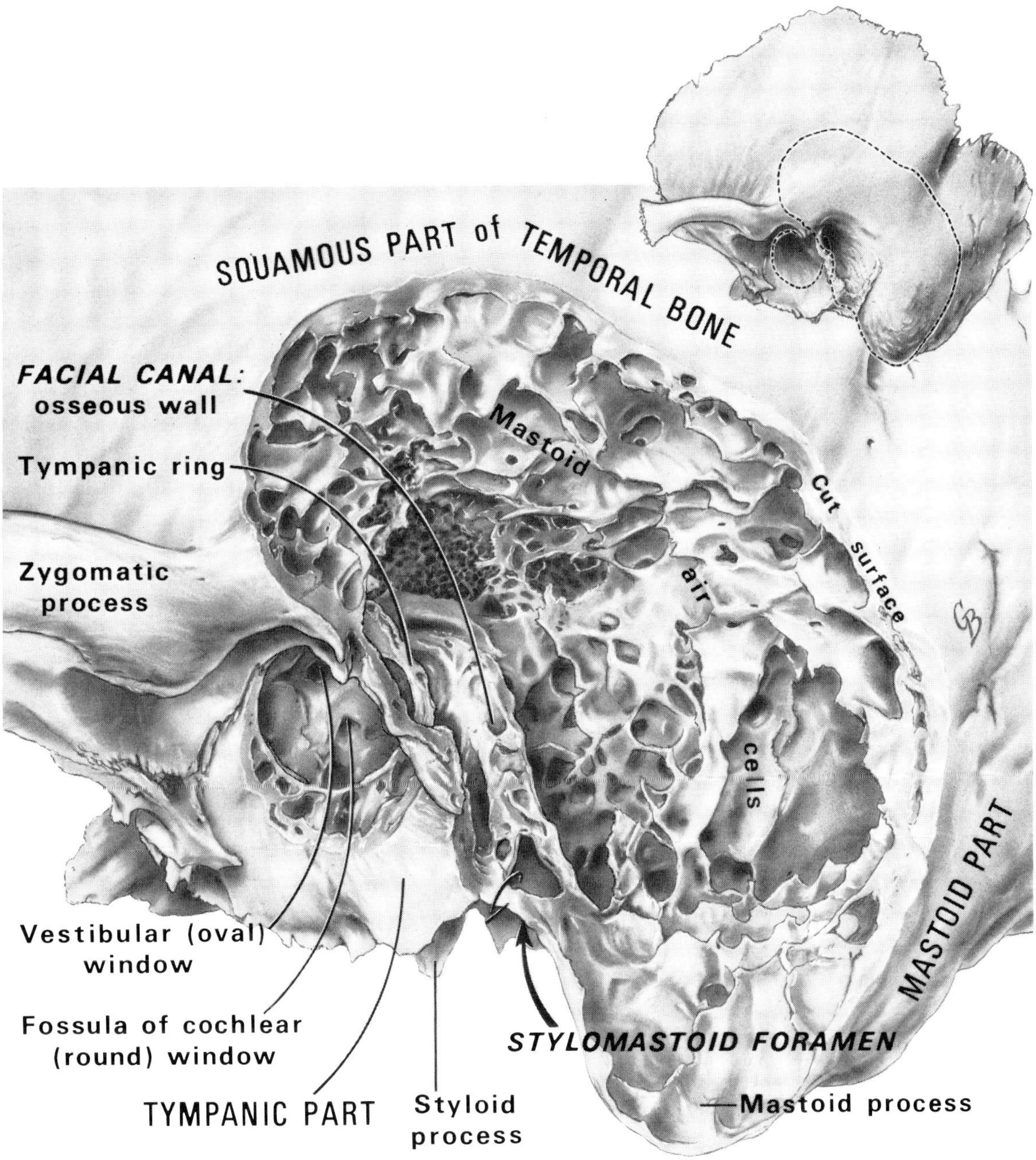

Figure III–32. MASTOID AIR CELLS AND RELATED ANATOMY, LATERAL VIEW OF A DISSECTED SPECIMEN.

The air cells of the mastoid process are shown in relation to the facial canal and the tympanic ring.

In the horizontal segment of its course (here out of view), the facial canal arches over the vestibular fenestra (oval window). The vertical segment descends in the posterior (or mastoid) wall of the tympanic cavity (see Figure III–11).

(From Anson: Trans. Amer. Acad. Ophthal. Otolaryng., 76:108–129, 1972.)

Figure III–33. MASTOID CAVITY IN A LEFT TEMPORAL BONE: COMPLETE EXENTERATION OF THE CELLS.

Demonstrating the relation of the facial canal to the lateral and posterior semicircular canals and of the latter to the sigmoid sulcus. Only the thin, immediately investing wall of bone remains on each of the structures named. This may serve as an example of a complete (simple) mastoidectomy.

The facial canal, in passing lateralward and downward, lies close to the mastoid wall of the tympanic cavity (see Figure III–3*b*). Surgically the tip cells are removed, with the facial canal as the anterior limiting boundary and the wall of the sigmoid sulcus serving as the posterior boundary. The sulcus, on the medial wall of the mastoid part of the temporal bone, curves from above and behind in a direction downward and forward. The floor of the space is elevated by the so-called digastric ridge. On the external surface of the mastoid process a corresponding depression occurs; this is the mastoid incisure (or digastric fossa of the older terminology). The sigmoid sulcus meets the "roof" of the cavity at an acute angle; externally the angle thus formed is represented by the junction of the middle with the posterior cranial fossa. The roof is the bone of the anterior surface of the petrous pyramid; it is covered by the meningeal layers of the cerebrum. A thorough understanding of the location and relationships of all these structures is necessary for safe cellular exenteration.

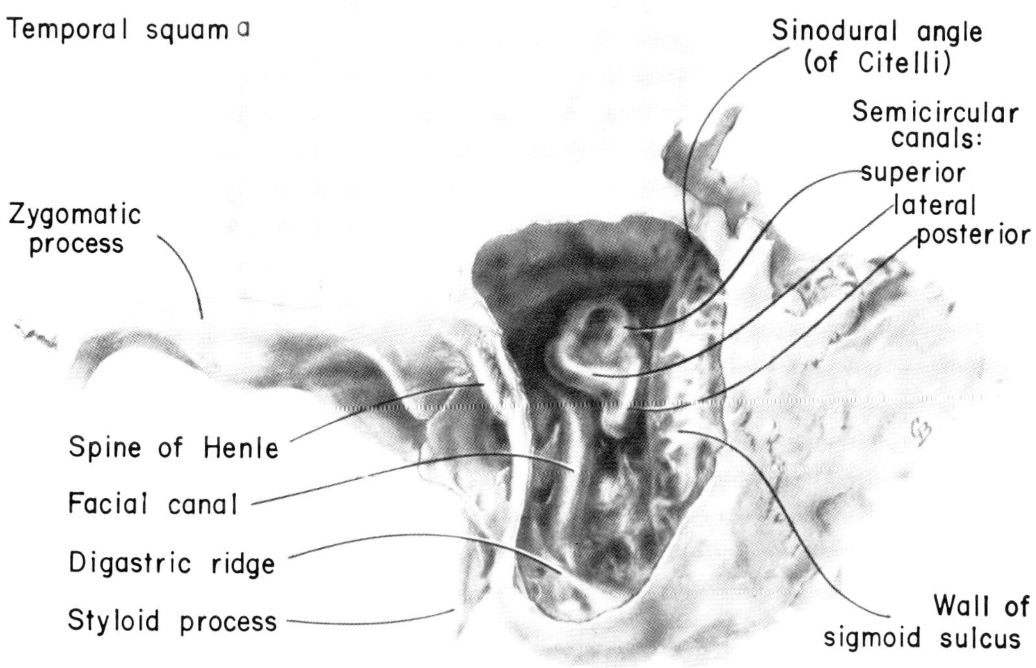

Figure III–33. See legend on the opposite page.

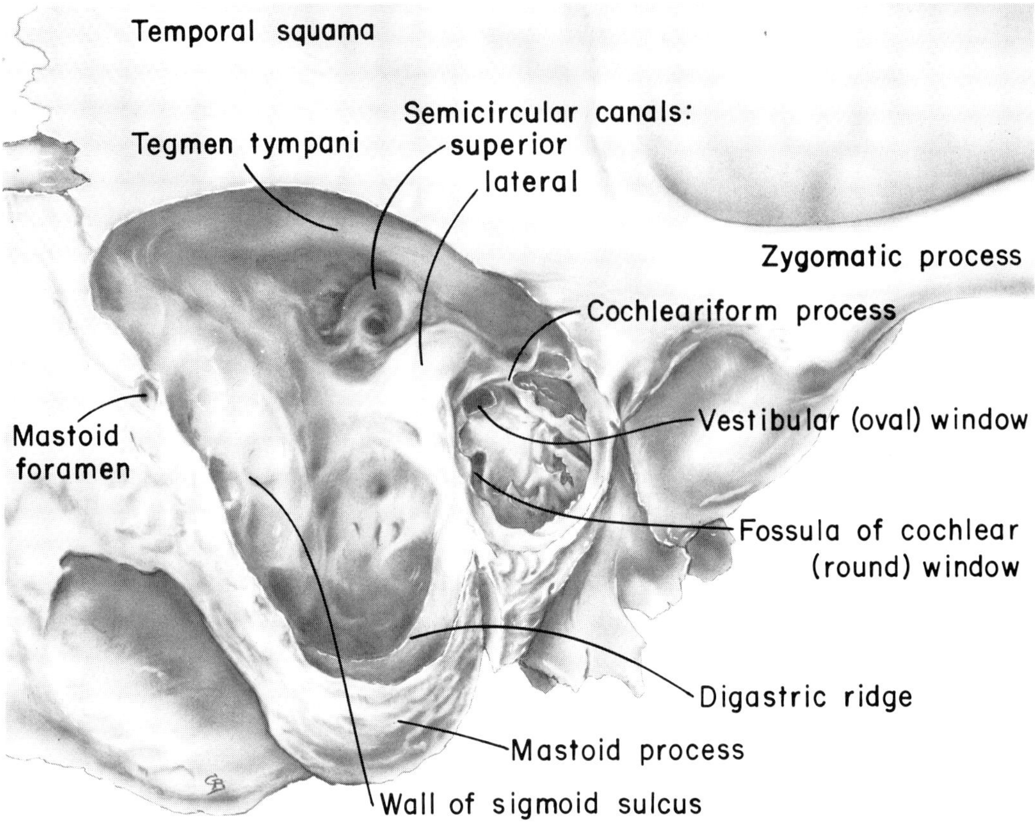

a

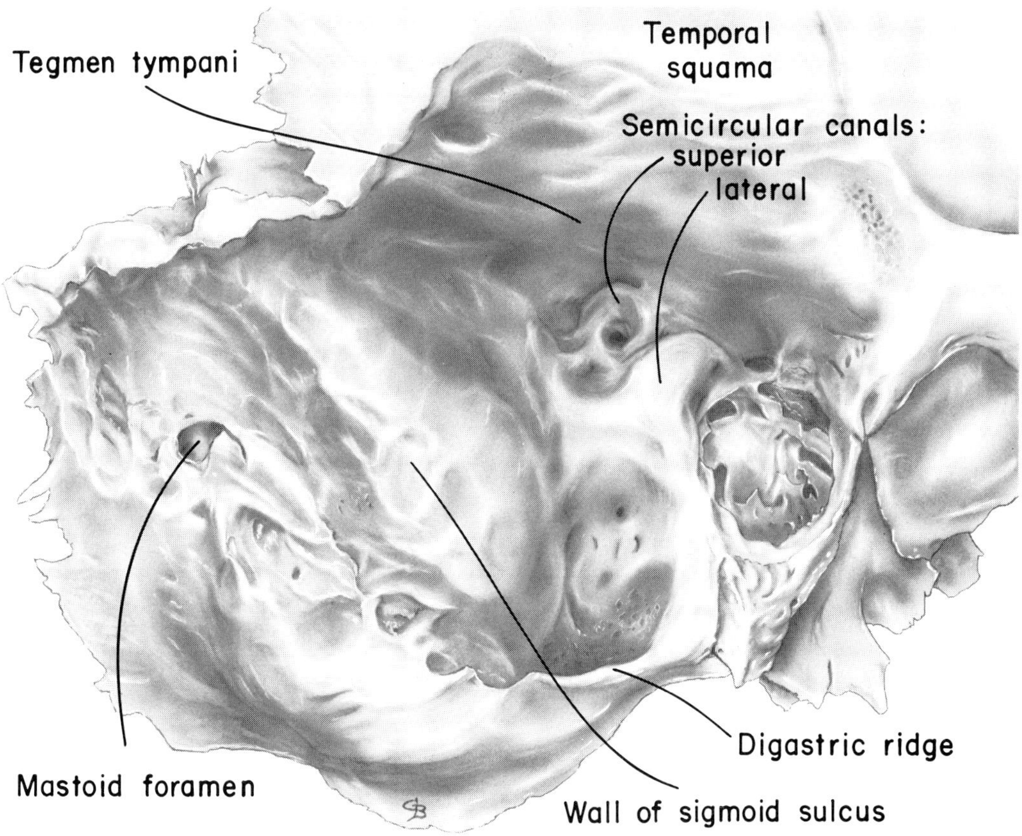

b

Figure III–34. See legend on the opposite page.

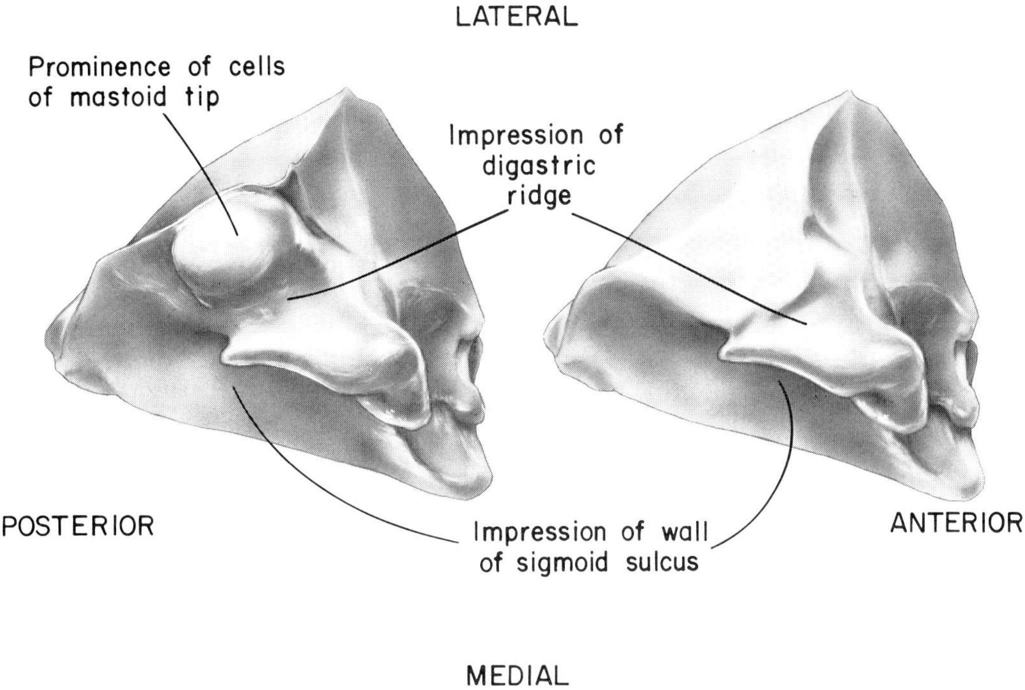

c

Figure III–34. FORM AND RELATIONSHIPS OF THE MASTOID CAVITY (RADIAL EXENTERATION).

a. Dissection of an extensively pneumatized temporal bone. The exposure is that of a radical mastoidectomy. In the middle ear the auditory ossicles have been removed, together with their muscles and ligaments. At surgery, the stapes and stapedius muscle would remain *in situ.*

Posteriorly the space is bounded by the wall of the sigmoid sulcus, superiorly by the *tegmen tympani*, and anteriorly by the prominence of the lateral semicircular canal. Inferiorly the floor is invaded by a ridge which, on the free surface of the mastoid process, is the impression for attachment of the digastric muscle. Above the prominence of the lateral canal the epitympanic recess communicates with the tympanic cavity proper.

b. Dissection continued by extensive "beveling." Beveling was not completed in sinodural angle to help retain perspective.

The mastoid foramen serves to transmit an emissary vein to the sigmoid venous sinus and the mastoid branch of the occipital artery to the *dura mater* of the posterior cranial fossa. The thin layer of periosteal bone that remains to separate the space of the mastoid space from the cranial cavity is sculptured by the gyri and sulci of the temporal lobe of the cerebrum. The space within the arc of the superior semicircular canal is frequently pneumatized. It is the site of the subarcuate fossa of fetal and early postnatal stages. On the anterior surface of the pyramid the canal produces the arcuate eminence (see Figure III–138*c*).

c. Size and form of the mastoid cavity in two unembalmed specimens of temporal bone. Demonstrated by the use of casts of the space prepared from specimens shown in the accompanying figures. Casts viewed from below. The sigmoid sulcus serves best as a guiding landmark. Beveling reduces the capacity of the cavity (from 8.4 to 6.6 cc.). The natural collapse of soft tissue would account for further reduction.

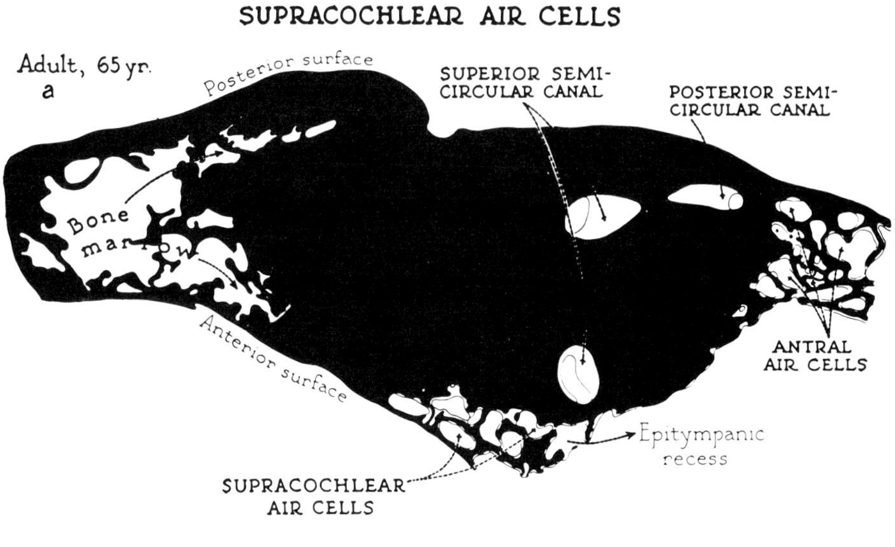

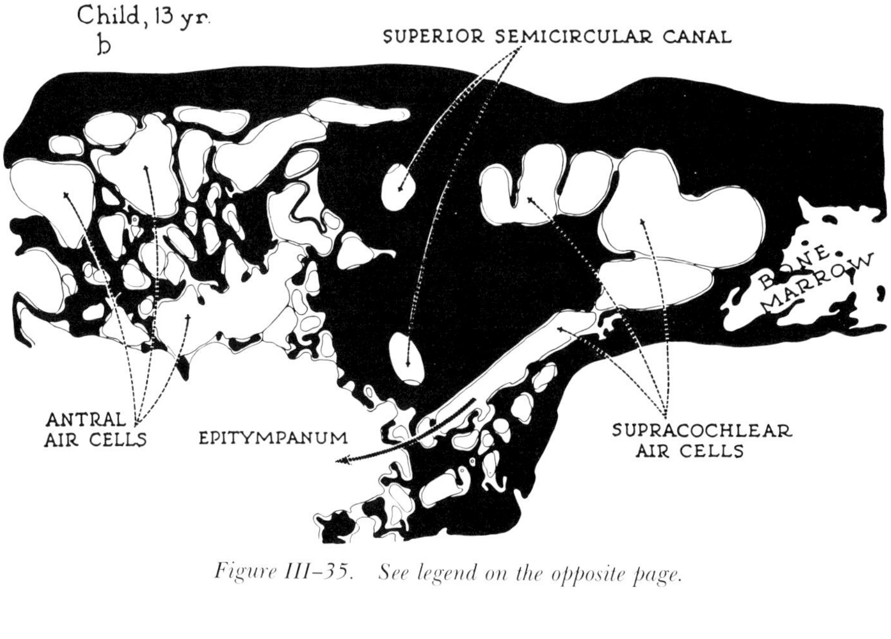

Figure III–35. See legend on the opposite page.

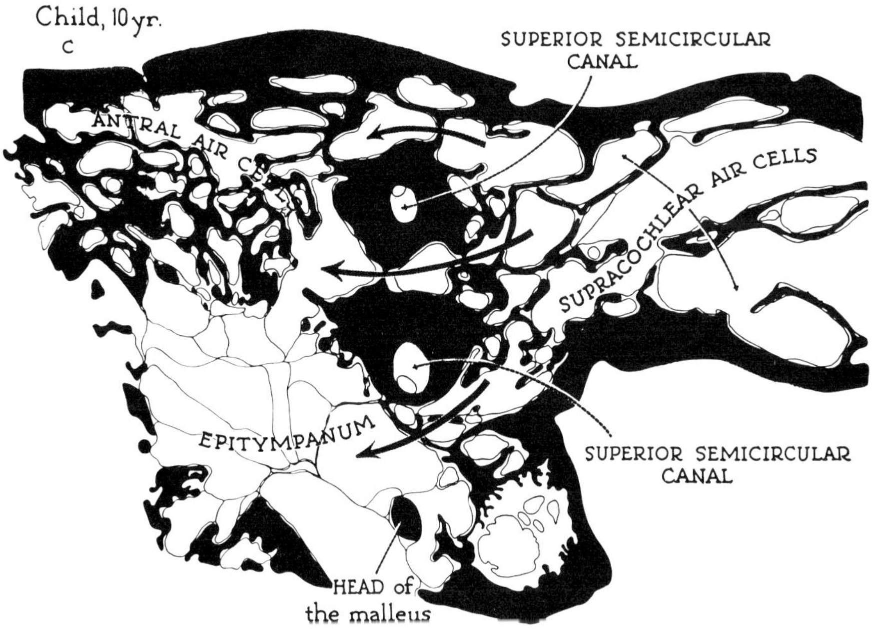

Figure III–35. Air cells of the petrous part of the temporal bone: variations demonstrated by selected examples.

a. From the left petrous bone of an adult male 65 years of age showing minimal extension of antral air cells around the forward turn of the superior semicircular canal.

b. From the right ear of a boy 13 years old. Example of an intermediate degree of antral extension around the forward turn of the superior semicircular canal, there forming a large group of supracochlear air cells.

c. Section from the right petrous bone of a girl 10 years old, showing extensive antral air cell infiltration of the otic capsule around the superior semicircular canal, to form a large group of supracochlear air cells on the medial aspect of the superior canal.

(From Stelter, Bast, and Anson: Quart. Bull., Northwestern Univ. Med. Sch., 34: 23–37, 1960.)

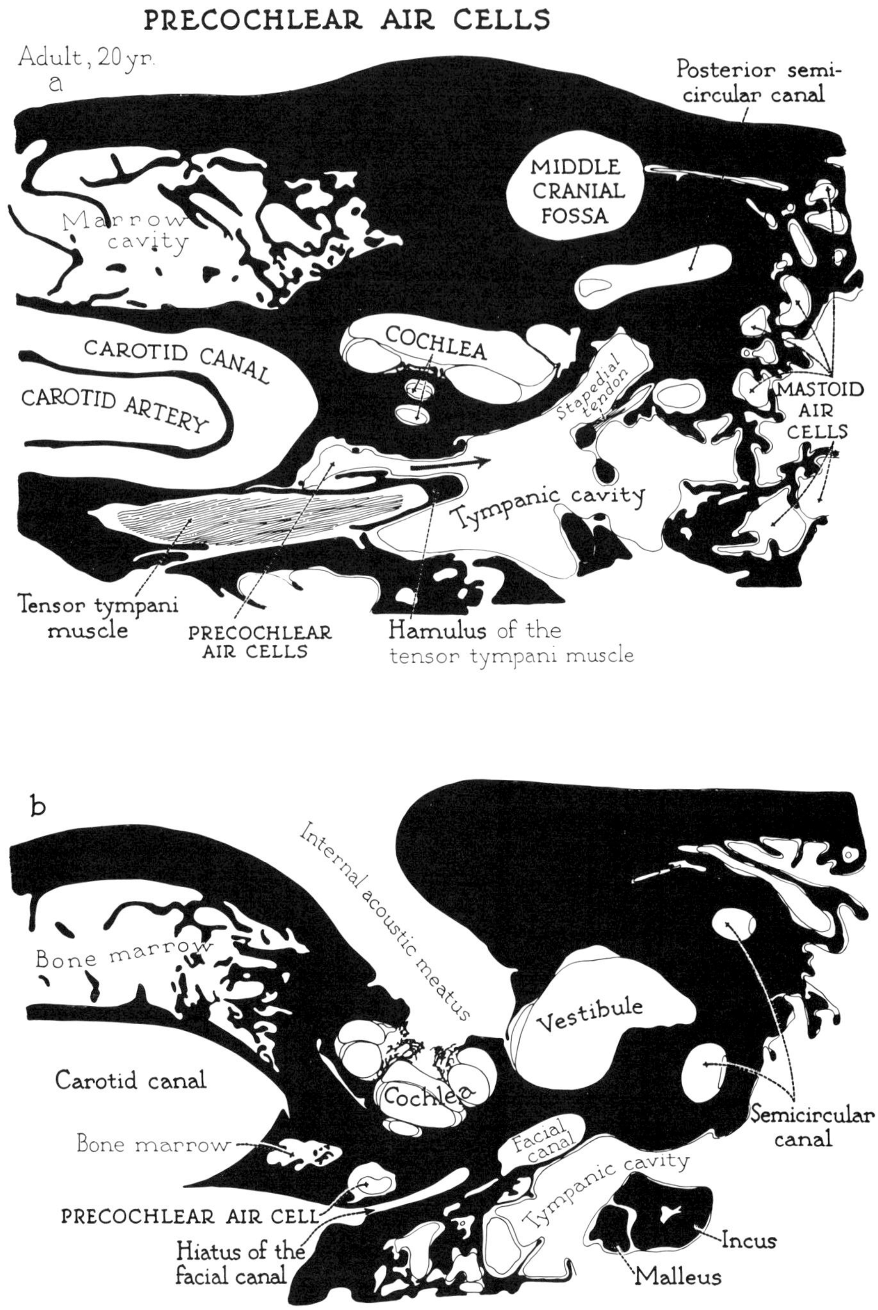

Figure III–36. AIR CELLS OF THE PETROUS PART OF THE TEMPORAL BONE; SELECTED EXAMPLES, CONTINUED. LEFT TEMPORAL BONE OF A FEMALE SPECIMEN 20 YEARS OLD.

a. Section at the transverse level of the communication (at arrow) of the precochlear air cell with the tympanic cavity at the level of the hamulus of the tensor tympani muscle.

b. An air cell situated on the lateral border of the carotid canal and anterior to the cochlea (this being precochlear).

(From Stelter, Bast, and Anson: Quart. Bull., Northwestern Univ. Med. Sch., 34:23–37, 1960.)

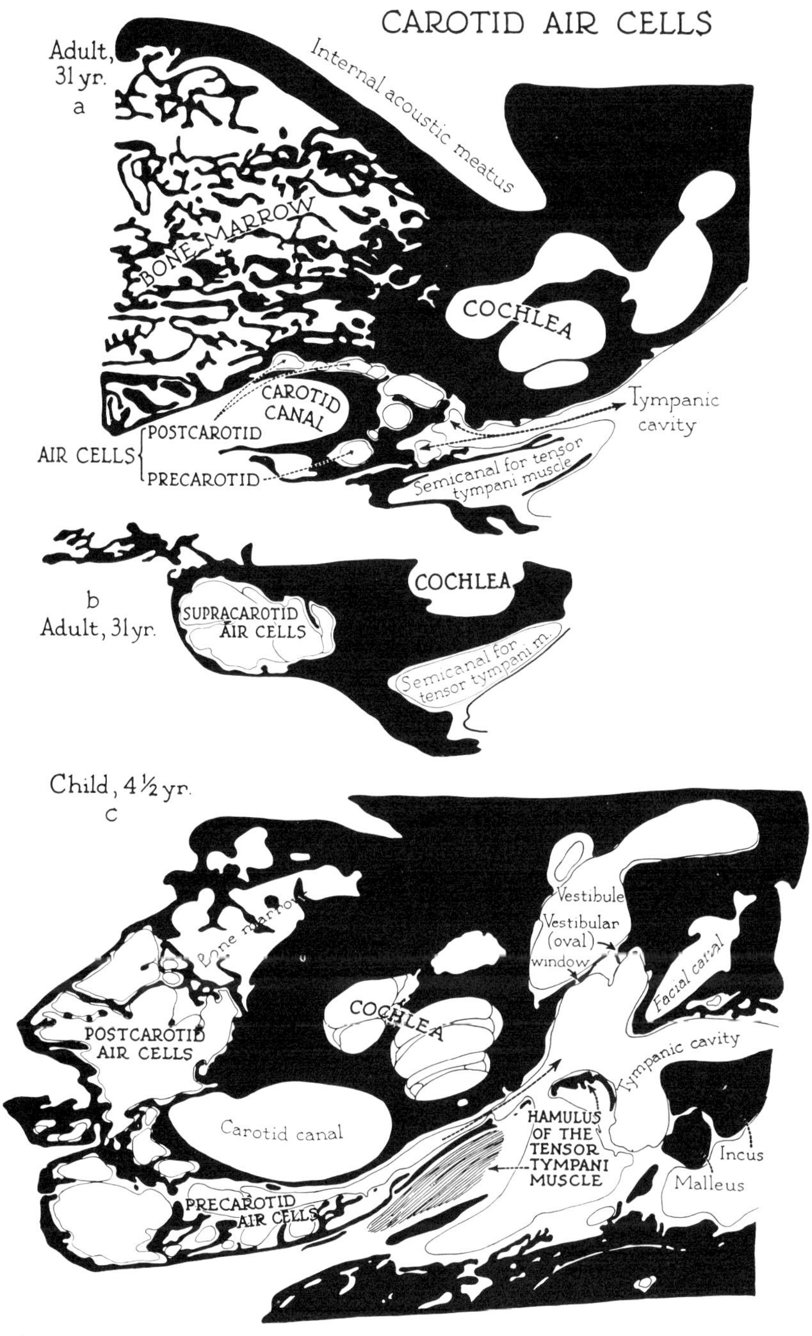

Figure III–37. Air cells of the petrous part of the temporal bone; selected examples, continued. Left petrous bone of (*a* and *b*) a 31-year-old male and (*c*) a child 4½ years of age.

a. Showing the communication of air cells in a precarotid and postcarotid position with the tympanic cavity at the level of the hamulus of the tensor tympani muscle. When precarotid cells are involved with disease, the tensor tympani muscle and its semicanal must be removed for adequate exposure.

b. Section in which a large air cell lies medial to the cochlea and overlies the carotid canal. These supracarotid air cells represent the superior extension of those which occupy a postcarotid position in *a.*

c. Section showing a large group of precarotid and postcarotid air cells and their communication with the tympanic cavity at the level of the hamulus of the tensor tympani muscle.

(From Stelter, Bast, and Anson: Quart. Bull., Northwestern Univ. Med. Sch., 34:23–37, 1960.)

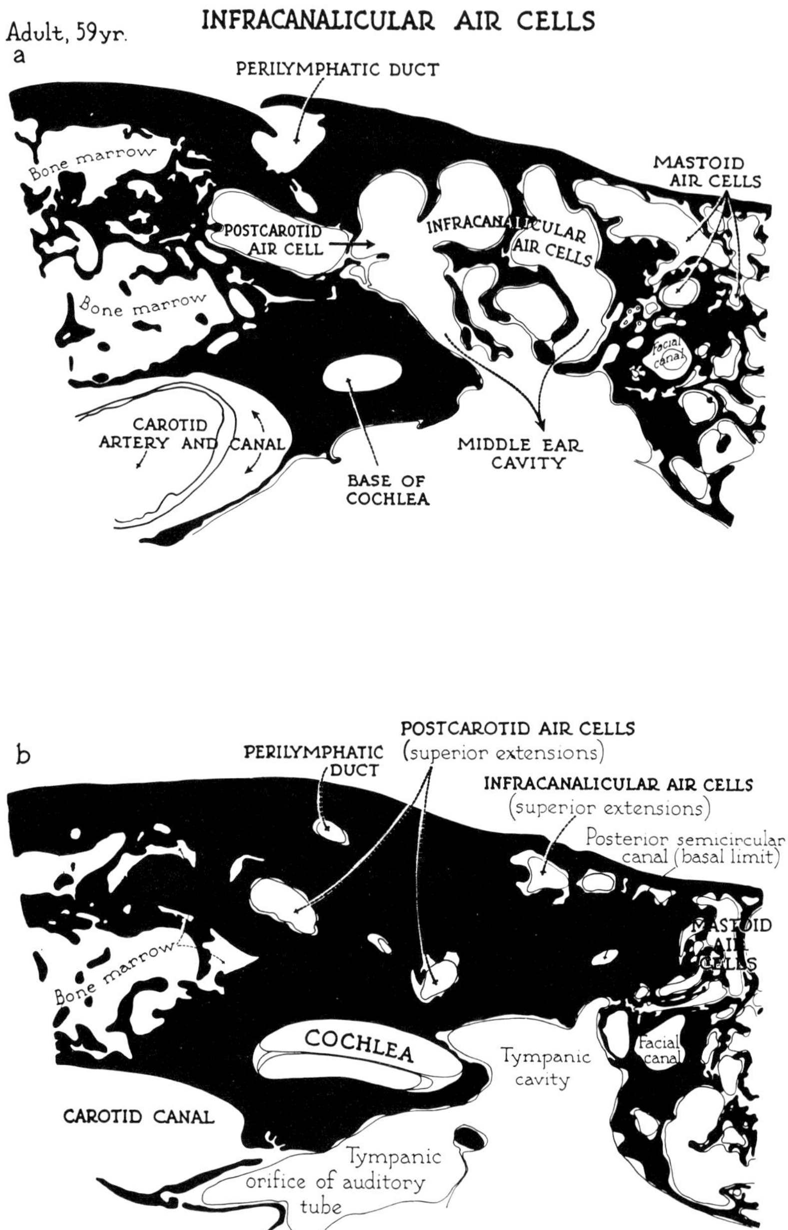

Figure III–38. AIR CELLS OF THE PETROUS PART OF THE TEMPORAL BONE; SELECTED EXAMPLES, CONTINUED. LEFT TEMPORAL BONE OF A MALE 59 YEARS OLD.

a. Showing the infracanalicular and postcarotid air cells which communicate with the posterior wall of the tympanic cavity inferior to the level of the semicircular canals.

b. Section at a more cranial level, in which the tympanic communication of the air cells is lost. The cells therefore appear as isolated units, posterior and medial to the tympanic cavity.

(From Stelter, Bast, and Anson: Quart. Bull., Northwestern Univ. Med. Sch., 34:23–37, 1960.)

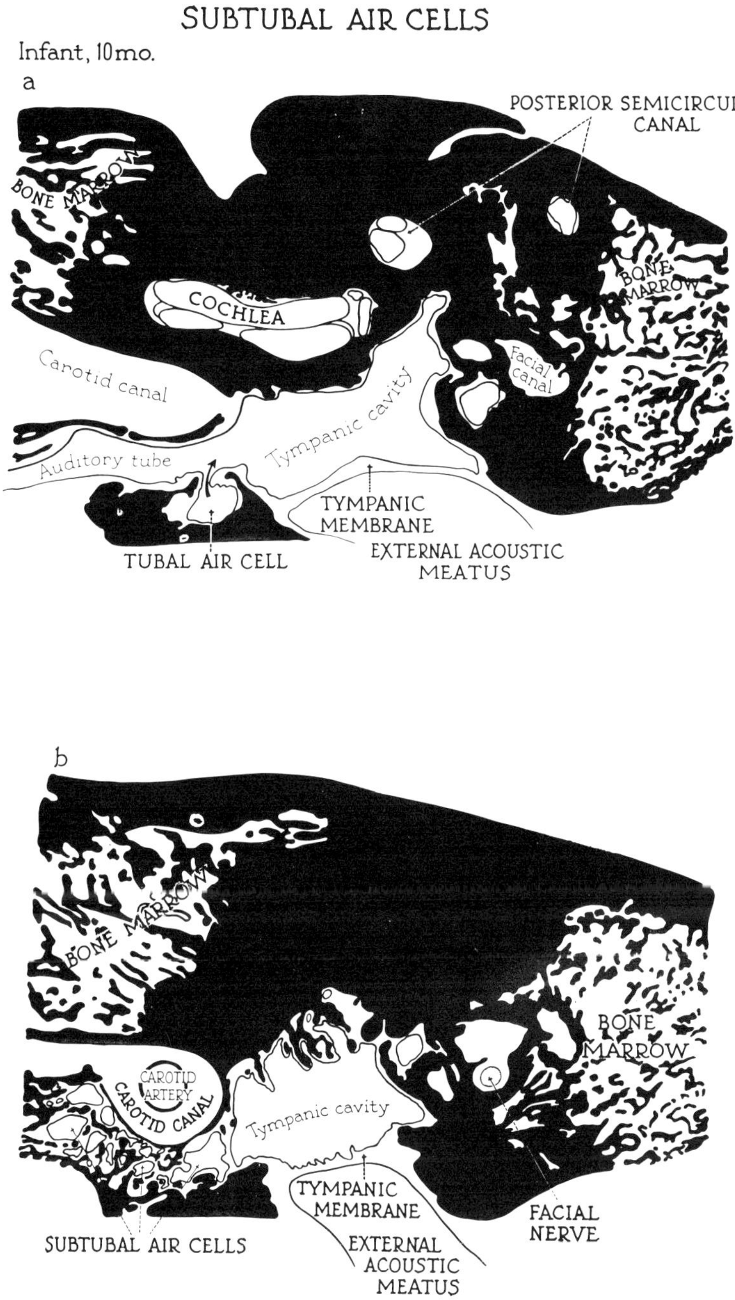

Figure III–39. AIR CELLS OF THE PETROUS PART OF THE TEMPORAL BONE; SELECTED EXAMPLES, CONCLUDED. LEFT TEMPORAL BONE OF AN INFANT 10 MONTHS OLD.

a. A section demonstrating an air cell's communication with the auditory tube, directly at its junction with the tympanic cavity.

b. Section at a more cranial level, showing the large group of air cells inferior to the auditory tube (that is, in subtubal location).

(From Stelter, Bast, and Anson: Quart. Bull., Northwestern Univ. Med. Sch., 34:23–37, 1960.)

Figure III–40. MEMBRANOUS LABYRINTH. A RECONSTRUCTION OF THE ENDOLYMPHATIC LABYRINTHINE SYSTEM, MEDIAL ASPECT. INFANT, 6 MONTHS OLD.

The membranous labyrinth is shown schematically in *a*, with the parts brought into the same plane. It is pictured in *b* as seen in a reconstruction prepared by the Born method (see also Figure III–44). In *c*, *d*, and *e*, details of macroscopic form are shown for the utricular (utriculoendolymphatic) duct (*c*), the ampullae of the semicircular ducts (*d*) and the rugose *saccus* of the endolymphatic duct (*e*). On the drawing of the entire reconstruction (*b*), numerals are placed in the areas shown in the regional drawings (*c*, *d*, and *e*) for purposes of reference.

The membranous labyrinth is a system of epithelial tubes invested by a thin layer of connective tissue and filled with a clear fluid, the endolymph. The tubes, of differing form, all communicate with one another, but are completely shut off from the outside. These tubes or canals lie within the osseous labyrinth, to the form of which they roughly correspond. They contain the terminations of the statoacoustic nerve that supply the maculae, the cristae, and the spiral organ (of Corti).

In the vestibule (of the osseous labyrinth), the membranous elements are the utricle and the saccule. Traditionally pictured as if they were droplet-shaped, characterless vesicles, these chambers actually possess distinctive form. The utricle communicates broadly with the common arm of the superior and posterior semicircular ducts; together they assume the form of an open **V**. The tube-shaped utricle, lying in the elliptical recess of the vestibule, is continuous with the three semicircular ducts. It is, in large part, fixed to the wall of the recess by connective tissue and by fibers of the utricular division of the vestibular nerve (see Figure III–50*b*); otherwise it is separated from the vestibular wall by the perilymphatic space. On its anterolateral surface is situated the utricular acoustic macula.

The saccule has the form of an elongate oval, the long axis of which parallels that of the utricle, to which vesicle it is contiguous. Whereas the utricle opens widely into its canalicular ducts, the saccule is connected with the anterior part of the system by narrow intermediary conduits, namely, the saccular and reuniting ducts. These enter and leave the saccule on the latter's inferior surface. The saccular acoustic macula is situated on the anteromedial surface of the saccule. As in the case of the utricle, the saccule is held firmly to the wall of the vestibule by connective tissue and bundles of nerve fibers (Figure III–57*c*). The saccule is connected with the utricle indirectly, through the saccular and the utricular (or utriculoendolymphatic) ducts; in the opposite direction (toward the cochlea) the connections are the reuniting duct (*ductus reuniens*) and the vestibular cecum, a cul-de-sac of the cochlear duct proper.

The endolymphatic duct, far from being a quill-like tube with a mushroom-shaped terminal expansion, is regionally modified in a constant fashion. The opening into the utricle, for example, is slitlike in form, the orifice being bounded by a folding of the apposed walls of the utricle and the endolymphatic duct (see Figure II–25*a*). The proximal part of the latter duct is expanded into a sinuslike enlargement that occupies the internal aperture of the vestibular aqueduct (Figure II–22*e*). Continuing toward the external aperture, the duct narrows into an isthmus. While still intraosseous, the duct becomes a flattened cecal dilatation, the endolymphatic sac. The *saccus* is prolonged beyond the aperture, to rest in a shallow impression on the posterior surface of the petrous pyramid (see Figures III–104 and III–105).

The cochlear part of the membranous labyrinth is formed by the cochlear duct. It begins in a recess of the vestibule, extends within the osseous spiral canal, through basal, middle, and apical coils, where it ends blindly in the cupular cecum. The cochlear duct is in large part triangular in cross section. Its outer wall is held by periosteal connective tissue to the osseous cochlea. It contains the spiral organ (*Cortii*), a highly differentiated structure that contains the termination of the cochlear nerve. The histological details are pictured in Figure III–56*a*.

Wisconsin Collection, series 121.

(From Anson, Harper, and Winch: Third Symposium on the Role of the Vestibular Organs in Space Exploration, NASA SP-152, pp. 125–146. Washington, D.C., U.S. Government Printing Office, 1968.)

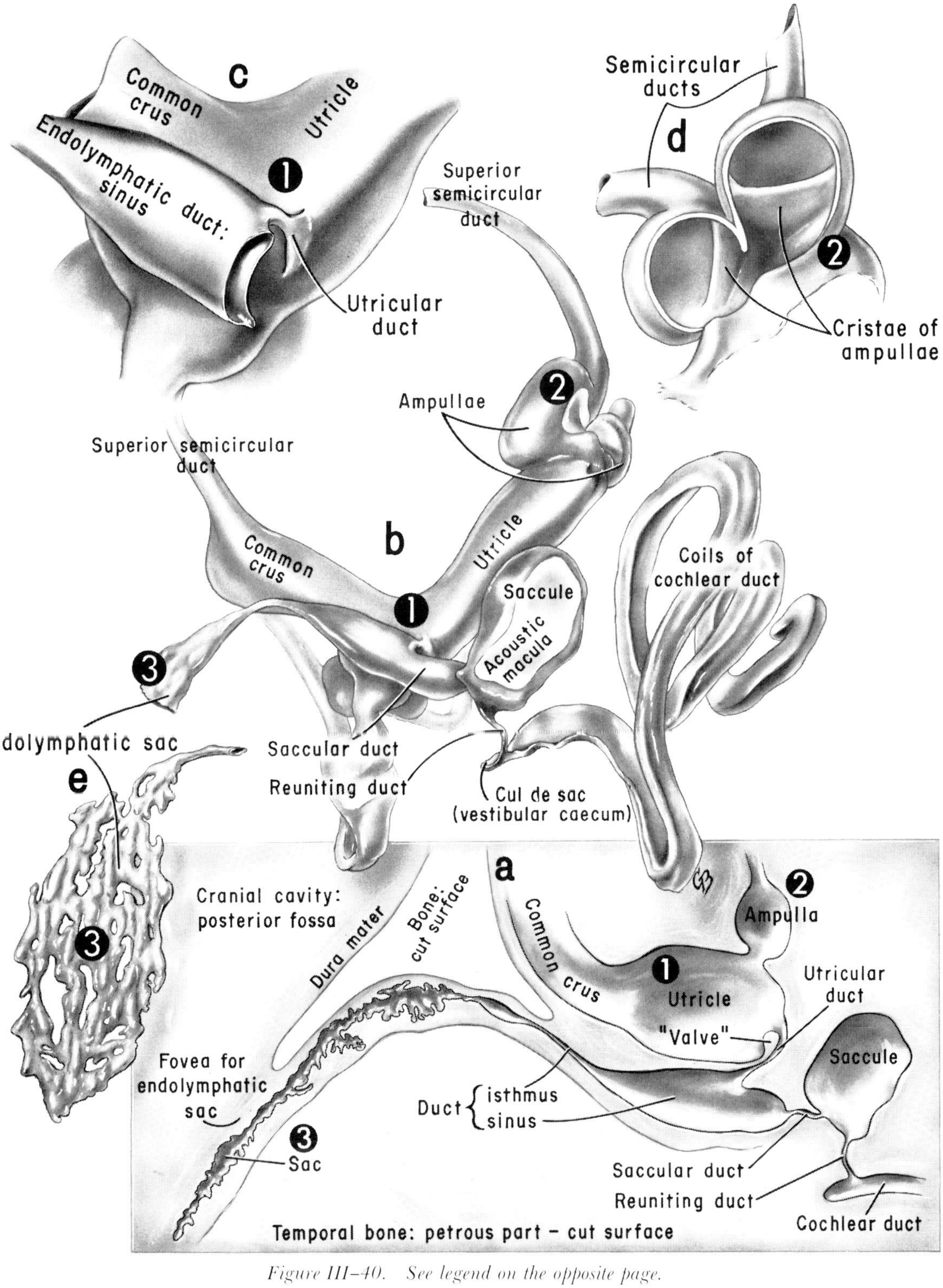

Figure III–40. See legend on the opposite page.

Figure III–41. MEMBRANOUS LABYRINTH AND RELATED ANATOMY, DEMONSTRATING ESPECIALLY THE SIZE AND RELATIONSHIPS OF THE ENDOLYMPHATIC SAC. RECONSTRUCTION PREPARED BY THE BORN METHOD. ADULT, 65 YEARS OF AGE.

The sac occupies a foveate impression on the posterior surface of the pyramid distal to the external aperture of the vestibular aqueduct. Typically, as in this instance, its long axis is directed anteroposteriorly (downward and backward). Within the distal segment of the aqueduct, the sac narrows in accommodation with the triangular form of the space (see gross dissections in Figures III–110 to III–115). Continuing as the constricted segment, or isthmus, of the endolymphatic duct, the duct is finally continuous with a sinuslike expansion that is lodged in the area of the elliptical recess of the vestibule (see section in Figure III–60*b*).

This proximal segment of the duct is continuous with the utricle through a communication (at arrow) that is guarded, so to speak, by the so-called utriculoendolymphatic valve (Figure II–25).

The endolymphatic sac is regularly either rugose or vesiculate (Figures III–61 and III–62). This feature of the epithelium could not be shown at the magnification used in preparing the reconstruction.

The following features are also of interest: position of the acoustic macula of the saccule (at asterisk); quill-like form of the *ductus reuniens;* continuity of the latter with the relatively capacious saccular duct; proximity of the sac to the sigmoid sulcus and jugular fossa; course of the cochlear aqueduct (or canaliculus) and the funnel-shaped character of its external aperture.

(From Anson. Arch. Otolaryng., 89:96–110, 1969.)

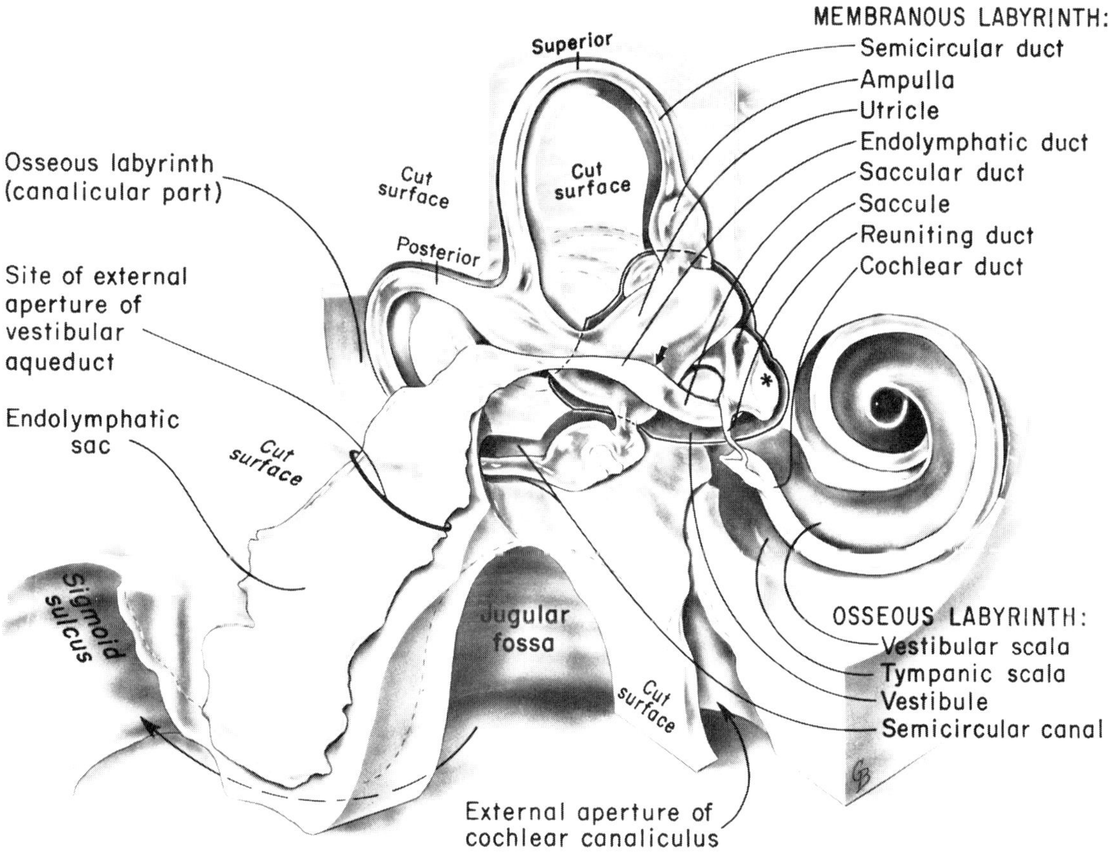

Figure III–41. See legend on the opposite page.

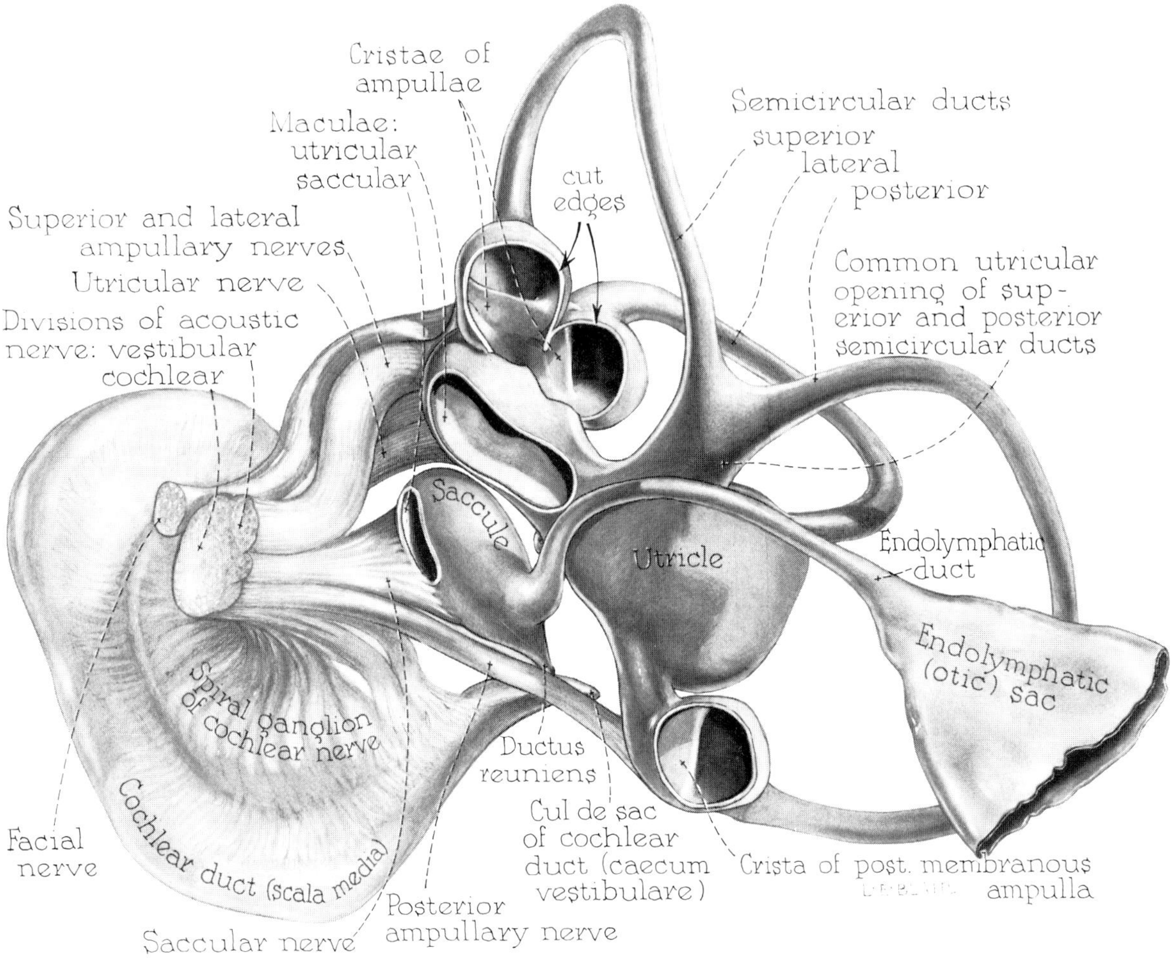

Figure III–42. BRANCHES OF THE EIGHTH CRANIAL (ACOUSTIC OR VESTIBULOCOCHLEAR) NERVE AND THE SENSORY ORGANS OF EQUILIBRIUM AND HEARING THAT ARE THEREBY INNERVATED. NEWBORN INFANT.

Reconstruction prepared from a serially sectioned temporal bone. Utricle, saccule and ampullae opened to show the sensory areas.

The eighth nerve, upon passing into the internal acoustic meatus with the seventh (facial) nerve and the nervus intermedius, divides into two branches, cochlear and vestibular. They enter separate areas at the fundus of the meatus in relation to the transverse crest (Figure III–134*a*).

The cochlear nerve, after going through the foraminous tract of the fundus, passes into the canals of the modiolus to form the elongate spiral ganglion. Therefrom, nerve fibers course through the osseous spiral lamina to the spiral organ of Corti (Figure III–120).

The vestibular nerve is interrupted by a ganglion at the bottom of the fundus. There it divides into upper and lower terminal branches. The upper branch passes through the wall that intervenes between the fundus and the vestibule, thus going from the superior vestibular area to the superior cribrose macula (Figure III–53); it divides in turn into the following nerves: the utricular, to the acoustic macula of the utricle; the superior ampullary, to the superior membranous ampulla; and the lateral ampullary, to the lateral membranous ampulla. The lower terminal branch divides into the following nerves: the saccular, which passes from the inferior vestibular area through the middle cribrose macula to the acoustic macula of the saccule (Figure III–57*c*); and the posterior ampullary, which passes into the singular foramen, whence it runs through a long canaliculus to the inferior cribrose macula.

Figure III–42 continues on the opposite page.

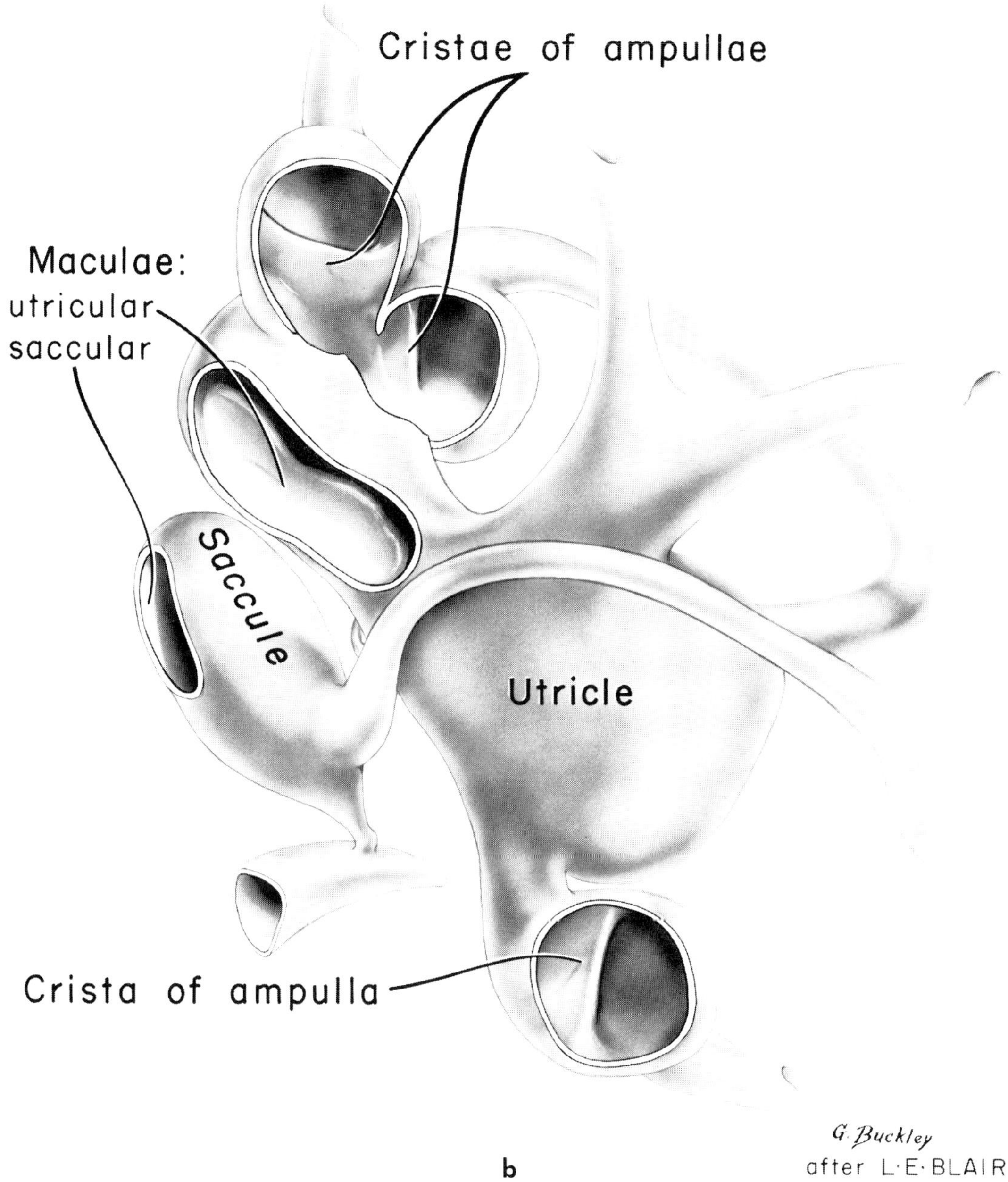

Figure III–42, Continued.

The acoustic macula of the utricle is a thickened area, oval in outline, on the anterolateral wall of the utricle (Figure III–50). The corresponding sensory area of the saccule, similarly oval, is situated on the saccule (Figure III–57*c*). Each receives filaments of the vestibular nerve; in each, the columnar epithelium has two kinds of cells: sensory (hair) and supporting cells. The surface of the macula is covered with a gelatinous otolithic membrane.

Each ampullary crista is an elongate shelf oriented transversely to the long axis of its semicircular duct. Histologically, a crista is generally similar to a macula, consisting of sensory and supporting cells. However, the crista is surmounted by a gelatinous mass, the cupula (not shown in the reconstruction, but pictured in Figures III–58*e* and III–59). Ciliary tufts of the hair cells project into this mass; the latter is similar to the otolithic membrane of a macula, except in the lack of otoconia.

(From Anson, Harper, and Winch: Arch. Otolaryng., 85:497–514, 1967.)

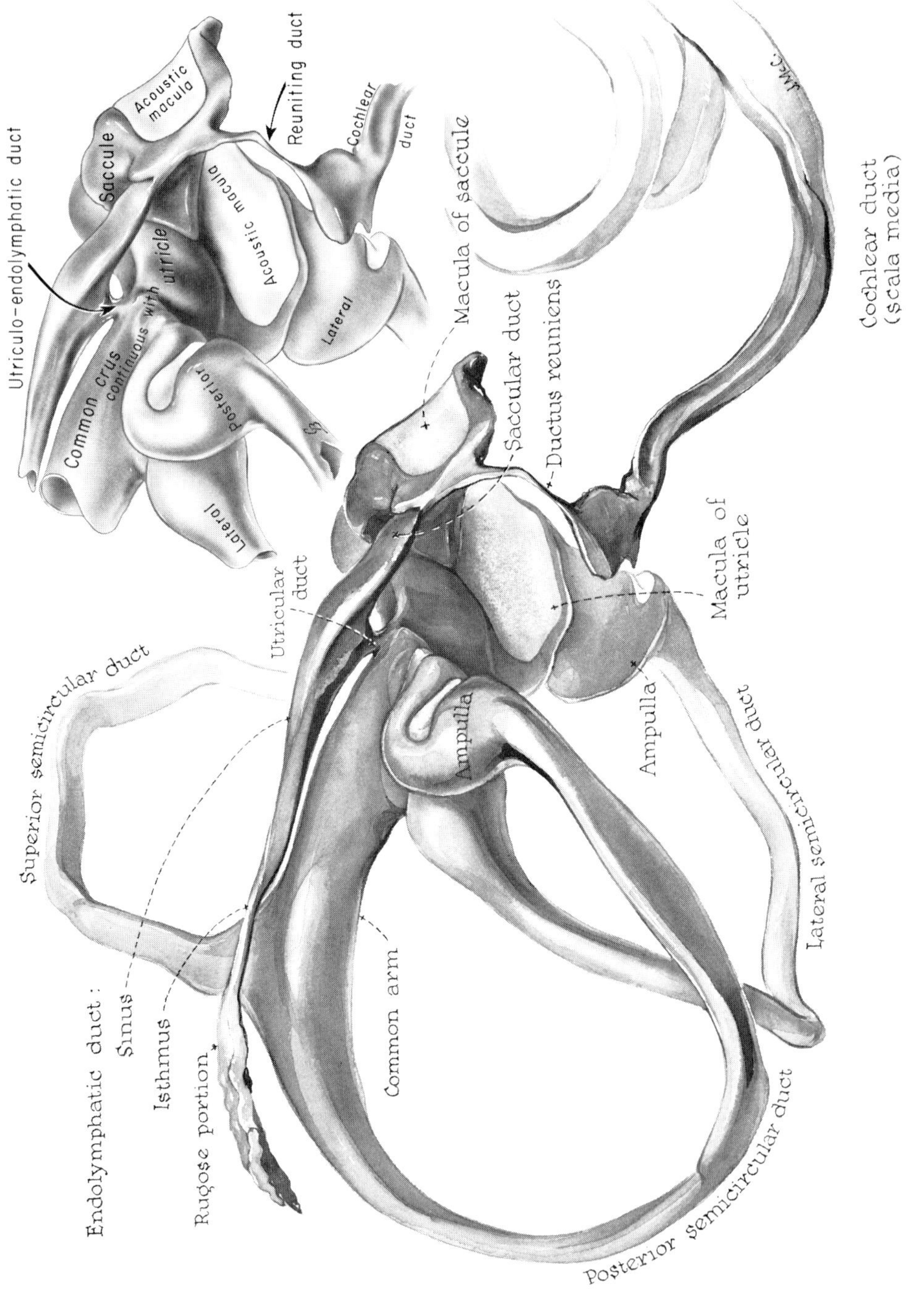
Utriculo-endolymphatic duct
Saccule
Acoustic macula
Reuniting duct
Cochlear duct
Acoustic macula
utricle
Lateral
Common crus
continuous with
Posterior
Lateral
Macula of saccule
Saccular duct
Ductus reuniens
Cochlear duct (scala media)
Macula of utricle
Utricular duct
Superior semicircular duct
Ampulla
Ampulla
Lateral semicircular duct
Endolymphatic duct:
Sinus
Isthmus
Rugose portion
Common arm
Posterior semicircular duct

Figure III–43. Membranous labyrinth. Infant, 6 months old. Reconstruction of the lumen of the epithelial duct system prepared by the Born method at a magnification of 37 diameters, inferomedial view. *Inset.* Detail of the area of the utricular, saccular and reuniting ducts.

Demonstrating especially the difference in form and capacity between the duct system of the utricular side and that of the saccular division of the membranous labyrinth. The utricle is widely continuous with the semicircular ducts. The saccule, on the contrary, communicates with the utricle and the cochlea through relatively small channels. Connection is made with the utricle beneath the valvelike fold that intervenes between the utricle and saccule. The saccule is brought into communication with the cochlear duct through the minute reuniting duct (*ductus reuniens*).

Explanatory Note: Because reconstructions of this type represent the space and not the wall of the epithelial duct system, the sensory area (maculae and cristae) appear to "invade" the lumen.

(From Anson, Harper, and Winch: Arch. Otolaryng., 85:497–514, 1967.)

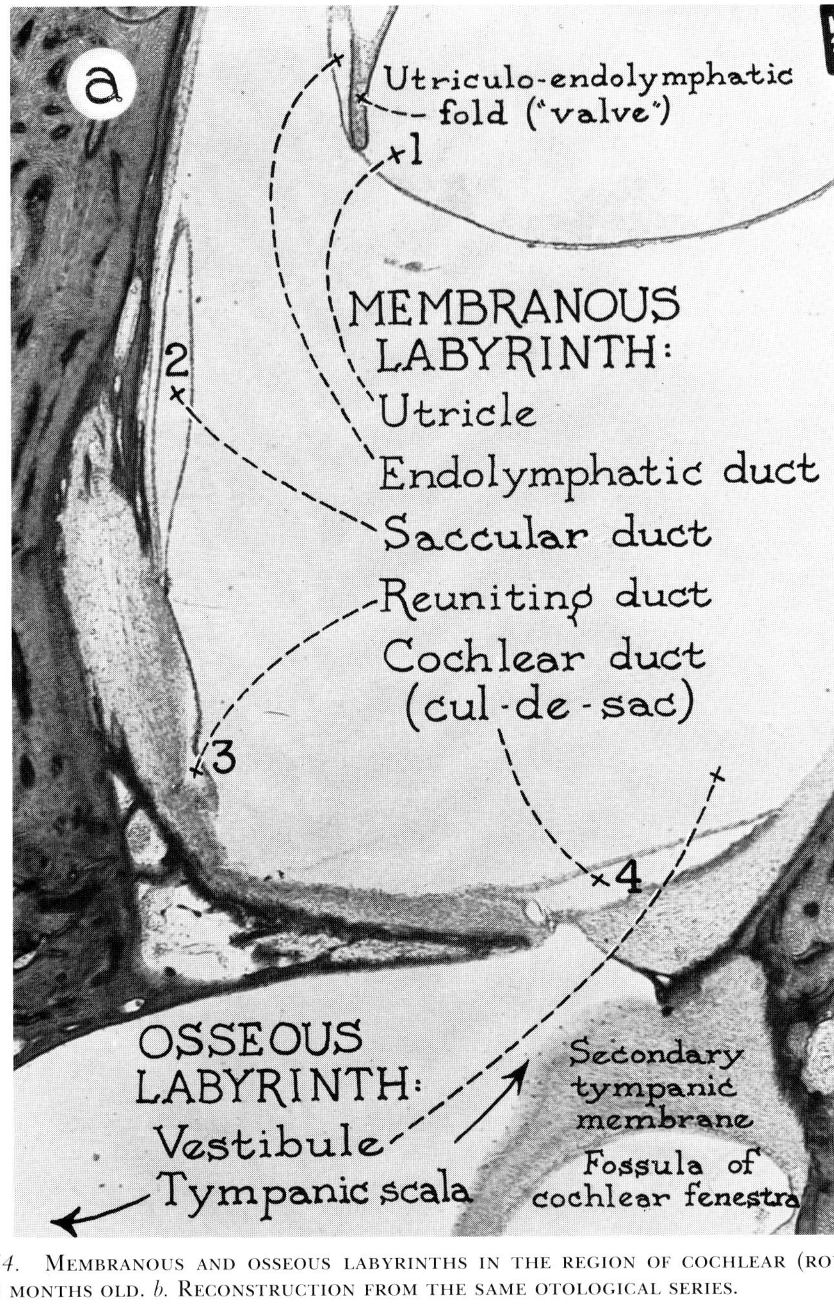

Figure III–44. Membranous and osseous labyrinths in the region of cochlear (round) window. *a.* Infant, 6 months old. *b.* Reconstruction from the same otological series.

a. Differing from the arrangement of structures in the area of the vestibular fenestra, in the region of the cochlear fenestra, the vestibule is separated from the tympanic cavity by the following: the secondary tympanic membrane; the tympanic scala of the cochlea; the membranous walls and contained space of the cul-de-sac (or *caecum vestibulare*) of the cochlear duct (the latter supported by the secondary osseous spiral). Within the vestibule, the cochlear duct is continuous with the sacculus through the reuniting duct (*ductus reuniens*) as an intermediary (the saccule is out of the plane of the section). The saccular duct becomes continuous in turn with the endolymphatic duct. Numerals indicate the succession of structures described in *b.*

Figure III–44 continues on the opposite page.

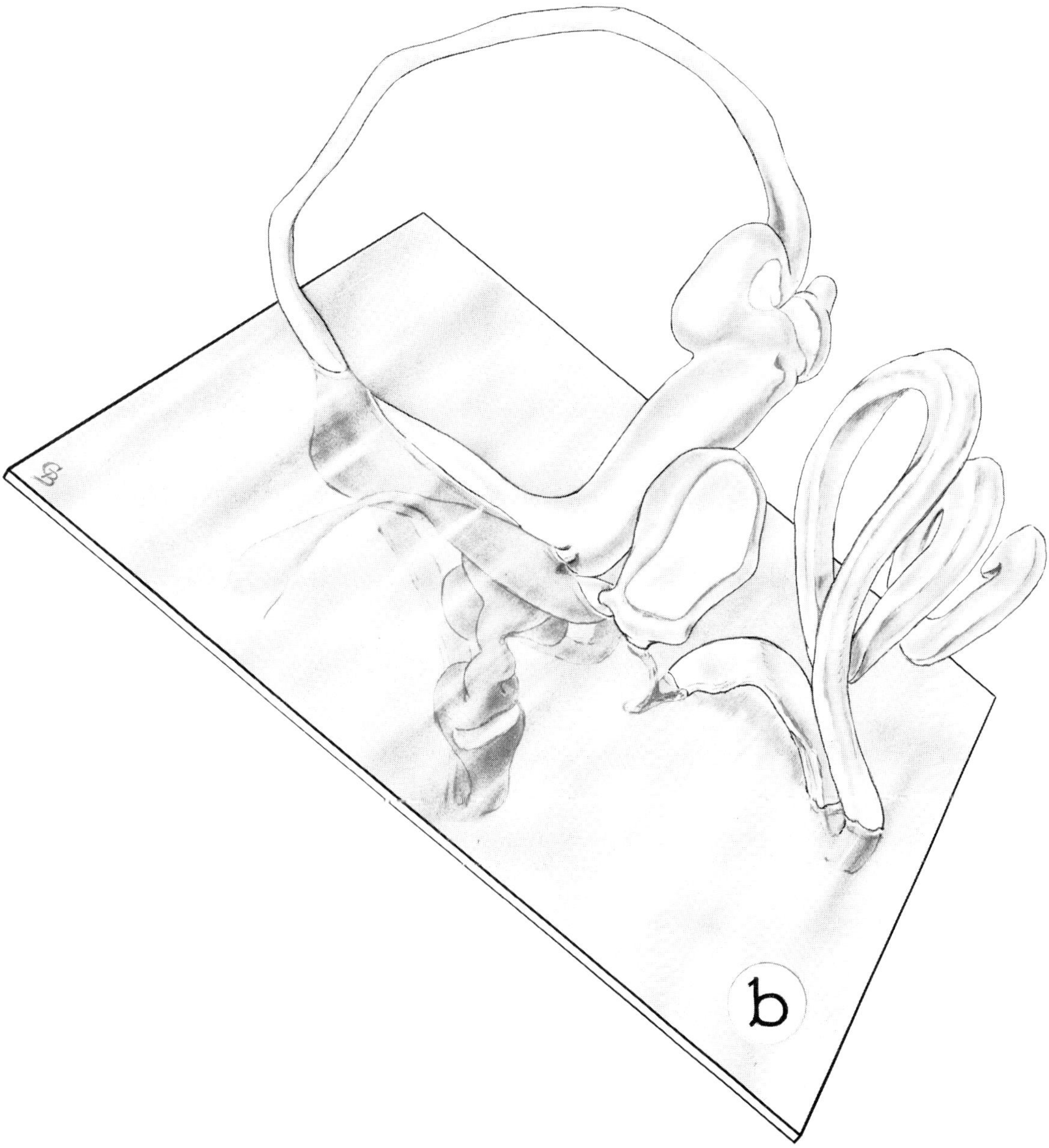

Figure III–44, Continued. MEMBRANOUS AND OSSEOUS LABYRINTHS IN THE REGION OF COCHLEAR (ROUND) WINDOW. *a.* INFANT, 6 MONTHS OLD. *b.* RECONSTRUCTION FROM THE SAME OTOLOGICAL SERIES.

b. The interposed plate is made to pass along the level of structures included in the photomicrograph (*a*). Reading from right to left, the parts of the membranous duct system are the following: cochlear duct; reuniting duct (*ductus reuniens*); saccular duct, at the inferior limit of the saccule; saccular duct in the area of its continuity with the sinuslike portion of the endolymphatic duct; and utricle.

Wisconsin Collection. *a*, transverse section, series 121, ×50.

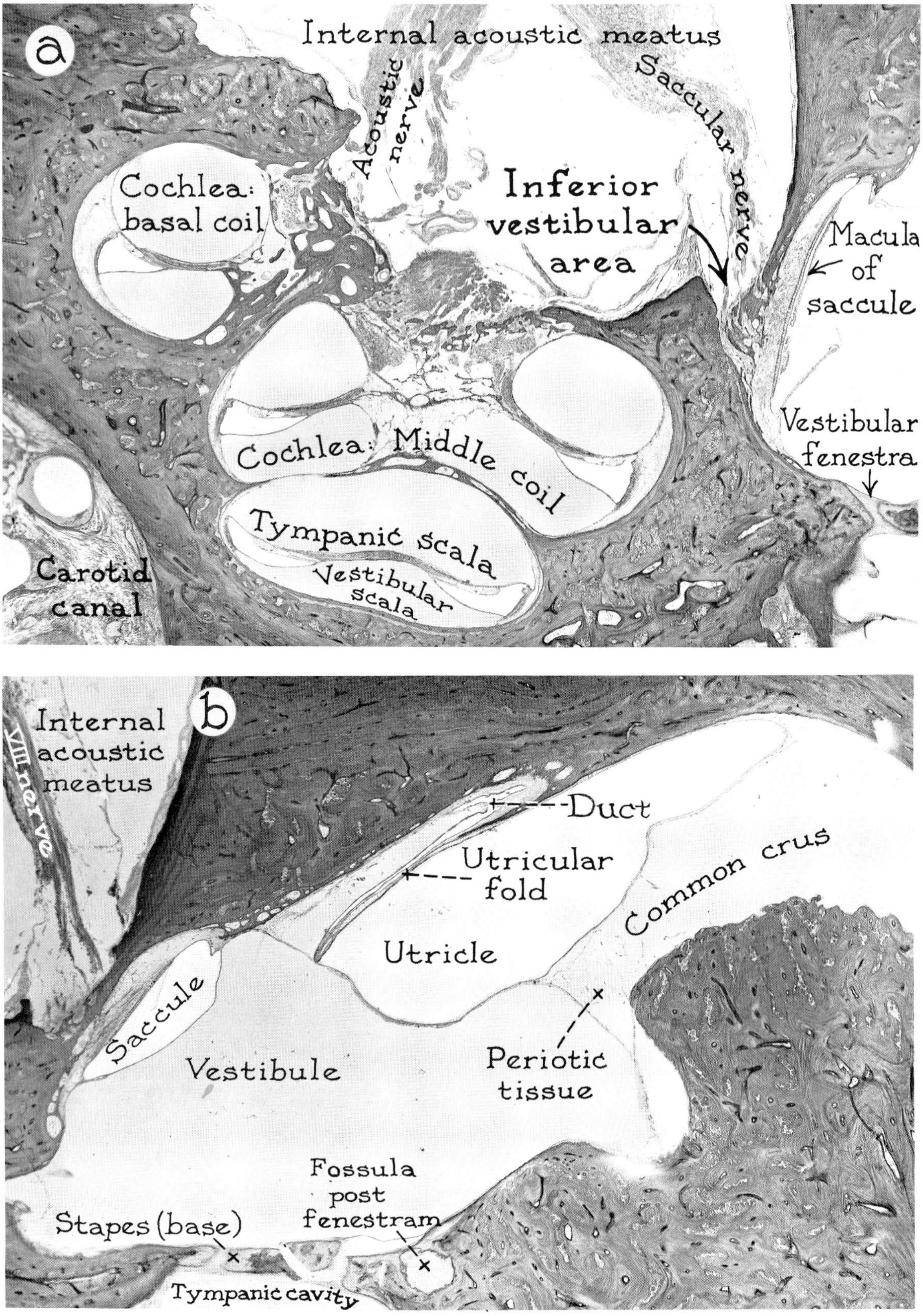

Figure III–45. See legend on the opposite page.

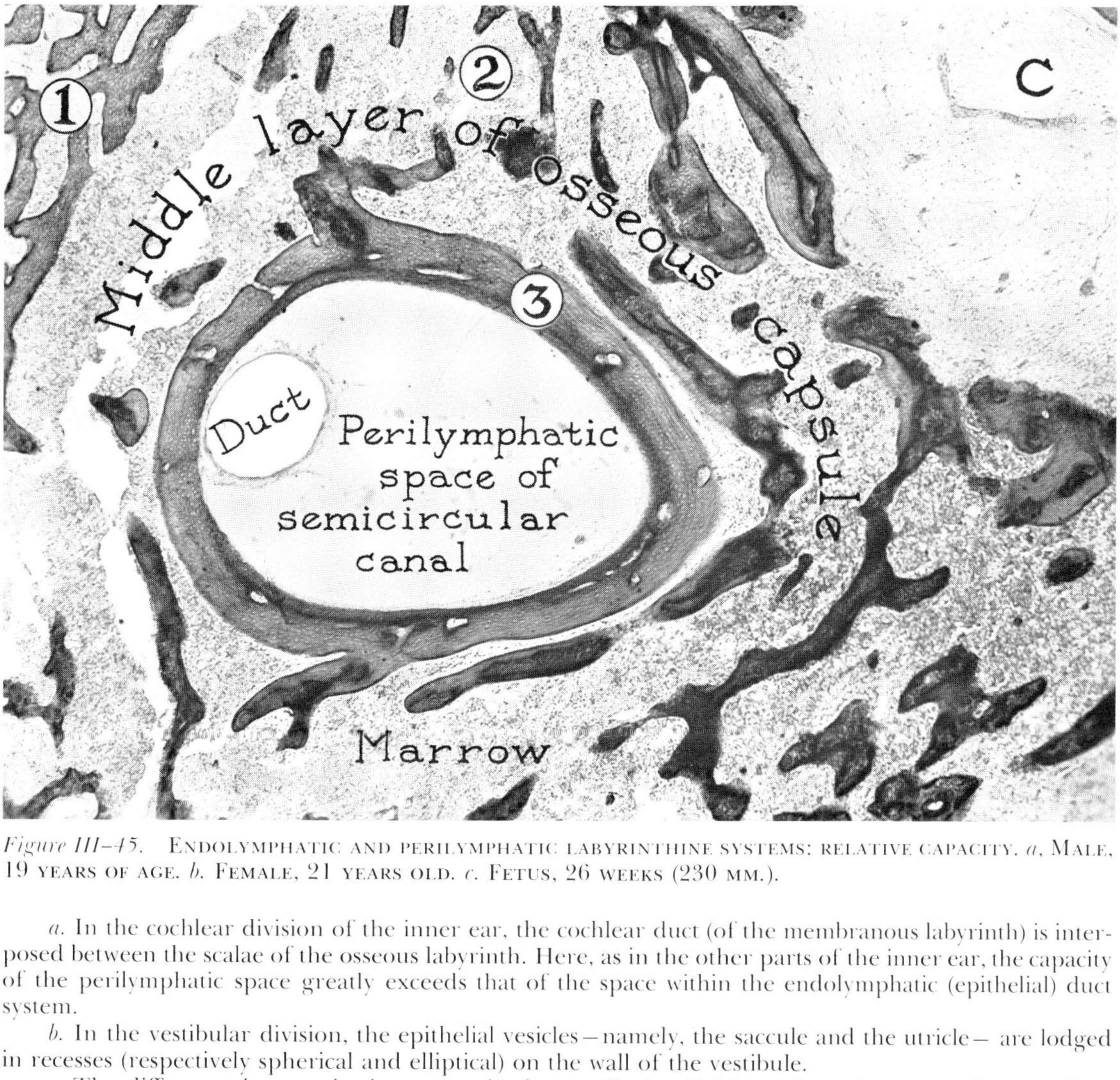

Figure III–45. ENDOLYMPHATIC AND PERILYMPHATIC LABYRINTHINE SYSTEMS: RELATIVE CAPACITY. *a*, MALE, 19 YEARS OF AGE. *b*. FEMALE, 21 YEARS OLD. *c*. FETUS, 26 WEEKS (230 MM.).

a. In the cochlear division of the inner ear, the cochlear duct (of the membranous labyrinth) is interposed between the scalae of the osseous labyrinth. Here, as in the other parts of the inner ear, the capacity of the perilymphatic space greatly exceeds that of the space within the endolymphatic (epithelial) duct system.

b. In the vestibular division, the epithelial vesicles—namely, the saccule and the utricle— are lodged in recesses (respectively spherical and elliptical) on the wall of the vestibule.

c. The difference in capacity is greatest in the canalicular division, where (except at the ampullary enlargements) the duct is very much smaller than the canal. It is to be noted that, whereas the duct systems appear mature, the encapsulating bone is still in a relatively primitive state. Numerals indicate the capsule layers (Figures II–6 and II–15*a*).

Transverse sections, Wisconsin Collection, series 29, 49, and 114, respectively. *a*, ×16; *b*, ×21; *c*, ×44.

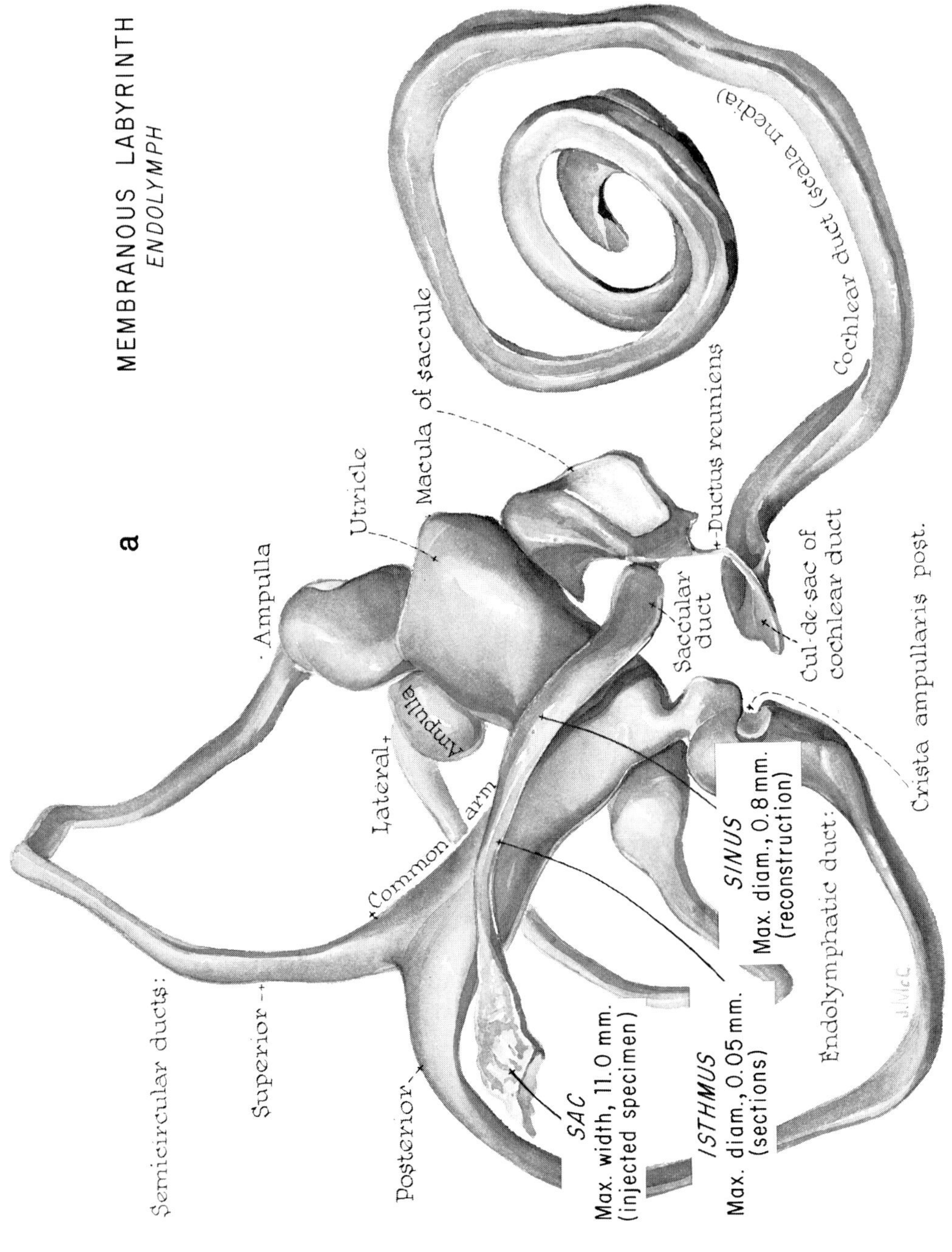
a
MEMBRANOUS LABYRINTH
ENDOLYMPH
Semicircular ducts:
Superior
Posterior
Common arm
Lateral
Ampulla
Ampulla
Utricle
Macula of saccule
Ductus reuniens
Saccular duct
Cul-de-sac of cochlear duct
Cochlear duct (scala media)
Crista ampullaris post.
Endolymphatic duct:
SAC
Max. width, 11.0 mm.
(injected specimen)
ISTHMUS
Max. diam., 0.05 mm.
(sections)
SINUS
Max. diam., 0.8 mm.
(reconstruction)
J. McC.

Figure III–46. MEMBRANOUS LABYRINTH, MEDIAL ASPECT. RECONSTRUCTION, BY THE BORN METHOD, OF THE LUMEN OF THE LABYRINTHINE SYSTEM. INFANT, 6 MONTHS OLD.

a. The form of the membranous labyrinth generally matches that of the osseous; however, in addition to being more capacious, the osseous labyrinth presents a common chamber, the vestibule, for the separate utricular and saccular parts of the membranous labyrinth (see *b*). The distal part of the endolymphatic sac is not included in this reconstruction (see Figure III–41).

Wisconsin Collection, series 121.

(From Anson, Harper, and Winch: Third Symposium on the Role of the Vestibular Organs in Space Exploration, NASA SP-152, pp. 125–146. Washington, D.C., U.S. Government Printing Office, 1968.)

Figure III–46 continues on the following page.

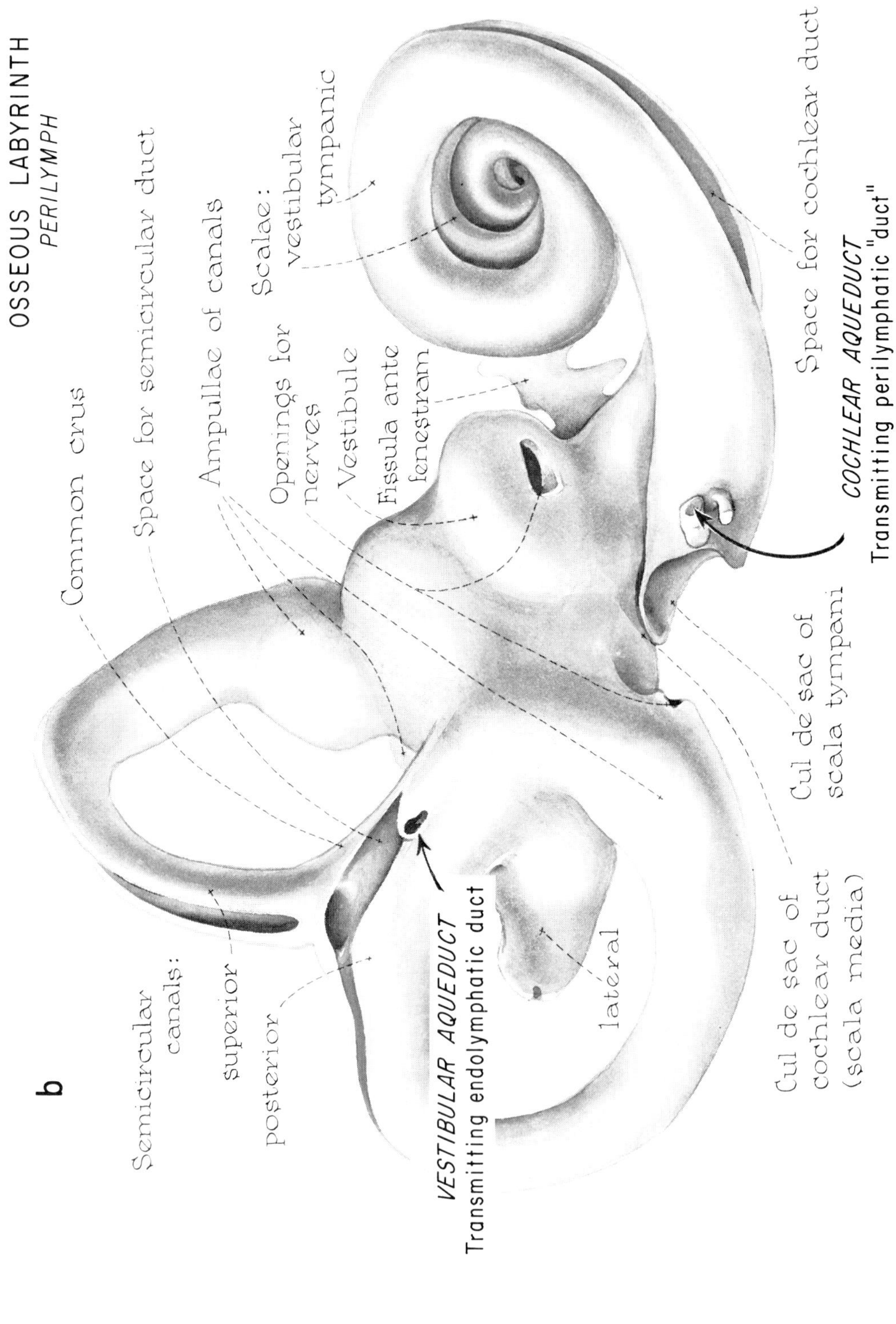
OSSEOUS LABYRINTH
PERILYMPH
b
Semicircular canals:
superior
posterior
lateral
Common crus
Space for semicircular duct
Ampullae of canals
Openings for nerves
Vestibule
Fissula ante fenestram
Scalae: vestibular
tympanic
Space for cochlear duct
COCHLEAR AQUEDUCT
Transmitting perilymphatic "duct"
Cul de sac of scala tympani
Cul de sac of cochlear duct (scala media)
VESTIBULAR AQUEDUCT
Transmitting endolymphatic duct

Figure III–46, Continued. OSSEOUS LABYRINTH, MEDIAL ASPECT. RECONSTRUCTION BY THE BORN METHOD. NEWBORN (4-DAY PREMATURE).

b. The perilymphatic spaces (cochlear, vestibular, and canalicular) are shown as a solid, with sulci representing the cochlear and semicircular ducts of the corresponding membranous duct system (shown in *a*).

The parts of the labyrinthine system are broadly confluent. The following spaces, of lesser capacity, occur as outpocketings or appendages: the cochlear canaliculus (with the so-called perilymphatic "duct"); the proximal part of the vestibular aqueduct; the fissula ante fenestram; and the fossula post fenestram (not in view). The secondary tympanic membrane would occupy the curving wall of the cul-de-sac of the scala tympani in the basal turn of the cochlea. The internal aperture of the cochlear canaliculus lies just within the *crista* for attachment of the membrane (see histology in Figure III–122*a*).

Wisconsin Collection, series 124.

(From Anson, Harper, and Winch: Third Symposium on the Role of the Vestibular Organs in Space Exploration, NASA SP-152, pp. 125–146. Washington, D.C., U.S. Government Printing Office, 1968.)

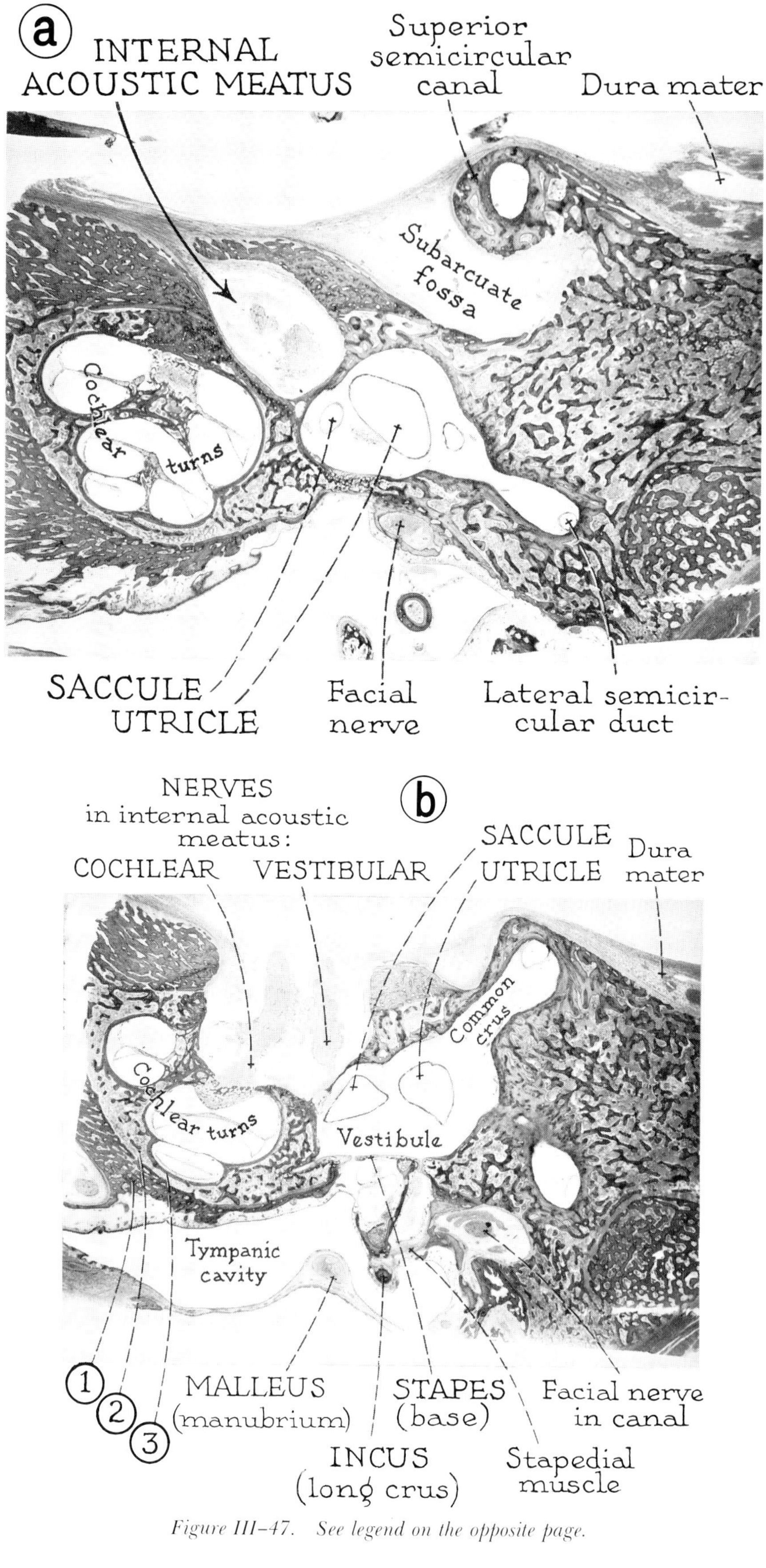

Figure III–47. See legend on the opposite page.

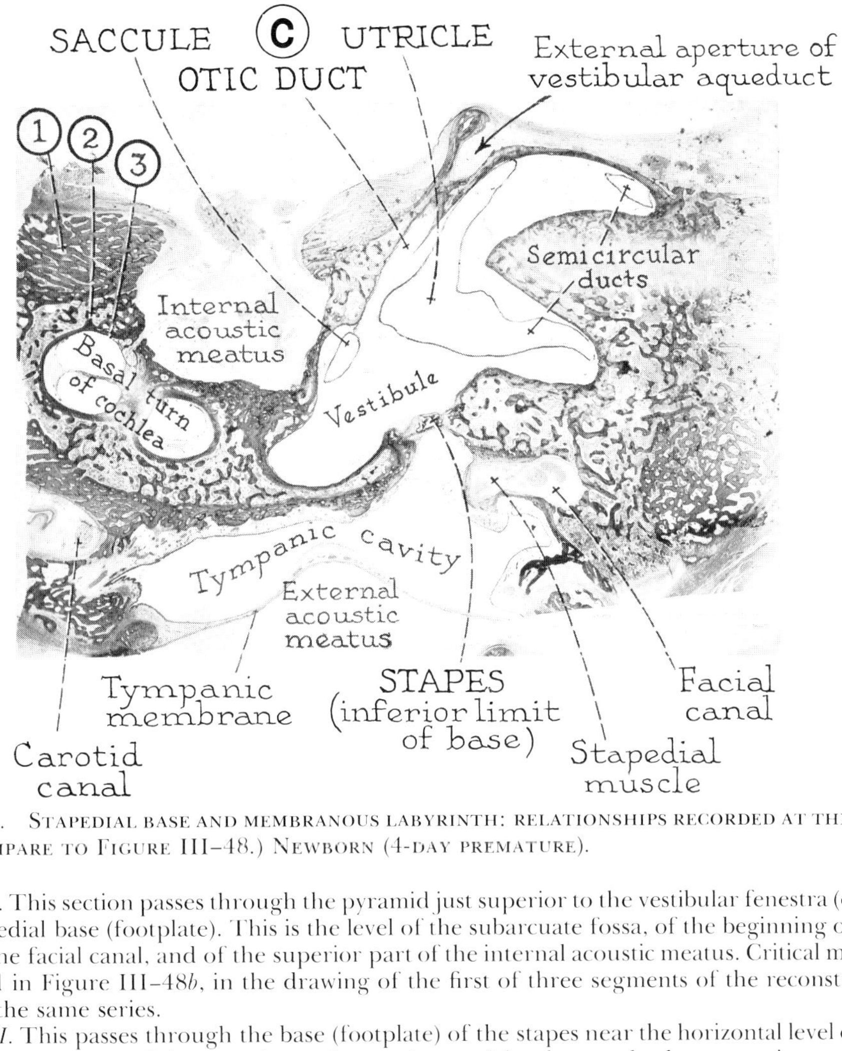

Figure III–47. STAPEDIAL BASE AND MEMBRANOUS LABYRINTH: RELATIONSHIPS RECORDED AT THREE SELECTED LEVELS. (COMPARE TO FIGURE III–48.) NEWBORN (4-DAY PREMATURE).

a. Level I. This section passes through the pyramid just superior to the vestibular fenestra (oval window) and the stapedial base (footplate). This is the level of the subarcuate fossa, of the beginning of the vertical segment of the facial canal, and of the superior part of the internal acoustic meatus. Critical measurements are recorded in Figure III–48*b*, in the drawing of the first of three segments of the reconstructions prepared from the same series.

b. Level II. This passes through the base (footplate) of the stapes near the horizontal level of its greatest width, the common crus of the superior and posterior semicircular canals, the tympanic membrane at the attachment of the manubrium of the malleus, and the stapedius tendon at the pyramidal eminence (cranial to the level of the muscle).

c. Level III. This passes through the inferior part of the stapedial footplate (and vestibular fenestra), the inferior part of the internal acoustic meatus, the basal turn of the cochlea, both apertures of the vestibular aqueduct and the endolymphatic (otic) duct, the stapedius muscle in the facial canal with the nerve, and the carotid canal. (For numerals in the primordial laminae of the capsule, see Figure II–6.)

Transverse sections, Wisconsin Collection, series 124. *a*, ×6.4; *b*, ×5.5; *c*, ×5.6.

(From Anson and Bast: Arch. Otolaryng., 71:188–206, 1960.)

Figure III–48. PARTS OF THE MEMBRANOUS LABYRINTH IN RELATION TO THE VESTIBULAR (OVAL) WINDOW.

a. This semischematic drawing is based upon a reconstruction prepared from a serially sectioned left temporal bone (newborn infant). The labyrinth is shown as if the medial wall of bone were transparent. The horizontal lines marked *I*, *II*, and *III* indicate the levels of the sections shown in the three succeeding parts of this figure.

The utricular and saccular portions of the membranous labyrinth occupy the vestibular division of the osseous labyrinth; they lie just medial to the vestibular (oval) window and the base (footplate) of the stapes. The lateral aspect of each, facing the stapes, is a free surface; on the opposite aspect both the utricle and the saccule are attached to the wall of the osseous labyrinth by periotic connective tissue and by the fibers of the vestibular nerve sent to the maculae. This means that the two membranous vesicles are partially supported by the perilymph in which they may be said to "float." A degree of mobility is contributed by this arrangement, in which portions of an epithelial duct system are provided with an almost circumambient fluid medium.

Despite the resiliency thus afforded, the short distance that intervenes between the footplate and the labyrinthine elements calls for caution in the several types of surgery involving the stapes. These distances can be considerably reduced by increased endolymphatic pressure or otosclerosis on the medial aspect of the footplate.

This intervening space will change from one transverse level to another in the same specimen, owing to the vesicular form of the two membranous chambers. Nor are the interdistances constant for all specimens.

At a transverse level near the superior margin of the oval window, in a representative otological series, the distance between the stapedial footplate and the saccule varied between 1.0 and 1.4 mm.; the corresponding distances for the utricle are 0.7 and 1.4 mm. In a group of 25 specimens, measured for comparative data, the shortest distance from the footplate to the saccule was 0.82 mm.; to the utricle, 0.38 mm.

At a level passing through the footplate at its maximum width, the shortest intervening distances were as follows: to the saccule, 1.4 mm.; to the utricle, the same. In the set of 25 specimens, the shortest intervening distances were as follows: to the saccule, 0.8 mm.; to the utricle, 0.2 mm.

The interdistances are slightly greater at a more inferior level, near the lower margin of the oval window. In the representative specimen, the distance to the saccule was 2.0 mm.; to the utricle it was 1.5 mm. A space of only 2.5 mm. separated the footplate from the cribrose macula in the wall of the spherical recess. Measurements made on the group of 25 specimens yielded the following information: the shortest distance (from the stapedial footplate) to the saccule was 0.38 mm.; to the utricle, 0.65 mm.

(Redrawn from Anson, Donaldson, Warpeha, and Winch: Laryngoscope, 75:1497–1517, 1965.)

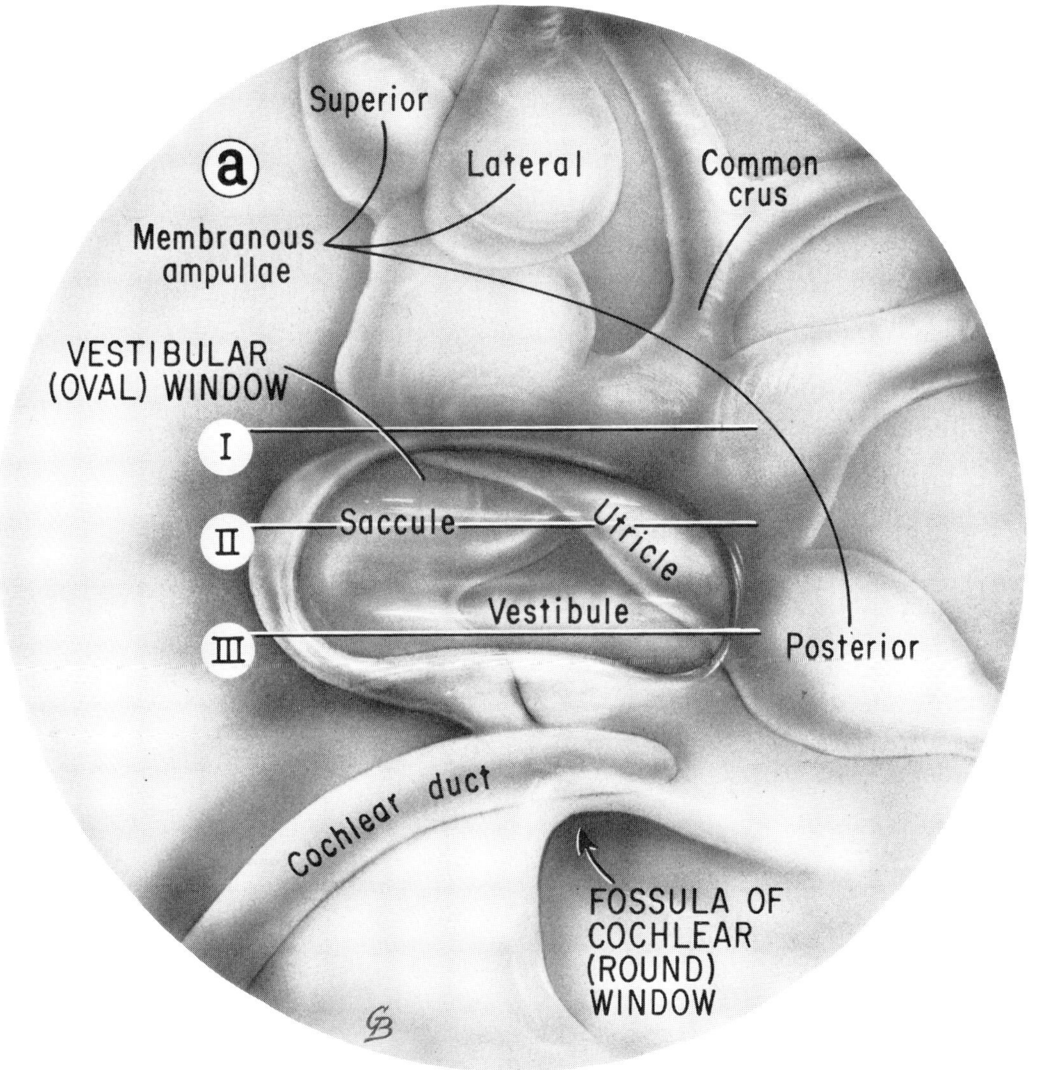

Figure III–48. See legend on the opposite page.

Figure III–48 continues on the following page.

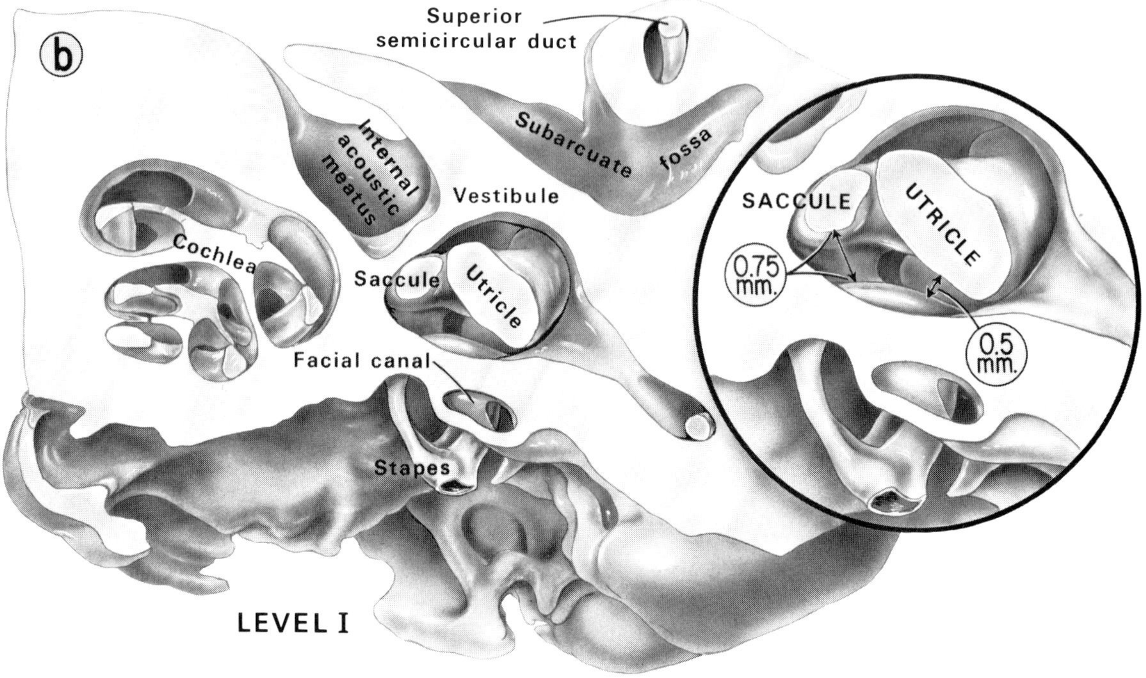

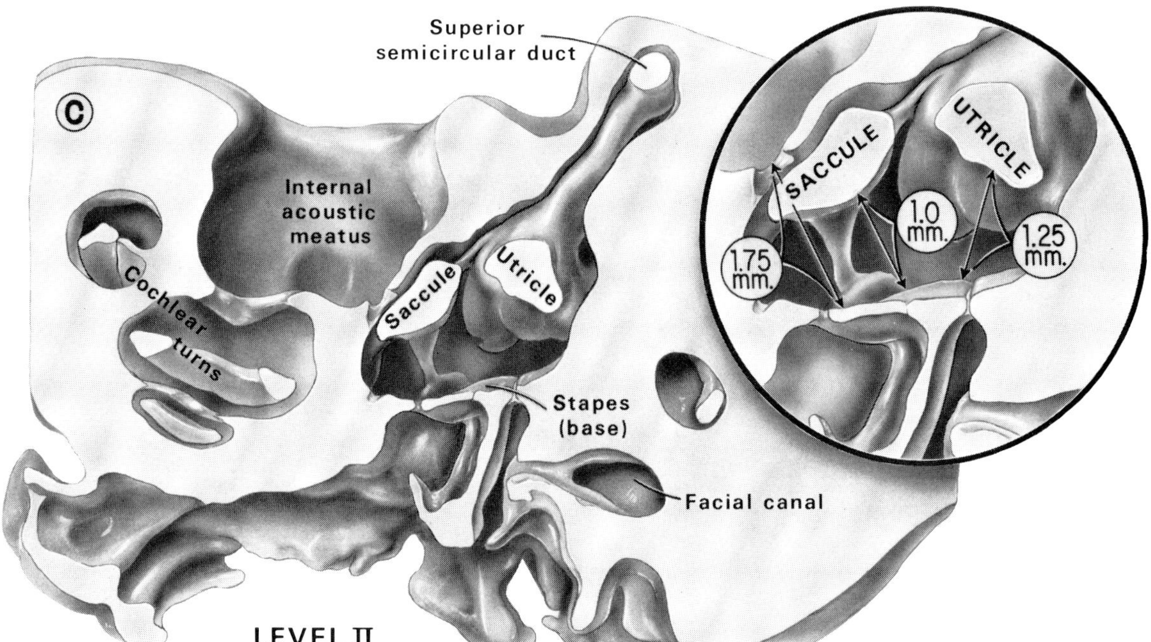

Figure III–48, Continued. See legend on the opposite page.

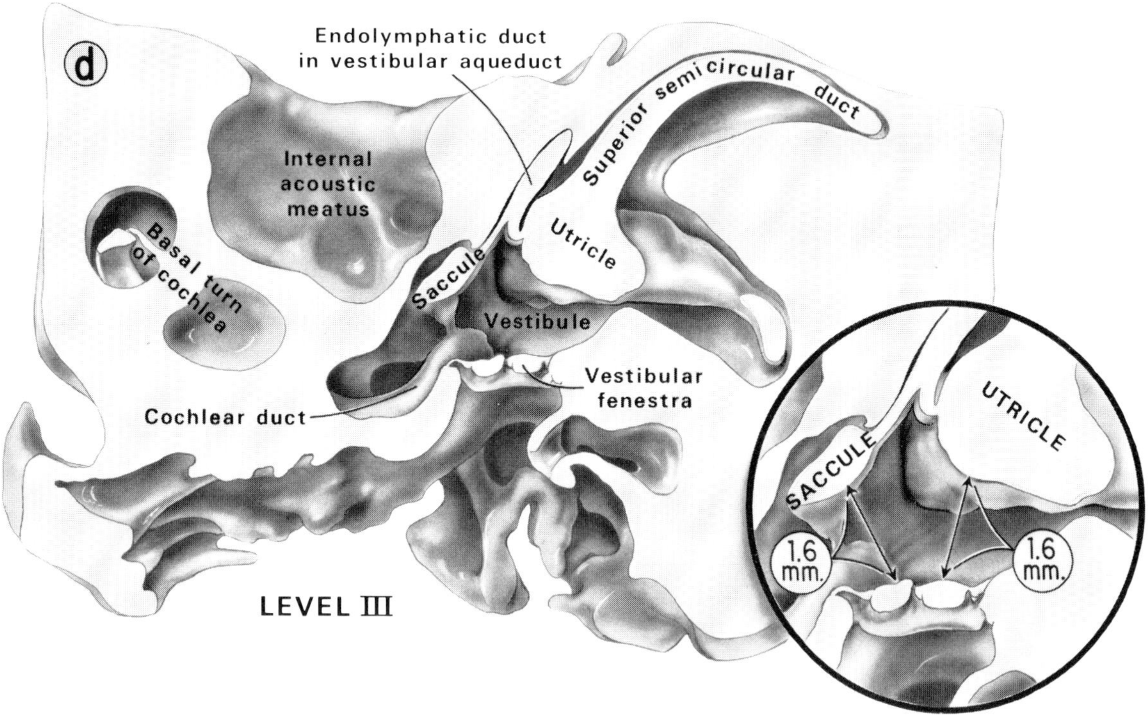

Figure III–48, Continued. RECONSTRUCTION DEMONSTRATING THE RELATION OF THE STAPEDIAL BASE (FOOTPLATE) TO THE SACCULE AND TO THE UTRICLE. THREE SEGMENTS IN SUPEROLATERAL VIEW. NEWBORN INFANT (4-DAY PREMATURE).

b. Level I. At this level, cranial to that of the stapes, the section at the free surface passed through the following: the cochlea near the modiolus; the subarcuate fossa and superior semicircular canal; the facial canal as it arches over the stapes; and the lateral semicircular canal. The interdistances are shown in the inset.

c. Level II. The section at the free surface of the reconstruction passed through the following structures: the cochlea and the internal acoustic meatus; the footplate and posterior crus of the stapes; the common crus; the facial canal (in vertical course); and the lateral semicircular canal. The distances between the footplate, the utricle, the saccule, and the cribrose macula of the saccule are recorded in the inset.

d. Level III. The section at the free surface passed through the following: the internal acoustic meatus near its floor; the basal turn of the cochlea near its lower limit; the vestibular fenestra (oval window); the vestibular aqueduct and endolymphatic duct; the superior and posterior semicircular canals; and the pyramidal eminence. The level is just superior to that of the *ductus reuniens* in communication with the saccule and the cochlear duct. The interdistances are shown in the inset.

Wisconsin Collection, series 124, left ear.

(Redrawn from Anson and Bast: Quart. Bull., Northwestern Univ. Med. Sch., 32:307–325, 1958.)

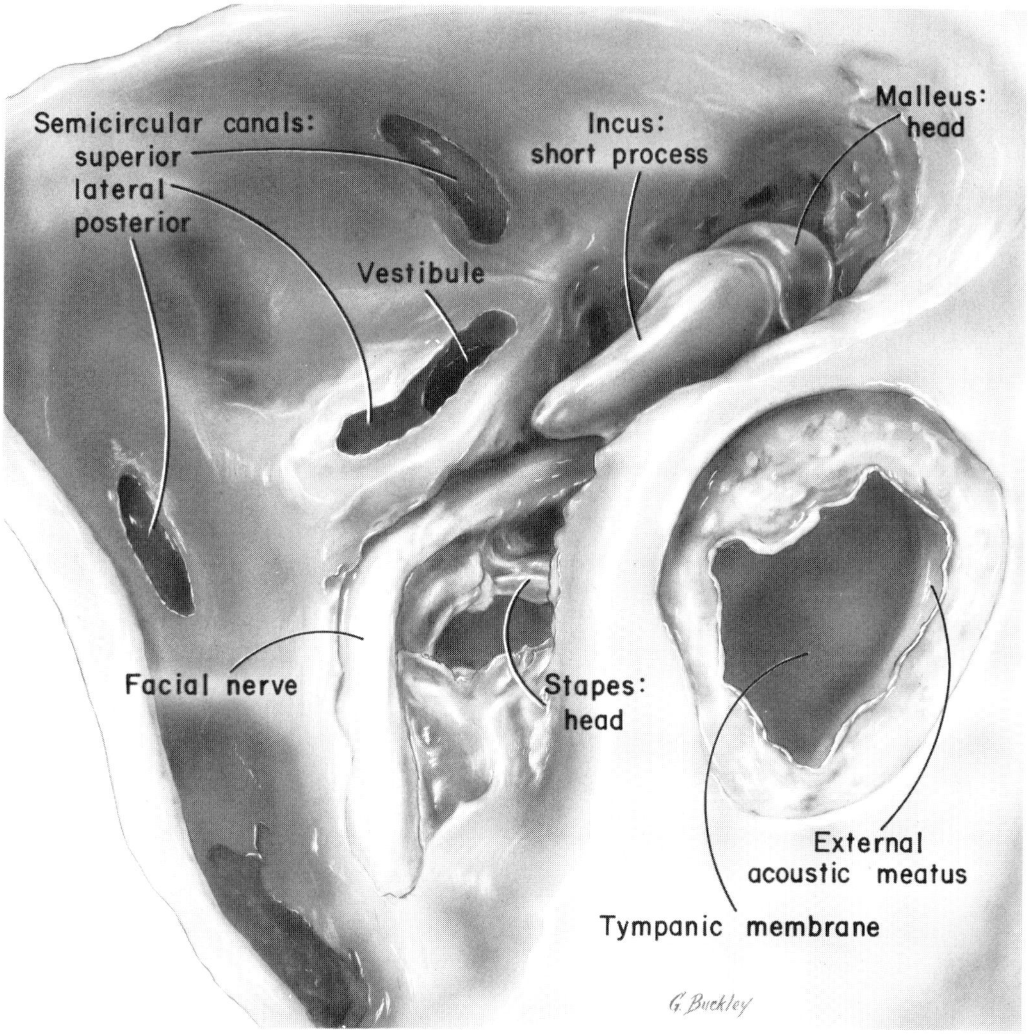

a

Figure III–49. ANATOMY OF THE MIDDLE AND INNER EAR, IN A TRANSTEMPORAL APPROACH TO THE INTERNAL ACOUSTIC MEATUS. FIRST IN A SERIES OF THREE DISSECTIONS OF AN UNEMBALMED RIGHT TEMPORAL BONE.

a. On the medial wall of the tympanic cavity the three semicircular canals have been opened. For purposes of orientation the distal part of the external acoustic meatus is retained.

The superior and posterior canals join at the common crus, the latter conjoined channel then continuing into the vestibule. Before dissection, the lateral semicircular canal causes a pronounced bulging on this medial, or labyrinthine, wall of the tympanic cavity; just below this is the prominence of the facial canal. Together they form the medial boundary of the epitympanic recess, occupied by the head of the malleus and the body of the incus.

Figure III–49 continues on the opposite page.

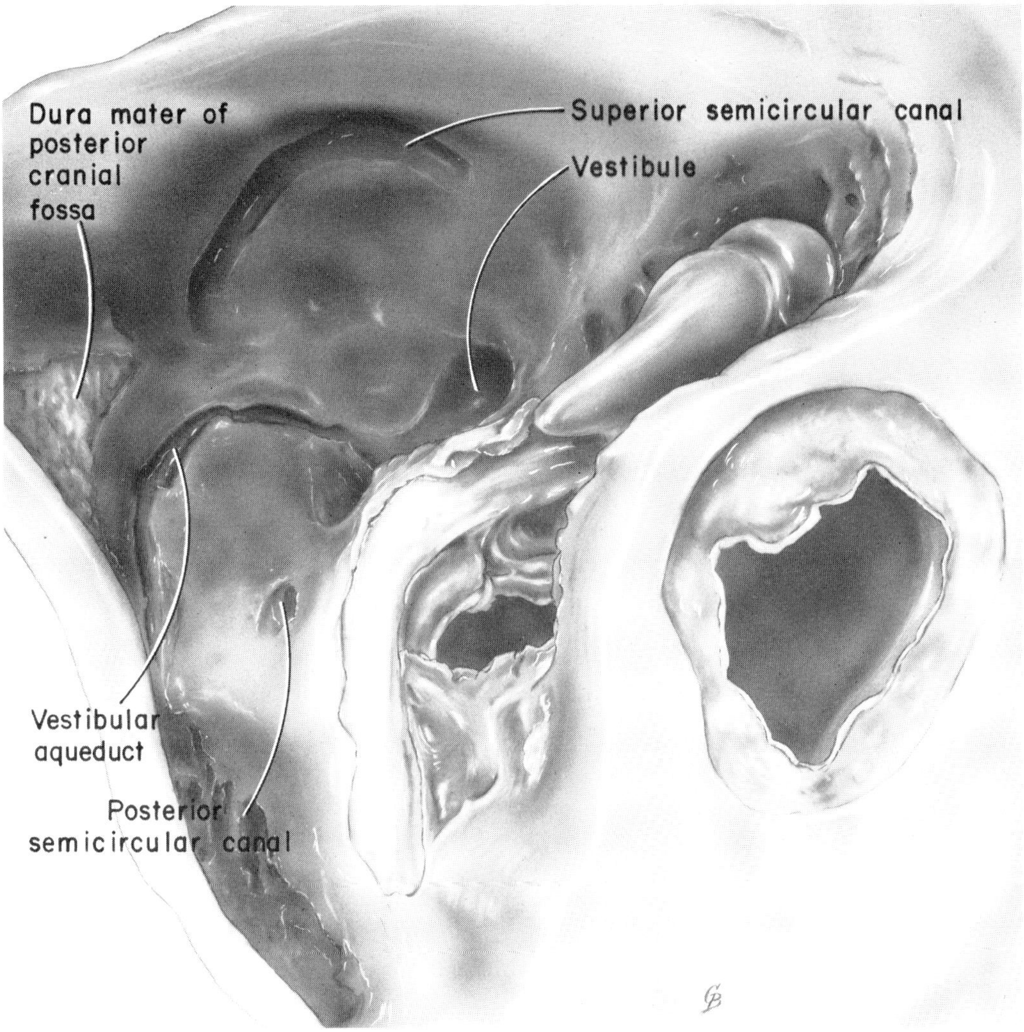

b

Figure III–49, Continued. STRUCTURES OF THE INNER EAR THAT ARE TOPOGRAPHICALLY IMPORTANT IN THE TRANSTEMPORAL APPROACH TO THE INTERNAL ACOUSTIC MEATUS. *b.* SECOND STAGE IN DISSECTION.

b. The bone around the lateral semicircular canal has been removed, the dissection then continued to the level of the vestibular aqueduct. An opening has been made into the posterior cranial fossa, the dural layer (of the cerebellum) exposed in the area between the superior petrosal and sigmoid venous sinuses.

The course of the vestibular aqueduct, in its proximal part, matches that of the common crus formed by the junction of the superior and posterior semicircular canals. Distally it departs therefrom, curving gently downward (Figures III–60*a*, III–101*b*, III–104 and III–106). The internal aperture is a small depression in the wall of the elliptical recess of the vestibule. The external aperture is a slit-shaped opening on the posterior surface of the petrous pyramid (see dissections in Figures III–110 to III–117). The contained endolymphatic sac is lodged in the dural covering of the bone (see sections in Figures III–61 and III–62).

Figure III–49 continues on the following page.

Figure III–49, Continued. STRUCTURES OF THE INNER EAR THAT ARE ENCOUNTERED IN THE TRANSTEMPORAL APPROACH TO THE INTERNAL ACOUSTIC MEATUS. *c.* THIRD STAGE IN DISSECTION.

c. This third stage is necessary for the removal of an acoustic neuroma or sectioning of the vestibular nerve by the transtemporal approach. Further removal of bone exposes the facial nerve and the two terminal divisions of the vestibular nerve in the internal acoustic meatus. The dural lining of the meatus and the related meningeal sheaths of the nerves have been opened, the cut edge drawn upward (at arrows). In the dissection a thin plate of bone remains (at asterisk) posterior to the meatus, separating the inner periosteal layer of the pyramid from the fossa of the cranial cavity. Just above this area the bone has been removed, exposing the dura mater of the cerebellum.

As the nerves approach the fundus of the internal acoustic meatus, the facial nerve and the superior, or upper, branch of the vestibular nerve pass to their areas above the level of the transverse crest; the inferior, or lower, branch of the vestibular nerve passes beneath the crest.

In this figure and in the two that precede it, the malleus and incus remain *in situ* as they extend into the epitympanic recess. The facial nerve is exposed through part of its horizontal and almost all of the vertical portion. The geniculum is out of view. In the vertical course, on the way to the stylomastoid foramen, the nerve is in close relation to the mastoid air cells, the intervening osseous wall of the canal sometimes being excessively thin.

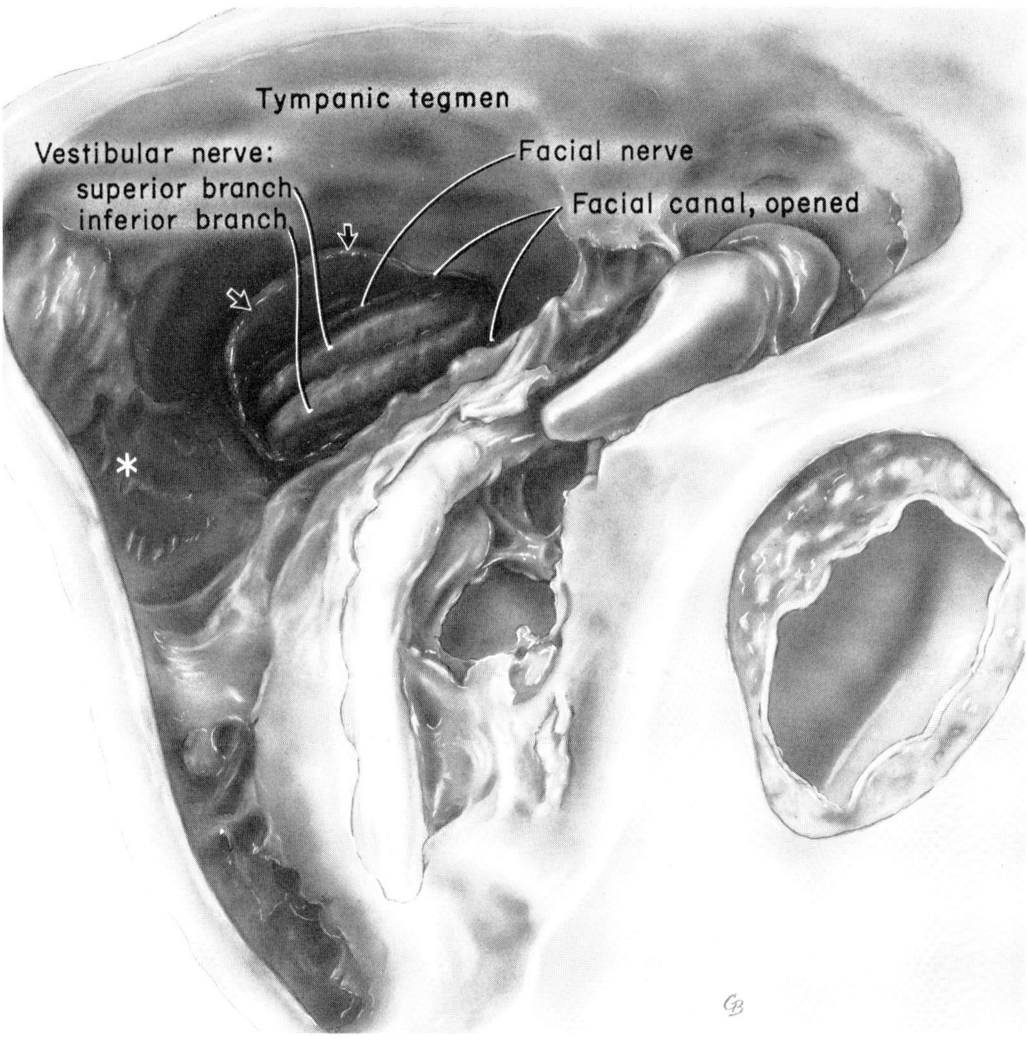

C

Figure III–49, Concluded. See legend on the opposite page.

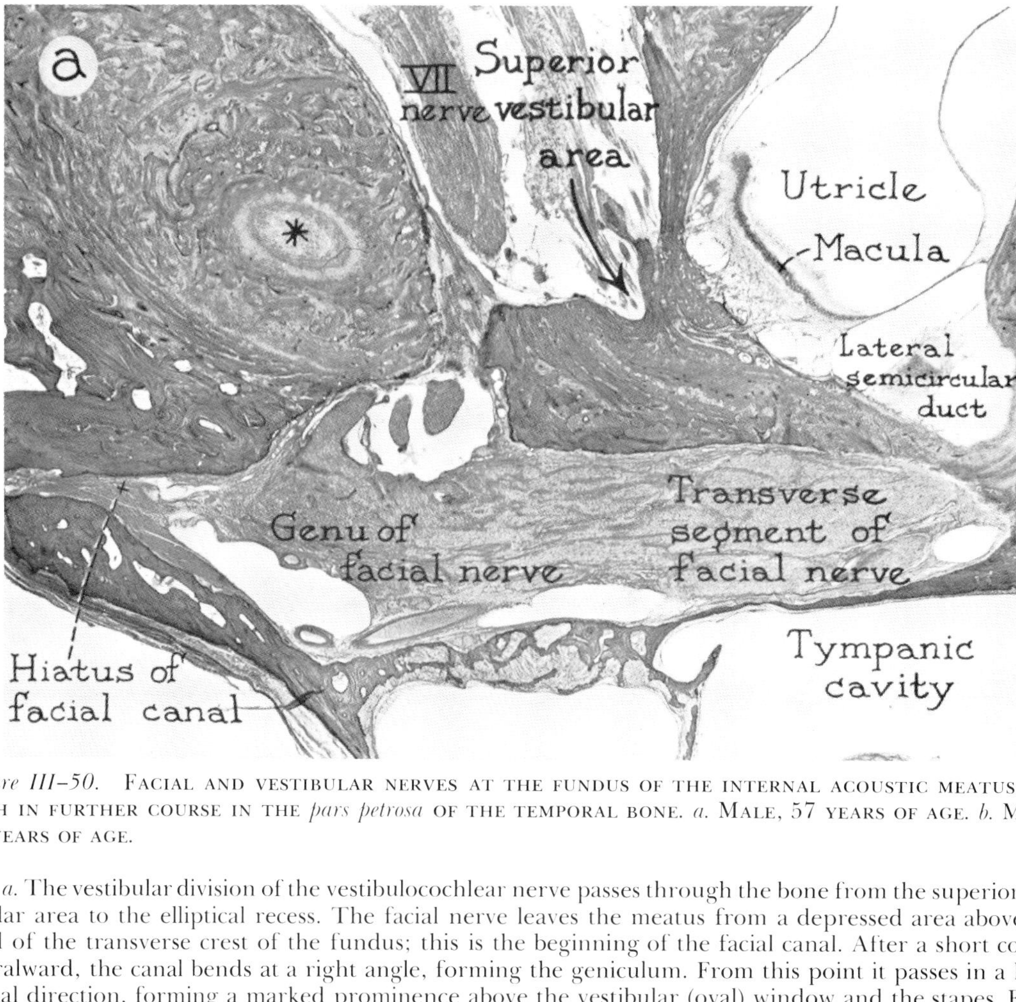

Figure III–50. FACIAL AND VESTIBULAR NERVES AT THE FUNDUS OF THE INTERNAL ACOUSTIC MEATUS AND EACH IN FURTHER COURSE IN THE *pars petrosa* OF THE TEMPORAL BONE. *a.* MALE, 57 YEARS OF AGE. *b.* MALE, 19 YEARS OF AGE.

a. The vestibular division of the vestibulocochlear nerve passes through the bone from the superior vestibular area to the elliptical recess. The facial nerve leaves the meatus from a depressed area above the level of the transverse crest of the fundus; this is the beginning of the facial canal. After a short course lateralward, the canal bends at a right angle, forming the geniculum. From this point it passes in a horizontal direction, forming a marked prominence above the vestibular (oval) window and the stapes. From the geniculum a short channel, the hiatus of the facial canal, passes medialward and forward transmitting the greater superficial petrosal nerve. The further course of the facial nerve is illustrated in Figures III–70 and III–78. Asterisk indicates the summit of the basal turn of the cochlea.

Figure III–50 continues on the opposite page.

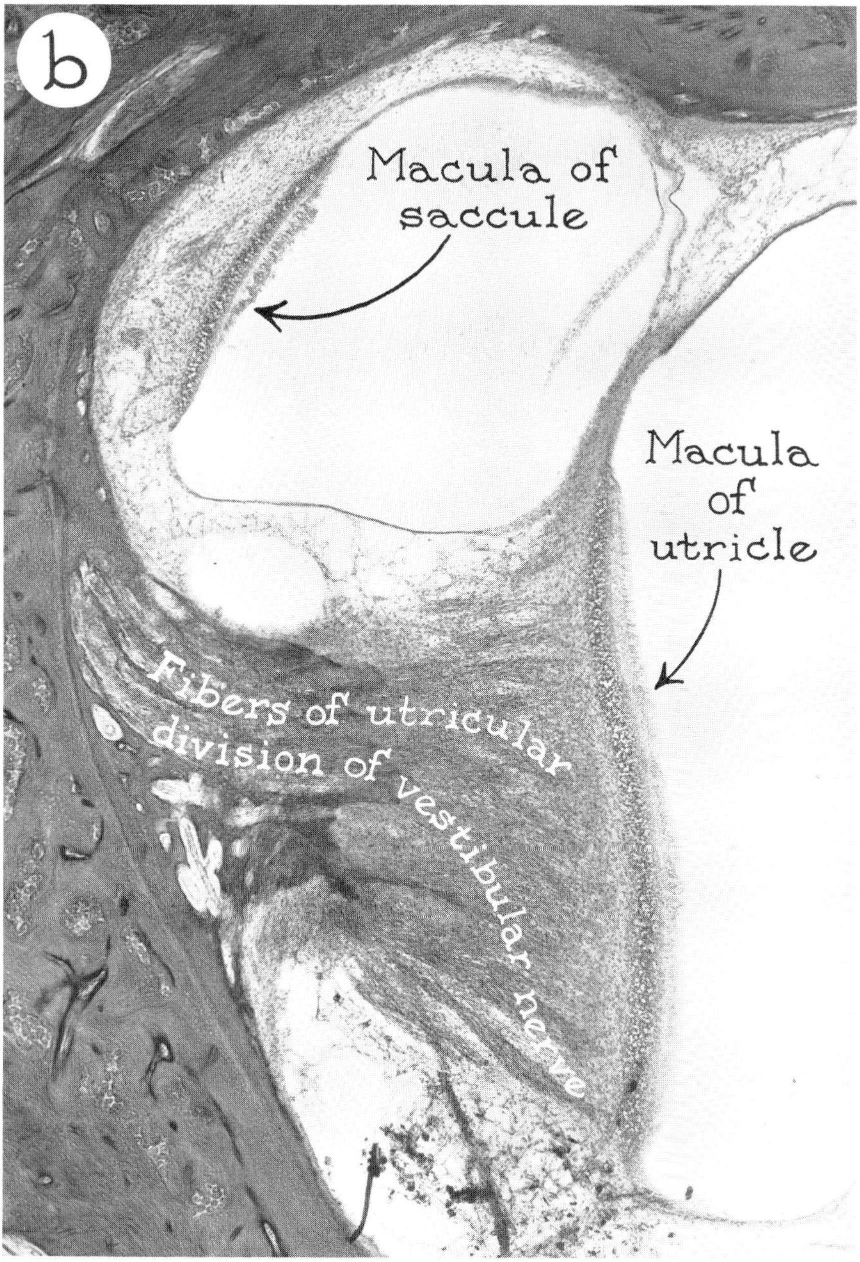

Figure III–50, Continued.

b. Innervation of the acoustic macula of the utricle. Showing the way in which fibers of the utricular branch of the superior or utriculoampullary division of the vestibular nerve pass through the superior cribrose macula to their termination in the acoustic macula of the utricle. Compare saccular innervation, Figure III–57*b*.

Transverse sections, Wisconsin Collection, series 32 and 29, respectively. *a*, ×13; *b*, ×43.

Figure III–51. INNERVATION OF THE MEMBRANOUS LABYRINTH: SPIRAL ORGAN (OF CORTI), MACULAE OF THE UTRICLE AND SACCULE, AND CRISTAE OF THE SEMICIRCULAR DUCTS. MALE, 19 YEARS OF AGE.

Showing the osseous channels for the cochlear and vestibular divisions of the vestibulocochlear nerve at the fundus of the internal acoustic meatus and on the walls of the vestibule and semicircular canals.

The cochlear nerve appears at the bottom of the internal acoustic meatus, with the ganglion (at asterisk), from which foramina carry bundles of the cochlear nerve directly to the basal turn and through the longitudinal canals of the modiolus to the middle and apical turns. The fibers of the utricular division of the vestibular nerve pass from the superior cribrose macula to the acoustic macula of the utricle.

The fibers of the saccular division of the nerve, in coursing from the inferior vestibular area of the fundus, emerge on the wall of the spherical recess of the vestibule to supply the acoustic macula of the saccule (Figure III–57*c*). The nerves to the cristae of the superior and lateral semicircular ducts pass through the superior cribrose macula of the vestibule (together with the utricular nerve) to the two ampullae (Figure III–54).

Transverse section, Wisconsin Collection, series 29. ×20.

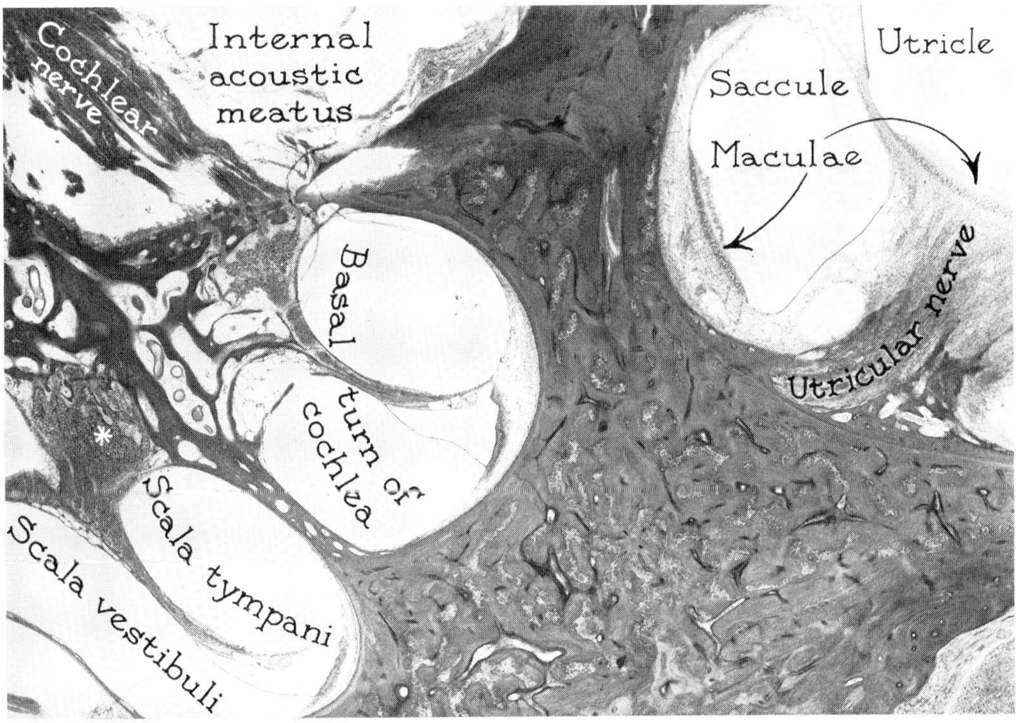

Figure III–51. See legend on the opposite page.

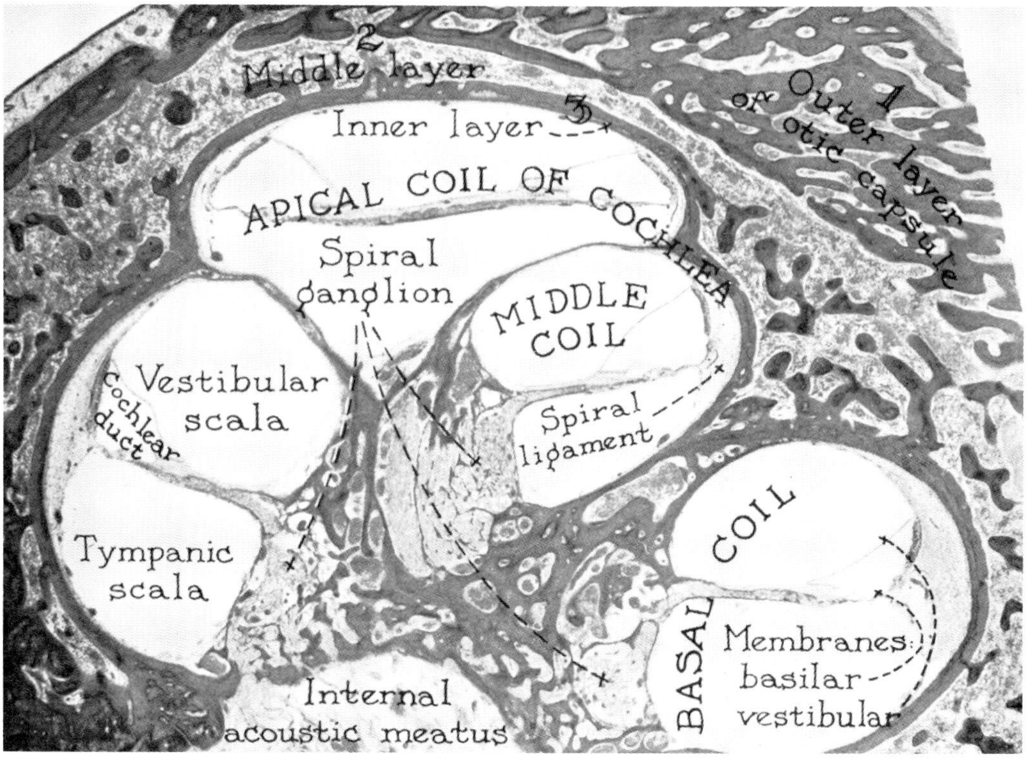

a

Figure III–52. LABYRINTHINE ANATOMY, COCHLEAR AND VESTIBULAR. *a.* NEWBORN INFANT (4-DAY PREMATURE). *b.* INFANT, 6 MONTHS OLD.

a. The cochlea forms the anterior part of the osseous labyrinth. Its shape is that of a low cone, with the axis disposed in the horizontal plane. The base is directed toward the fundus of the internal acoustic meatus (see Figure III–51); the apex, or cupola, toward the semicanal for the tensor tympani muscle (see Figures II–21*c* and II–34*d*). The inferior wall is shared with the upward-directed curvature of the carotid canal (Figure III–18). The cochlea contains a spirally wound canal that begins in the anteroinferior part of the vestibule at the cochlear fenestra (round window) (see Figure III–94) and ends blindly at the apex. The space of the cochlea, around which the spiral canal is coiled, consists of spongy bone, the modiolus or spindle. This spindle forms the inner wall of the canal; the outer wall is the compact bone of the capsule; it is connected with the spindle by thin lamellae of bone which constitute septa between the coils. The modiolus is hollowed out on the surface that faces the fundus, there forming the cochlear area. The modiolus is perforated by longitudinal canals that run parallel to the axis. At the apex it becomes compact bone, the lamina of the modiolus, around which the apical turn curves.

Midway between the septa that divide the cochlear space into coils, a delicate bony plate (the osseous spiral lamina) passes part way into the lumen dividing it incompletely into the vestibular and tympanic scalae. Separation is completed by the interposition of the membranous cochlear duct (Figures III–55 and II–25). The breadth of the spiral lamina decreases from the base toward the apex, corresponding generally to diminution in size of the cochlear canal. The osseous spiral lamina ends in the apical coil in a free, projecting process, the hamulus. At this point, the fresh state, the cochlear duct terminates at the helicotrema, and the scalae establish their sole connection (being elsewhere separated from one another by the membranous duct). The layers of capsular bone are numbered *1* to *3*.

Figure III–52 continues on the opposite page.

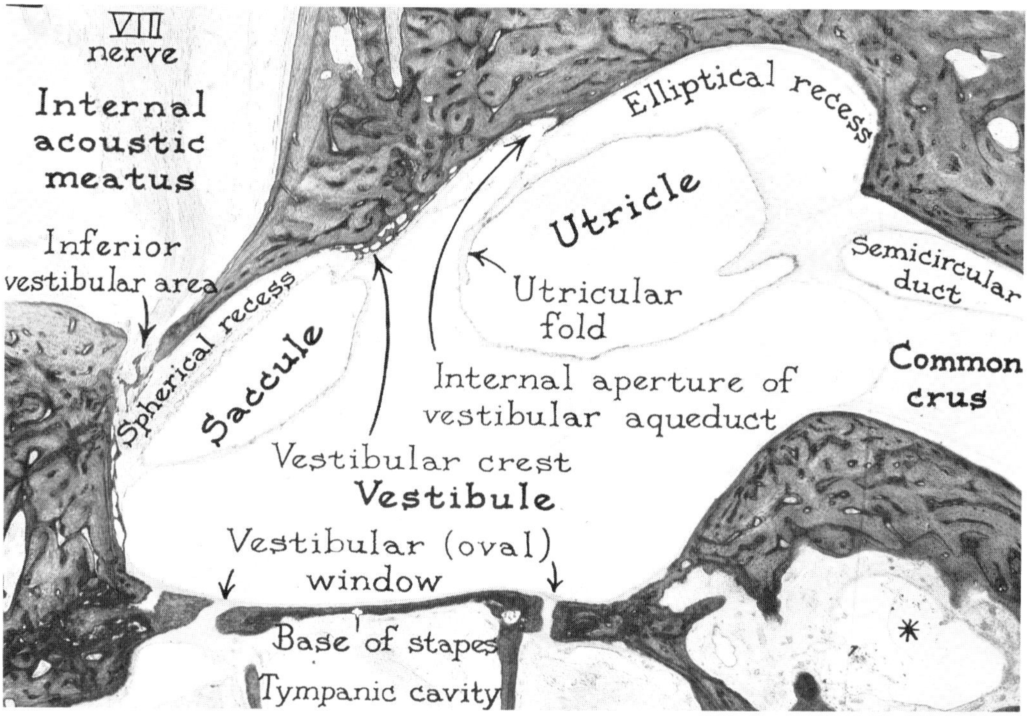

b

Figure III–52, Continued.

b. The vestibule is the middle part of the osseous labyrinth. The vestibule is continuous with the cochlea anteriorly and with the semicircular canals posteriorly. Its medial wall helps to form the fundus of the internal acoustic meatus; the vestibular window is seen on the lateral (or tympanic) wall. Two small depressions are present on the medial wall. The more posterior of the two, the elliptical recess, serves for reception of the utricle; the anterior member of the pair, the spherical recess, receives the saccule (see Figure III–57*b* for additional detail). The saccule is firmly attached to the bone of its recess by connective tissue and by bundles of the saccular nerve emerging from the middle cribrose macula; otherwise it is separated from the walls of the vestibule by the relatively capacious periotic space. Like the saccule, the utricle is anchored to the wall of its recess (Figure III–53*b*). The remainder of the surface is free, except where slender strands of periotic tissue cross the perilymphatic space. Asterisk indicates part of the tympanic cavity.

Transverse sections, Wisconsin Collection, series 124 and 121, respectively. *a*, ×21; *b*, ×20.

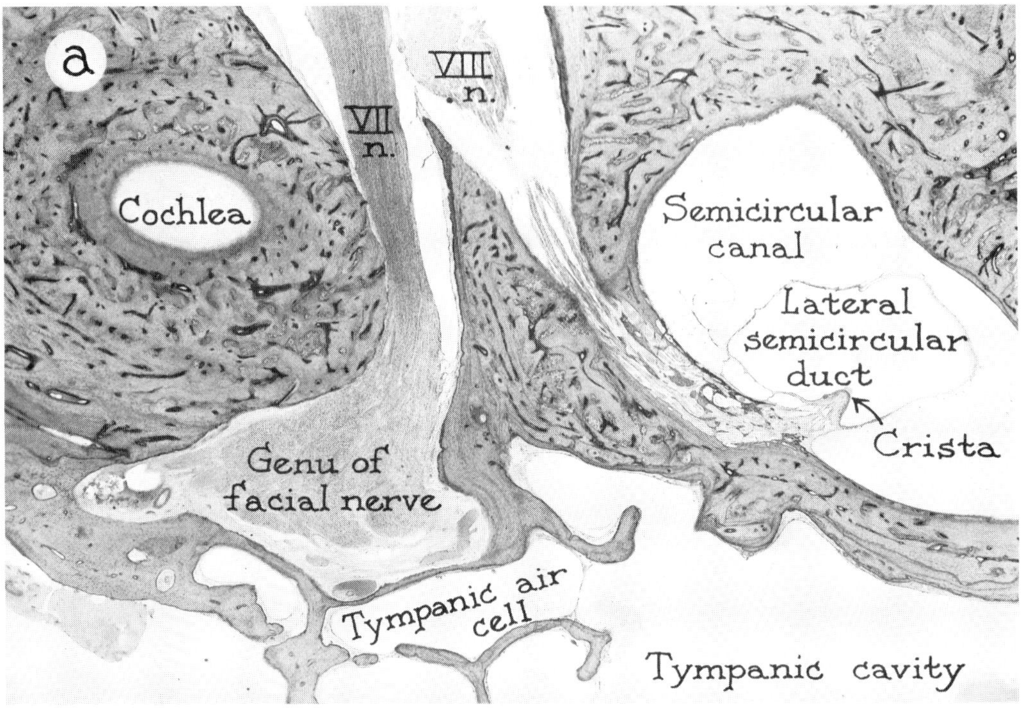

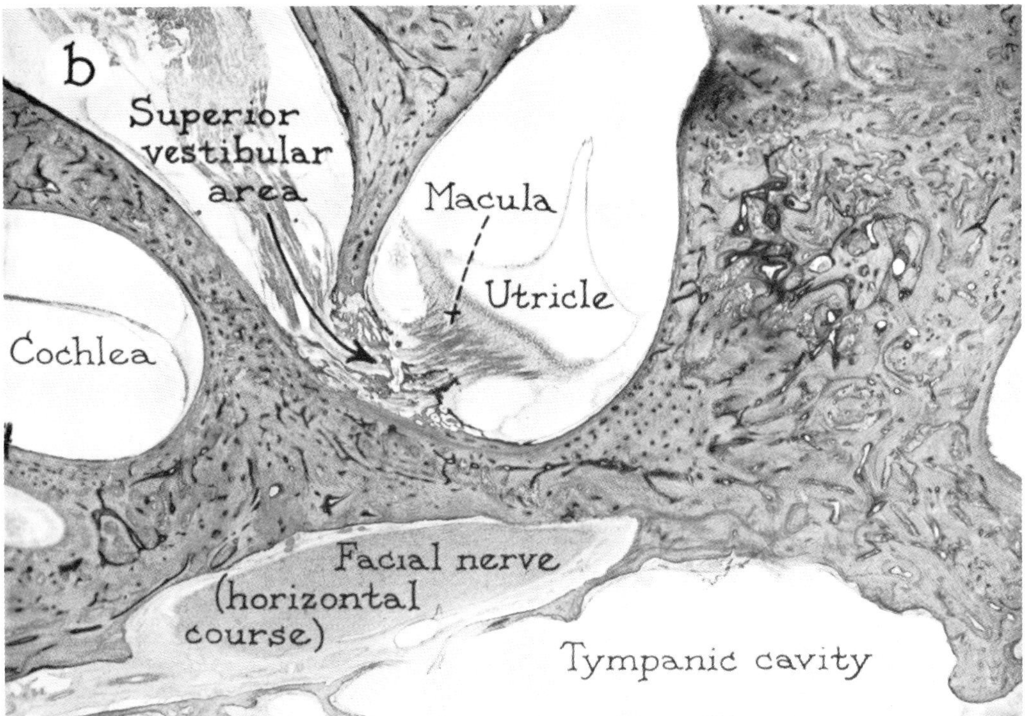

Figure III–53. See legend on the opposite page.

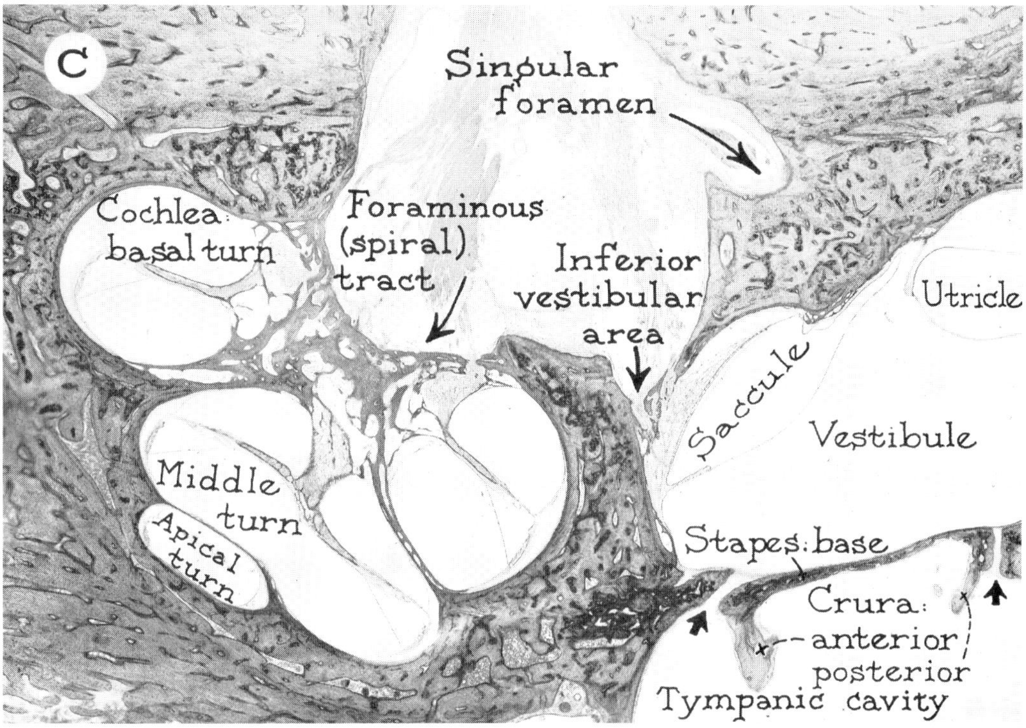

Figure III–53. FACIAL NERVE AND COCHLEAR AND VESTIBULAR DIVISIONS OF THE VESTIBULOCOCHLEAR NERVE IN RELATION TO THEIR CHANNELS AND FORAMINA IN THE PETROUS PART OF THE TEMPORAL BONE. *a* AND *b*. FEMALE, 38 YEARS OF AGE. *c*. INFANT, 10 WEEKS OLD.

a. The facial nerve is sectioned in its course from the internal acoustic meatus to the *geniculum* of the facial canal. The passageway for the lateral ampullary branch of the vestibular nerve is shown from the superior vestibular area of the fundus of the meatus to the superior cribrose macula of the vestibule, and thence to the crista of the semicircular duct.

b. The facial nerve is shown just distal to the knee, where it extends backward and lateralward in the horizontal part of its course. The utricular nerve, derived from the upper terminal branch of the vestibular nerve, passes with the lateral ampullary nerve from the fundus to the vestibule; it terminates in the acoustic macula of the utricle, where the latter occupies the elliptical recess.

c. The cochlear division of the vestibulocochlear nerve is sectioned as its fibers pass from the fundus of the internal acoustic meatus through the spiral foraminous tract into the modiolus. The saccular nerve, from the lower terminal branch of the vestibular, passes out from the inferior vestibular area of the fundus through the middle cribrose macula of the vestibule; it ends in the acoustic macula of the saccule, as the latter is lodged in the spherical recess (see also Figure III–57*c*). The posterior ampullary nerve here begins its course through a relatively long canaliculus on the way to the inferior cribrose macula on the anterior wall of the posterior osseous ampulla. The margins of the vestibular fenestra (oval window) are indicated by the unlabeled arrows.

Transverse sections, Wisconsin Collection, series as follows: *a* and *b*, 24; *c*, 83. *a*, *b*, and *c*, ×12.

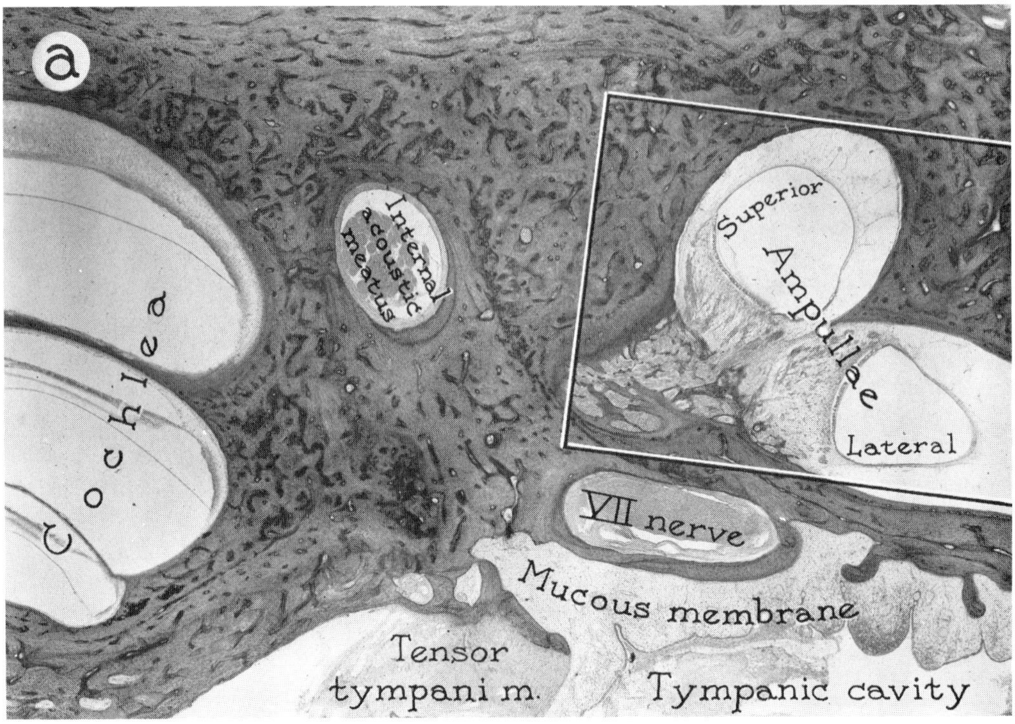

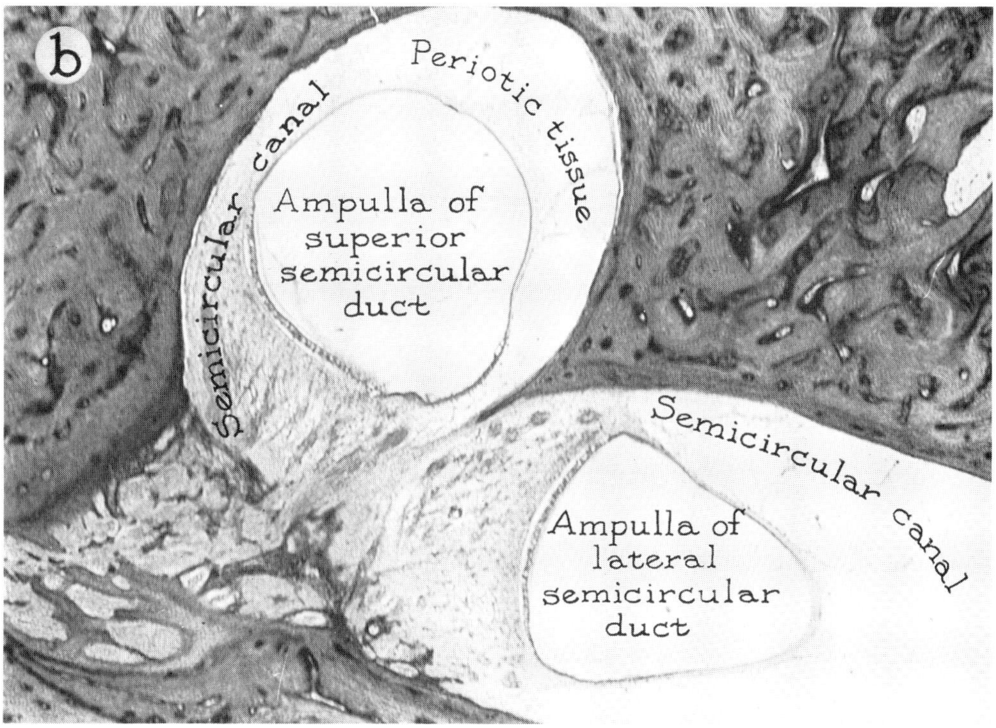

Figure III–54. See legend on the opposite page.

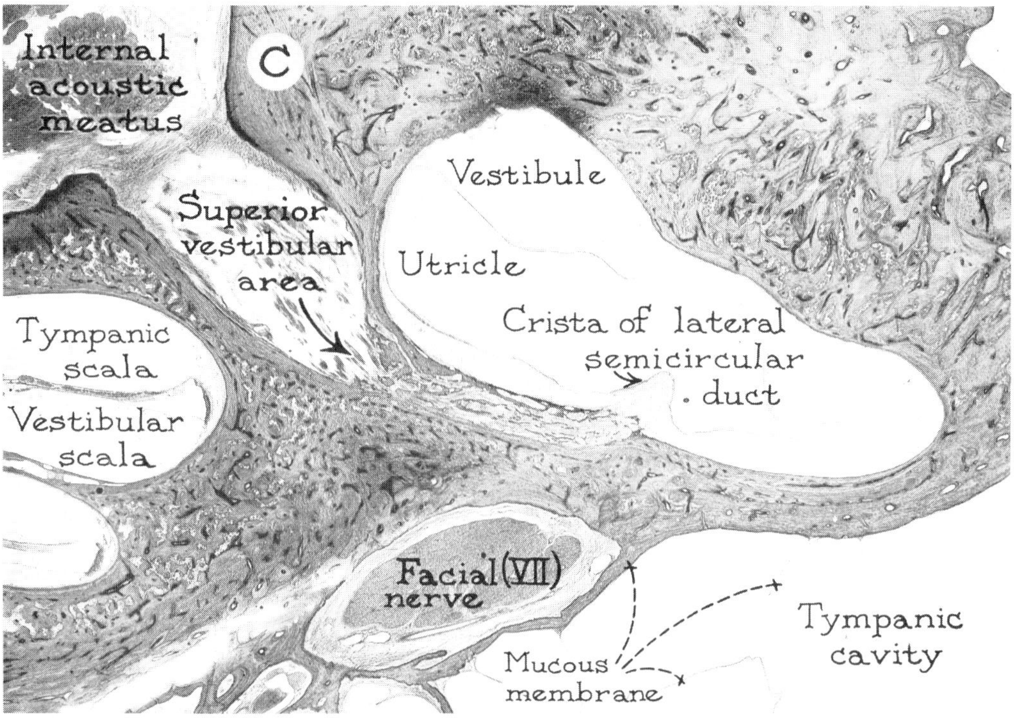

Figure III–54. The membranous ampullae, corresponding osseous dilatations, ampullary cristae, and nerves of supply; the utricle, acoustic macula, and vestibular nerve. *a* and *b*. Infant, 6 months old. *c* to *f*. Male, 19 years of age.

a. Ampullae of the superior and lateral semicircular ducts, at the level of innervation by branches of the vestibular nerve. Section at the level of the facial canal, internal acoustic meatus, and cochlea.

b. Ampullae of the superior and lateral semicircular ducts, the analogous enlargements of the osseous labyrinth, and the nerves of sensory supply. The area is that which is blocked in the preceding figure. The upper of the two terminal branches of the vestibular nerve passes from the inferior vestibular area of the internal acoustic meatus, supplies the cristae of these ampullae and the macula of the utricle (shown in Figure III–50).

c. Crista of the lateral semicircular duct and acoustic macula of the utricle. The vestibular nerve, leaving the ganglion in the internal acoustic meatus, passes from the superior vestibular area to the superior cribrose macula on the wall of the elliptical recess. Emerging from the foramina, the nerve bundles supply the acoustic macula. Other fibers pass to the crista of the duct. Shown also are the cochlea, the facial canal in its horizontal course, and the tympanic cavity.

Figure III–54 continues on the following page.

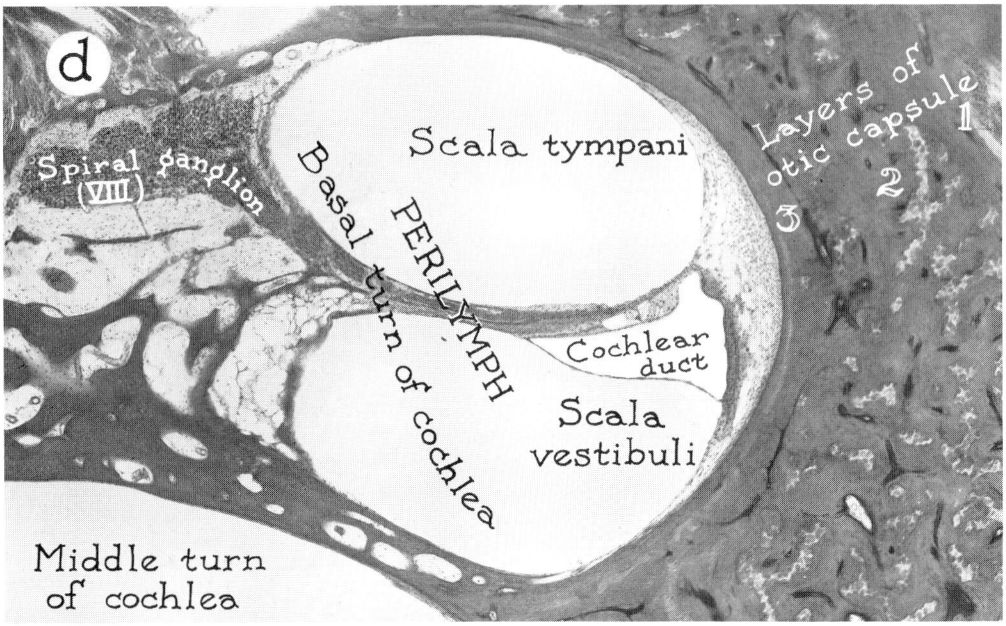

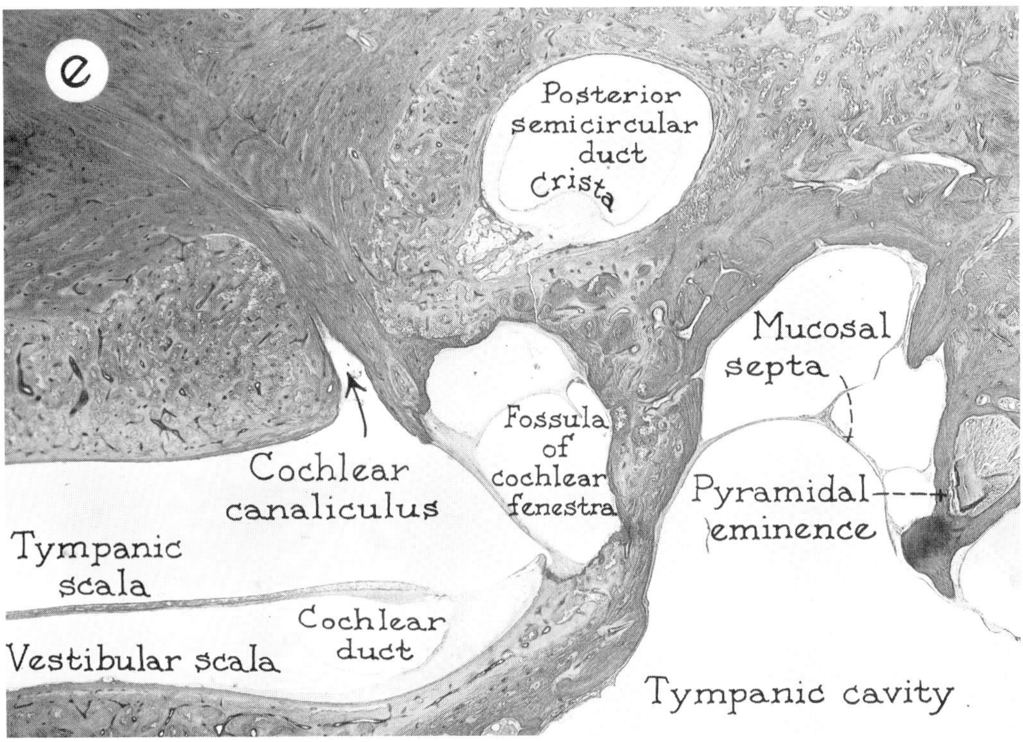

Figure III–54, Continued. See legend on the opposite page.

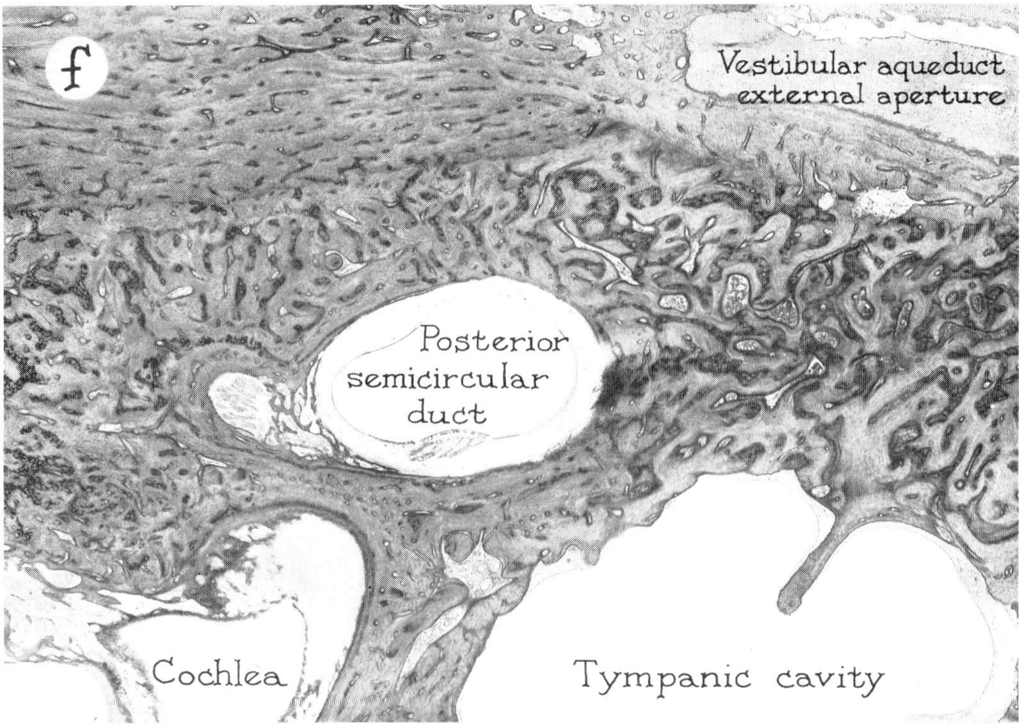

Figure III–54, Continued. COCHLEAR AND VESTIBULAR DIVISIONS OF THE VESTIBULOCOCHLEAR NERVE.

d. The cochlear nerve, after entering the foraminous spiral tract, is continued in the spiral canal of the modiolus as the spiral ganglion. Its peripheral fibers pass from the modiolus through the osseous spiral lamina to reach the hair cells in the spiral organ of Corti, about which the fibers arborize.

e and *f.* The lower terminal branch of the vestibular nerve divides into the saccular nerve and the posterior ampullary nerve. The latter nerve leaves the internal acoustic meatus through a relatively large opening, the singular foramen, situated below the transverse crest. It traverses a greater distance than do the nerves to the other ampullae. The ampulla of the posterior semicircular canal is placed inferiorly, and opens into the lower part of the vestibule, where six or eight small apertures, making up the inferior cribrose macula, transmit the nerve fibers to the sensory endings in the *crista* of the membranous ampulla.

Transverse sections, Wisconsin Collection, series as follows: *a* and *b*, 121; *c* to *f*, 29. *a*, ×17; *b*, ×34; *c*, ×12; *d*, ×35; *e*, ×15; *f*, ×18.

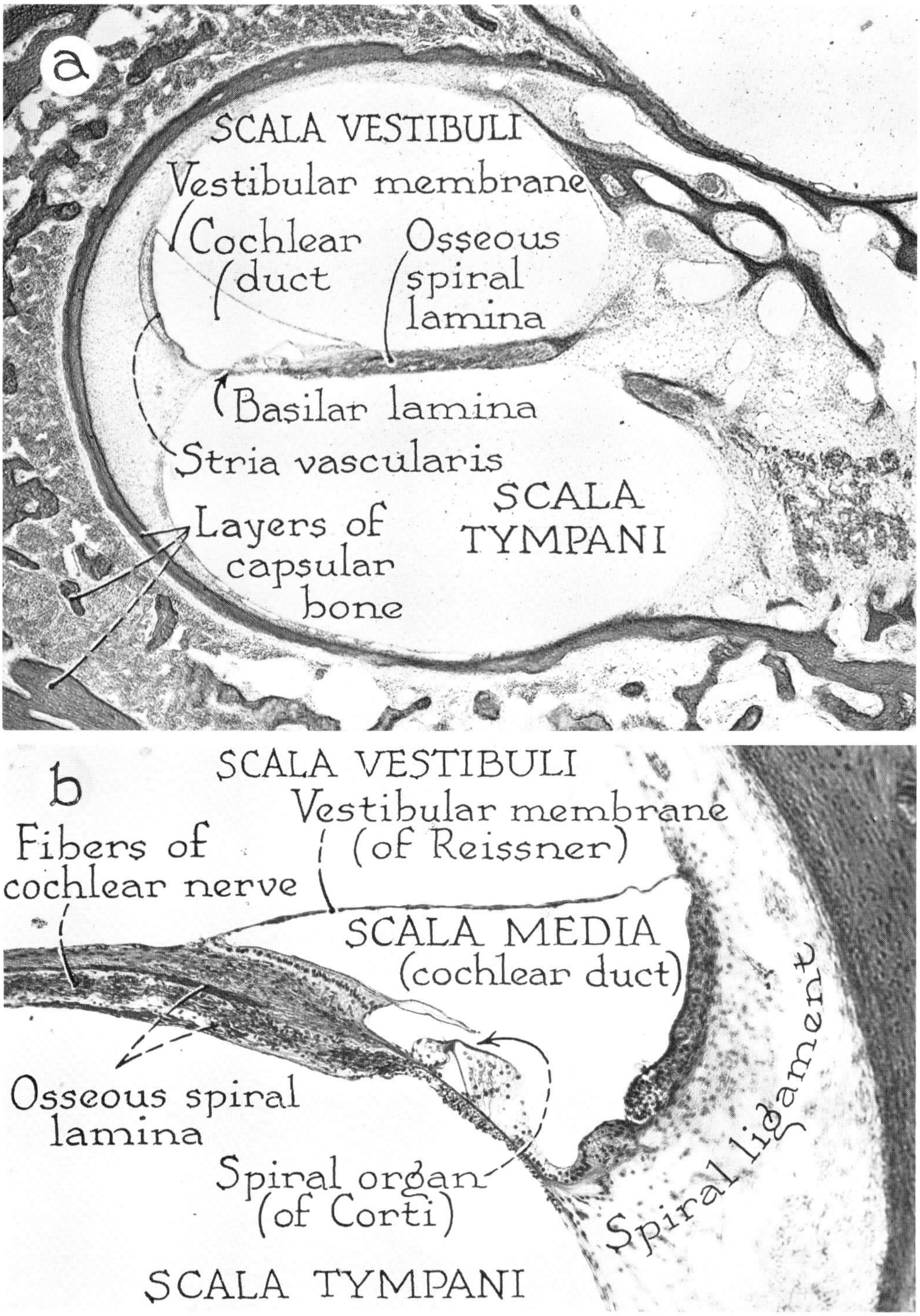

Figure III–55. Cochlea: section through one coil and detail of the cochlear duct. *a.* Fetus of 23 weeks (202 mm.). *b.* Male, 19 years of age.

a. Cochlear duct, perilymphatic scalae, and surrounding osseous capsule. The labyrinthine systems for the endolymph and perilymph in the cochlear division of the ear, like those in the canalicular part, have already attained adult dimensions (see Figure II–32*c*). In contrast, however, the surrounding capsule has not kept pace in progress toward histological adulthood; the middle layer consists of scattered islands of intrachondral bone and primitive marrow.

b. Showing the cochlear duct, the membranes and ligament that form its boundaries and the histology of its specialized floor, the elements constituting the spiral organ (*Cortii*). The capsule has attained petrous character.

Transverse sections, Wisconsin Collection, series 70 and 29, respectively. *a*, ×47; *b*, ×113.

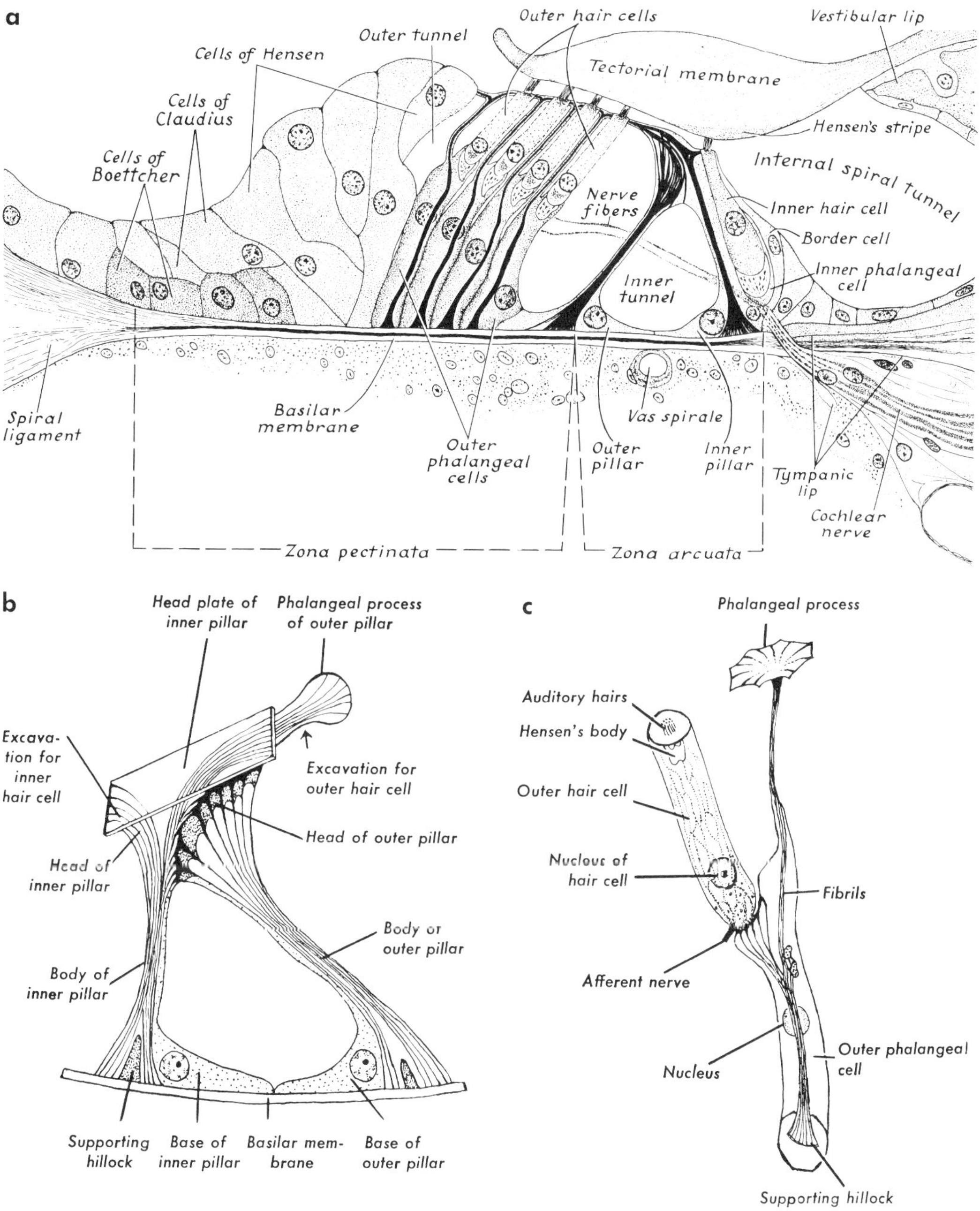

Figure III–56. SPIRAL ORGAN (*Cortii*): HISTOLOGICAL STRUCTURE.

a. Radial transection of the organ of Corti, taken from the first turn of the human cochlea. *b.* The inner and outer pillar cells shown diagrammatically. *c.* The supporting cells of Deiters and the associated outer hair cells in diagram.

The spiral organ is a specialized arrangement of epithelial cells which extends throughout the length of the cochlea. It is composed of hair cells, which are receptors for sound, and cells of other various forms which serve to support these sensory elements. The supportive cells are the following: inner and outer pillars, inner and outer phalangeal cells, and cells of Hensen.

(From Bloom and Fawcett: A Textbook of Histology, 9th ed. Philadelphia, W. B. Saunders Co., 1968.)

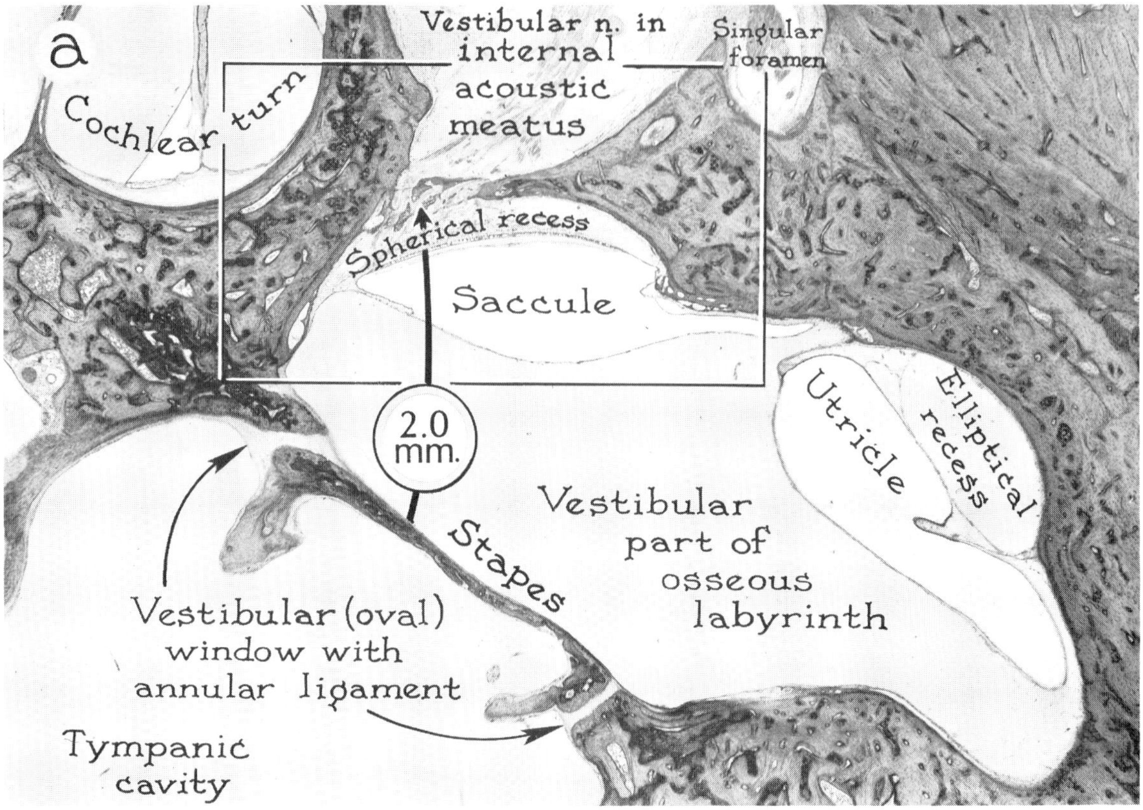

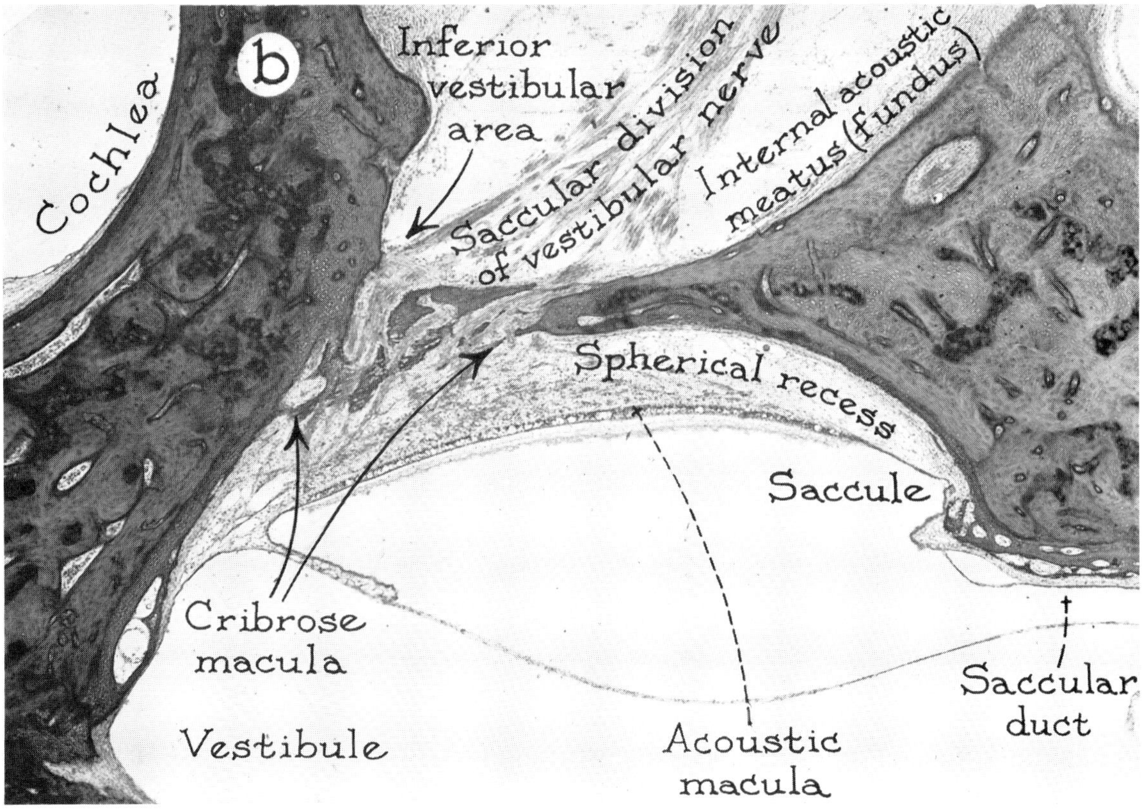

Figure III–57. See legend on the opposite page.

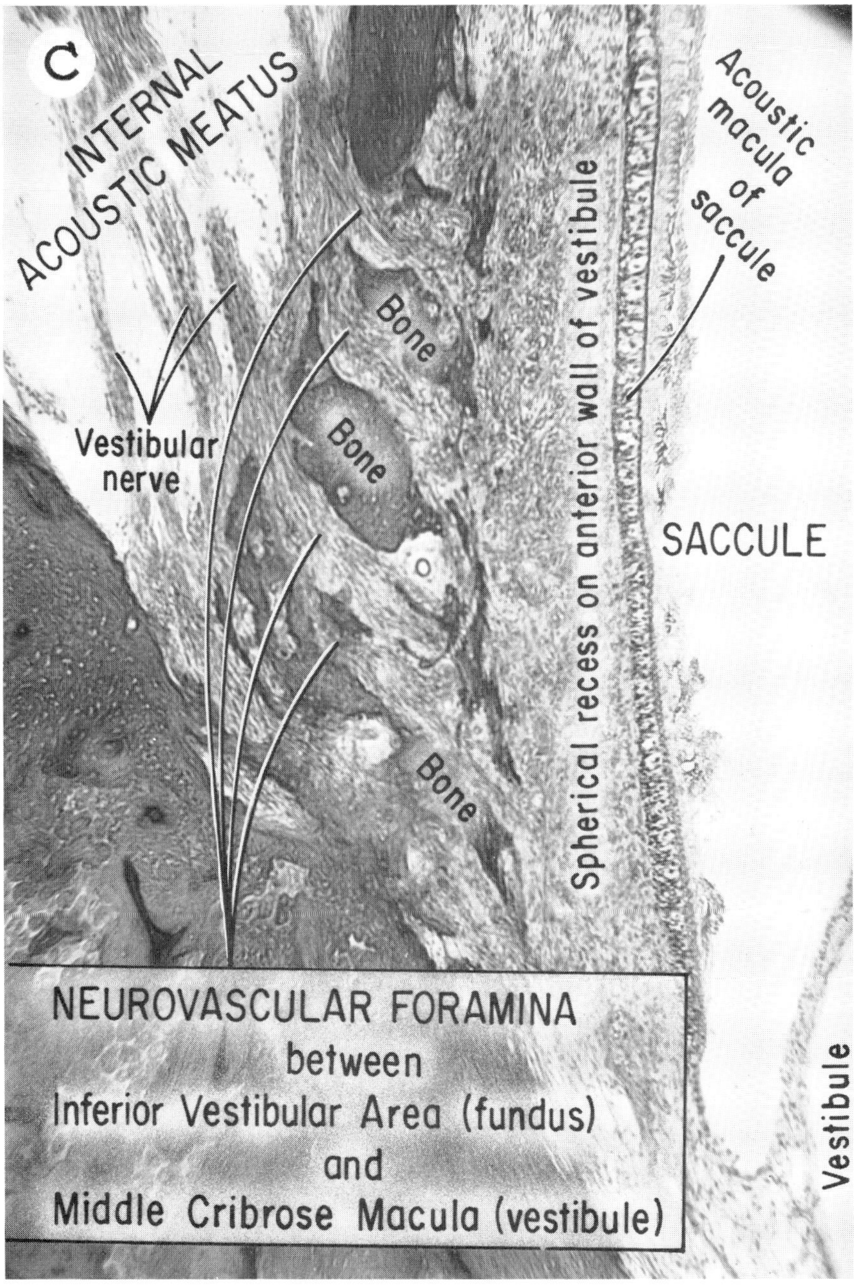

Figure III–57. SENSORY ELEMENTS OF THE MEMBRANOUS LABYRINTH: POSITION, INNERVATION AND BLOOD SUPPLY OF THE SACCULE. *a* and *b*. INFANT, 10 WEEKS OLD. *c*. INFANT, 6 MONTHS OLD.

a and *b*. The saccule, lodged in the spherical recess of the vestibule, receives fibers of the vestibular nerve and branches of the internal auditory blood vessels through foramina that pass from the inferior vestibular area of the fundus of the internal acoustic meatus and the cribrose macula of the vestibule. The distance between the anterior part of the stapedial footplate and the cribrose macula is recorded in the photomicrograph. The rectangular area outlined in *a* is shown at higher magnification in *b*.

c. Showing the neurovascular foramina in the wall between the meatus and the vestibule.

Transverse sections, Wisconsin Collection, series 83 and 121, respectively. *a*, ×18; *b*, ×44; *c*, ×34.

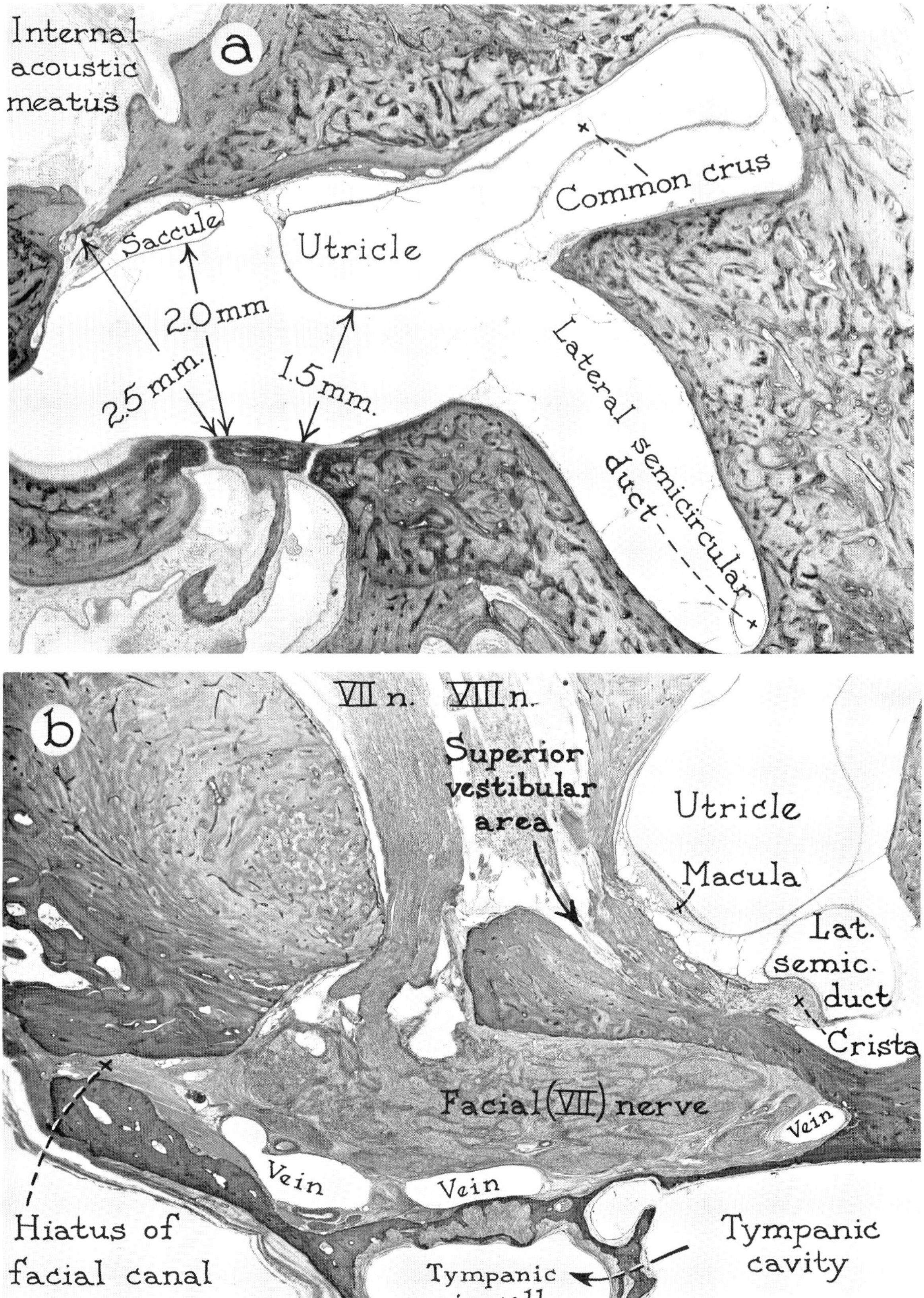

Figure III–58. See legend on the opposite page.

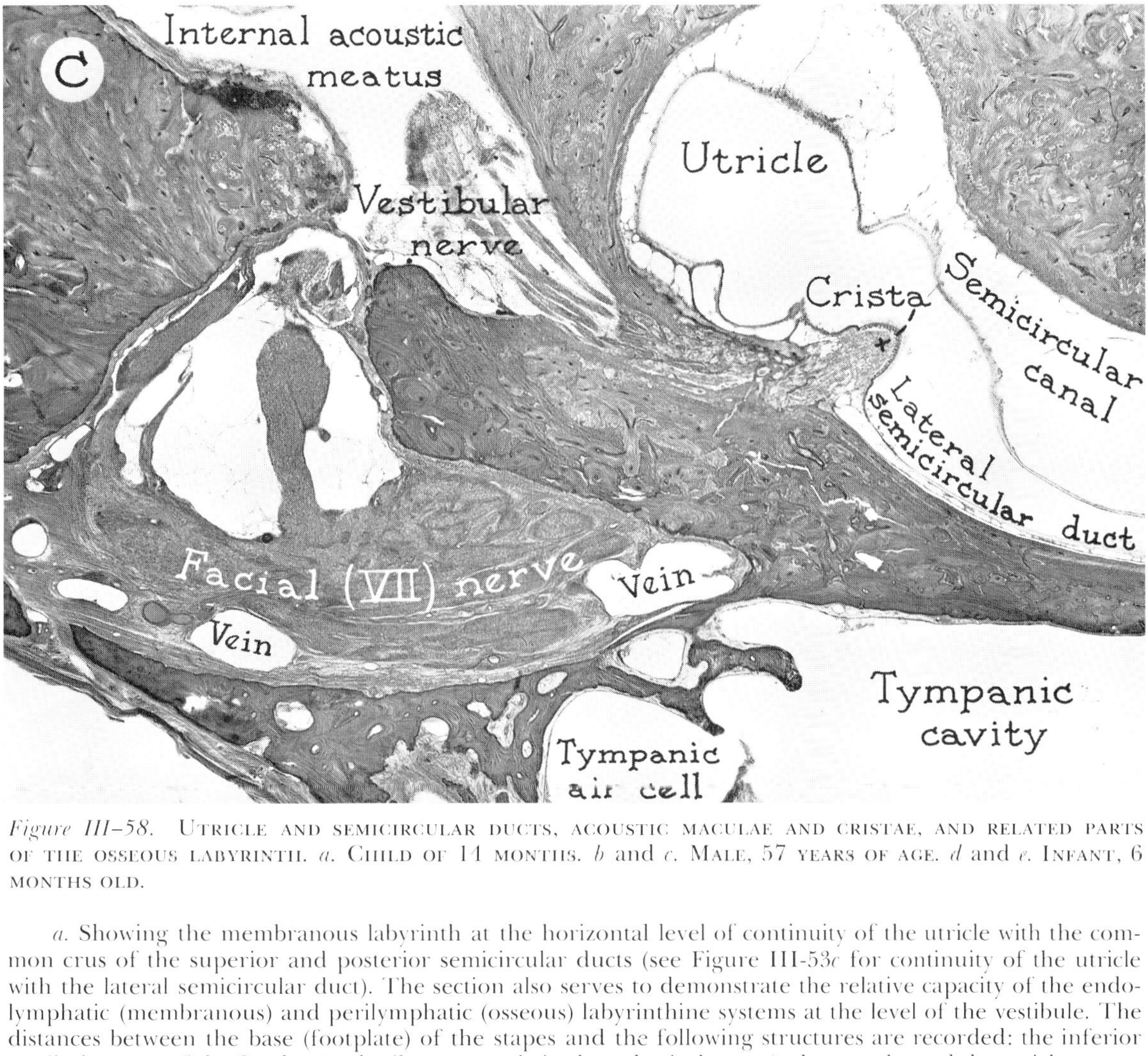

Figure III–58. UTRICLE AND SEMICIRCULAR DUCTS, ACOUSTIC MACULAE AND CRISTAE, AND RELATED PARTS OF THE OSSEOUS LABYRINTH. *a.* CHILD OF 14 MONTHS. *b* and *c.* MALE, 57 YEARS OF AGE. *d* and *e.* INFANT, 6 MONTHS OLD.

a. Showing the membranous labyrinth at the horizontal level of continuity of the utricle with the common crus of the superior and posterior semicircular ducts (see Figure III-53*c* for continuity of the utricle with the lateral semicircular duct). The section also serves to demonstrate the relative capacity of the endolymphatic (membranous) and perilymphatic (osseous) labyrinthine systems at the level of the vestibule. The distances between the base (footplate) of the stapes and the following structures are recorded: the inferior vestibular area of the fundus (and cribrose macula in the spherical recess), the saccule, and the utricle.

b. The utricle is shown at the level of the acoustic macula; the lateral semicircular duct is sectioned through the ampulla. The fibers of the vestibular division of the eighth (acoustic or vestibulocochlear) nerve are sectioned where they pass through the foraminous wall between the superior vestibular area of the fundus and the cribrose maculae of the vestibule. The photomicrograph also demonstrates the relation between the eighth and seventh cranial nerves at the fundus of the internal acoustic meatus, as well as the latter nerve in the geniculum of the facial canal where it is closely related to the labyrinth medially and the tympanic cavity (and air cells) laterally.

c. At this level in the same series, the utricle is broadly continuous with the lateral semicircular duct through the intermediation of the latter's ampulla.

Figure III–58 continues on the following page.

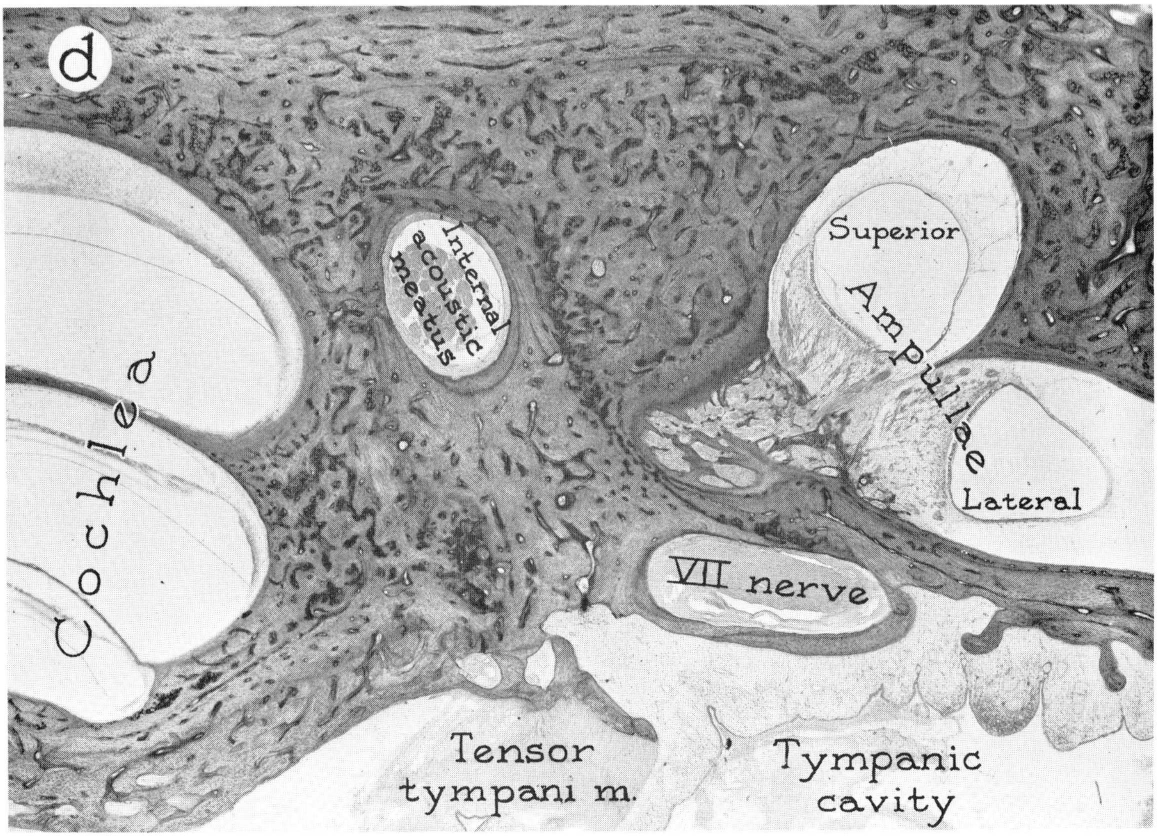

Figure III–58, Continued. SEMICIRCULAR DUCTS AND RELATED STRUCTURES.

d. The ampullary parts of the superior and lateral semicircular ducts are shown at the level at which their cristae receive fibers of the vestibular nerve through the cribrose macula. The section passes through the superior part of the internal acoustic meatus and the facial canal in its horizontal segment.

Figure III–58 continues on the opposite page.

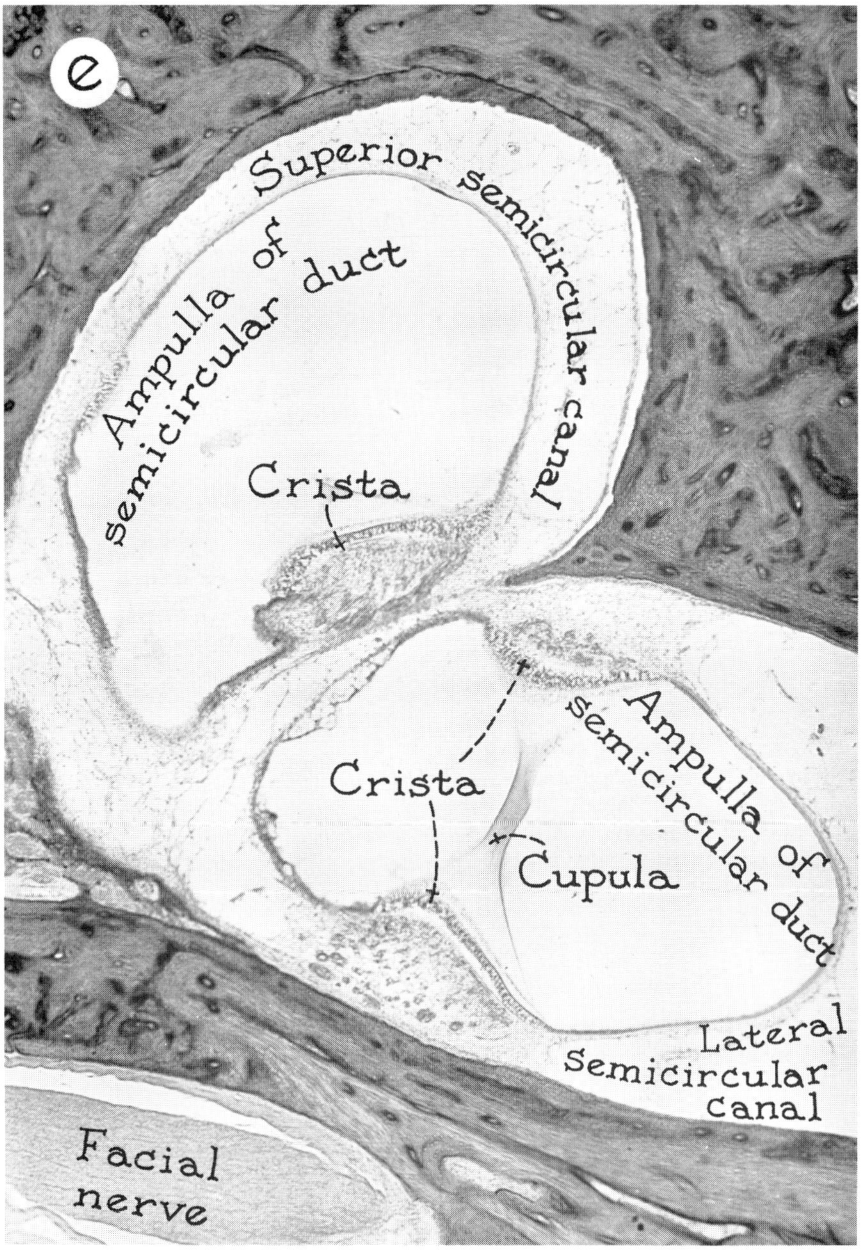

Figure III–58, Concluded.

e. Showing the cristae of the two ampullae. The crista of the lateral ampulla is sectioned through the cupula.

Transverse sections, Wisconsin Collection, series 93, 32, and 121, respectively. *a*, ×16; *b*, ×13; *c*, ×16; *d*, ×18; *e*, ×44.

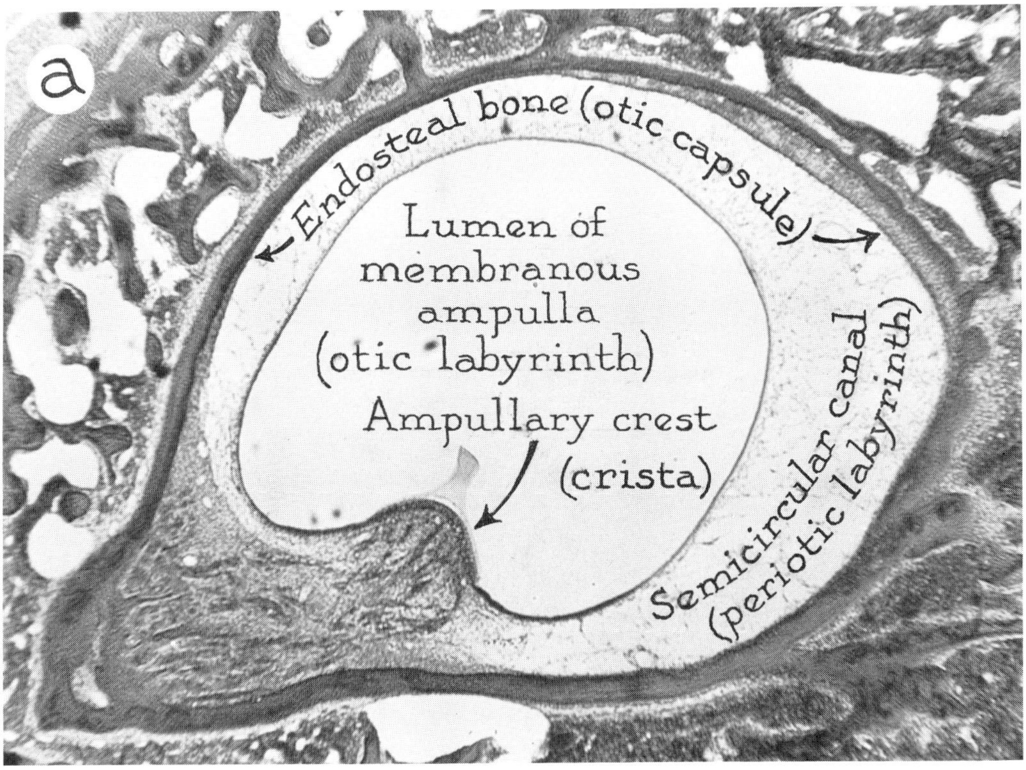

Figure III–59. SEMICIRCULAR DUCT AND CANAL: GENERAL STRUCTURE AND HISTOLOGICAL DETAIL. FETUS OF 23 WEEKS (202 MM.).

a. Semicircular duct, surrounding canal of the perilymphatic labyrinth and encompassing wall of capsular bone. Some periotic connective tissue occupies the perilymphatic space, as a remnant of the embryonic reticulum. The membranous labyrinth has attained maximum size. The surrounding perilymphatic space is bounded by a layer of endosteal (inner periosteal) bone which determines the adult dimensions of the osseous labyrinthine system. The middle layer, however, is still fetal in respect to histological structure (see Figure III–55*a* on the cochlea).

Figure III–59 continues on the opposite page.

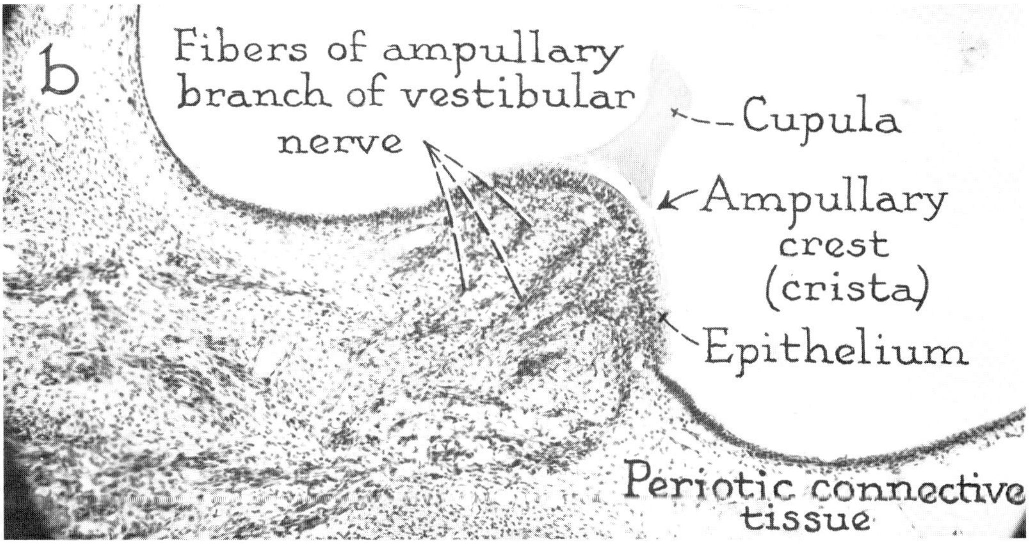

Figure III–59, Continued.

b. Histological structure of the crest in the ampullary enlargement of the duct. Here the epithelium is thickened to produce the characteristic elevation of the duct, the *crista*. The lining epithelium elongates to columnar type, in which flask-shaped sensory hair cells are distributed among supporting cells. The hair cells, enmeshed in a material of gelatinous consistency, form the cupula (here shrunken, owing to the use of reagents).

Transverse sections, Wisconsin Collection, series 70. *a*, ×40; *b*, ×93.

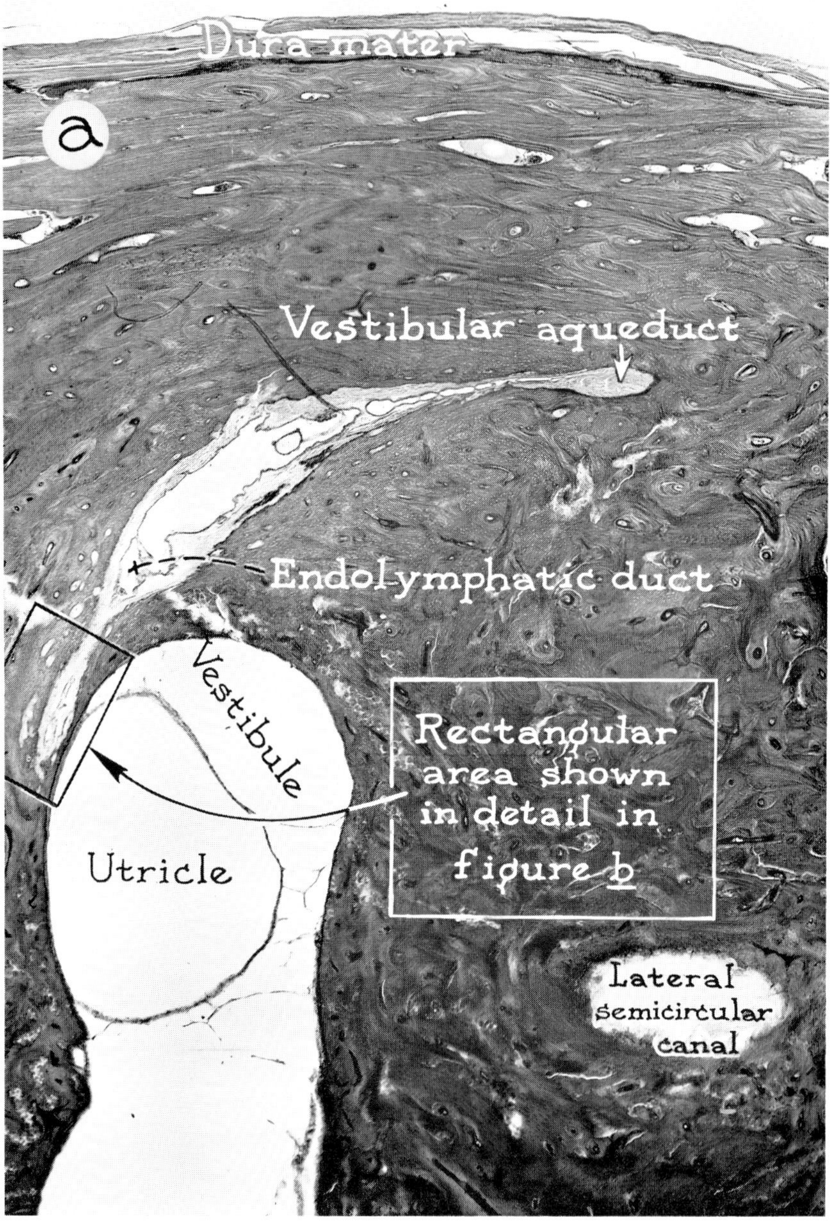

Figure III–60. ENDOLYMPHATIC DUCT, SAC, AND RELATED ANATOMY: TOPOGRAPHY AND DETAIL. MALE, 62 YEARS OF AGE.

a. Showing the curving course of the vestibular aqueduct, from a point near the internal aperture to a level approximately midway between the two apertures, together with the contained duct and sac.

Figure III–60 continues on the opposite page.

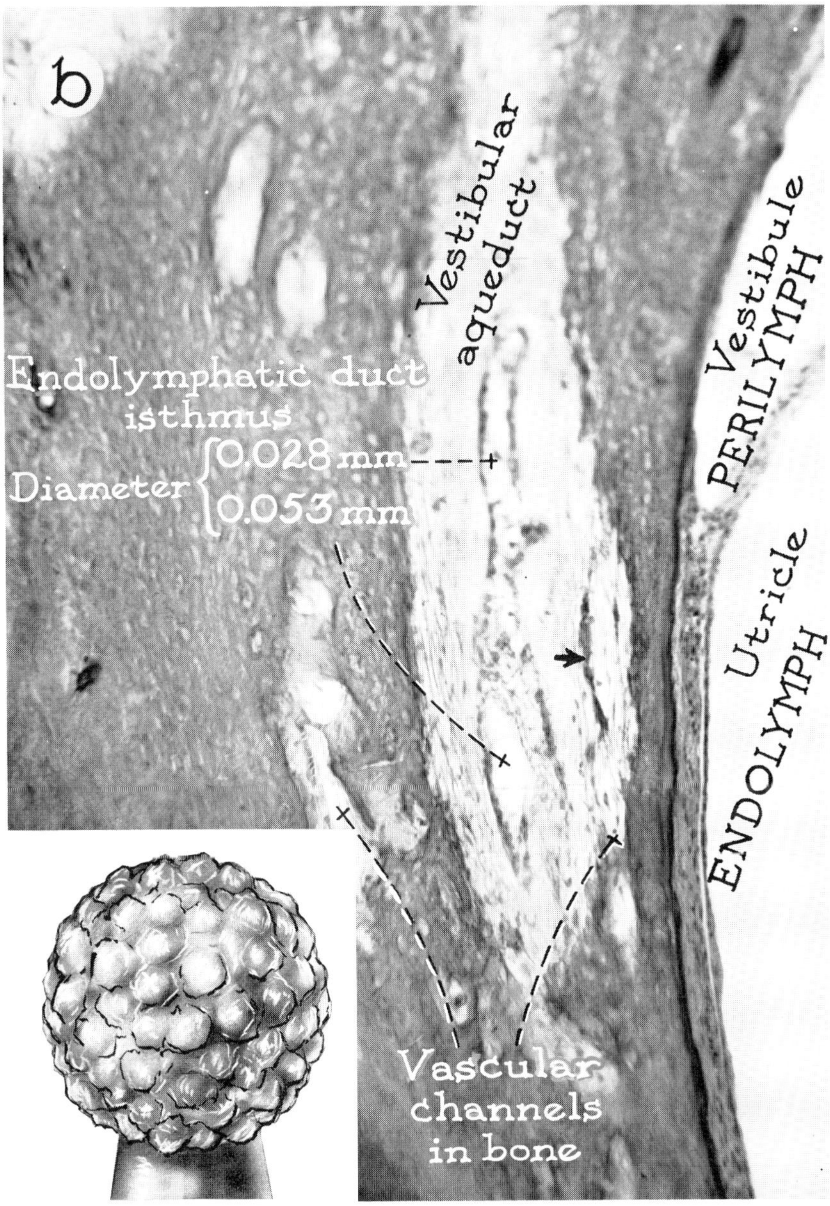

Figure III–60, Continued.

b. Histological detail of the segment outlined as a rectangular area in *a*. Measurements are given. *Inset:* Diamond burr, 1.3 mm., demonstrating the size of this instrument in relation to the diameter of the duct. Unlabeled arrow indicates blood vessel.

Transverse section, Wisconsin Collection, series 13. *a*, ×22; *b*, ×177.

(From Anson, Warpeha, and Rensink: Ann. Otol., 77:538–607, 1968.)

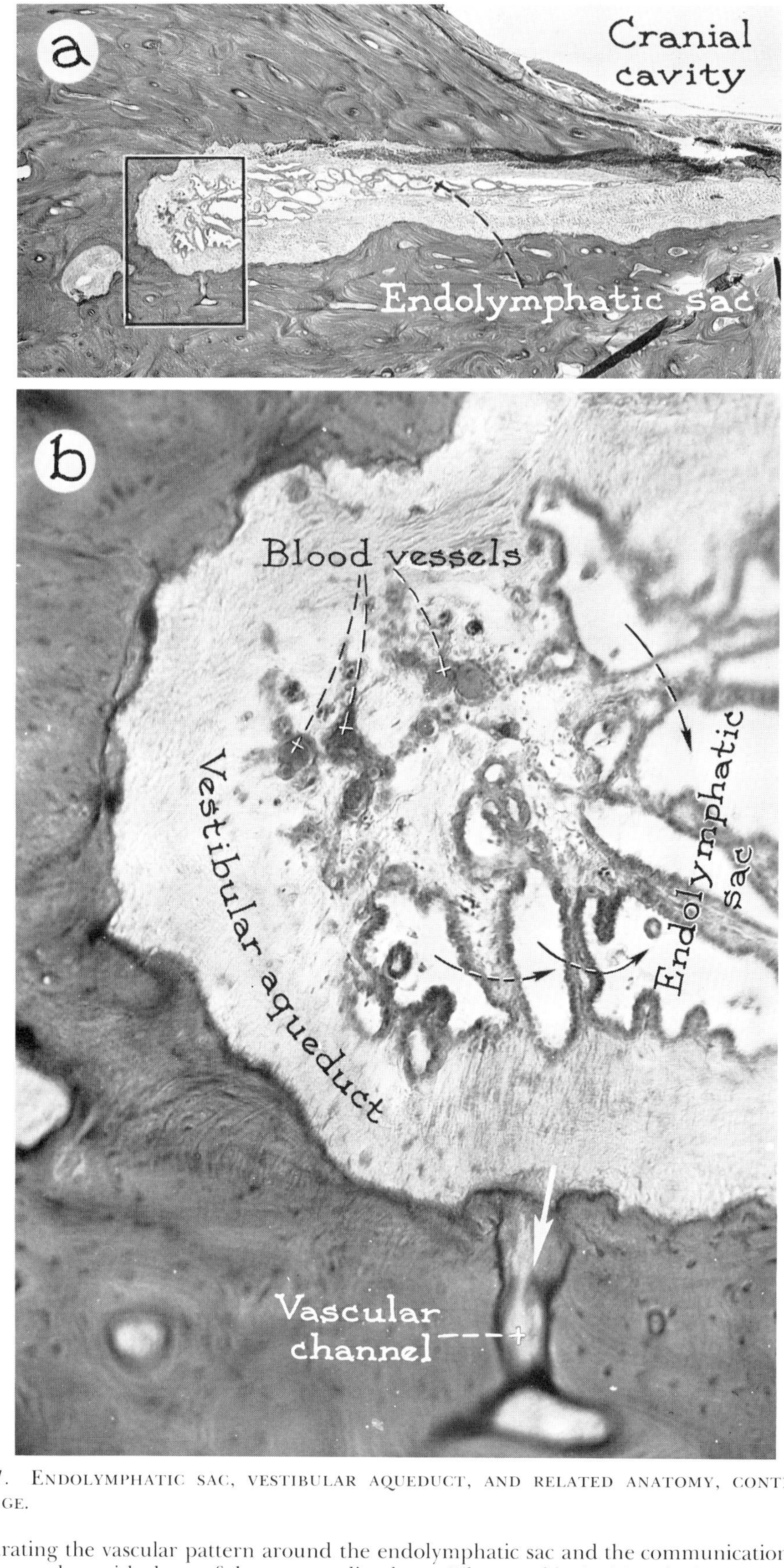

Figure III–61. ENDOLYMPHATIC SAC, VESTIBULAR AQUEDUCT, AND RELATED ANATOMY, CONTINUED. MALE, 62 YEARS OF AGE.

Demonstrating the vascular pattern around the endolymphatic sac and the communication of the blood vessels in the aqueduct with those of the surrounding bone. The area blocked in *a* is shown at higher magnification in *b*.

Transverse section, Wisconsin Collection, series 13. *a*, ×18; *b*, ×154.

(From Anson, Warpeha, and Rensink : Ann. Otol., 77:538–607, 1968.)

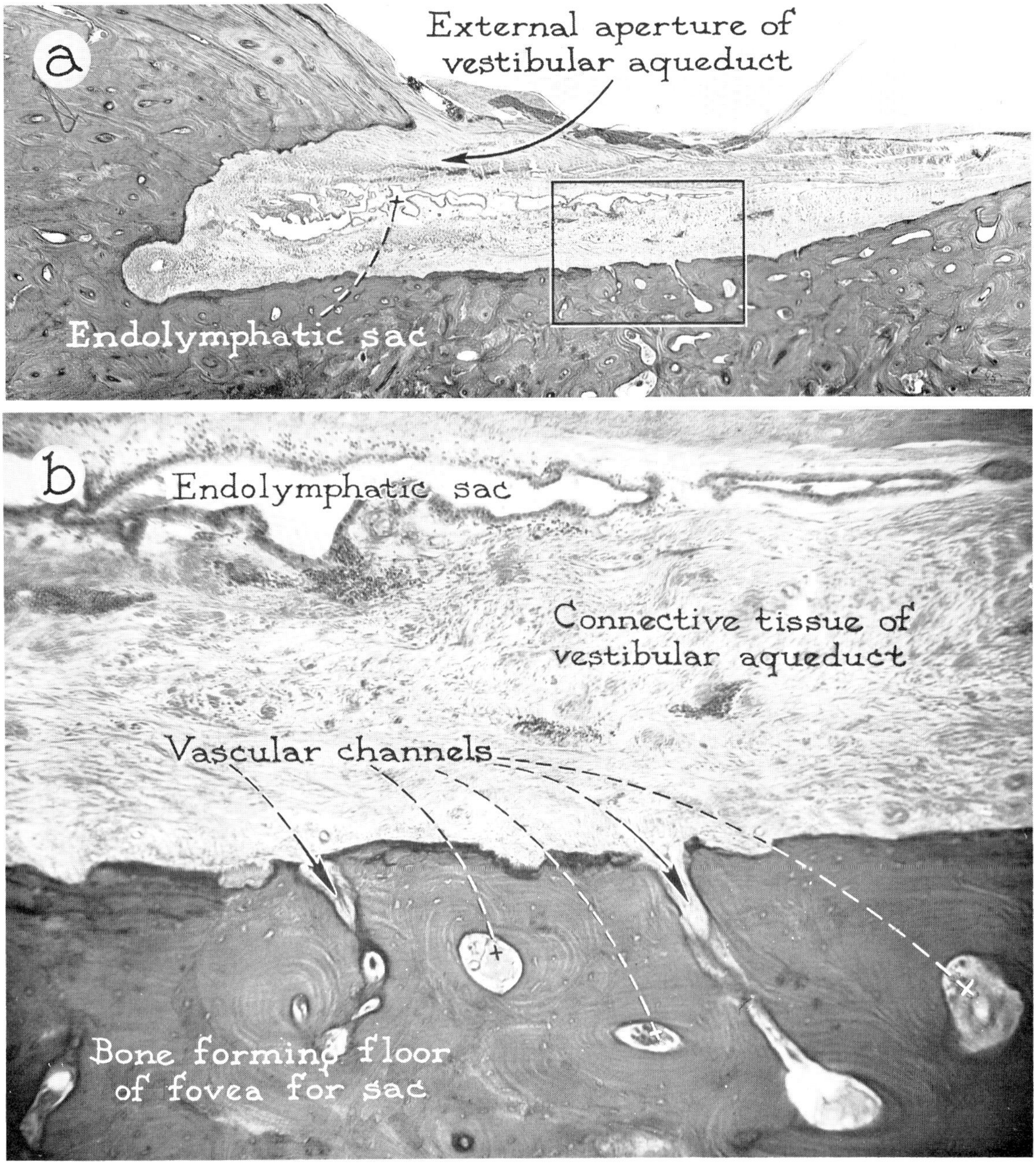

Figure III–62. ENDOLYMPHATIC SAC, VESTIBULAR AQUEDUCT, AND RELATED ANATOMY, CONCLUDED. MALE, 62 YEARS OF AGE.

The histology at the more distal level. The sac occupies the foveate impression on the posterior surface of the pyramid, just distal to the external aperture. The area blocked in figure *a* is shown at higher magnification in *b*.

Arteries and veins that supply the contents of the vestibular aqueduct come from vascular channels in the surrounding bone as well as directly from the cranial cavity through the external aperture of the aqueduct. Arteries of the latter group are derived from the internal auditory artery. The corresponding veins terminate in the transverse or the inferior petrosal sinus.

Transverse section, Wisconsin Collection, series 13. *a*, ×22; *b*, ×132.

(From Anson, Warpeha, and Rensink: Ann. Otol., 77:538–607, 1968.)

Figure III–63. TEMPORAL BONE, MEDIAL SURFACE: NEURAL AND VASCULAR STRUCTURES, EMPHASIZING THE ANATOMICAL RELATIONSHIPS AT AND NEAR THE APERTURES WHERE THE FACIAL (VII CRANIAL) NERVE BEGINS AND ENDS ITS COURSE THROUGH THE TEMPORAL BONE.

The pore of the internal acoustic meatus is situated approximately at the center of the posterior surface of the pyramid. It transmits the facial and acoustic (vestibulocochlear) nerves, the nervus intermedius, the internal auditory branch of the basilar artery, and the corresponding veins (which end in the superior petrosal sinus or the transverse sinsus). The stylomastoid foramen is situated between the styloid and mastoid processes. It transmits the stylomastoid vessels as well as the facial nerve.

The transverse sinus occupies a sulcus on the mastoid part of the temporal bone, this portion being termed sigmoid sinus. These veins receive blood from the superior and inferior petrosal sinuses of the *dura mater* and from the mastoid and other emissary veins. The transverse sinus continues into the internal jugular vein. At the origin, on the base of the skull the vein is dilated as the superior bulb. The bulb occupies a fossa of variable depth on the inferior surface of the pyramid (see Figure III–131).

The large circular aperture of the carotid canal, transmitting the internal carotid artery and carotid plexus of nerves, lies in front of the jugular fossa. The canal ascends at first vertically; then making a bend, it runs horizontally forward and medialward, to an internal aperture at the apex of the pyramid.

Two additional openings appear on the posterior surface, namely, the subarcuate fossa and the external aperture of the vestibular aqueduct, the former just below the superior petrosal sinus, the latter above and anterior to the sigmoid part of the transverse sinus. Both are important in otological surgery. The subarcuate fossa serves as a vascular route between meninges and bone, transmitting branches of the internal auditory artery which are sometimes large enough to be consequential in the extirpation of an acoustic nerve tumor. The aperture of the aqueduct is the site of emergence of the endolymphatic sac from an intraosseous to an intradural position. In the latter situation it may be approached through a mastoid dissection.

(From Anson, Donaldson, Warpeha, and Rensink: Ann. Otol., 79:710–727, 1970.)

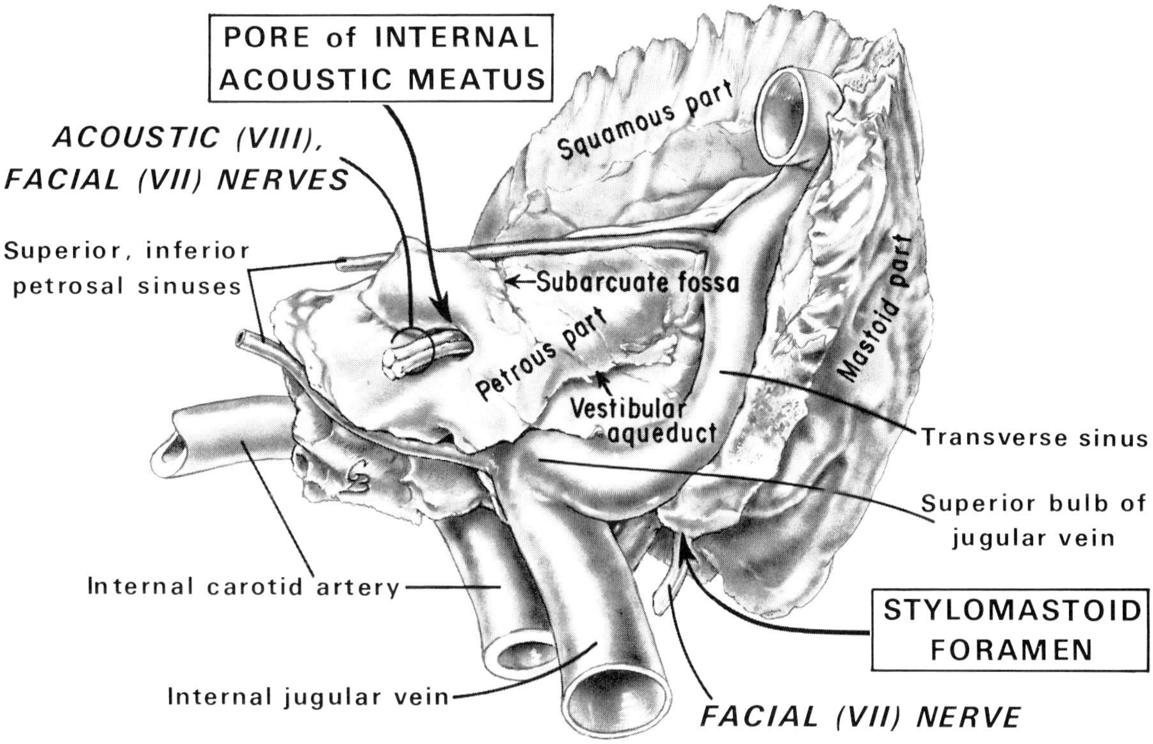

Figure III–63. See legend on the opposite page.

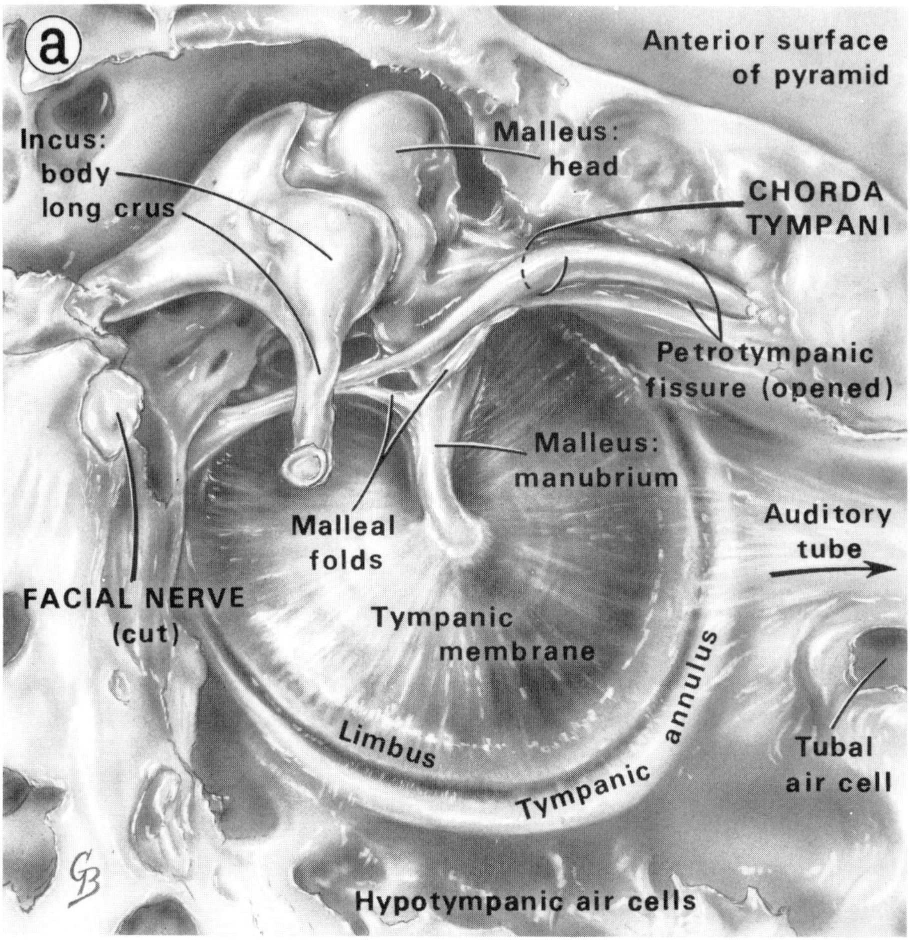

Figure III–64. CHORDA TYMPANI IN RELATION TO THE FACIAL NERVE, AUDITORY OSSICLES, OSSICULAR FOLDS, AND TYMPANIC MEMBRANE: LEFT TEMPORAL BONE, UNEMBALMED SPECIMEN. DISSECTIONS VIEWED FROM WITHIN.

a. The mucous membrane is intact; the stapes has been removed.

Figure III–64 continues on the opposite page.

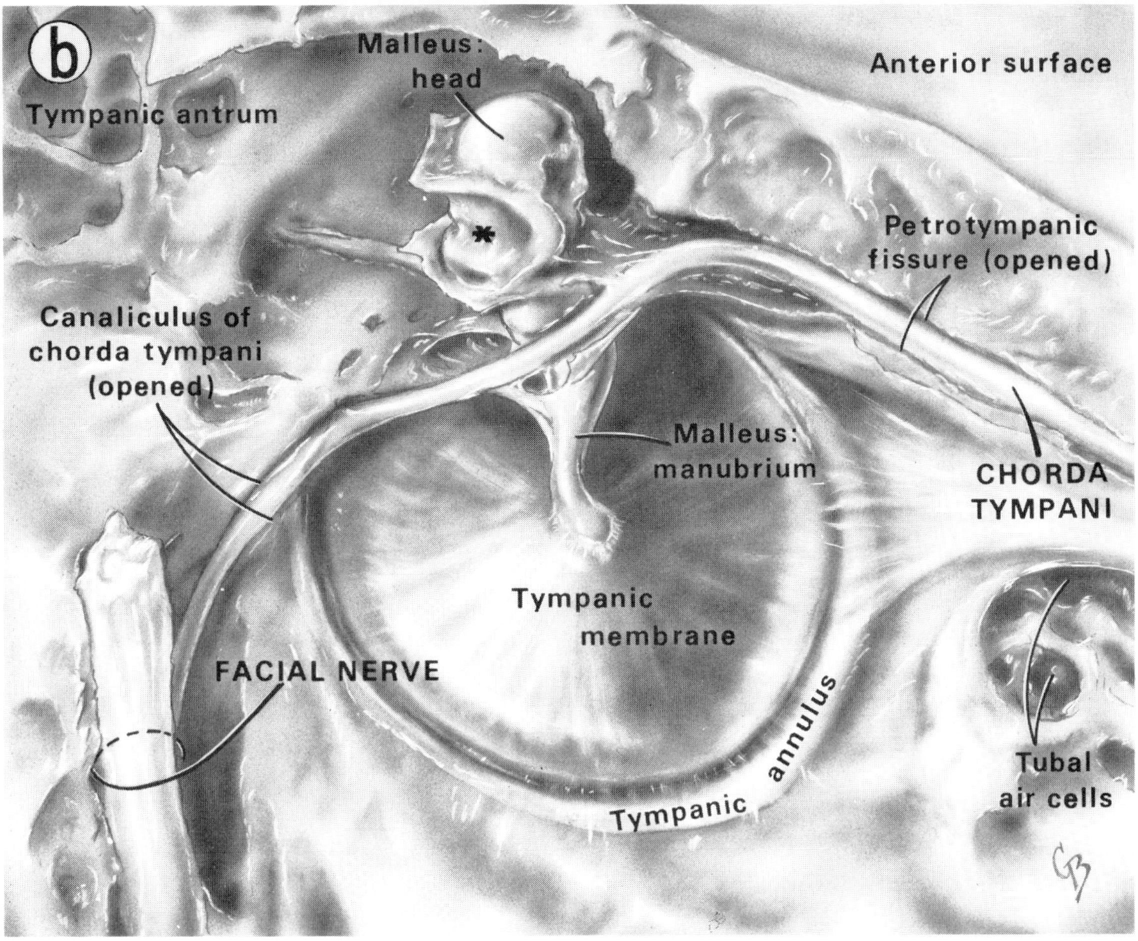

Figure III–64, Continued.

b. The incus has been excised and the mucosal lining of the middle ear dissected away. The relation of the chorda tympani to the facial nerve is demonstrated by opening the canal; the course of the chorda in the petrotympanic fissure is demonstrated in both stages of the dissection. Asterisk indicates the articular surface.

Chorda Tympani. The chorda arises from the facial (VII) nerve in the facial (Fallopian) canal. It then ascends at an acute angle through the tympanic canaliculus of the chorda to an aperture on the posterior wall of the tympanic cavity *(b)*. Invested by mucous membrane in the form of two *plicae*, the posterior and anterior malleal folds, it crosses the tympanic cavity. In this segment of its course, the chorda tympani passes between the long crus of the incus and the manubrium of the malleus *(a)*. Reaching the aperture of the petrotympanic fissure *(Glaseri)*, it descends in that osseous channel to the inferior surface of the tympanic part of the temporal bone.

Tympanic Cavity. The middle ear, consisting of tympanic cavity and auditory tube, is shown as viewed from within; that is, as the observer would face the lateral or membranous wall—the large part of which is occupied by the tympanic membrane (*a* and *b*). The space is continuous with the tympanic antrum and the epitympanic recess (*a*).

Auditory Ossicles, Ligaments, Folds. The malleus, largest of the three small ear bones, lies farthest lateralward and forward. The upper, club-shaped part, the head, is situated in the epitympanic recess, to whose roof it is attached by the superior malleal ligament. The neck of the ossicle is continued forward as the anterior process *(Folii)*. To this process is attached the anterior malleal ligament (covered by a correspondingly named fold of mucous membrane). It passes into the petrotympanic fissure with the chorda tympani. The manubrium of the malleus, directed downward in the form of a thin rod, is fastened to the tympanic membrane *(a* and *b)*. It is crossed by the chorda tympani near the area of junction of the manubrium with the neck of the ossicle near the site of attachment of the tendon of the tensor tympani muscle.

The body of the incus is attached to the roof of the epitympanic recess by the superior incudal ligament; the short crus, directed horizontally backward, is anchored to the wall of the incudal fossa. The ligament is invested by tympanic mucous membrane *(a)*. The long crus descends parallel to the manubrium of the malleus (but medially thereto); it ends in a foveate impression, the lenticular process, for articulation with the head of the stapes.

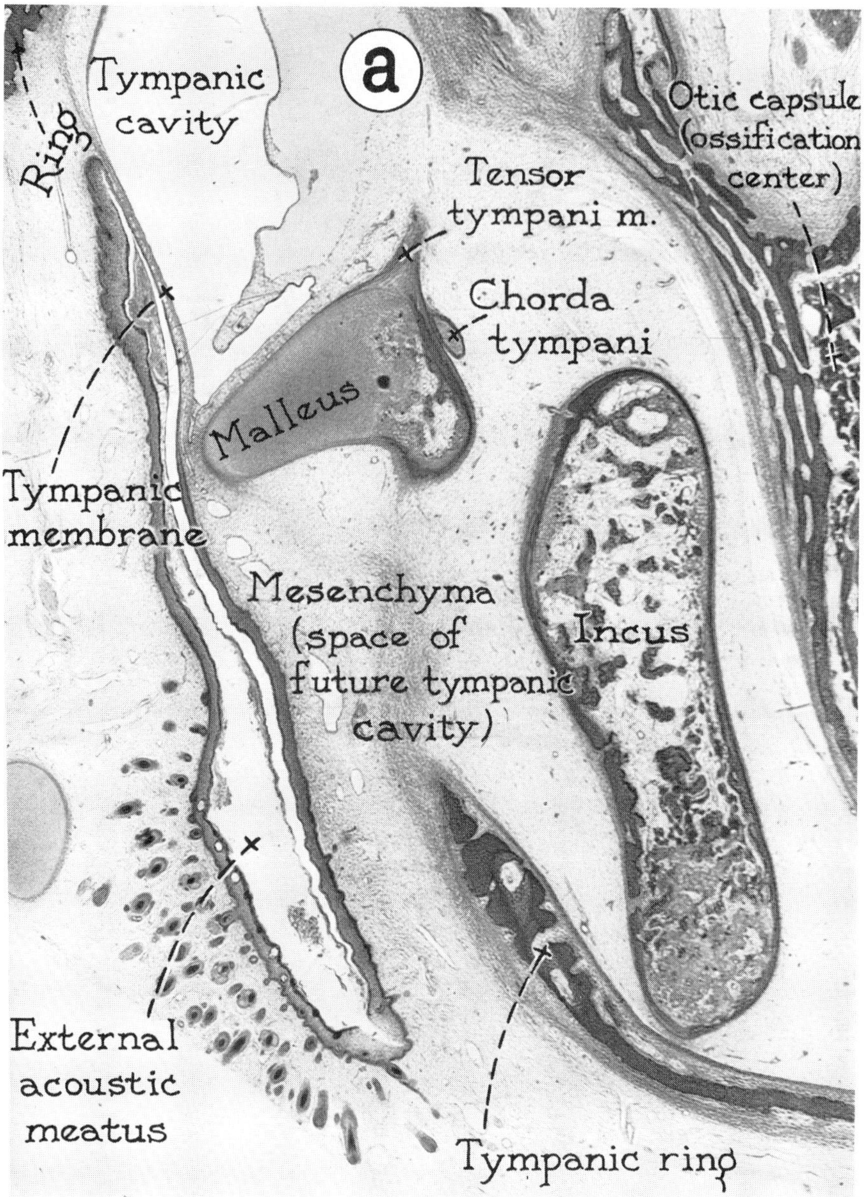

Figure III–65. CHORDA TYMPANI: FETAL AND ADULT ANATOMY. *a.* FETUS OF 21 WEEKS (183 MM.). *b* to *h.* MALE, 19 YEARS OF AGE.

a. In the fetal stage at which bone formation in the ossicles and the otic capsule is well under way, the relation of the chorda tympani to the auditory ossicles is established. The nerve lies in mesenchyma—here the primordial tissue of the submucosal lining of the tympanic cavity (compare *d* and *e*).

b. In the adult temporal bone, the chorda tympani arises in the facial canal. Ascending, it leaves the canal, traversing its own channel, the canaliculus of the chorda tympani. At the level illustrated, the nerve passes from the canaliculus at the *iter.*

c. The nerve is then lodged in the mucous membrane on the posterior (mastoid) wall of the tympanic cavity.

Figure III–65 continues on the opposite page.

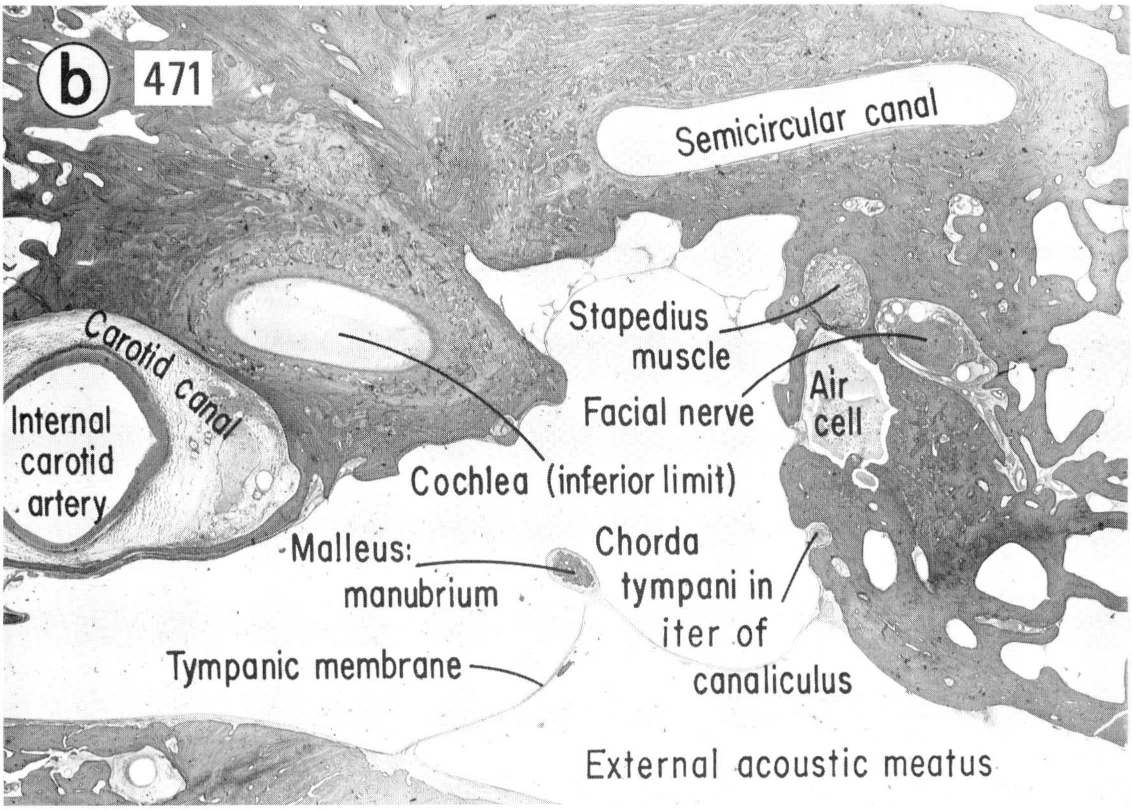

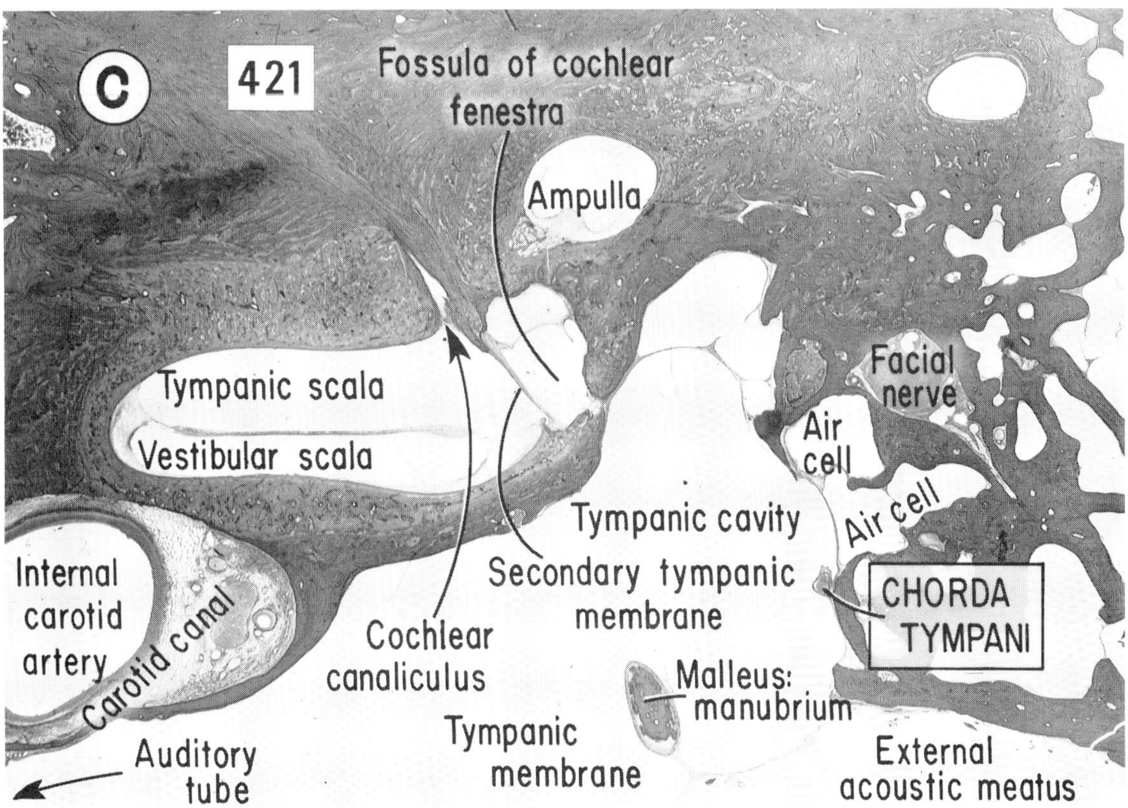

Figure III–65, Continued. *See legend on the opposite page.*

Figure III–65 continues on the following page.

Figure III–65, Continued. PROGRESSIVE STEPS IN THE COURSE OF THE CHORDA TYMPANI TOWARD THE PETROTYMPANIC FISSURE.

d and *e*. The nerve, invested by mucous membrane, advances in an anterior direction to the auditory ossicles, passing between the long process of the incus and manubrium of the malleus. The area blocked in *d* is shown at higher magnification in *e*. In *e* a vascular channel is indicated by an arrow.

Figure III–65 continues on the opposite page.

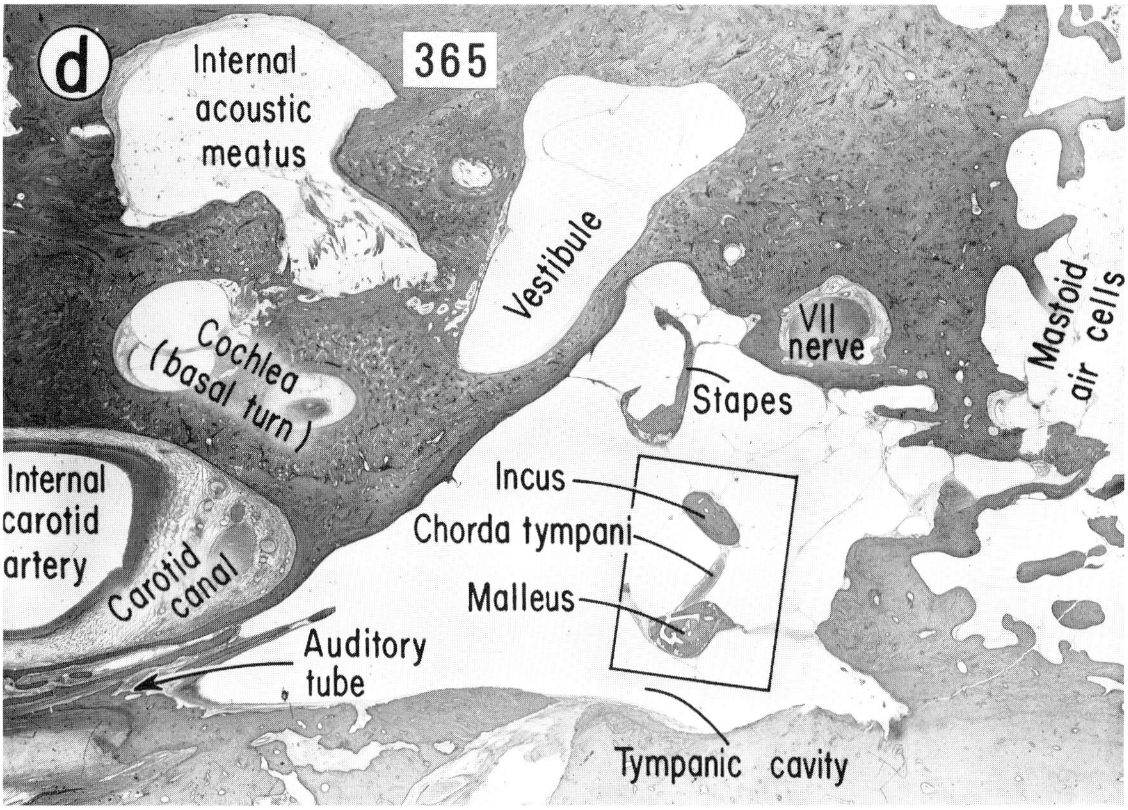

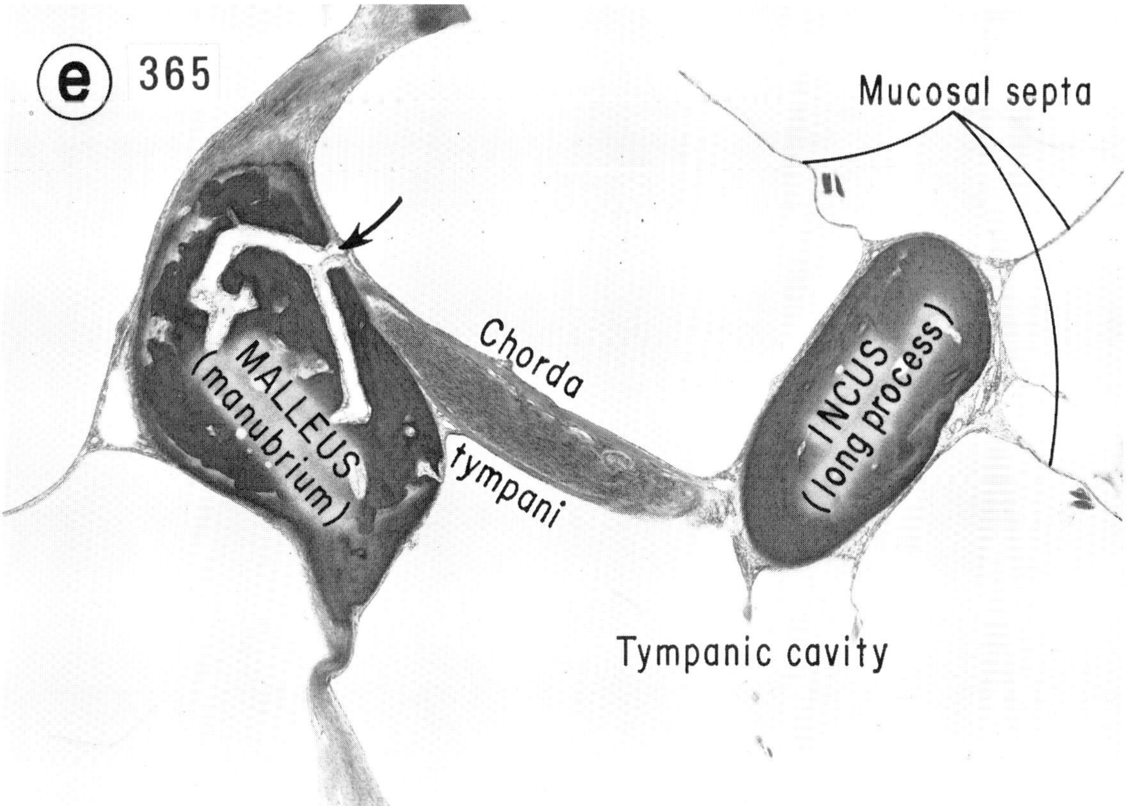

Figure III–65, Continued. See legend on the opposite page.

Figure III–65 continues on the following page.

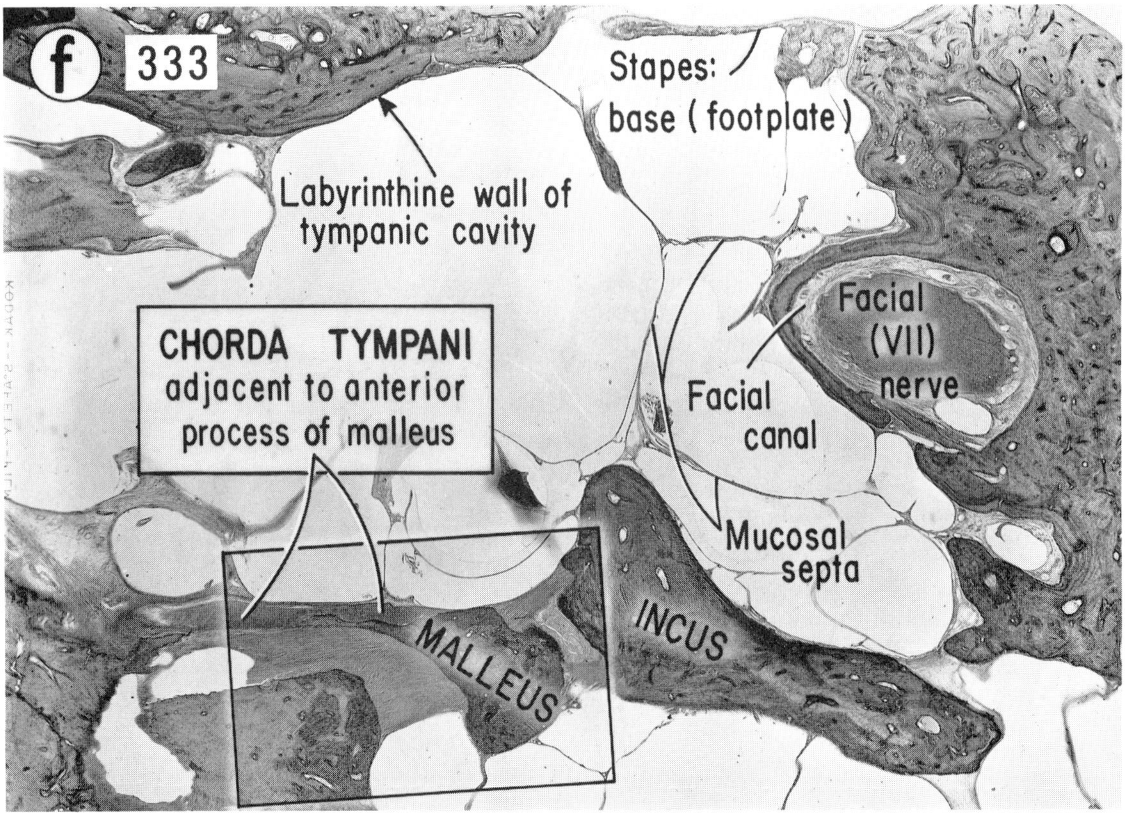

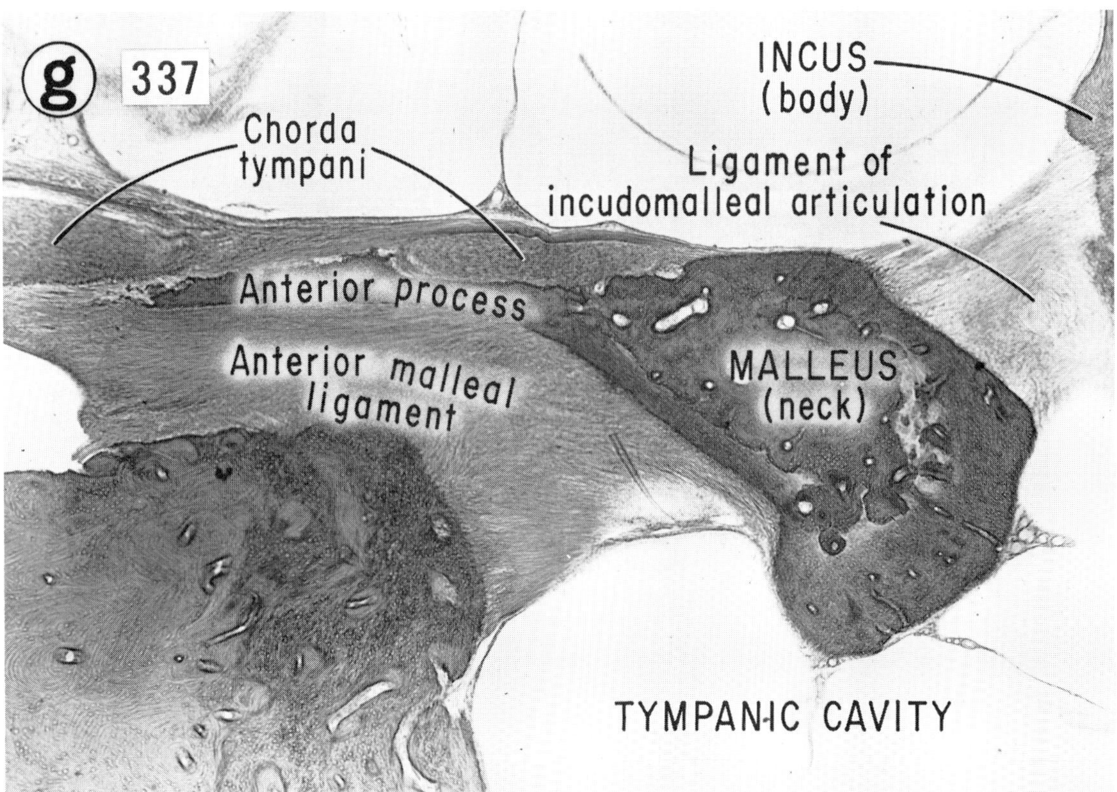

Figure III–65, Continued. See legend on the opposite page.

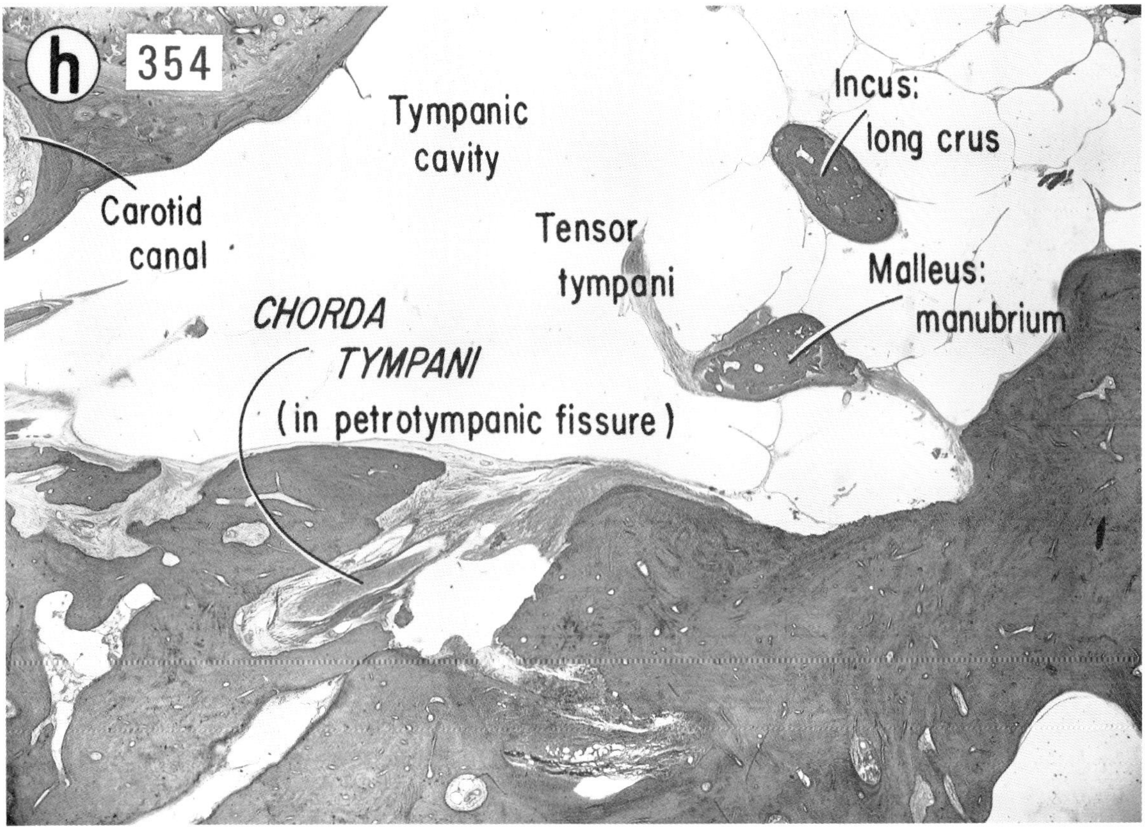

Figure III–65, Concluded.

f and *g*. In further course, the chorda passes through the posterior and anterior malleal folds, along the anterior process of the malleus toward the aperture of the petrotympanic fissure. The rectangular area outlined in *f* is shown at higher magnification in *g* (adjacent section).

h. The nerve enters the petrotympanic fissure at the anterior *iter*.

Transverse sections, Wisconsin Collection, series follows: 21; *b* to *h*, 29. *a*, ×27; *b*, ×8; *c*, ×8; *d*, ×7; *e*, ×37; *f*, ×13; *g*, ×36; *h*, ×12.

(*b* to *h*, with some added labels, from Anson, Donaldson, and Shilling: Ann. Otol., 81:616–631, 1972.)

Figure III–66. COURSE OF THE FACIAL NERVE AND CHORDA TYMPANI SHOWN IN DIAGRAM.

a. The facial nerve, the source of the chorda tympani, passes from an origin in the brain (at *1*) to the facial area of the fundus of the internal acoustic meatus (*2*), there entering the geniculum of the facial canal (*3*). The facial nerve then descends through its canal (*4*) to emerge from the temporal bone at the stylomastoid foramen (*5*). Its fibers are distributed chiefly to the muscles of facial expression (*6*).

The chorda tympani leaves the trunk of the facial nerve (at *7*). After a slightly recurrent course upward in its canaliculus, it crosses the tympanic cavity (*8*) to descend to the neck in the petrotympanic fissure to join the lingual nerve (*9* and *10*).

b. From the chorda, sensory fibers are distributed to the anterior two-thirds of the tongue (*11*).

In the tympanic cavity, the chorda tympani leaves its canaliculus at the *iter chordae posterius.* Invested by mucuous membrane it crosses to the ossicles, passing between the long crus of the incus and the manubrium of the malleus. Continuing its course anteriorward, it passes along the tympanic membrane to the *iter chordae anterius*, there entering the petrotympanic fissure (see Figure III–64).

Figure III–66 continues on the opposite page.

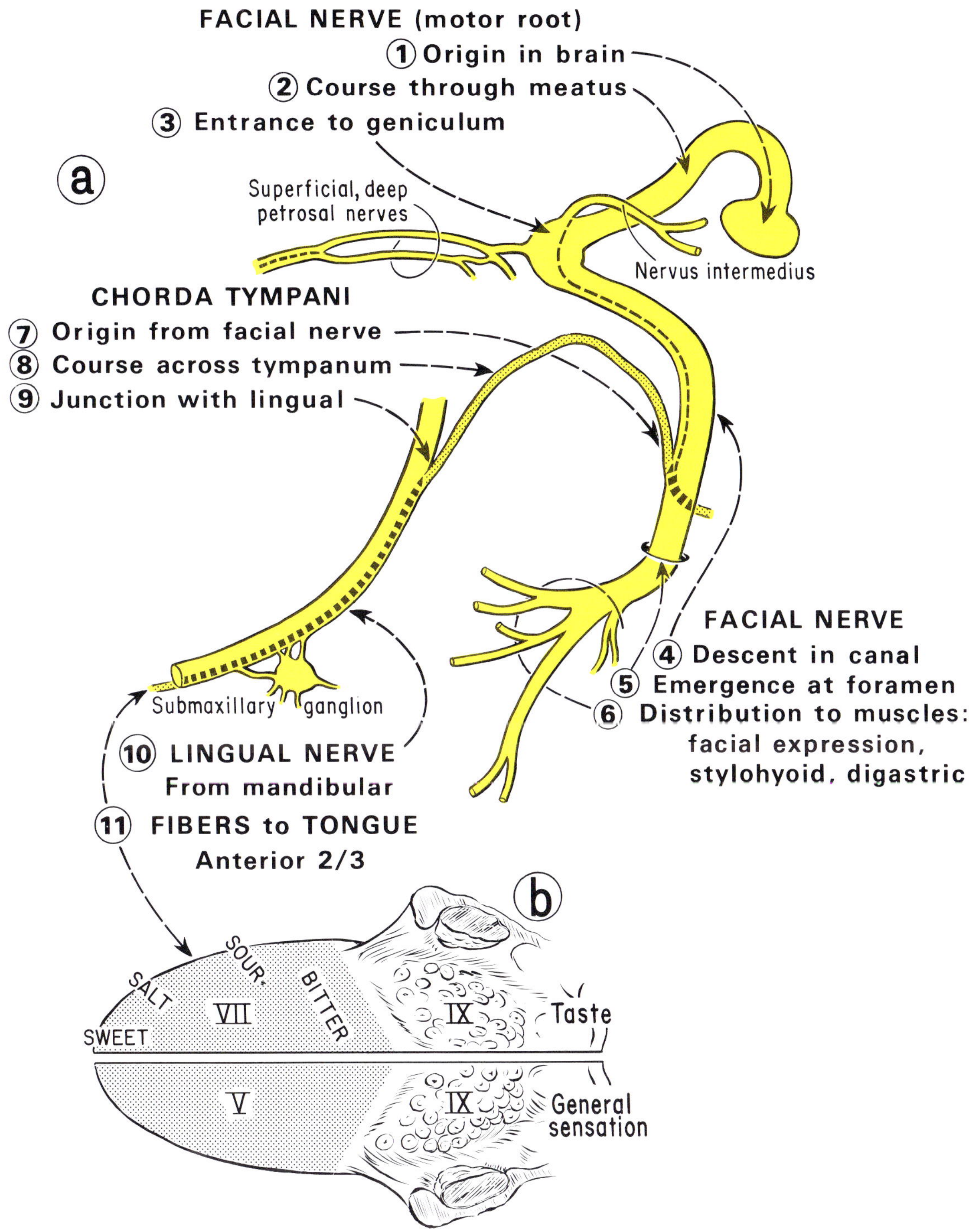

Figure III–66. See legend on the opposite page.

Figure III–66 continues on the following page.

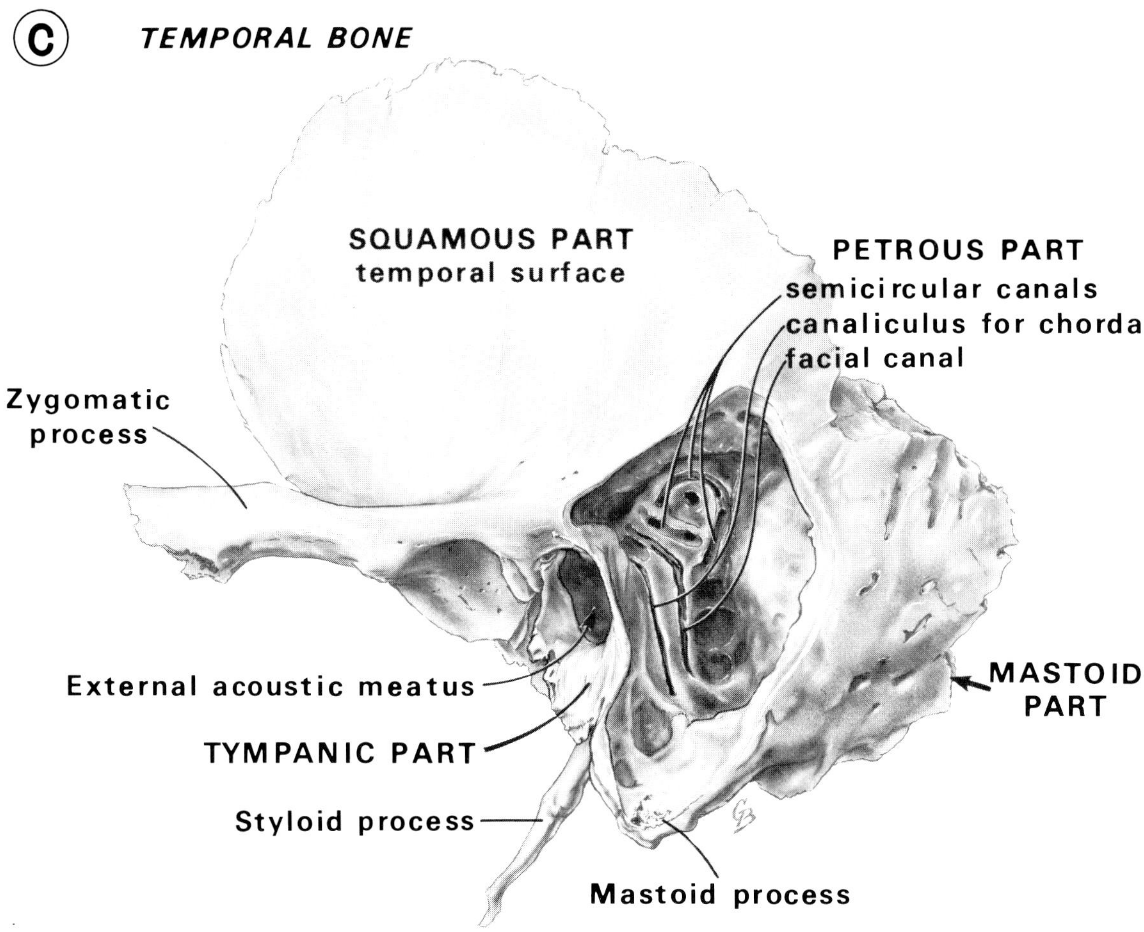

Figure III–66, Continued. Canal of the facial nerve and canaliculus of the chorda tympani.

c. The entire temporal bone, dissected to show the two channels. Posterolateral view. Bone was first removed in an area roughly corresponding to the extent of the mastoid air cells. Next, the dissection was carried forward, medialward, and upward. Above, air cells remain in relation to the tegmen; anteriorly, the two channels are opened as they traverse the mastoid (posterior) wall of the tympanic cavity; the osseous shell of each of the semicircular canals has been removed. Details of anatomic structure and relationship are shown in *d.*

Figure III–66 continues on the opposite page.

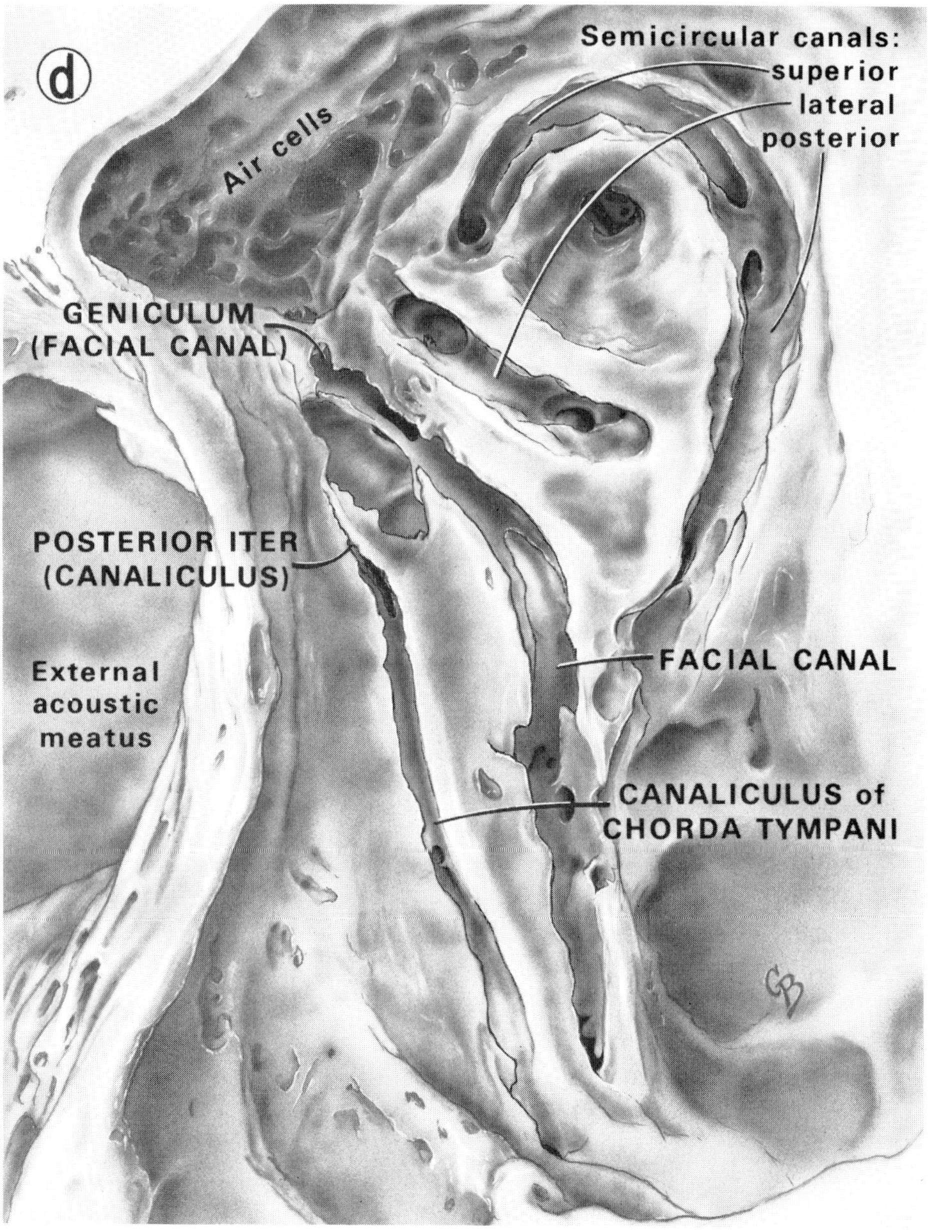

Figure III–66, Continued.

d. The facial canal lies close to the lateral semicircular canal in the superior part of its course. In descent, it changes direction from horizontal to vertical. Typically, the chorda tympani is given off as the facial nerve nears the stylomastoid foramen. In the specimen pictured here, the chorda arose in the cervical region—its channel then remaining independent of the facial canal. The two channels are shown as they follow a parallel course which ends on the inferior surface of the *pars petrosa.*

Dissection by Dr. Bruce B. Shilling.

Figure III–66 continues on the following page.

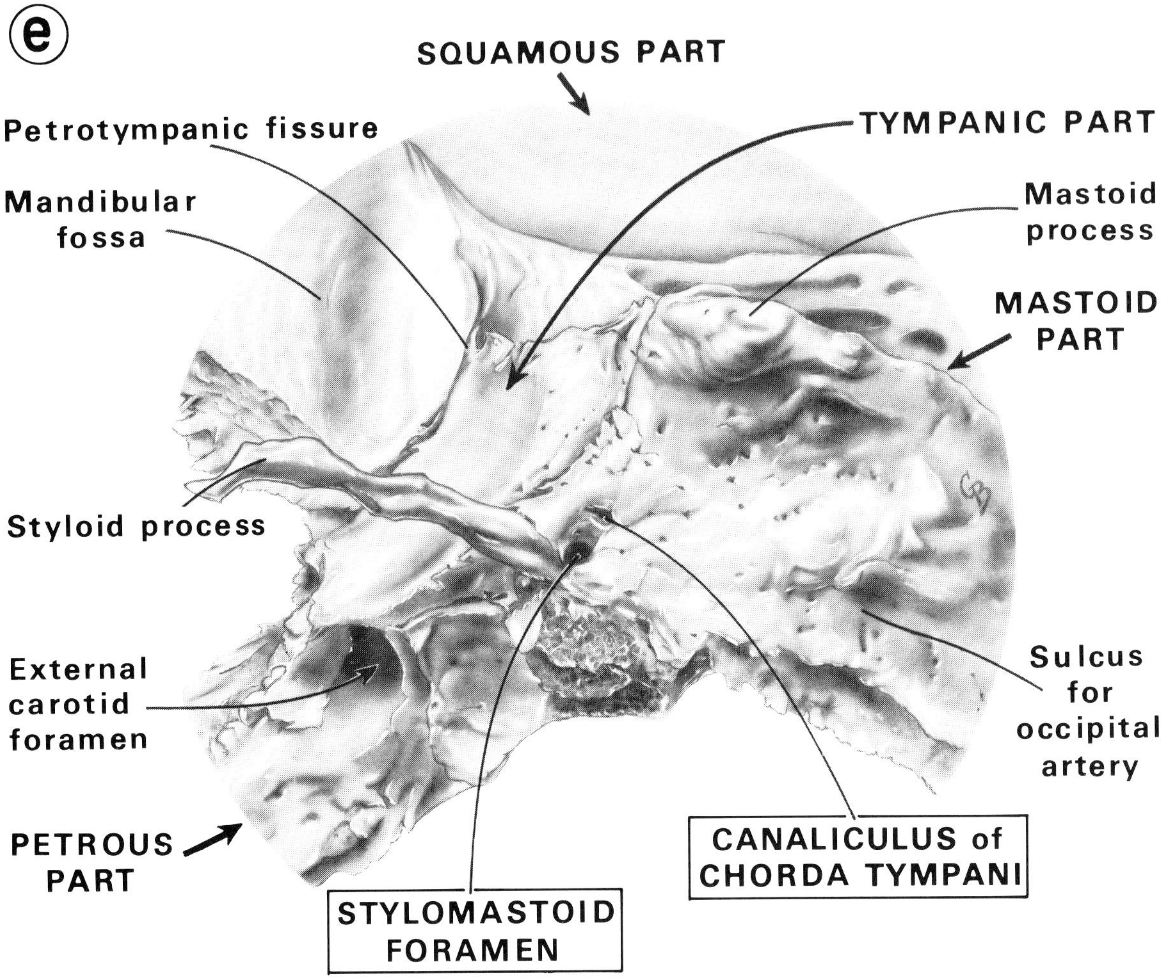

Figure III–66, Continued. CANAL OF THE FACIAL NERVE AND CANALICULUS OF THE CHORDA TYMPANI.

e. The specimen seen in inferolateral view. The stylomastoid foramen is shown just behind the styloid process. The aperture of the canaliculus appears close to the foramen, posterior thereto. In the natural state, a chorda of this less frequent type, could be closely related to the stylohyoid and stylopharyngeal muscles.

The following elements of the skull are also shown: the tympanic, squamous and mastoid parts of the temporal bone; the mastoid process; the mandibular fossa and petrotympanic fissure; and the external aperture of the carotid canal.

Figure III–66 continues on the opposite page.

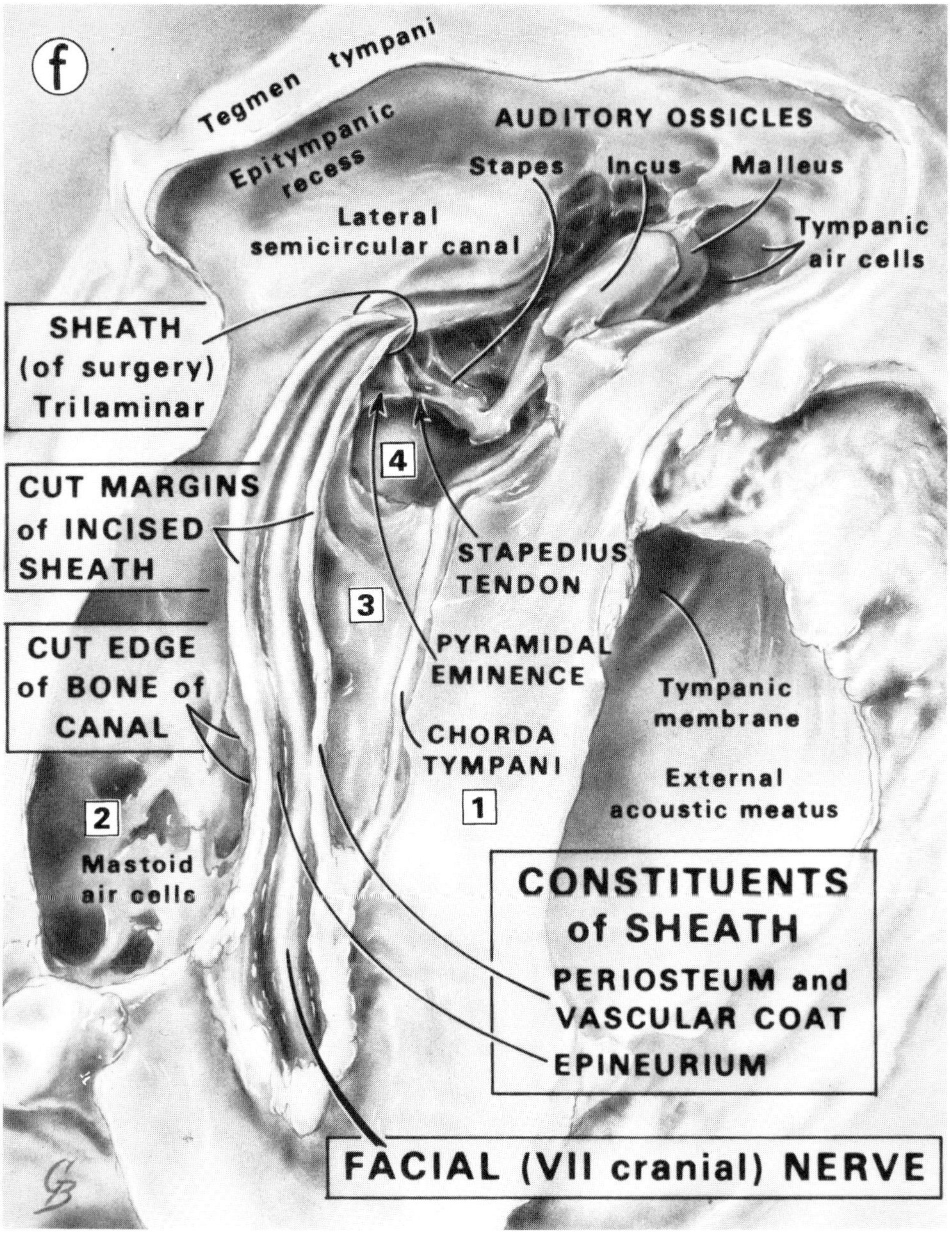

Figure III–66, Concluded.

f. The facial nerve, chorda tympani and related anatomy, in a dissection of an unembalmed specimen, from the mastoid cavity. The auricle has been removed, the external acoustic meatus opened, the bone of the tympanic part of the temporal bone exposed (at numeral *1*). Posteriorly (reader's left, at *2*) appear mastoid air cells. In the process of exenteration, the bone lodging the facial nerve and the chorda tympani has been dissected away (at *3*). On the middle ear side, this would be the posterior (mastoid) wall of the tympanum. Cranialward this wall has been removed (at arrows), giving a view of the tympanic cavity, the auditory ossicles, and the widened space of the facial recess (at *4*). In the caudal portion of the dissection, the sheath of the exposed facial nerve has been opened by a longitudinal cut; in the cranial portion, the nerve is shown at the level of the geniculum as it arches over the stapes. The chorda tympani is seen as it passes between the incus and the malleus.

(From Anson, Donaldson, and Shilling: Ann. Otol., 81:616–631, 1972.)

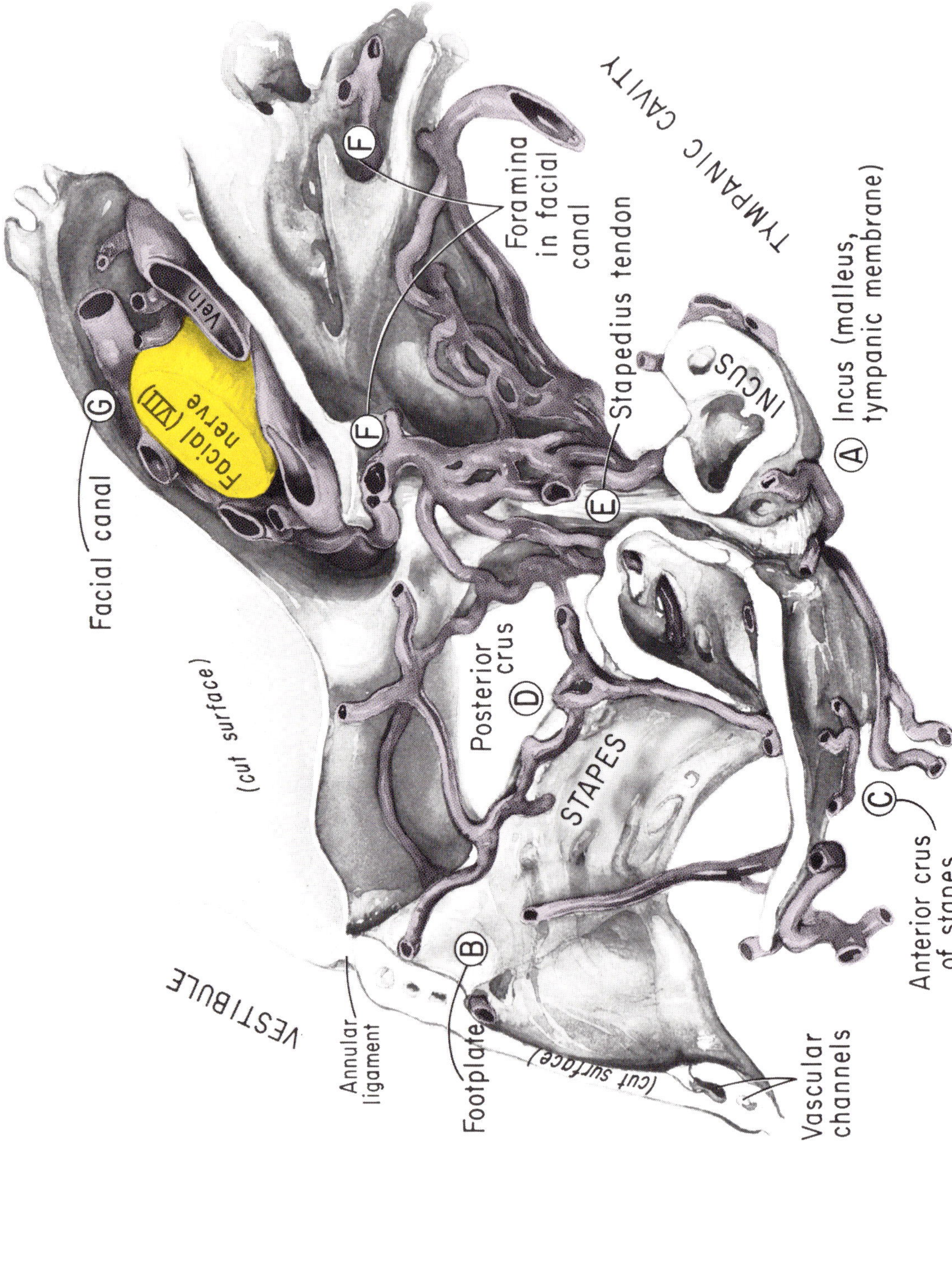
TYMPANIC CAVITY
Foramina in facial canal
F
F
Stapedius tendon
E
INCUS
A
Incus (malleus, tympanic membrane)
Vein
Facial (VII) nerve
G
Facial canal
(cut surface)
Posterior crus
D
STAPES
C
Anterior crus of stapes
B
VESTIBULE
Annular ligament
Footplate
(cut surface)
Vascular channels

Figure III–67. BLOOD SUPPLY OF THE FACIAL NERVE, AUDITORY OSSICLES AND TYMPANIC MUCOUS MEMBRANE. SHOWN BY A RECONSTRUCTION OF THE VEINS PREPARED BY THE BORN WAX-PLATE METHOD. NEWBORN (4-DAY PREMATURE).

The facial canal transmits blood vessels not only to the contained facial nerve and stapedius muscle but also to the surrounding bone and to structures in the tympanic cavity. Using the venous pattern as the guide, veins are here followed from the circumneural plexus in the canal (*G*), through vascular foramina (*F*), along the stapedius tendon (*E*), to the stapes (*B*, *C*, *D*), and to the incus (*A*). Branches continue to the malleus and the tympanic mucous membrane.

Blood vessels to the structures in the middle ear and to the mucous membrane are most prominent as they envelop the stapedius tendon (see Figure III–26*a* and III–69*b*). In the stapes they are most evident in the base (footplate), where they enter circumferentially arranged foramina. In the malleus and incus the vascular channels are uniformly distributed through the bone.

The veins shown in the reconstruction, like the arteries which they accompany, course through the investing mucous membrane, contiguous to the structures that they vascularize. Additional supply comes from arterial branches and venous tributaries which are transmitted by numerous mucosal septa (Figures III–10*a* and III–22*b*). Communications are established with the constituents of the tympanic plexus derived from internal maxillary and ascending pharyngeal sources.

Transverse sections, Wisconsin Collection, series 124.

(After Anson, Donaldson, Warpeha, and Winch: Laryngoscope, 77:1269–1294, 1967.)

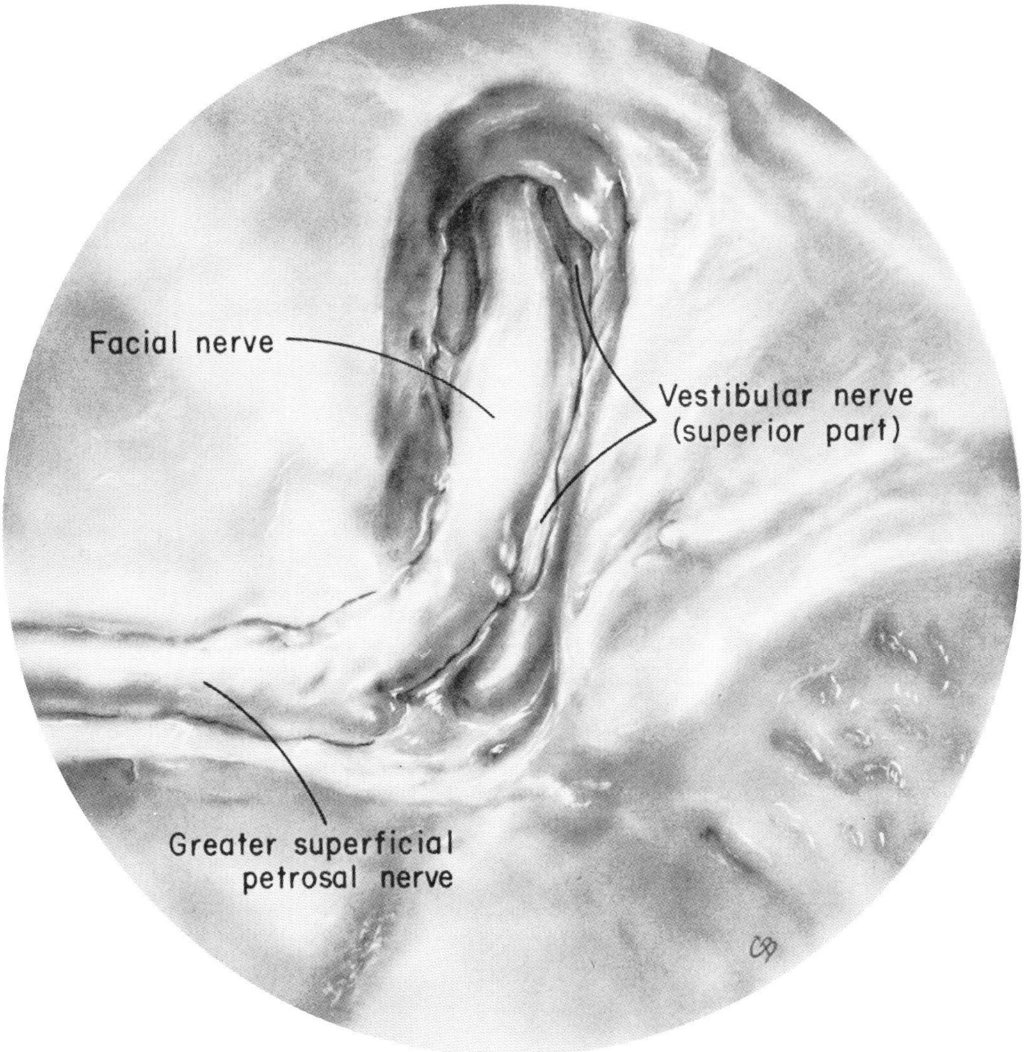

a

Figure III–68. NEURAL CONTENTS OF THE INTERNAL ACOUSTIC MEATUS, FACIAL CANAL, AND HIATUS OF THE LATTER.

a. Dissection of an unembalmed specimen, a left temporal bone. The opened channels are seen in superior view. The facial nerve is exposed, beginning with the point of its passage from the cranial cavity through the *porus* of the meatus. The upper, or superior, branch of the vestibular division of the vestibulocochlear nerve lies posterior to the facial nerve and has not been completely uncovered. The greater superficial petrosal nerve arises at the facial knee, or *geniculum*, and passes through the *hiatus canalis facialis.* The upper branch of the vestibular nerve will continue to the superior vestibular area of the fundus (here out of view).

Figure III–68 continues on the opposite page.

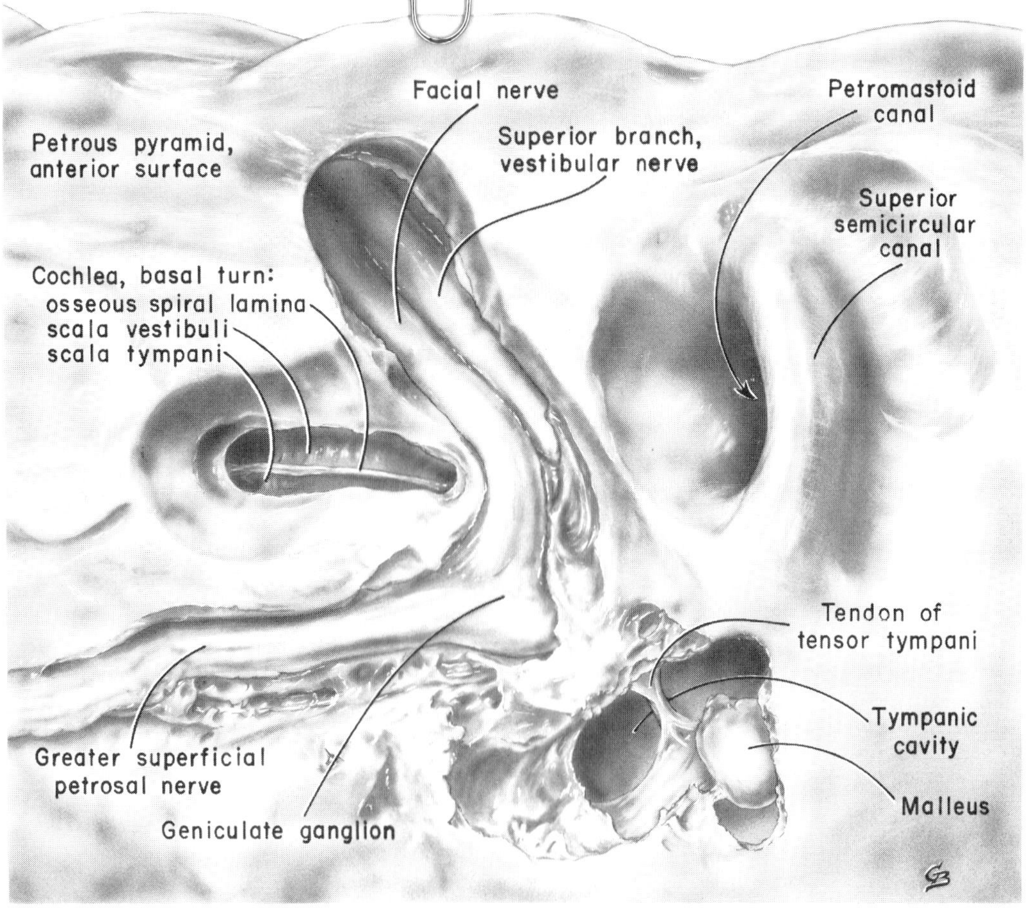

b

Figure III–68, Continued. INTERNAL ACOUSTIC MEATUS: ITS COURSE AND CONTENTS.

b. Demonstrating especially the surgically important relationship of the contained nerves to cochlear, canalicular, and tympanic structures. Dissection of an unembalmed specimen of left temporal bone, viewed from above; that is, as if toward the floor of the middle cranial fossa. In such an exposure, the greater superficial petrosal nerve is identified first; next, it is followed into the hiatus of the facial canal. After the geniculate ganglion has been identified, the internal meatus is opened.

In an anterior direction from the meatus the basal coil of the cochlea is seen; in a posterior direction the dissection has been carried into the pneumatized bone situated beneath the superior semicircular canal. The *tegmen tympani* has been removed in order to reveal the head of the malleus in the epitympanic recess. The ridge at the top of the figure is the angle separating the anterior and the posterior surfaces of the petrous pyramid. In the meatus the nerves have been freed of their meningeal investments, which reach as far as the fundus.

The upper, or superior, terminal branch of the vestibular nerve lies to the posterior side of the facial nerve as it courses toward the superior vestibular area of the fundus on the way to the utricle and to the superior and lateral membranous ampullae. The facial nerve takes a slightly curving course toward the knee (*geniculum*), the concavity of the flexure being an accommodation to the basal turn of the cochlea. At the geniculate ganglion, the greater superficial petrosal nerve arises from the facial nerve, and enters (as is here demonstrated) the *hiatus canalis facialis*. The main nerve, passing in the opposite direction, takes an arciform course over the vestibular window (here out of view). The most familiar landmark on the anterior surface of the pyramid is the *eminentia arcuata*. Situated somewhat lateralward from the middle of that aspect of the pyramid, it is caused mainly by the superior semicircular canal. In this instance, as is commonly the case, a tract of air cells, termed petromastoid, passes through the arch and becomes continuous with the tympanic antrum. Here they are entered from above, by dissection. In the fetus and infant the space occupied by the cells and their trabeculate walls is the subarcuate fossa, a route of invasion of the bone by arteries and veins that are offsets of the meningeal vessels.

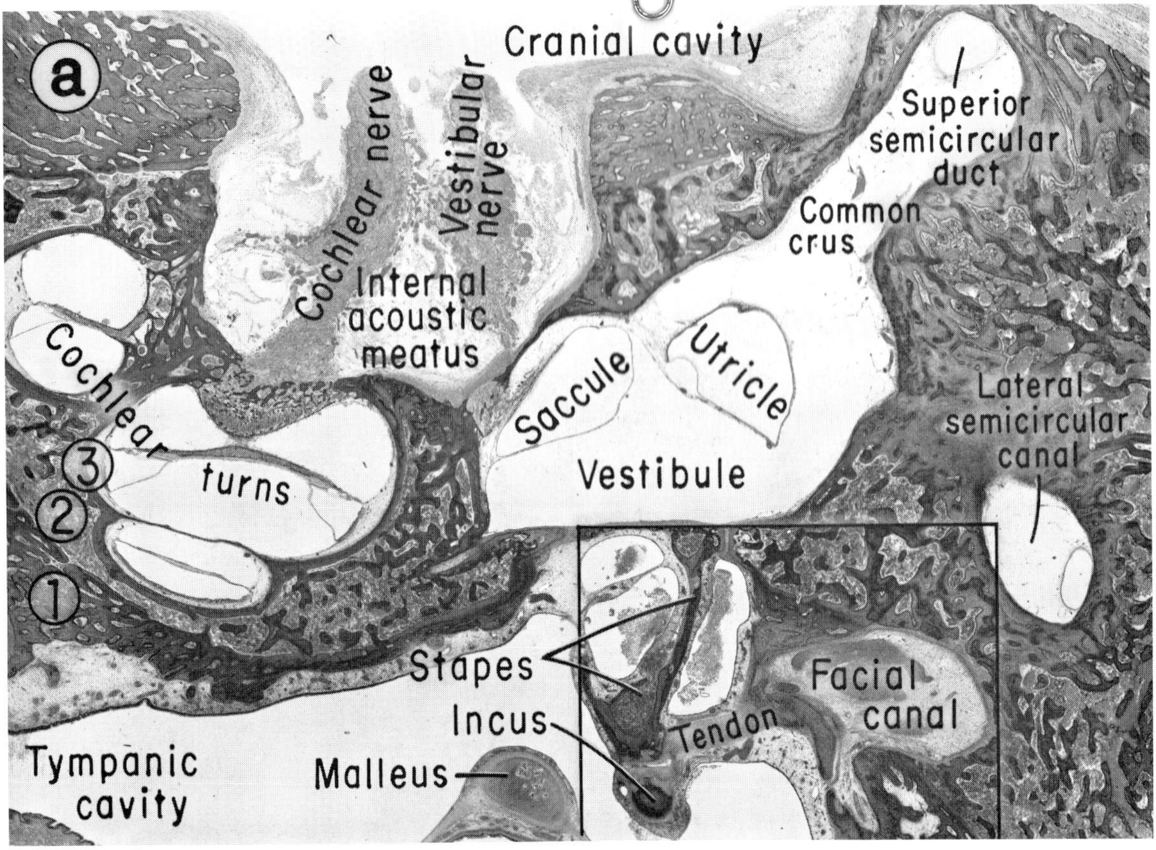

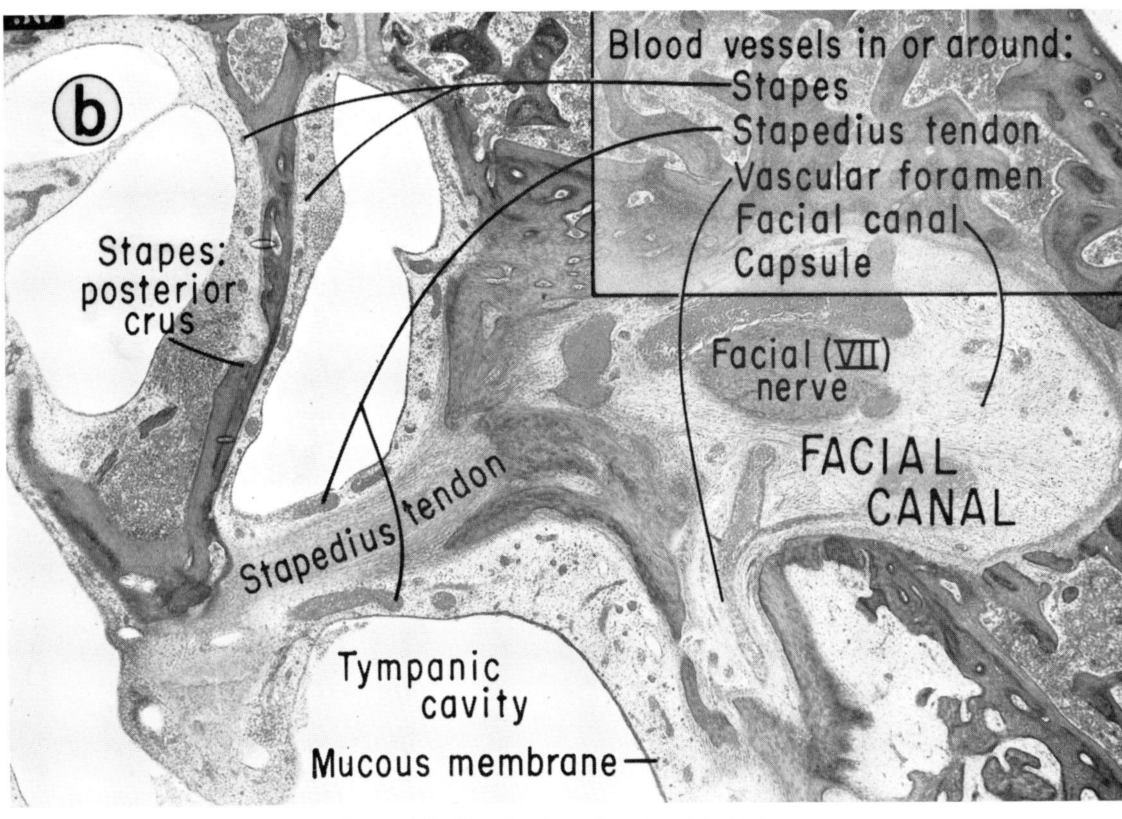

Figure III–69. See legend on the opposite page.

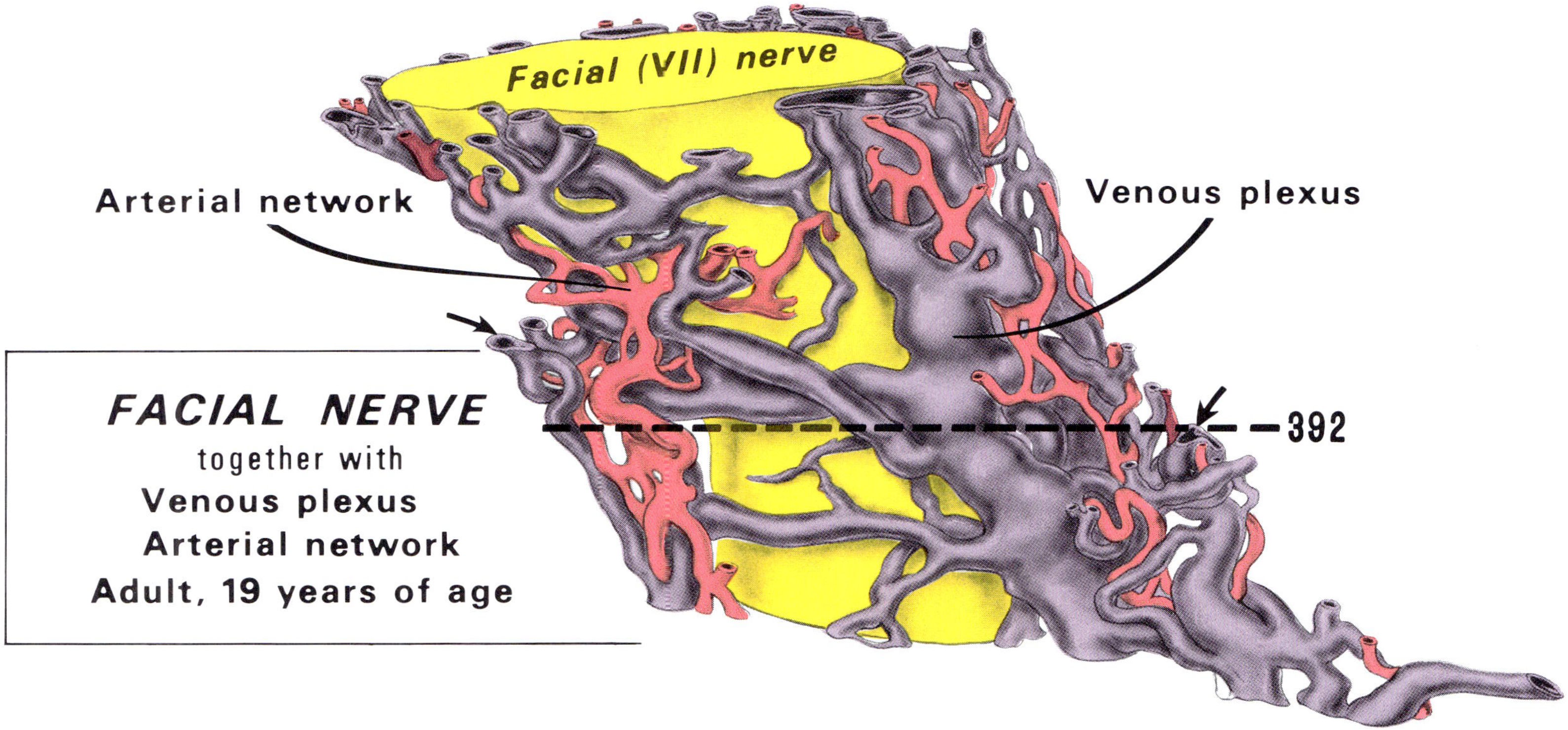

c

Figure III–69. ROUTES REGULARLY FOLLOWED BY ARTERIES AND VEINS WITHIN THE FACIAL CANAL IN PASSING BETWEEN THE CANAL AND THE MIDDLE EAR. *a* and *b*. NEWBORN INFANT (4-DAY PREMATURE). *c*. MALE, 19 YEARS OF AGE.

a. Topographical relations. Details of anatomy in the area blocked are shown in *b*.

b. The vessels leaving or entering the canal reach the stapes, then the incus and the malleus by way of the pyramidal eminence (around and within the stapedius tendon) and through separate foramina in the wall of the canal.

c. Showing, by means of a reconstruction, the plexiform arrangement of the capacious veins and the complex system of intercommunicating arteries that surround the nerve. Arrows indicate the points of continuity of the circumneural vessels with those that occur in vascular channels of the surrounding bone. The approximate level of section 392 is indicated in the drawing of the specimen in Figure III–72.

Transverse sections, Wisconsin Collection, series as follows: *a* and *b*, 124; *c*, 29. *a*, ×14; *b*, ×29.

(*a* and *b* from Anson: Trans. Amer. Acad. Ophthal. Otolaryng., 73:17–38, 1969. *c* from Anson, Warpeha, Donaldson, and Rensink: Ann. Otol., 79:710–720, 1970.)

Figure III–70. FACIAL CANAL: DEHISCENCE. MALE, 54 YEARS OF AGE.

The facial canal is dehiscent (at arrow) in its vertical course. On the opposite wall, an otosclerotic lesion has replaced normal bone in the area of the fissula ante fenestram (see Figure III–126).

This section also passes through the following: stapedial footplate; tensor tympani muscle, tendon, and manubrium of the malleus; cochlea (near the modiolus); internal acoustic meatus (throughout its length); tympanic membrane; and external acoustic meatus.

Courtesy of Dr. C. M. Kos.

Transverse section, Iowa Otological Collection, series 583.R. × 4.

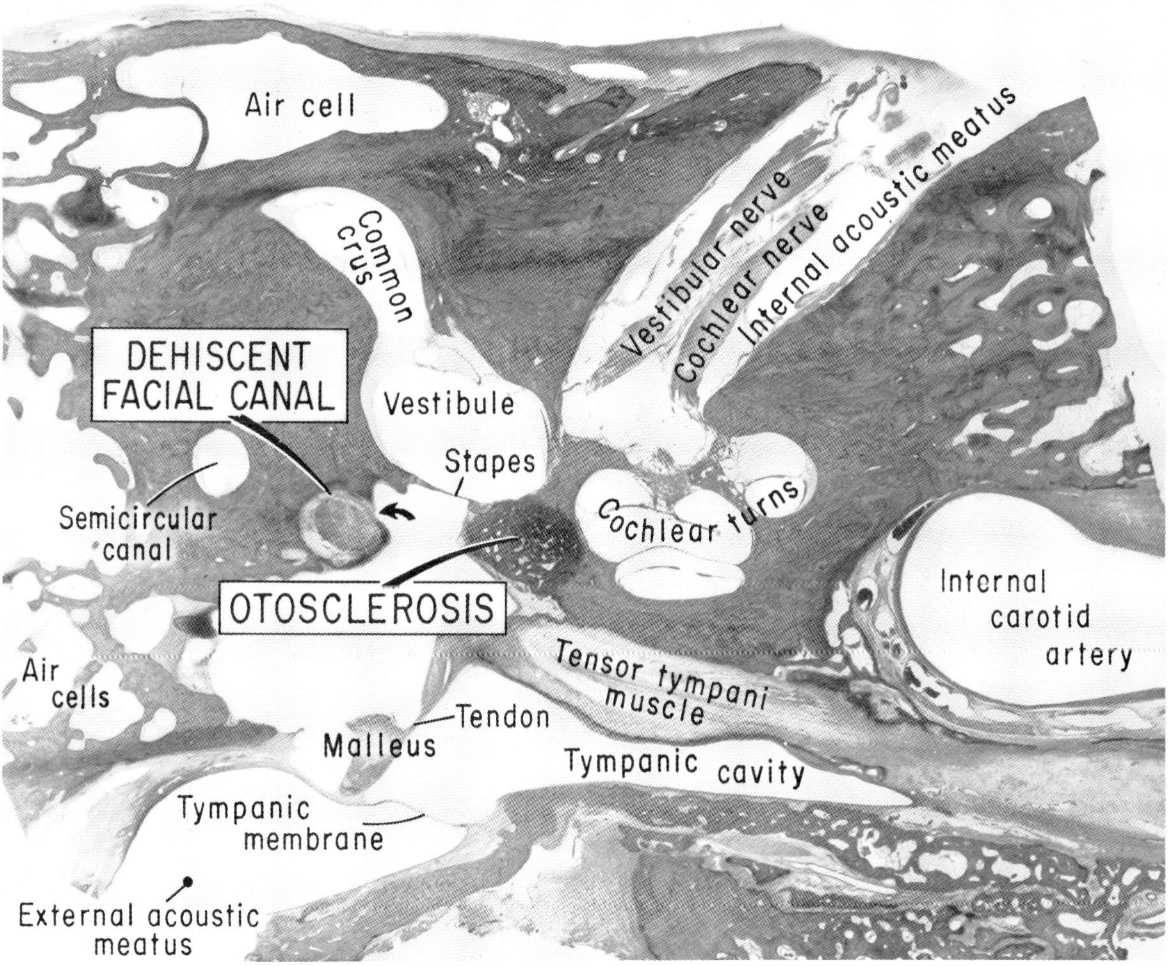

Figure III–70. See legend on the opposite page.

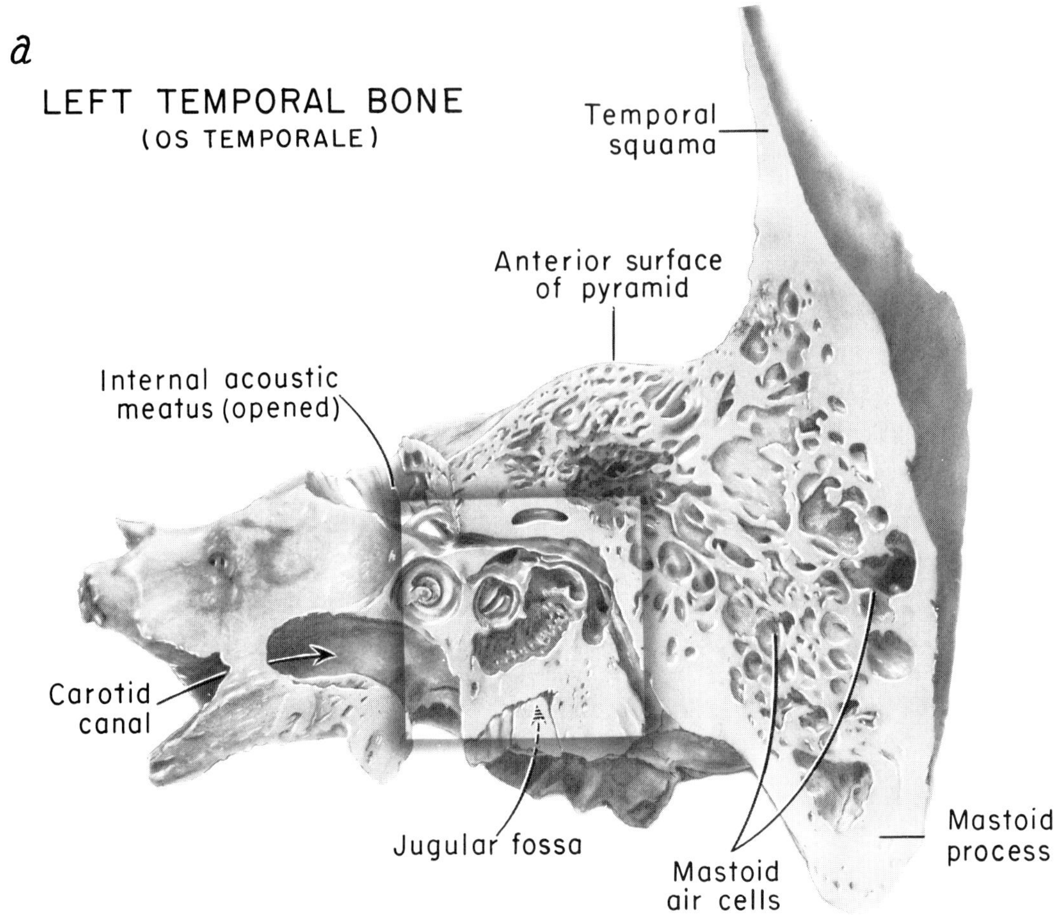

Figure III–71. FACIAL CANAL AND RELATED STRUCTURES, SHOWN IN A GROSS SECTION OF TEMPORAL BONE IN THE PLANE OF THE LONG AXIS OF THE TYMPANIC CAVITY.

The "roof" of the internal acoustic meatus has been removed (between the small unlabeled arrows); similarly, the tympanic wall of the fossula of the cochlear window has been dissected away, so that the tympanic and vestibular scalae are seen through the artificial opening and the natural fenestra.

a. The detailed anatomy of the blocked portion is depicted in the following figure.

This important surgical area, measuring only 2 cm. by 2 cm., is surrounded by the following structures: the fossa for the jugular vein, the canal for the internal carotid artery, and the air cells of the epitympanic space and the mastoid portion of the temporal bone.

b. Details of anatomy immediately related to the facial canal in the quadrilateral area blocked in the preceding topographical figure.

The following structures are demonstrated: the cochlea, the internal acoustic meatus, the lateral semicircular canal and vestibular window (above and below the facial canal), and the cochlear window.

Figure III–71 continues on the opposite page.

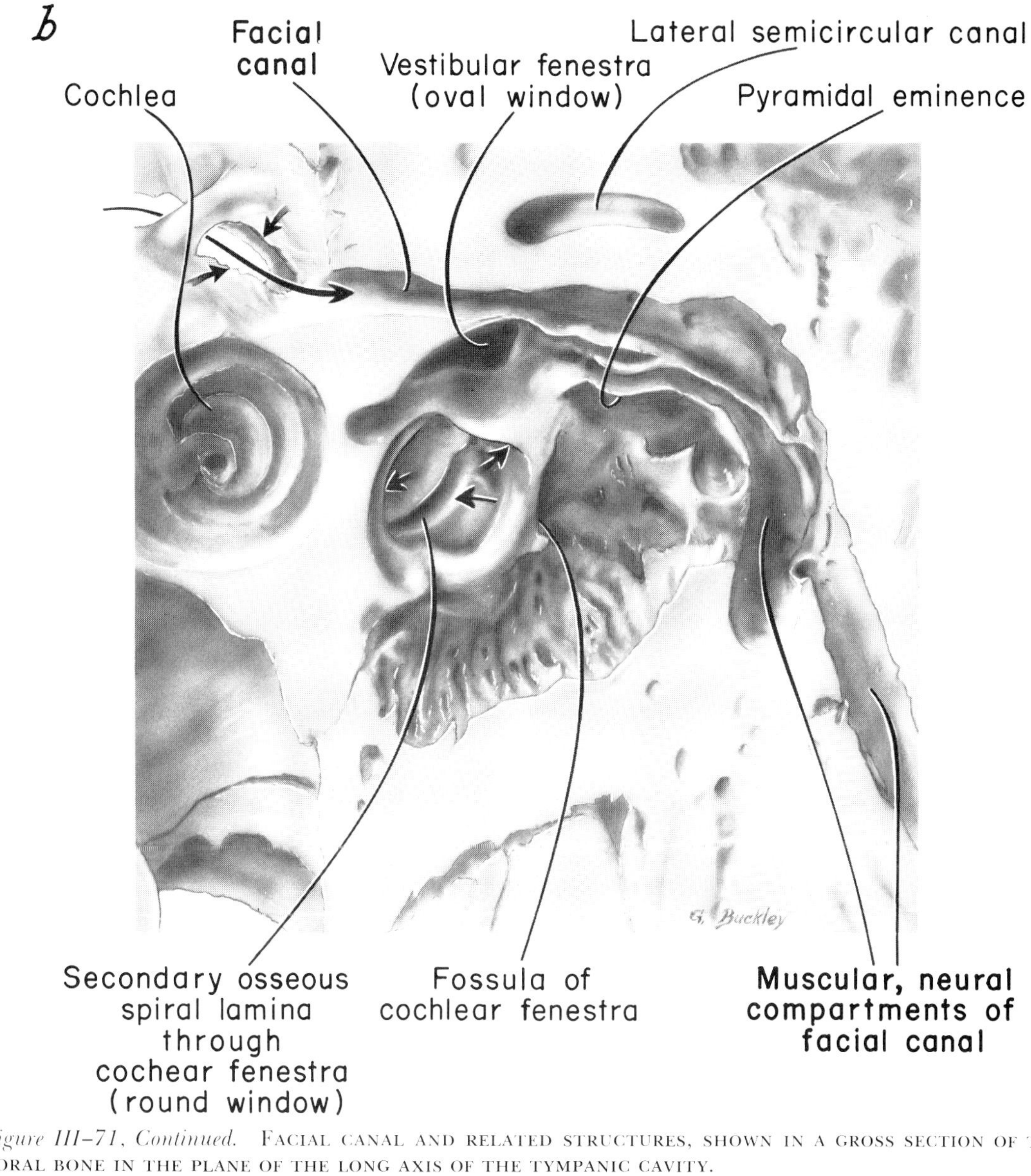

Figure III–71, Continued. FACIAL CANAL AND RELATED STRUCTURES, SHOWN IN A GROSS SECTION OF TEMPORAL BONE IN THE PLANE OF THE LONG AXIS OF THE TYMPANIC CAVITY.

The course of the facial nerve may be traced from the internal acoustic meatus (where a bridge of bone marks the *porus acusticus internus*), through the *area n. facialis* of the fundus, to the *geniculum* (knee) of the facial canal; then, horizontally backward and continuing in the facial canal, the nerve passes lateralward, finally downward, on the way to emergence at the stylomastoid foramen. The channel for the facial nerve is matched, in the superior half of its course, by a semicanal for the stapedius muscle. Thus, the facial canal, as a whole, may be said to contain two compartments, at times incompletely separated. A portion of the *sinus tympani* is seen beneath the compartment for the stapedius muscle and its tendon.

Dissection by Dr. Raymond L. Warpeha.

(From Anson, Harper, and Warpeha: Ann. Otol., 72:713–734, 1963.)

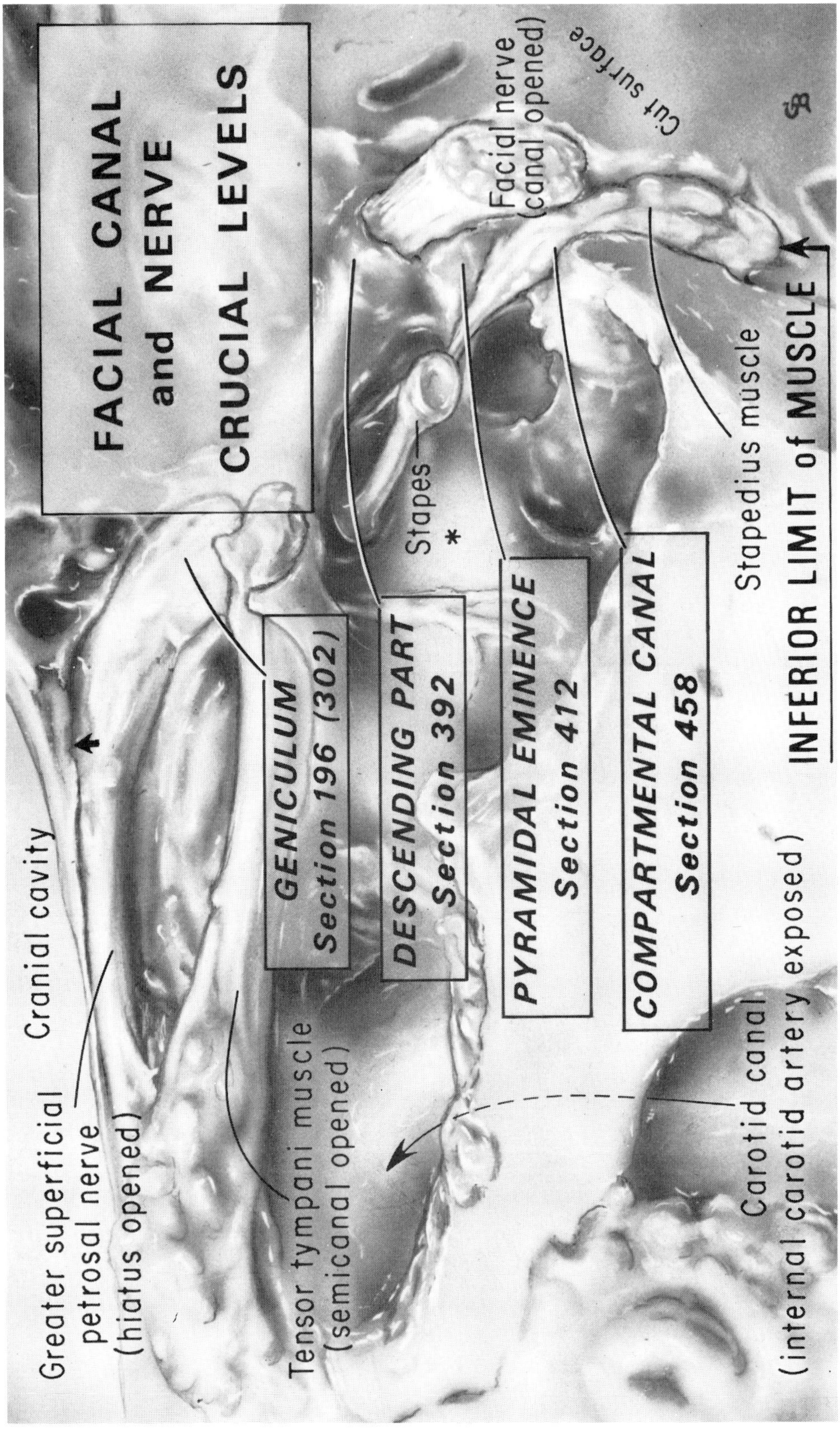
FACIAL CANAL
and NERVE
CRUCIAL LEVELS
GENICULUM
Section 196 (302)
DESCENDING PART
Section 392
PYRAMIDAL EMINENCE
Section 412
COMPARTMENTAL CANAL
Section 458
INFERIOR LIMIT of MUSCLE
Greater superficial
petrosal nerve
(hiatus opened)
Cranial cavity
Tensor tympani muscle
(semicanal opened)
Stapes
*
Facial nerve
(canal opened)
Cut surface
Stapedius muscle
Carotid canal
(internal carotid artery exposed)

Figure III–72. FACIAL CANAL, NERVE, AND RELATED STRUCTURES ON THE LABRYINTHINE WALL OF THE TYMPANIC CAVITY.

In this dissection of an unembalmed specimen of a left temporal bone, four levels are indicated. They record the approximate location of the photomicrographs in the figures which follow. The facial canal, the hiatus of the facial canal, and the semicanal of the tensor tympani muscle have been opened; the facial nerve has been transected. The site of the promontory is indicated by an asterisk.

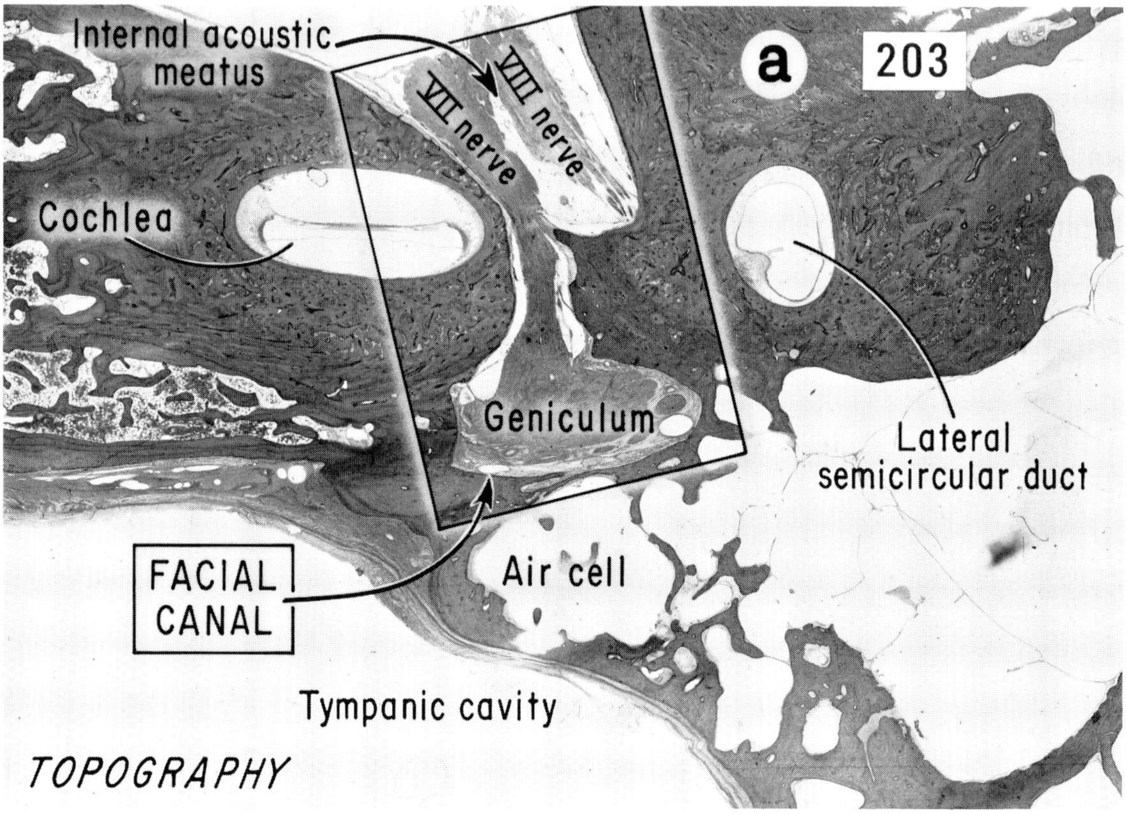

Figure III–73. Fundus of the acoustic meatus and the geniculum of the facial canal: contents and related anatomical structures. Male, 19 years of age.

a. Showing the facial canal and the inferior vestibular area of the fundus of the internal acoustic meatus and the geniculum of the facial canal. Tympanic air cells are present in the wall of the facial canal. The area blocked appears at higher magnification in the following figure (*b*).

Figure III–73 continues on the opposite page.

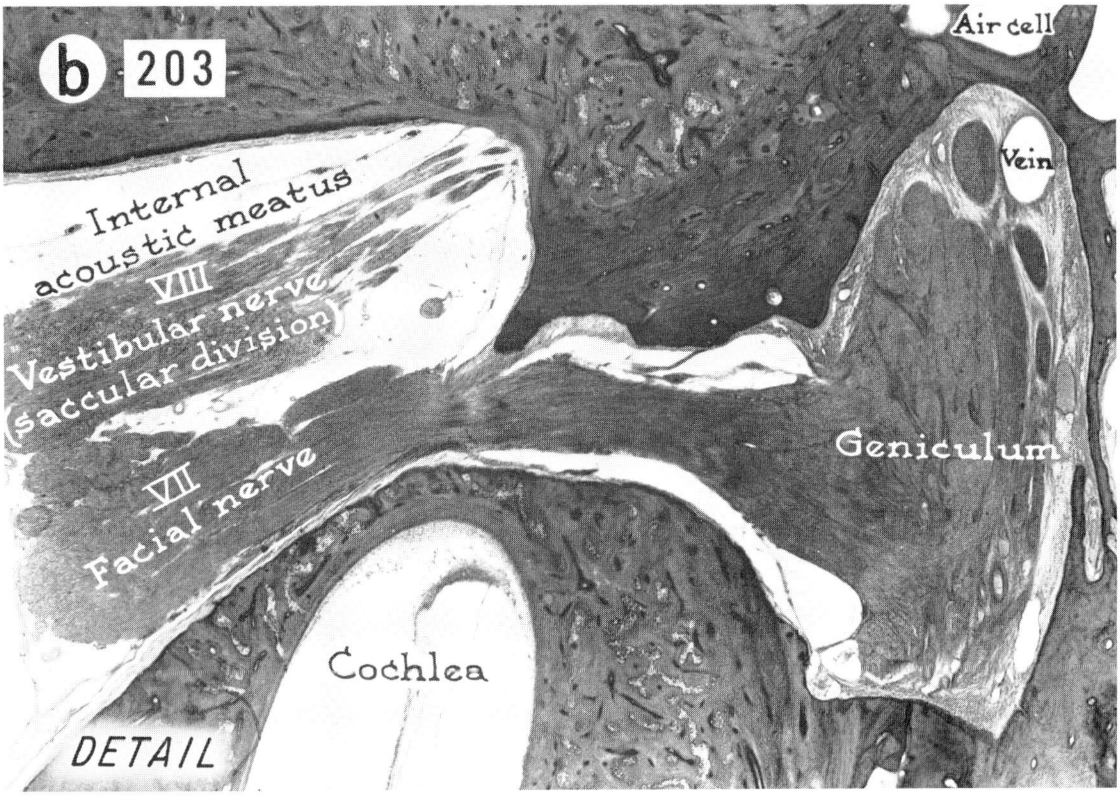

Figure III–73, Continued.

b. The lower terminal branch of the vestibular nerve is sectioned en route to the vestibular area of the fundus. The facial nerve, in passing from the facial area of the fundus to the facial canal, thereby completes its course from the posterior cranial fossa to the labyrinthine wall of the tympanic cavity.

Explanatory Note: These figures serve to demonstrate, respectively, topography and detail, at the same time establishing the orientation of the sections that follow in Figure III–74 (*a* to *i*).

Transverse section (203), Wisconsin Collection, series 29, left temporal bone. *a*, ×7; *b*, ×18.

(*a* from Anson: Trans. Amer. Acad. Ophthal. Otolaryng., 76:108–129, 1972.)

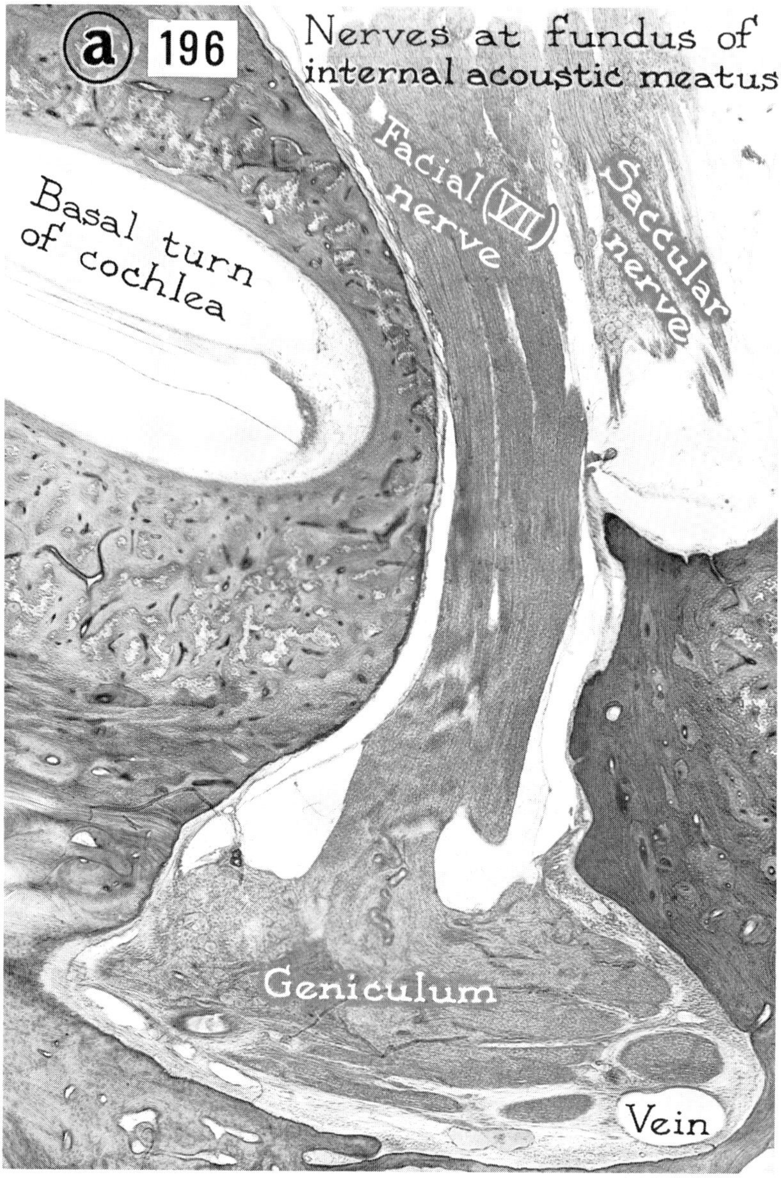

Figure III–74. FACIAL CANAL, CONTENTS, AND RELATED ANATOMY: TRANSVERSE SECTIONS IN CRANIOCAUDAL SUCCESSION AT NINE SELECTED LEVELS. MALE, 19 YEARS OF AGE.

a. The facial (VII cranial) nerve passes from the fundus of the internal acoustic meatus into the genicular part of the facial canal. At the same horizontal level the saccular division of the acoustic (VIII cranial) nerve is sectioned on the way to the inferior vestibular area of the fundus. Vessels accompany the facial nerve as it passes from the meatus into the facial canal.

b. Here the nerve, having emerged from the fundus (indicated by the arrow), has turned in a posterior direction in the beginning (genicular) part of its horizontal course. This is the level of origin of the greater (superficial) petrosal nerve.

c. The facial canal occupies the labyrinthine wall of the tympanic cavity, separated from the latter by an excessively thin plate of bone. Medial to it lies the lateral semicircular canal.

Figure III–74 continues on the opposite page.

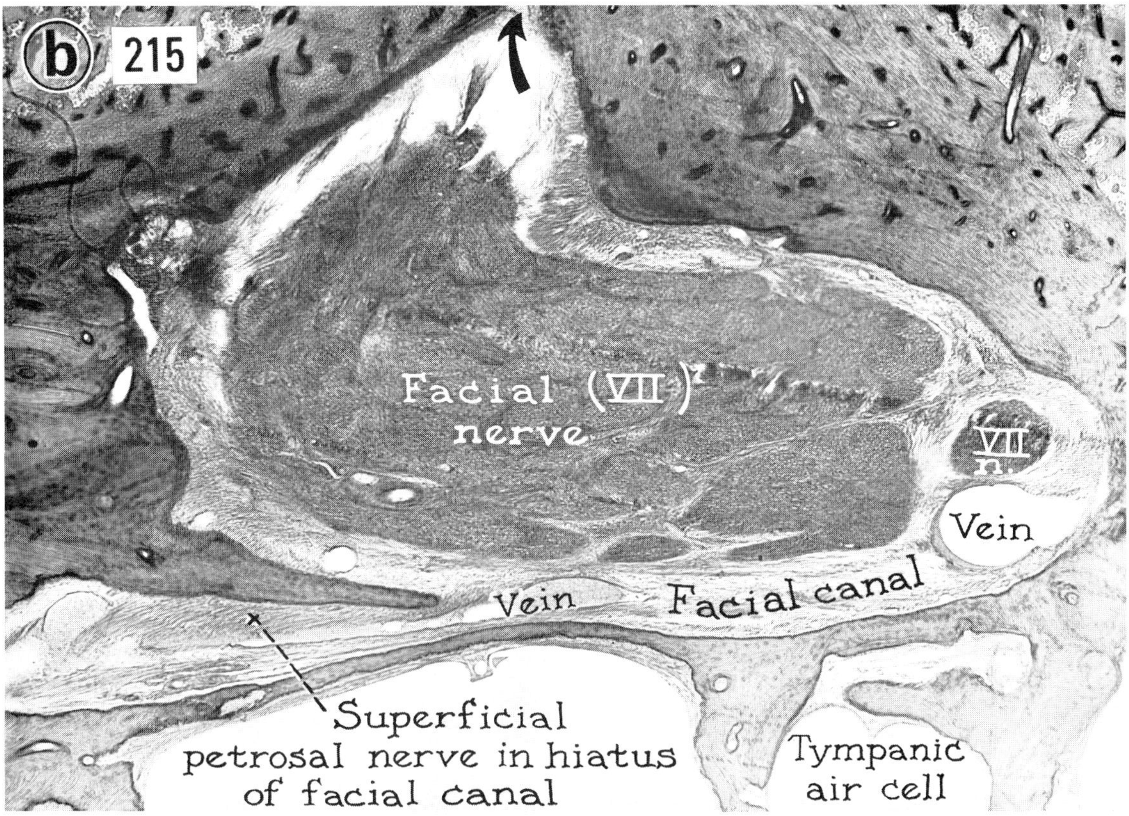

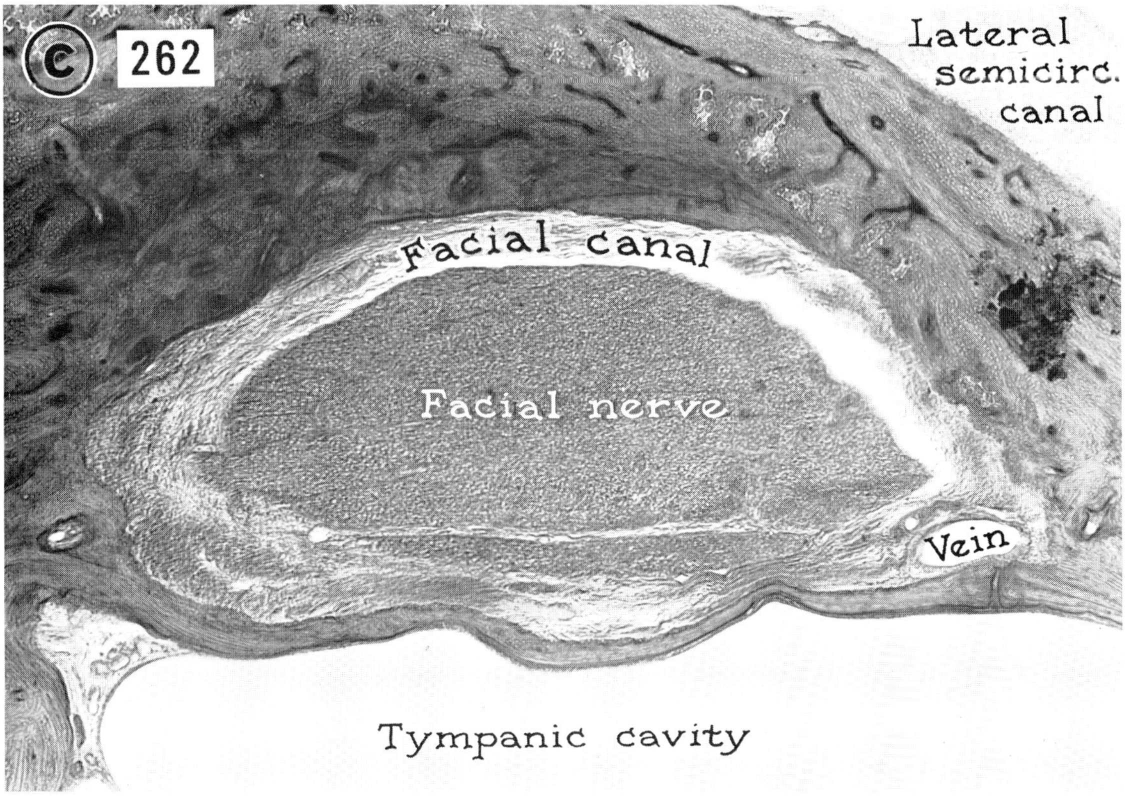

Figure III–74, Continued. *See legend on the opposite page.*

Figure III–74 continues on the following page.

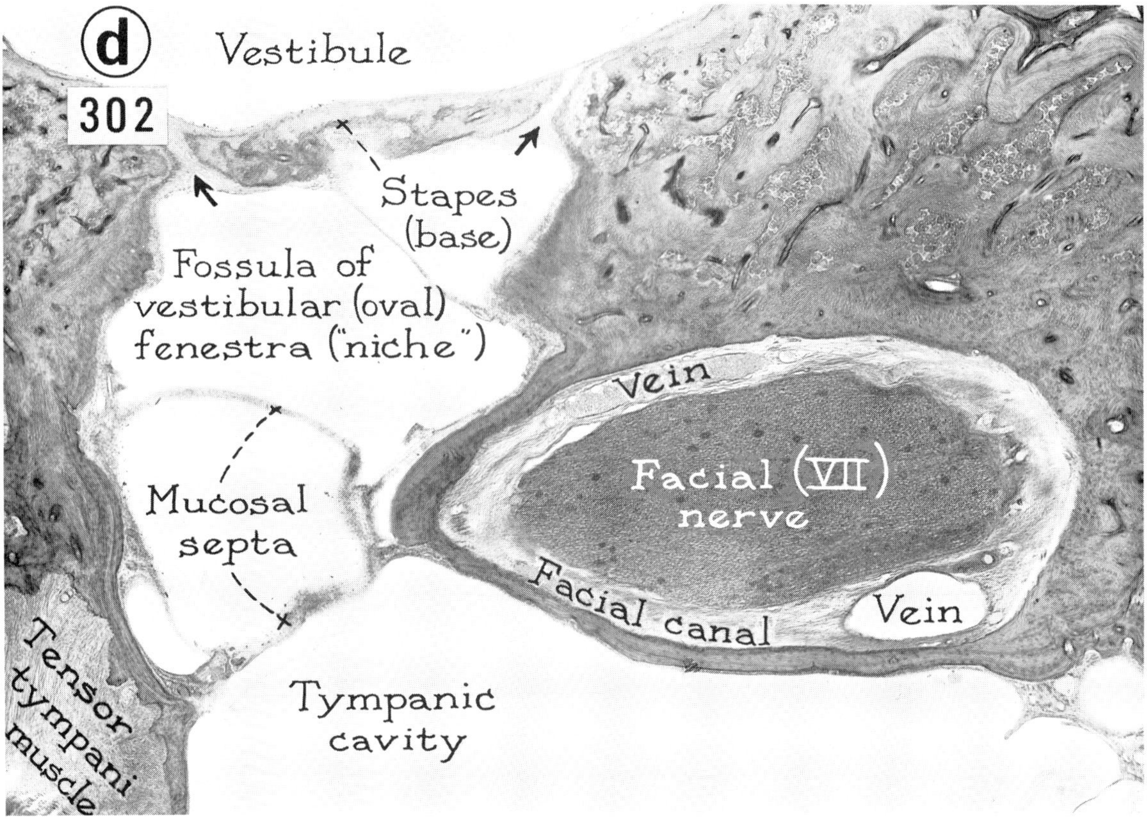

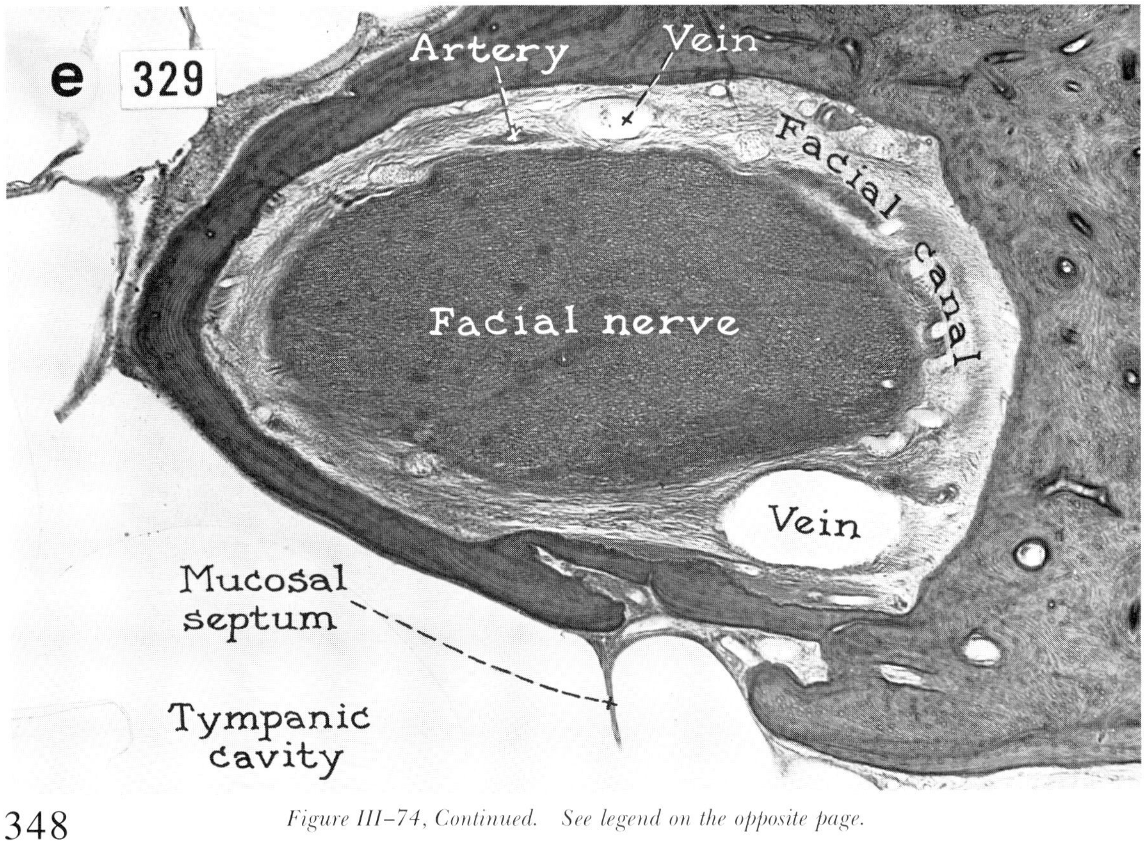

Figure III–74, Continued. See legend on the opposite page.

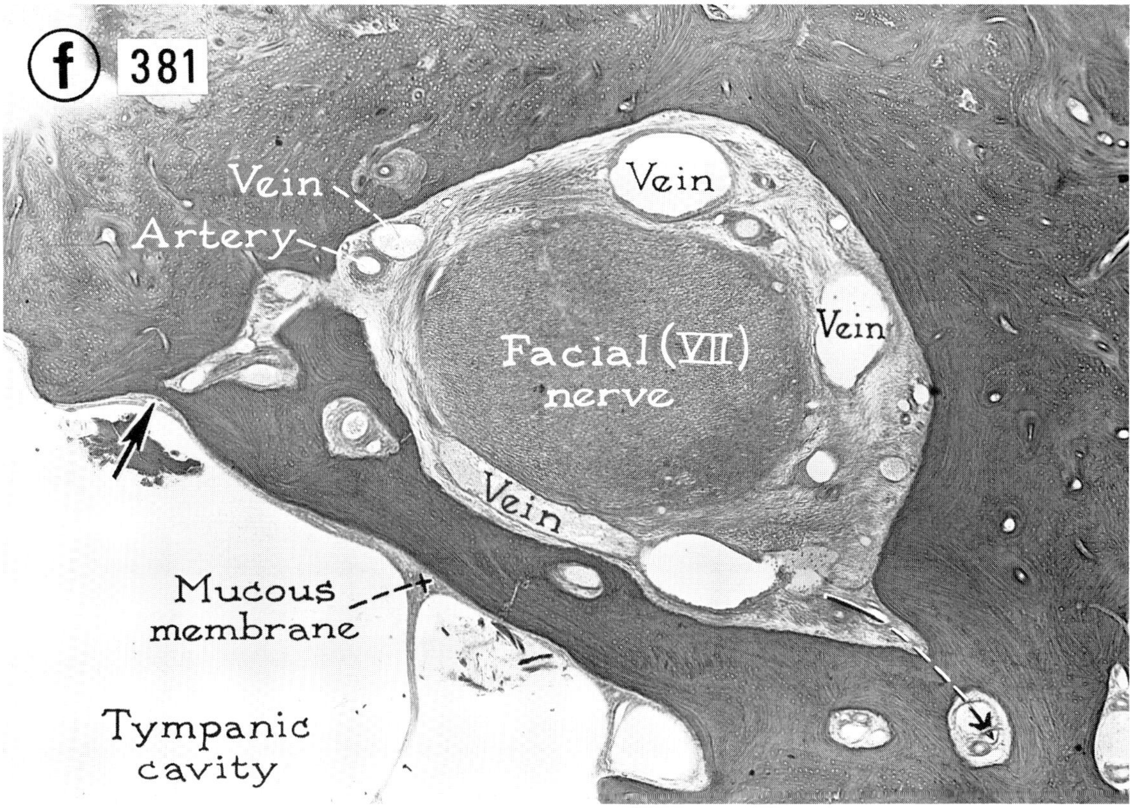

Figure III–74, Continued. FACIAL CANAL, CONTENTS, AND RELATED ANATOMY: LEVELS IN SUCCESSION CAUDALWARD.

d. In continuation of its course in a posterior direction, the nerve is carried medial to the vestibular (oval) window at arrows and the base (footplate) of the stapes. Thereby, a fossula is formed between the ossicle and the facing surface of the jutting prominence produced by the facial canal. The canal is in the path of direct horizontal approach to the stapes. As the canal approaches the level at which it changes from a horizontal to a vertical course, the tissue external to the epineurium becomes more vascular; in this investing tissue, veins are far more prominent than arteries.

e. Blood vessels become a more striking feature of the structure of the canal as progress is made toward the stylomastoid foramen.

f. At a level just cranial to that of the pyramidal eminence, communications between the lumen of the facial canal and channels in the surrounding bone become an added feature of anatomy. Thereby vascular interdependence is established between the nerve and its surrounding tissue on the one hand and the otic capsule on the other (arrow at lower right). Through the vascular channels as intermediaries, connection continues to the mucous membrane (arrow at upper left). Distribution is even wider than these photomicrographs show, since the blood vessels in the mucosal investment of the tympanic cavity are carried to the auditory ossicles and the tympanic membrane.

Figure III–74 continues on the following page.

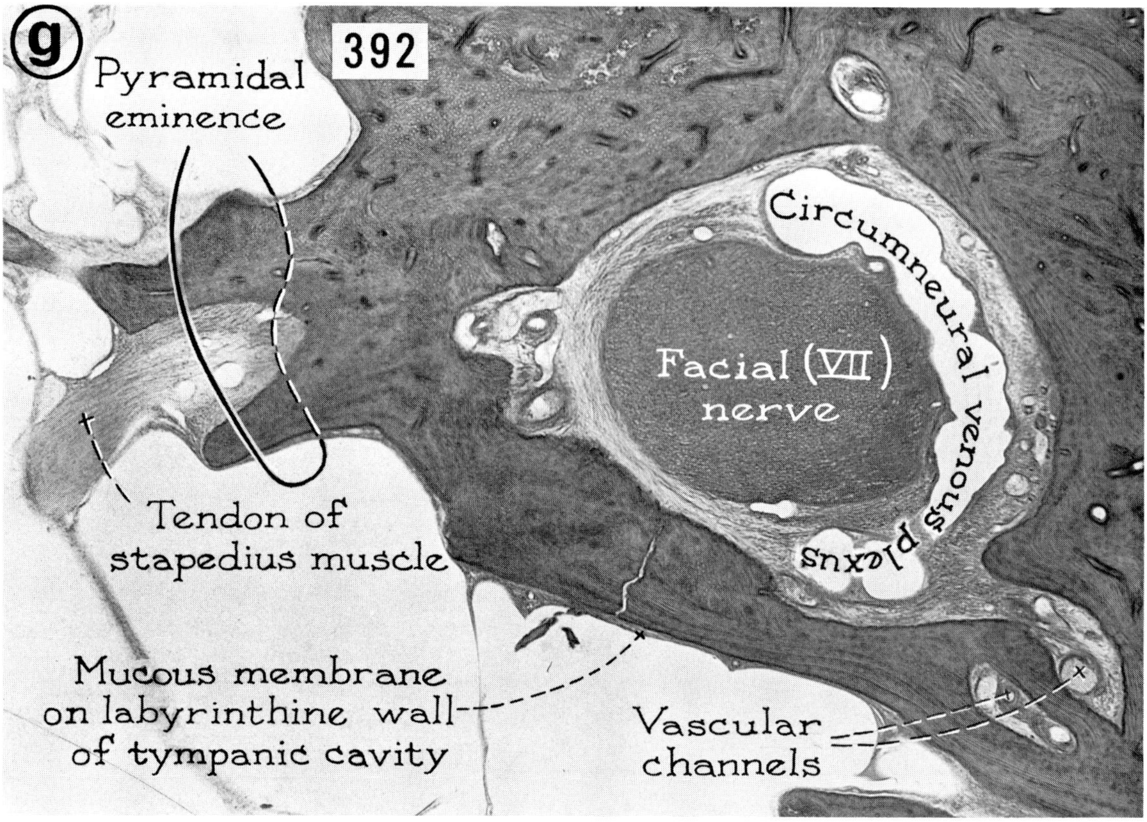

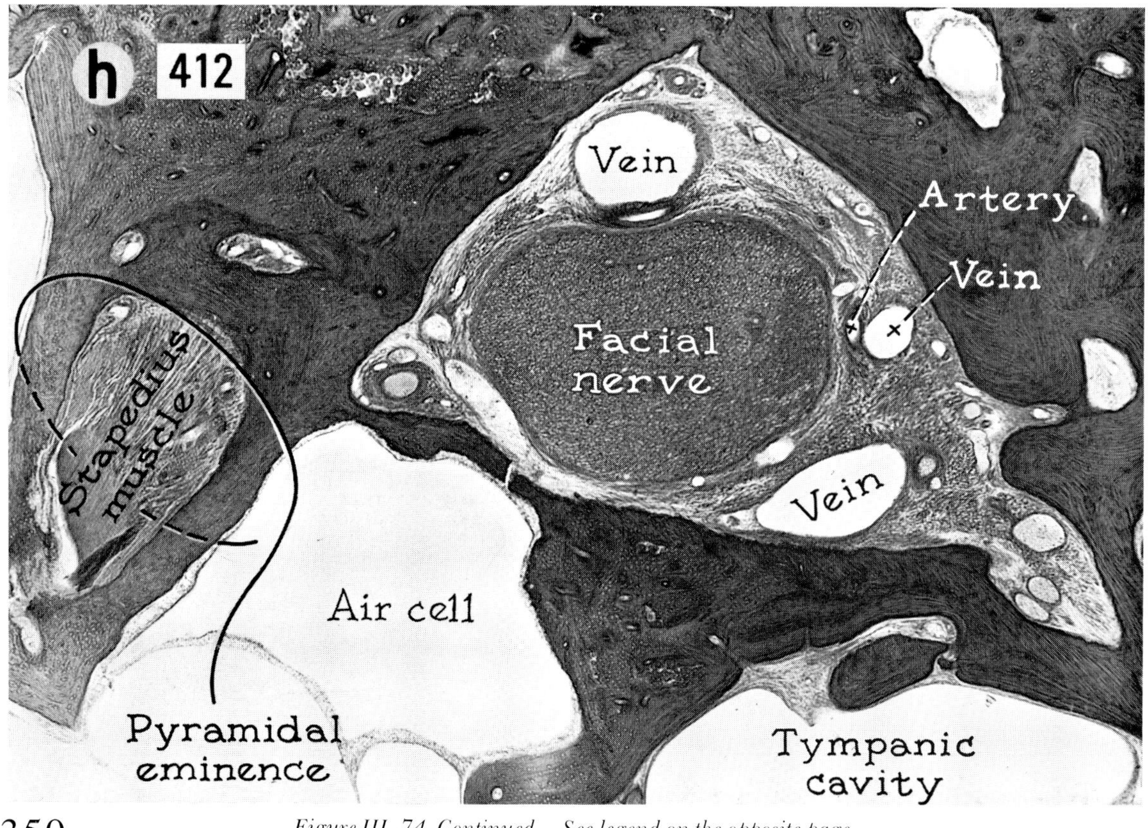

Figure III–74, Continued. See legend on the opposite page.

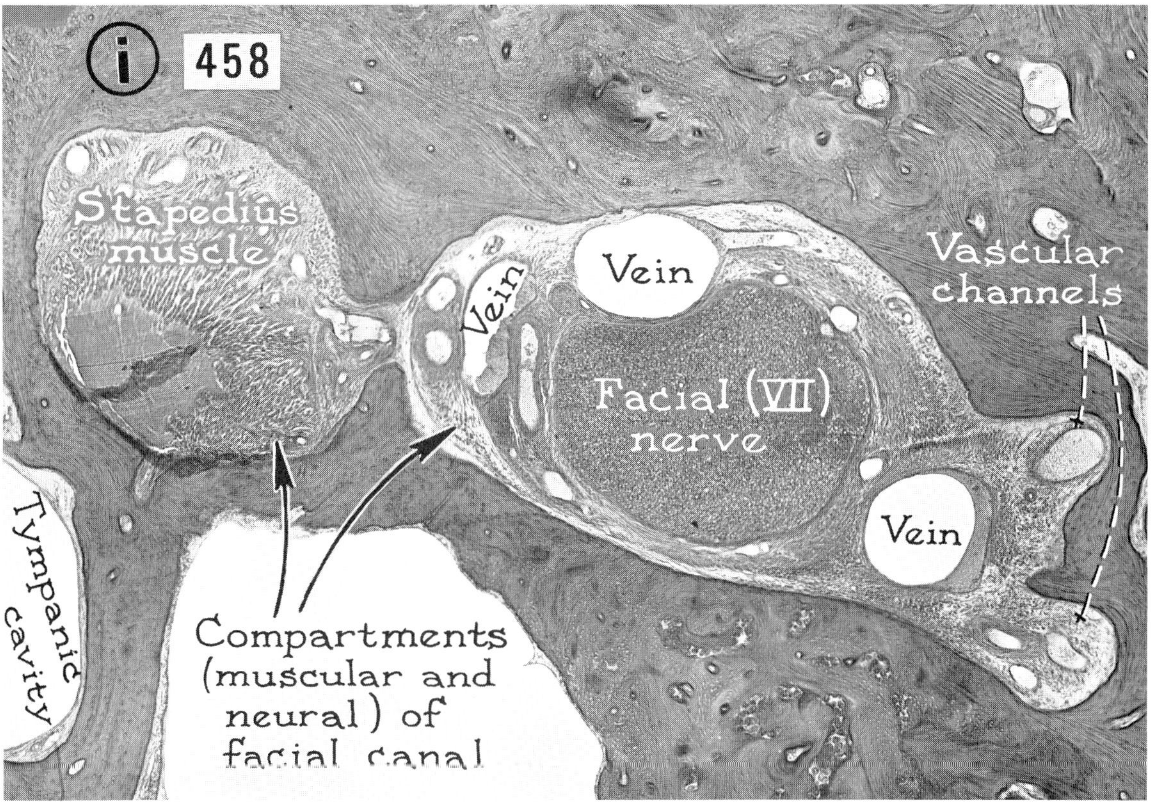

Figure III–74, Concluded. FACIAL CANAL, CONTENTS, AND RELATED ANATOMY: LEVELS IN SUCCESSION CAUDALWARD.

g. Vascularity becomes an even more arresting feature, as the canal nears the vertical part, owing, assumedly, to augmentation in supply from below, by the stylomastoid artery and the vein. At this level the circumneural plexus of veins surrounds more than one-half of the facial nerve. The supply is shared with the surrounding bone. It is shown that connections are made not only between the vessels in the canal (around the nerve) and those that supply the bone of the *pars petrosa* but also between the former and the auditory ossicles by way of the stapedius tendon (see reconstruction, Figure III–67).

h. At a level slightly below that of the section in the preceding figure, the arteries and veins with the canal appear to special advantage, as do their communications with vessels in the surrounding bone.

i. Resuming the demonstration of the histology of the canal and contents at selected levels, a third feature of structural importance becomes evident, namely, a compartmental arrangement of the space of the canal. The entire facial canal is subdivided into two "semicanals": one for the muscle, the other for the nerve and accompanying blood vessels.

Transverse sections, Wisconsin Collection, series 29, left ear. The section number in the series is recorded at the upper left in each photomicrograph. *a*, ×22; *b*, ×33; *c*, ×40; *d*, ×30; *e*, ×42; *f*, ×37; *g*, ×39; *h*, ×36; *i*, ×40.

(*a* to *i* from Anson, Donaldson, Warpeha, Rensink, and Shilling: Arch. Otolaryng., 97:201–213, 1973.)

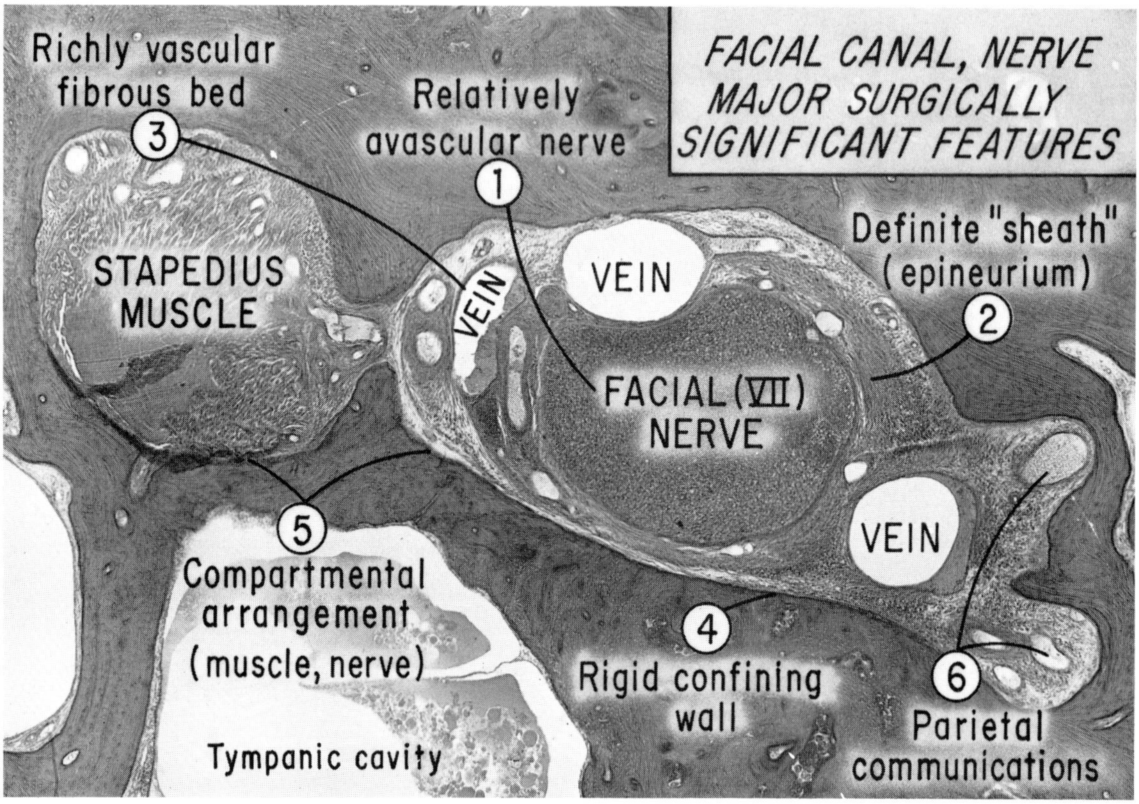

Figure III–75. DEMONSTRATING SIX STRUCTURAL FEATURES CONSIDERED TO BE IMPORTANT IN THE PATHOGENESIS AND SURGICAL CORRECTION OF BELL'S PALSY. ADULT, 19 YEARS OF AGE.

The six features are indicated by labels numbered in succession from the nerve to the tympanic cavity; that is, from within outward.

1. A relatively avascular nerve (in the normal state). *2.* A definite coat qualifying for the term "sheath" (at least, in the anatomical use of the term). *3.* A connective tissue layer between the periosteum (or endosteum) and epineurium, containing a rich arterial supply and an even more evident system of venous drainage consisting of large vessels that are constituents of a circumneural plexus. *4.* A wall of bone, the tortuous "rigid" canal. *5.* Division of the whole canal into compartments, meaning further complication in anatomic relationships. *6.* Vascular channels in the bone that bring the contents of the facial canal into close relationship with surrounding tissue of the petrous air cells and marrow spaces and of the mucous membrane that lines the middle ear cavity. *Note:* This summarizing illustration is section 458 of the set shown in Figure III–74. In representing a level below Figure III–74*h*, it serves to complete the craniocaudal set to a level below the pyramidal eminence.

Transverse section, Wisconsin Collection, series 29, left temporal bone. ×40.

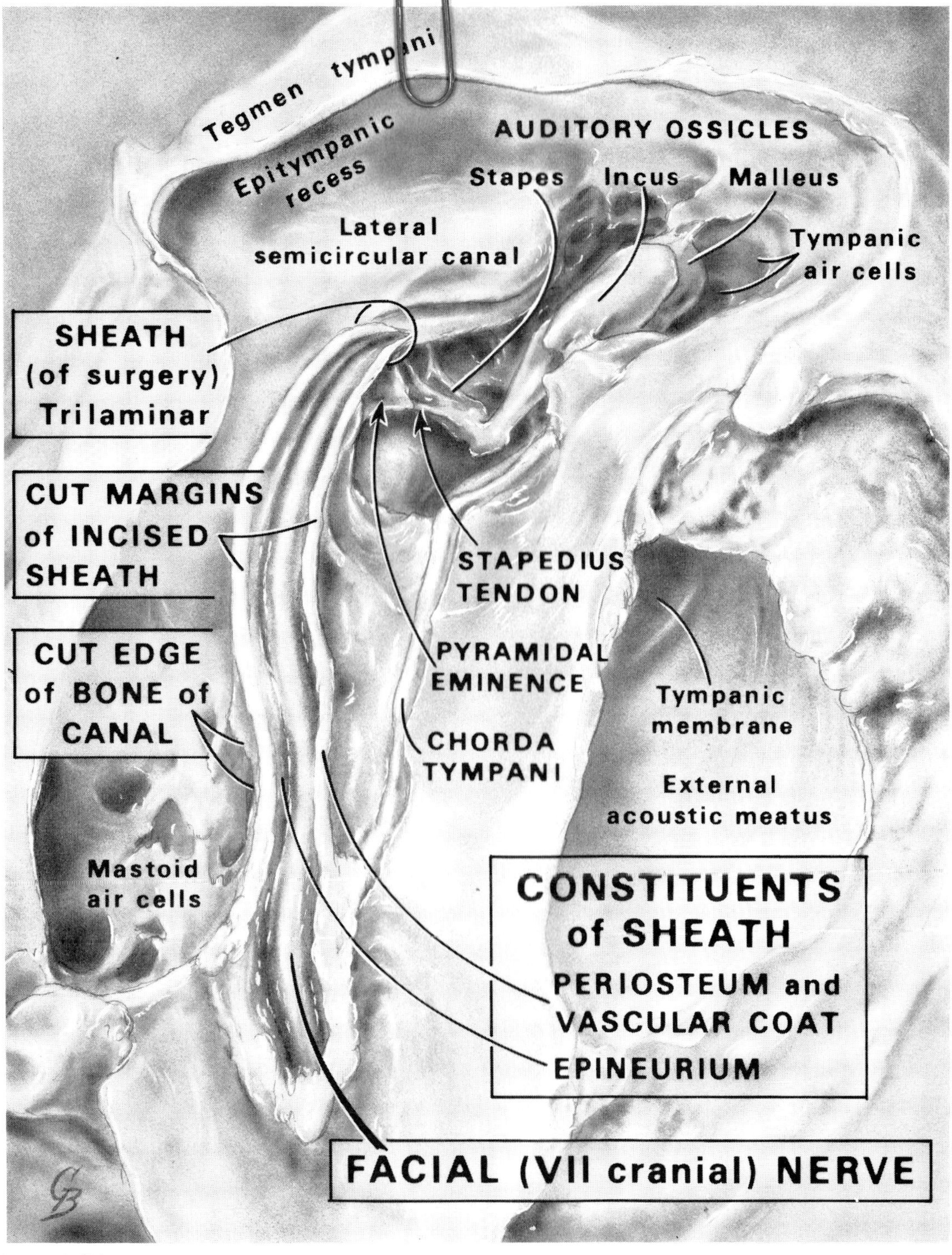

Figure III–76. FACIAL NERVE, ITS SHEATH, AND RELATED ANATOMY: DISSECTION OF AN UNEMBALMED SPECIMEN, LATERAL VIEW.

The sheath of the facial nerve has been exposed and incised lengthwise through most of its course from the level of junction of the horizontal segment with that of the vertical segment distalward to a point near the stylomastoid foramen. The sheath remains intact proximally toward the geniculum. The investments are shown as they constitute the "sheath" of otologic surgery.

The following additional features are demonstrated: course of the facial nerve above the vestibular (oval) window and stapes; presence of air cells in the labyrinthine wall of the tympanic cavity around the canal in its horizontal segment; course of the nerve in the posterior wall of the tympanic cavity where it is related to the mastoid air cells; and origin and course of the chorda tympani.

(From Anson, Donaldson, Warpeha, and Rensink: Ann. Otol., 79:710–727, 1970.)

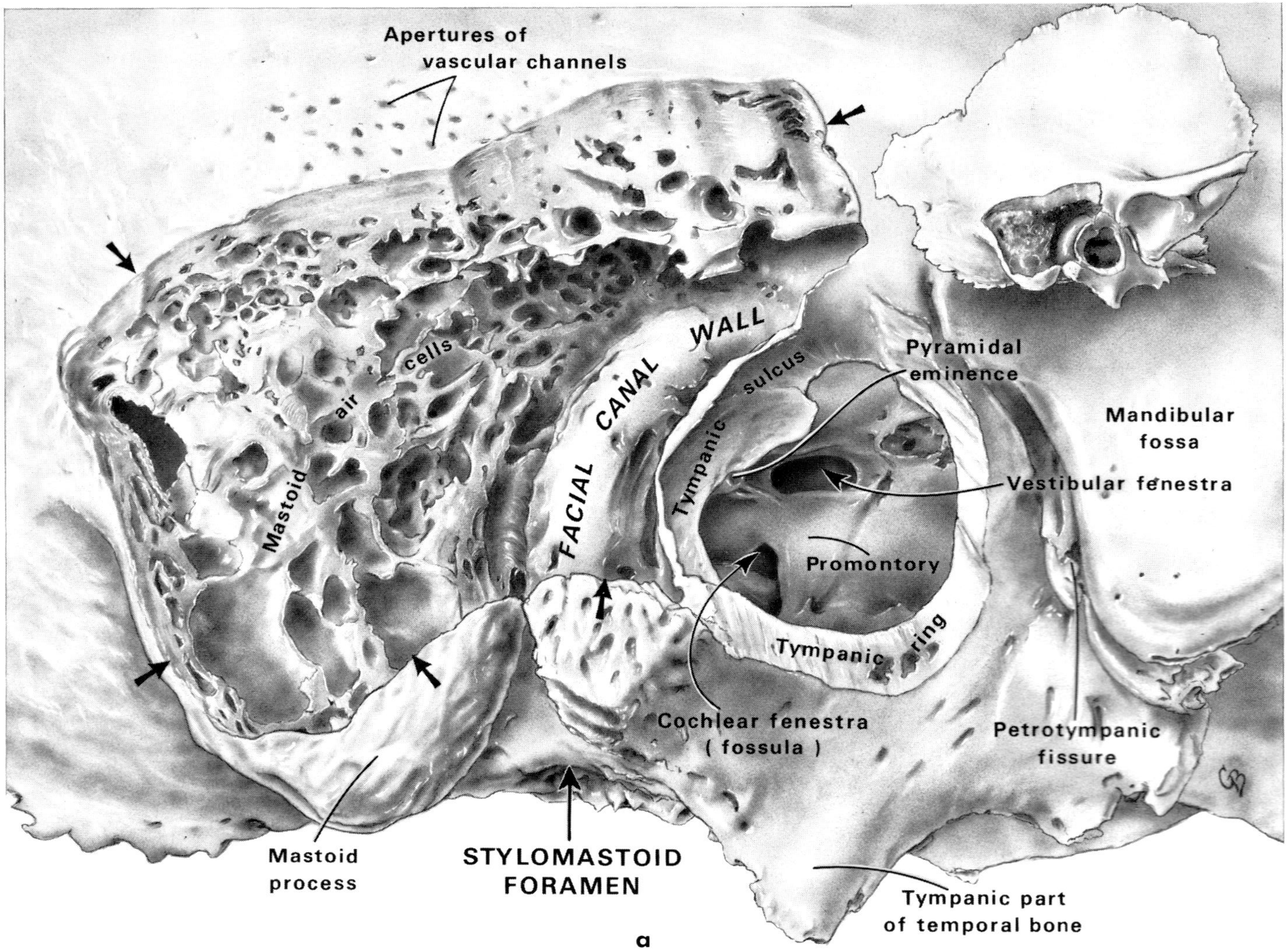

a

Figure III–77. TEMPORAL BONE: DISSECTION SHOWING THE LABYRINTHINE WALL OF THE MIDDLE EAR, TYMPANIC ANNULUS, AND MASTOID SPACES IN RELATION TO THE FACIAL CANAL. *Inset.* RECORDING THE AREA PICTURED IN THE MAIN FIGURE.

a. The vestibular (oval) window is evident in lateral view (seen through the ring); the cochlear (round) window lies concealed in a fossula. The facial canal descends to the stylomastoid foramen in the mastoid wall of the tympanic cavity. The air cells, extensively pneumatizing the mastoid process, are exposed. The curving course of the facial canal is demonstrated.

Dissection by Dr. Raymond L. Warpeha.

Figure III–77 continues on opposite page.

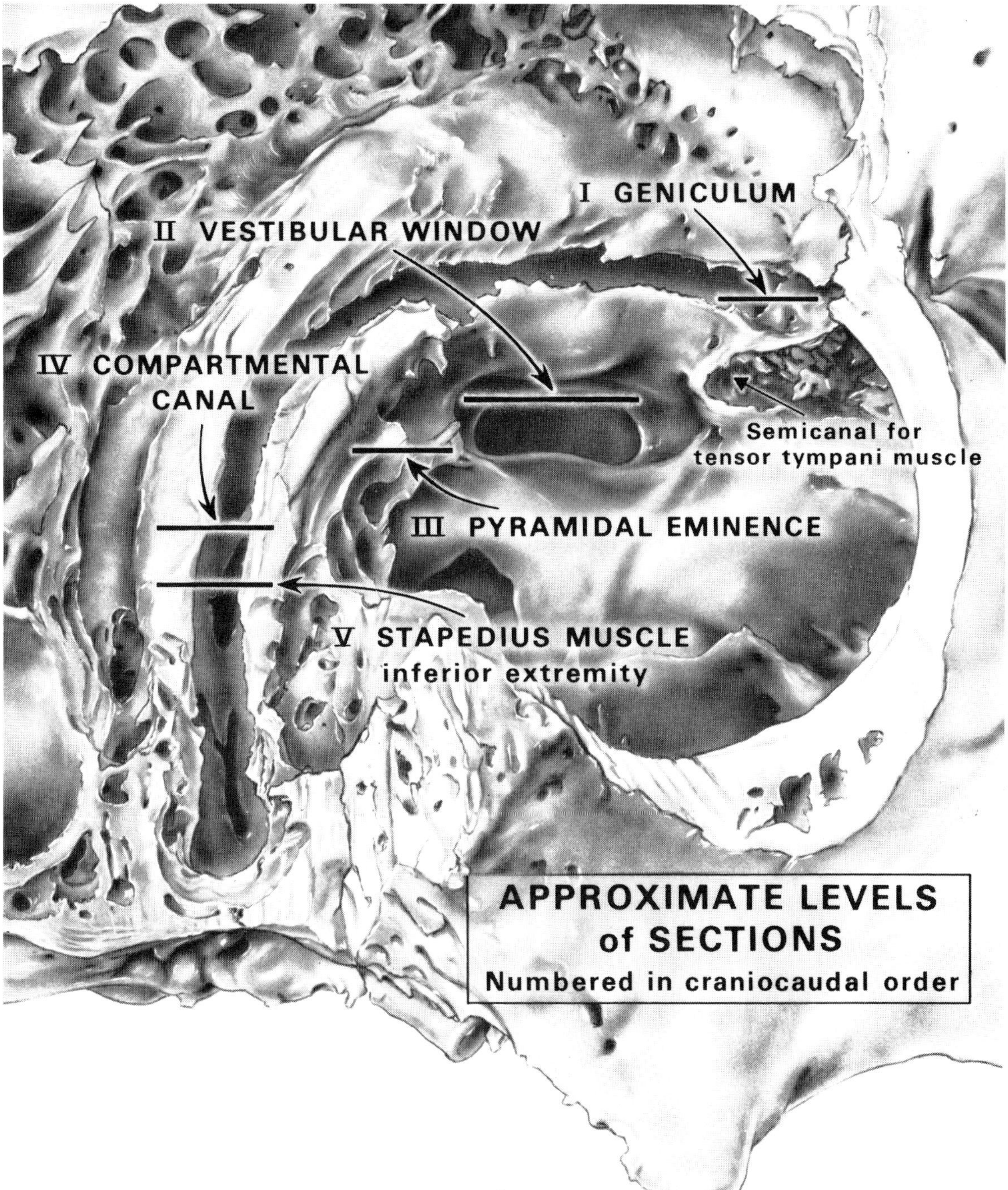

Figure III–77, Continued. FACIAL CANAL AND RELATED STRUCTURES, FROM THE LEVEL OF THE GENICULUM TO A POINT JUST ABOVE THE STYLOMASTOID FORAMEN.

b. The opened canal is shown as it arches over the vestibular (oval) window and descends in the mastoid wall of the tympanic cavity. The topographical markers (*I* to *V*) indicate the approximate levels of the transverse sections in the figures which follow.

Dissection by Dr. Raymond L. Warpeha.

(*b* from Anson, Donaldson, Warpeha, and Rensink: Ann. Otol., 79:710–727, 1970.)

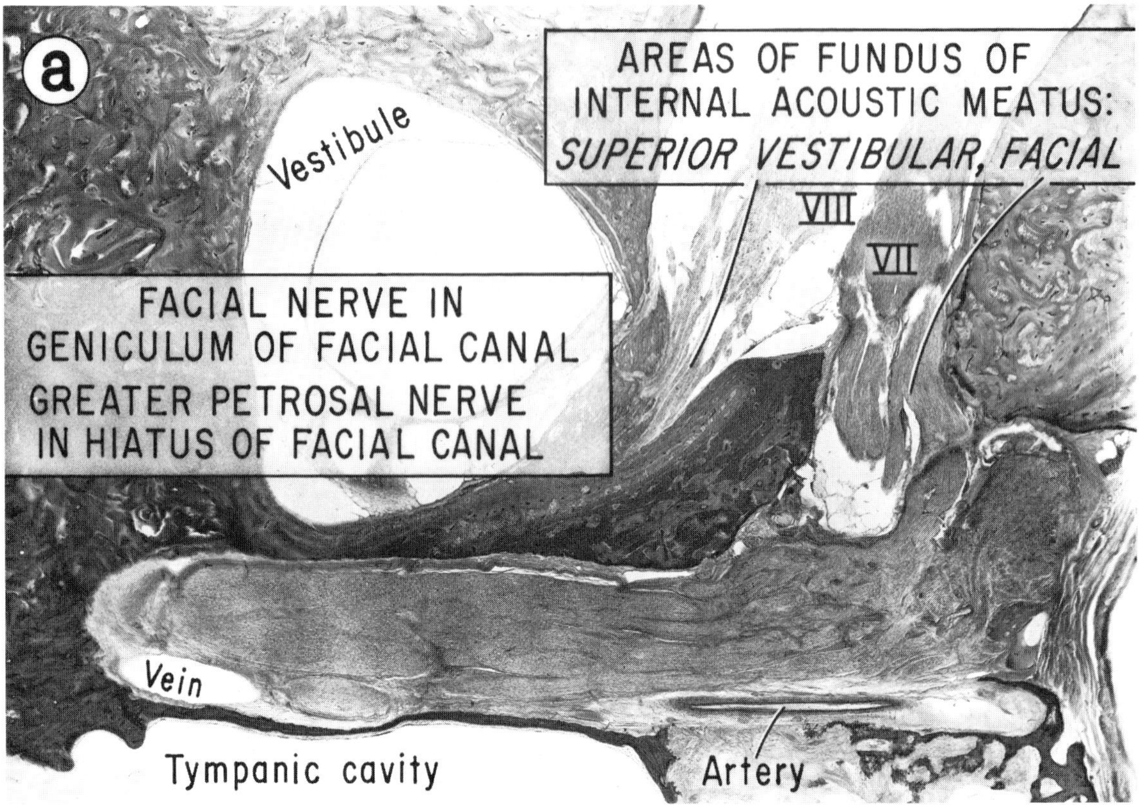

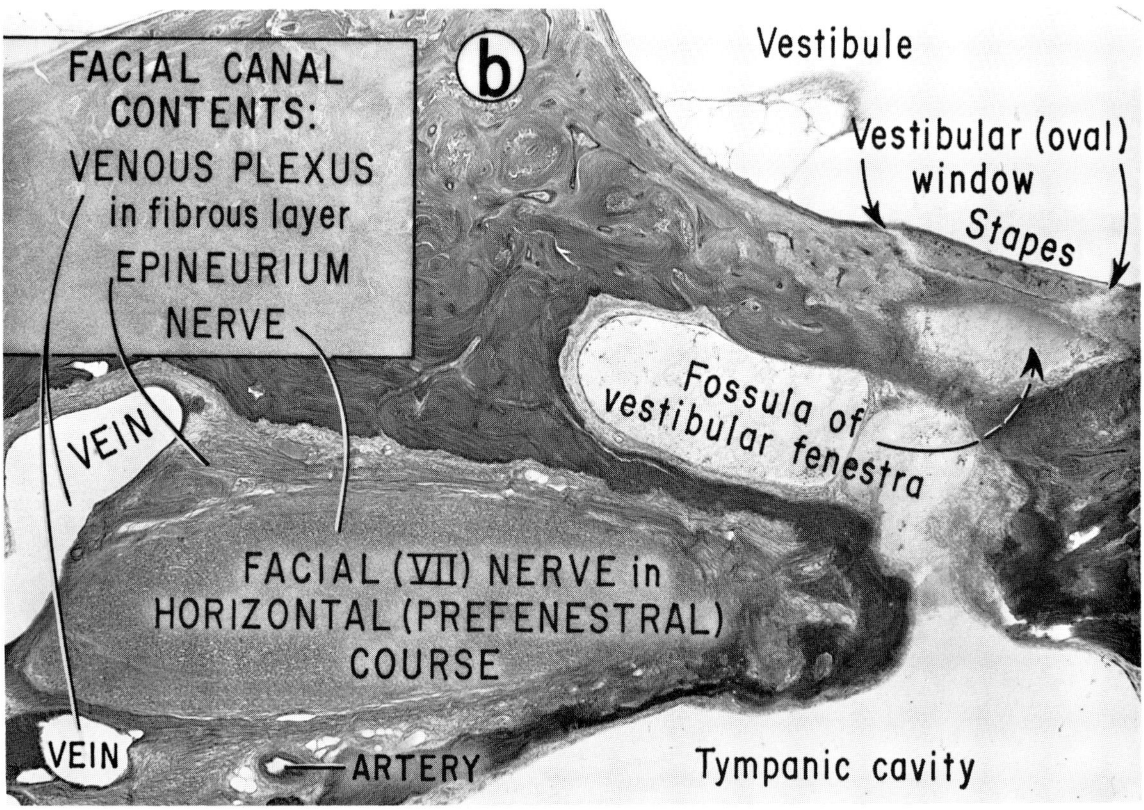

Figure III–78. See legend on the opposite page.

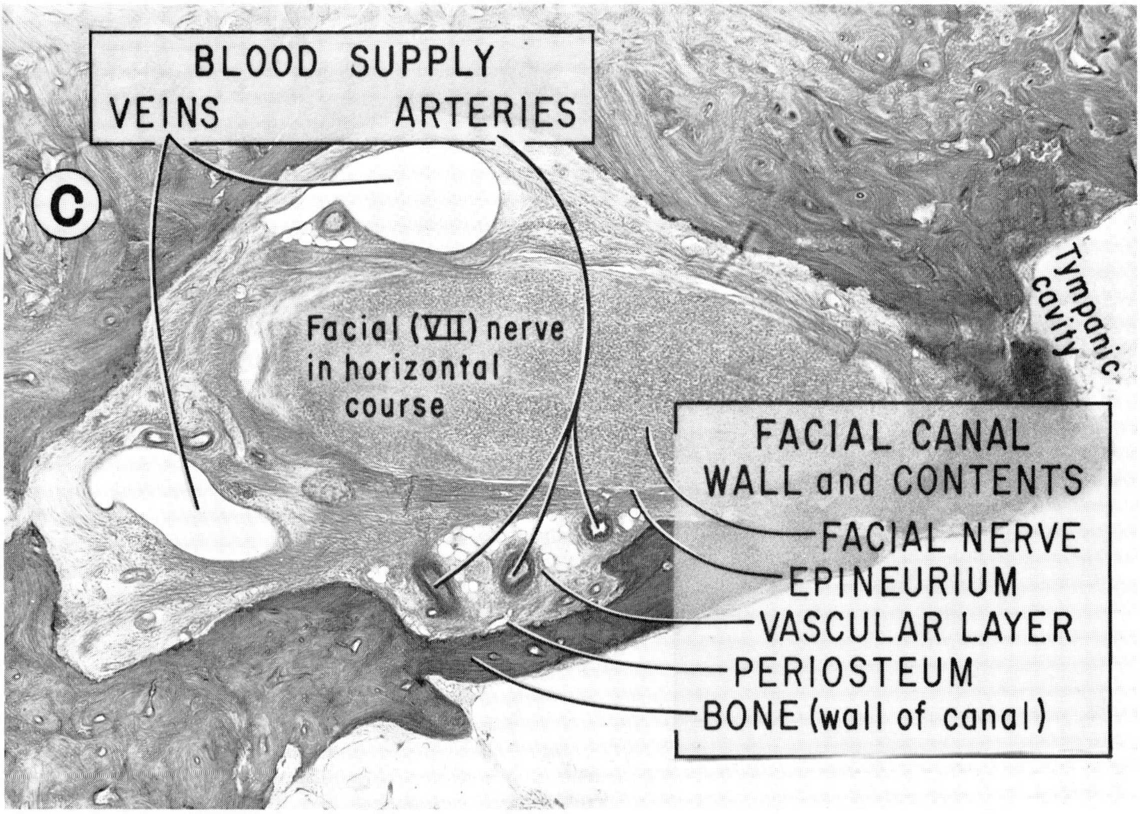

Figure III–78. FACIAL CANAL AND CONTENTS: TRANSVERSE SECTIONS IN CRANIOCAUDAL SUCCESSION. ADULT, 57 YEARS OF AGE.

a. Level I (section 285). The facial nerve (medial to the vestibule) courses horizontally from the geniculum, along the labyrinthine wall of the tympanic cavity. In this position, its branch, (at right), the greater (superficial) petrosal nerve, is entering the hiatus of the facial canal. The acoustic (VIII), or vestibulocochlear, nerve is passing through the foraminous partition that separates the superior vestibular area of the fundus of the internal acoustic meatus from the superior cribrose macula of the elliptical recess (on the wall of the vestibule).

b. Level II (section 330). Bending at a right angle, the facial nerve passes horizontally lateralward in front of the vestibular fenestra (oval window) and the latter's fossula. Here, as in fact throughout the course of the nerve, the surrounding connective tissue is richly vascular. Capacious veins (part of a circumneural plexus) accompany the smaller and less numerous arteries.

c. Level III (section 340). Continuing posteriorly, the nerve approaches the beginning of a curving course into vertical descent to the stylomastoid foramen on the inferior surface of the temporal bone. This level is cranial to that of the pyramidal eminence.

Figure III–78 continues on the following page.

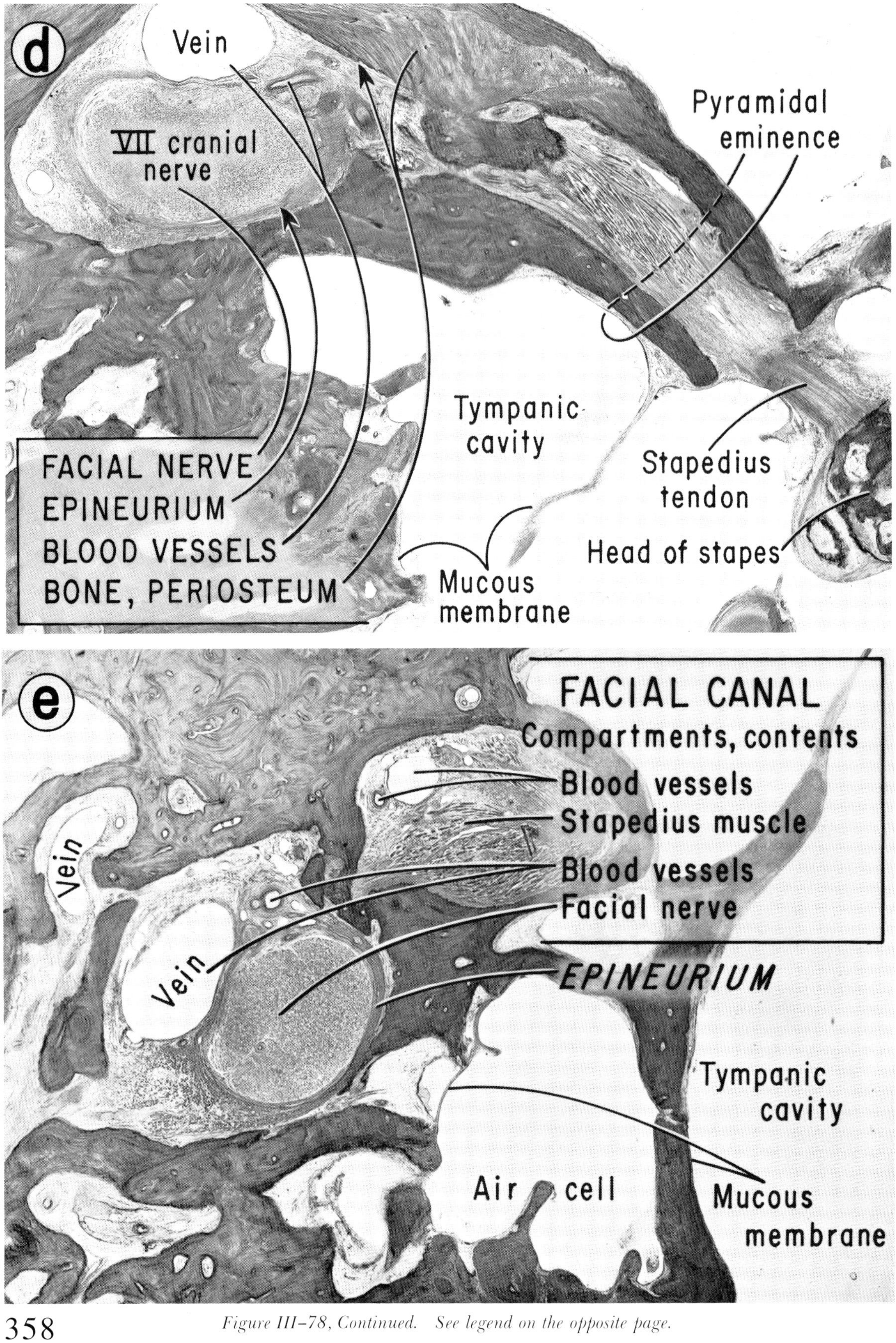

Figure III–78, Continued. See legend on the opposite page.

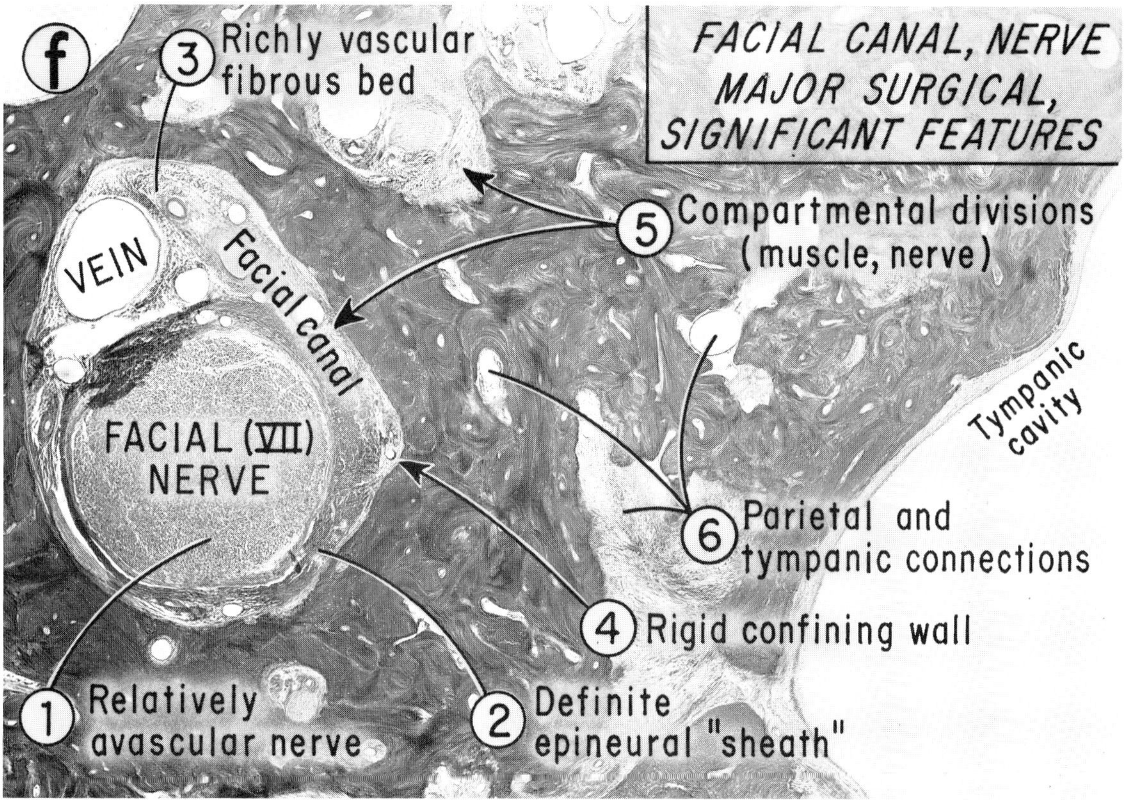

Figure III–78, Continued. FACIAL CANAL AND CONTENTS

d. Level IV (section 385). The stapedius muscle, having ascended through its special compartment in the facial canal, leaves the latter through the pyramidal eminence. At the tip of the eminence it emerges from the canal to cross the tympanic cavity (invested by mucous membrane) for an insertion on the head of the stapes. The facial nerve is enveloped in a definite epineural sheath. Between the epineurium and the periosteal lining of the osseous canal the space is occupied by vascular connective tissue. The veins are capacious, the arteries relatively small.

e. Level V (section 455). Just below the level of the pyramidal eminence the stapedius muscle and the facial nerve occupy separate compartments in the general space of the facial canal. Both nerve and muscle are lodged in vascular connective tissue. The wall of each compartment on its tympanic side (middle ear) is related to large air spaces. The blood vessels, at this and at more caudal levels, lie external to a fibrous sheath.

f. Below V (section 556). Approximately midlength in the intracapsular course of the stapedius, the compartmental arrangement is especially striking. The veins of the plexus are large, the sheath definite.

Transverse sections, Wisconsin Collection, series 32, right temporal bone. *a*, ×15; *b*, ×22; *c*, ×22; *d*, ×23; *e*, ×28; *f*, ×29.

(*a*, *b*, *d*, and *e* adapted from Anson, Donaldson, Warpeha, and Rensink: Ann. Otol., 79:710–727, 1970.)

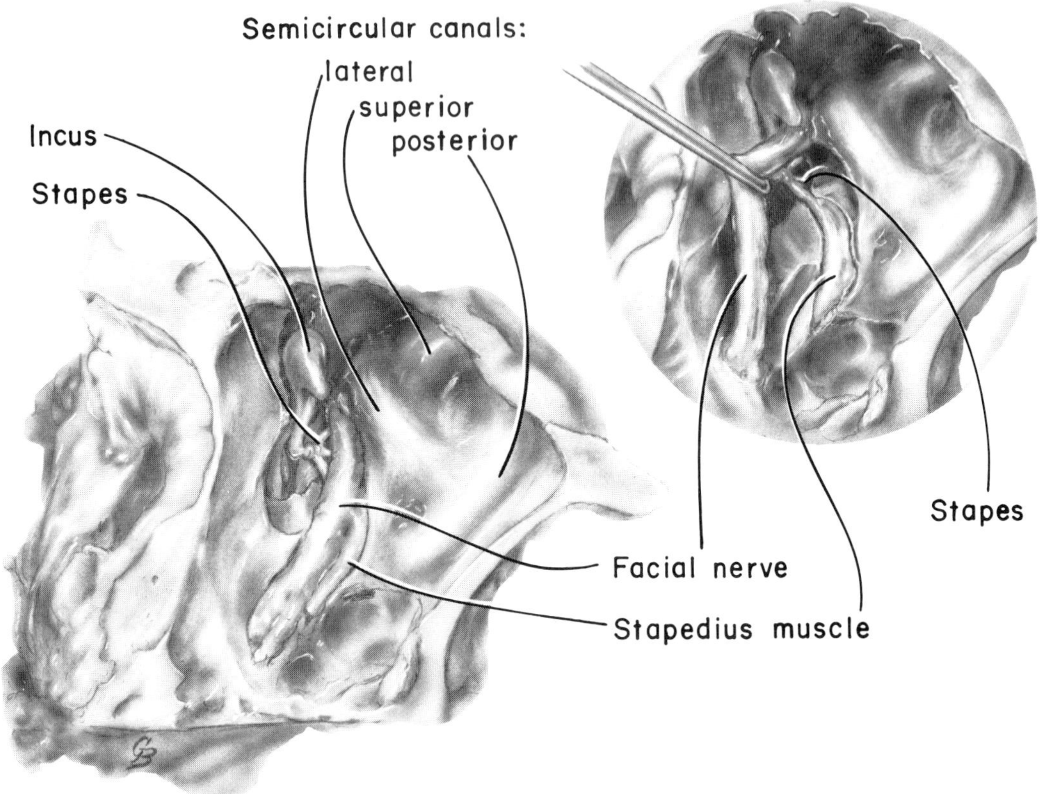

Figure III–79. FACIAL NERVE AND STAPEDIUS MUSCLE: DISSECTION OF AN UNEMBALMED SPECIMEN, LATERAL VIEW OF A LEFT TEMPORAL BONE.

The facial canal has been opened throughout its length, from the geniculum to the stylomastoid foramen. The contained nerve and the stapedius muscle are thereby exposed. In the figure to the lower left both structures lie *in situ*; in the illustration at the upper right the nerve has been retracted in order to show the muscle. The dissection is essentially a mastoidectomy, with access to the tympanum achieved by removing the facial sinus cells to expose the posterior sinus (suprapyramidal recess, facial sinus). In the specimen, the soft tissues of the external acoustic meatus remain at the reader's left; the bone at the lower right is the wall of the sigmoid sulcus (from which the vein has been removed). Below, the stylomastoid foramen is concealed by the digastric ridge.

The stapedial muscle occasionally lies anterior to the facial nerve in the canal. Usually it is medial to the nerve, from which it is separated by an incomplete partition (see section in Figure III–75). The lateral (or "horizontal") semicircular canal is directed lateralward and backward, forming the *prominentia* on the wall of the epitympanic recess. The other two canals run in approximately vertical planes. The superior canal gives rise to the *eminentia arcuata* on the anterior surface of the petrous pyramid; the posterior canal, longest of the three, lies almost parallel to the posterior surface of the pyramid.

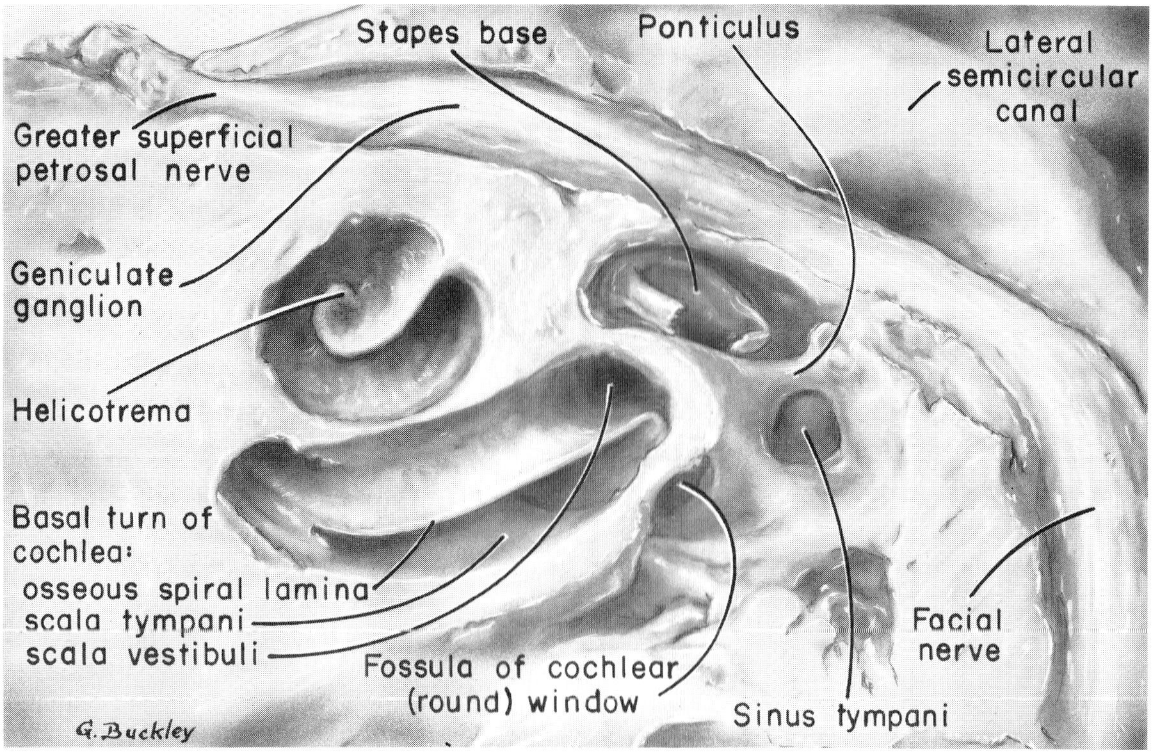

Figure III–80. THE RELATION OF THE FACIAL NERVE TO THE COCHLEA AND THE STAPES AND THE RELATION OF THE STAPES TO THE PONTICULUS AND THE TYMPANIC SINUS. DISSECTION OF AN UNEMBALMED SPECIMEN.

The facial canal has been opened, the stapes cut across the crura, and the scalae shown in the apical and basal coils. The facial nerve is shown in its horizontal and vertical portions (see description of the preceding figure). The ponticulus of the promontory, here shown in its medial part, connects the medial wall of the cavity with the pyramidal eminence. The tympanic sinus appears as a deep fossa on the medial wall of the tympanic cavity, just in front of and below the pyramidal eminence. Its space is continuous with the fossula of the cochlear (round) window.

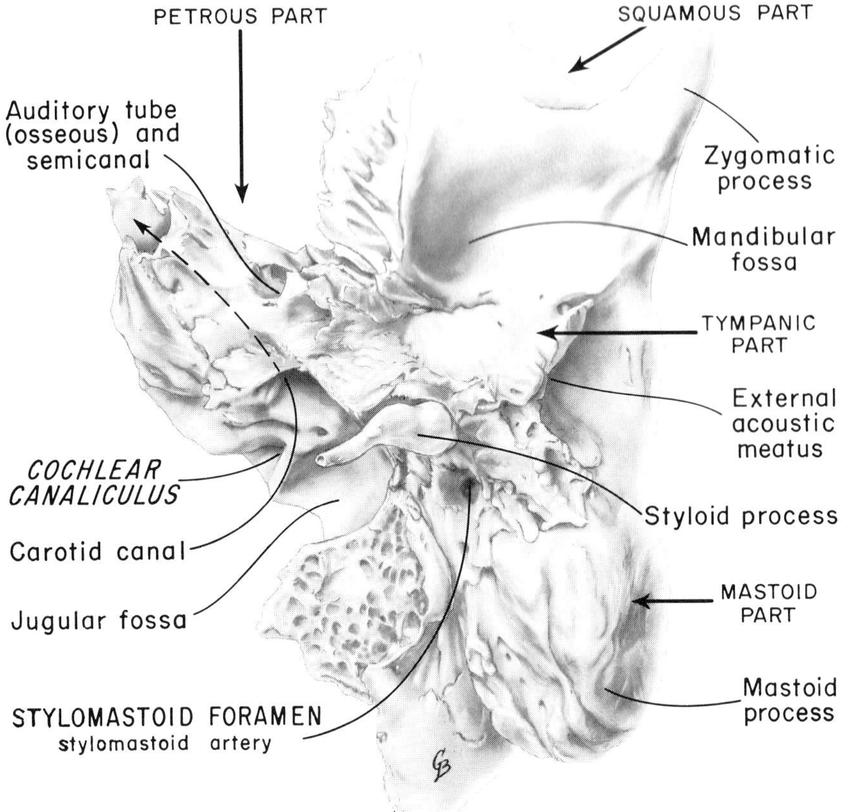

Figure III–81. STYLOMASTOID FORAMEN AND RELATED STRUCTURES. LEFT TEMPORAL BONE, INFERIOR SURFACE.

The stylomastoid foramen, for transmission of the facial nerve and stylomastoid vessels, is situated just behind the styloid process; the latter is partially covered in front by a sheathlike extension of the tympanic part of the temporal bone.

The thick, downward-directed mastoid process is situated to the lateral side and behind the foramen. It presents a smooth depression, the mastoid incisure, for attachment of the digastric muscle, and further medianward a sulcus for the occipital artery (see also Figure III–119).

The styloid process holds a topographically important position in relation to the jugular bulb and the carotid canal, being lateral to the former and posterior to the latter. In addition, it is just anterior to the stylomastoid foramen for transmission of the facial nerve. The process, when present, is shielded by a downward-directed portion of the tympanic part of the temporal bone. Contrary to common opinion, this osseous spine is undependable as a surgical landmark, since it was not only wholly absent in 58 of 150 cranial halves examined, but concealed by the *vagina processus styloidei* in more than 20 others—a length of approximately 1 cm. often being required to bring the process downward beyond the free edge of the sheath. The distribution is as follows: absence, 58; length from 0.1 to 0.9 cm., 18 processes; length from 1.0 to 1.9 cm., 40; from 2.0 to 2.9 cm., 19; from 3.0 to 3.9 cm., 14; from 4.0 to 4.2 cm. (maximum length), 1 process. It is, perhaps, important to add that bilateral dissimilarity is the rule in the matter of length; and in respect to absence, it may be recorded that in 18 skulls total absence was unilateral, while in 20 the styloid process was wanting on both sides.

RAMI OF FACIAL (VII) NERVE

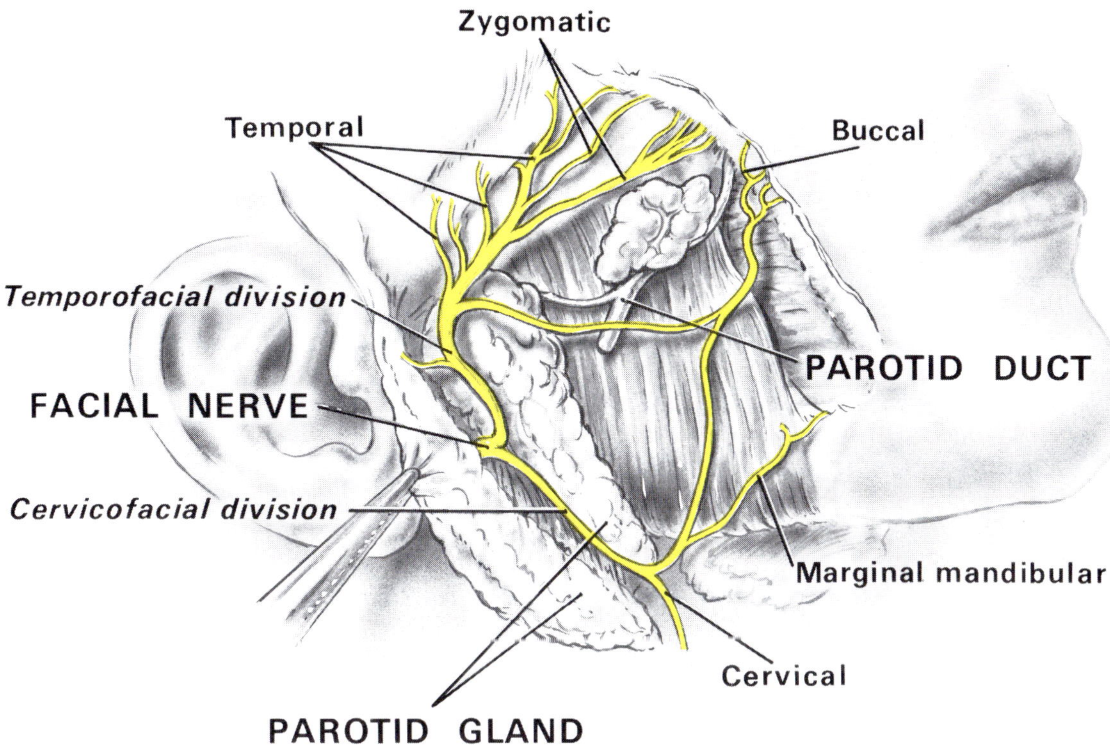

Figure III–82. FACIAL NERVE AND PAROTID GLAND: PATTERN OF DIVISION FOR INNERVATION OF THE FACIAL MUSCULATURE.

The main trunk of the facial nerve, upon emerging from the stylomastoid foramen, passes forward between the laminae of the parotid gland. Within the substance of the gland the trunk separates into temporofacial and cervicofacial divisions, which then branch into temporal, zygomatic, buccal, marginal mandibular, and cervical rami. Together they supply the muscles of facial expression, from the frontalis of the scalp to the platysma in the neck. Intercommunications are frequent and highly variable (see figure following).

Proximal to the point of ramification into the five large rami, the facial nerve gives off three, and sometimes four, small branches. One, the nerve to the stapedius muscle, arises before the nerve leaves the skull (in the facial canal); the other three are the posterior auricular, the nerve to the posterior belly of the digastric, and the lingual branch.

(Redrawn from Davis, Anson, Budinger, and Kurth: Surg. Gynec. Obstet., 102:384–412, 1956.)

Figure III–83. FACIAL NERVE: MAJOR TYPES OF BRANCHING AND INTERCOMMUNICATION, WITH PERCENTAGE OCCURRENCE OF EACH PATTERN. FROM RECORDS ON 350 CERVICOFACIAL HALVES.

Schematically shown, as of the right side of the head. Note that types III, IV, V, and VI together represent almost 70 per cent of specimens. *Type I*, Absence of anastomosis between the branches of the two divisions (temporofacial and cervicofacial) of the facial nerve; although regularly pictured, actually a least common type. *Type II*, Anastomoses within the temporofacial division. *Type III*, Anastomosis between chief divisions. *Type IV*, Two anastomotic loops within the temporofacial part. *Type V*, Two loops from the cervicofacial division, intertwined with branches of the temporofacial. *Type VI*, Extensive intermixture.

(From Davis, Anson, Budinger, and Kurth: Surg. Gynec. Obstet., 102:384–412, 1956.)

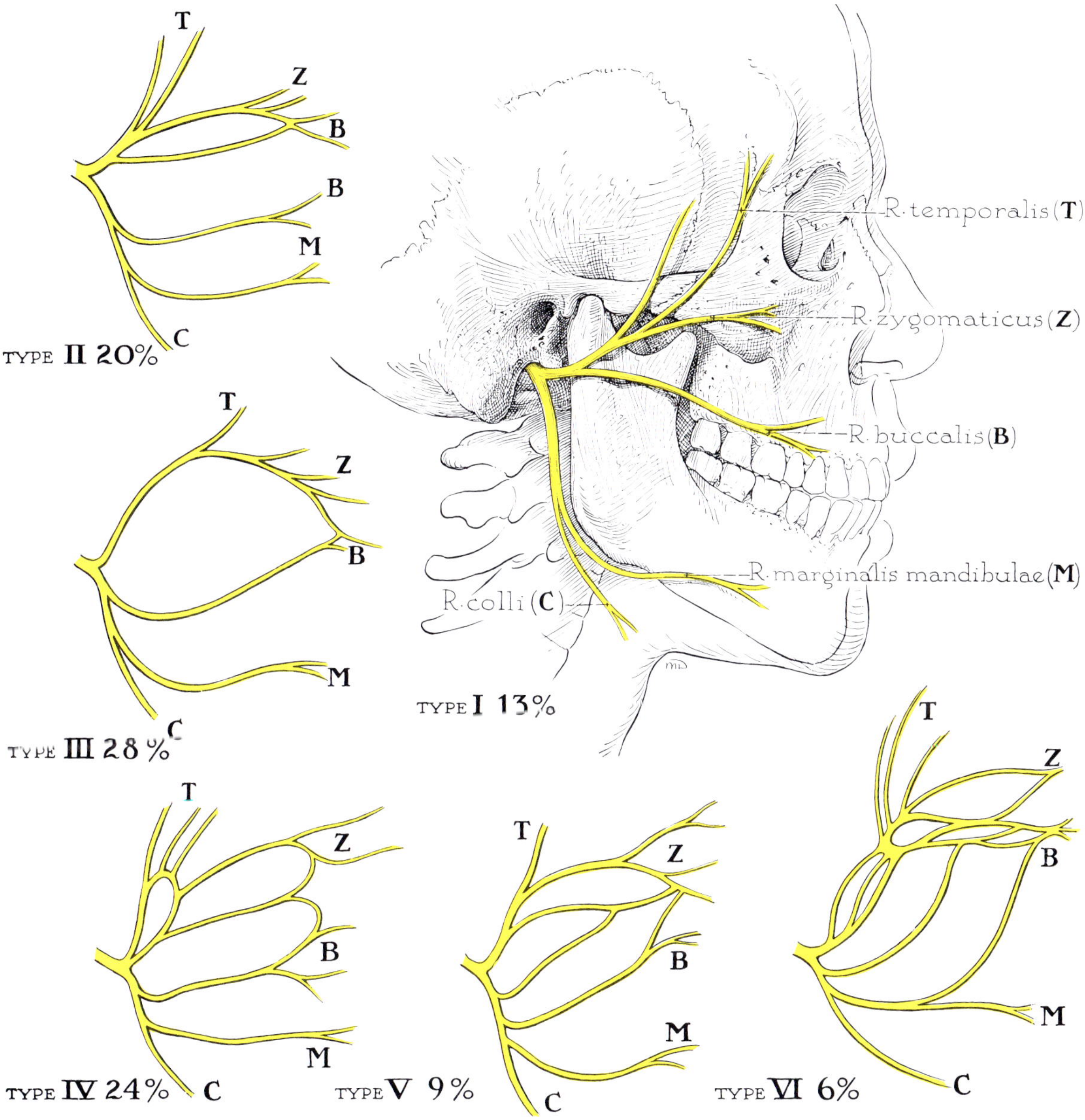

Figure III–83. See legend on the opposite page.

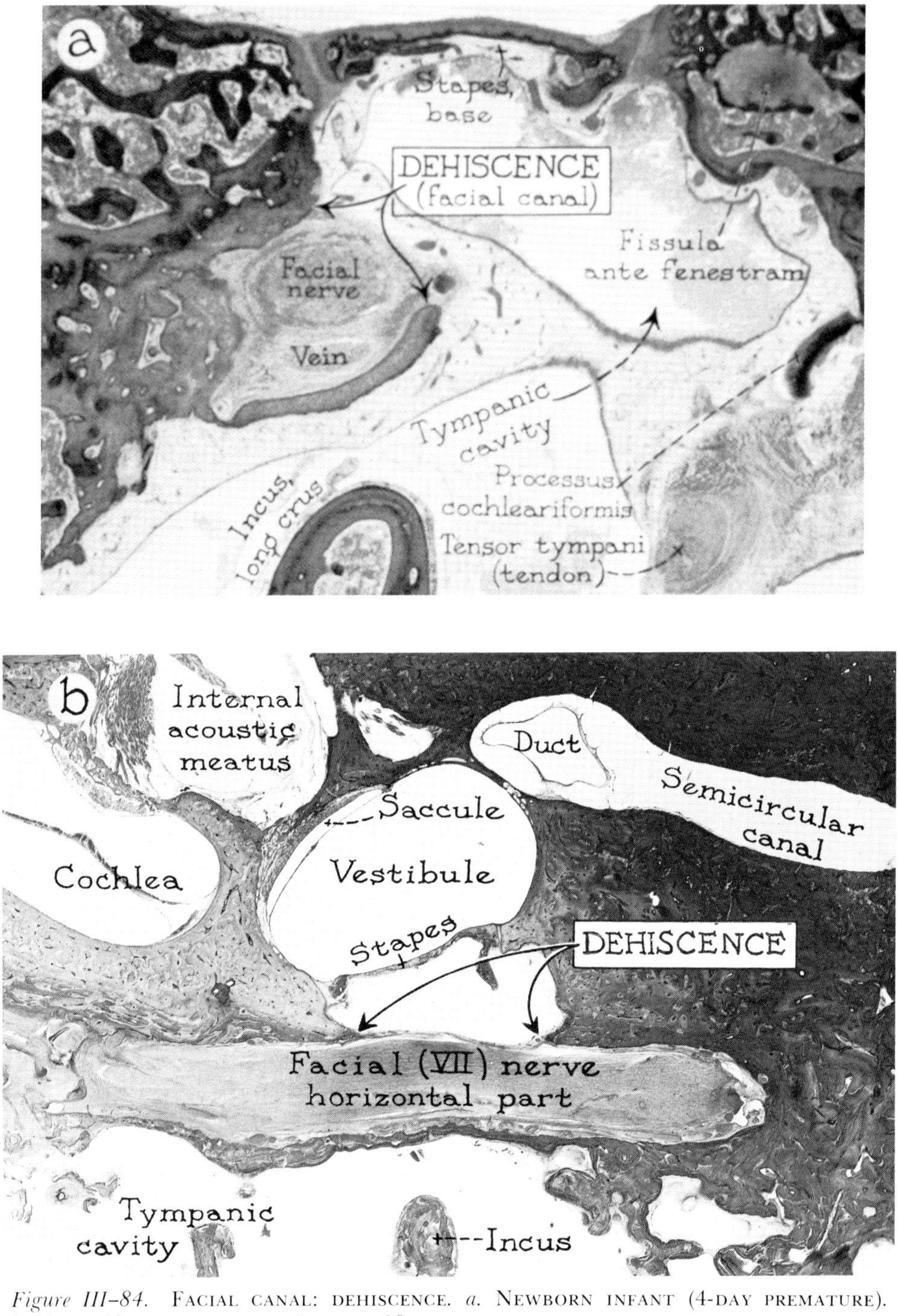

Figure III–84. FACIAL CANAL: DEHISCENCE. *a.* NEWBORN INFANT (4-DAY PREMATURE). *b.* MALE, 40 YEARS OF AGE. *c.* INFANT, 10 WEEKS OLD.

a. The wall is deficient in the vertical segment of its course, where it forms the posterior boundary of the fossula of the vestibular fenestra (stapes "niche").

b. Dehiscence in the horizontal segment, facing the vestibular window and the stapes.

Figure III–84 continues on the opposite page.

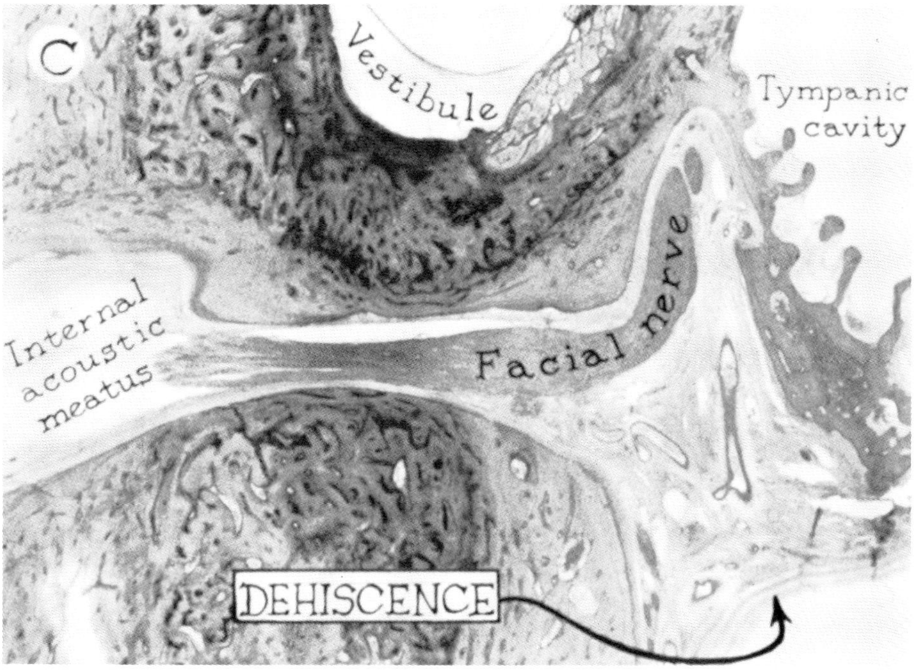

Figure III–84, Continued.
c. Defect in the hiatus of the facial canal.
Transverse sections, Wisconsin Collection, series 124, 18, and 83, respectively. *a*, ×24; *b*, ×11; *c*, ×20.

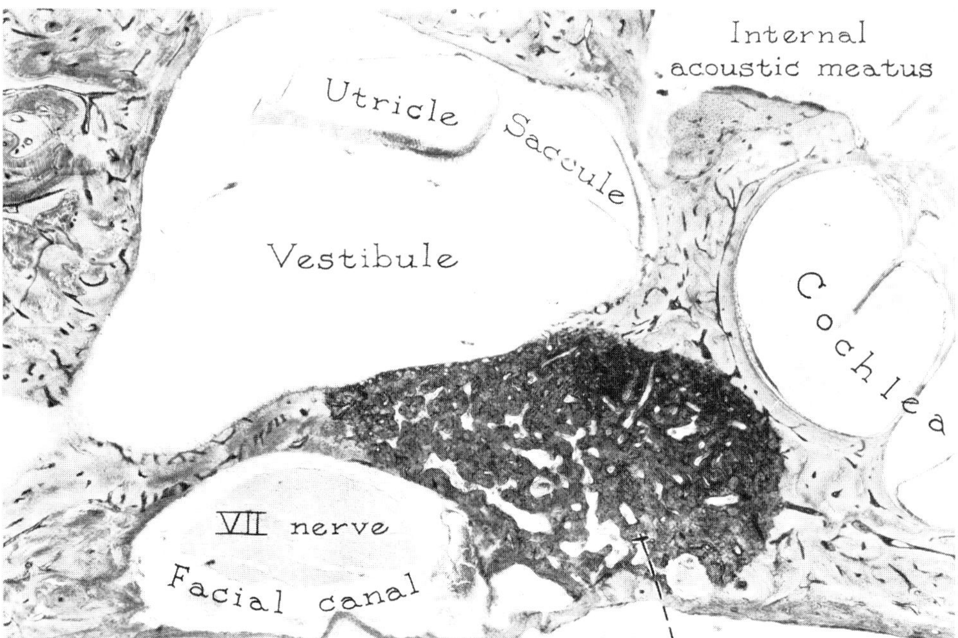

Figure III–85. FACIAL CANAL: OTOSCLEROSIS. MALE, 54 YEARS OF AGE.

In this case, the otosclerotic bone had replaced the normal bone of the anterior wall of the facial canal and the walls of the adjacent areas of the vestibule and of the tympanic cavity. The pathological bone replaced the middle, but not the inner, layer of the cochlear capsule (see laminae in Figures II–34, II–35, and III–88).

Transverse section, Iowa Collection, series 583. ×17.

(From Anson, Harper, and Warpeha: Ann. Otol., 72:713–734, 1963.)

Figure III–86. OSSEOUS LABYRINTH: A RECONSTRUCTION OF THE PERILYMPHATIC LABYRINTHINE SYSTEM, TO INCLUDE THE TRANSCAPSULAR APPENDAGES, LATERAL AND INFERIOR ASPECTS.

The bony labyrinth, here represented as the contained perilymphatic space, consists of three parts: the middle, the vestibule; the cochlear, situated anteromedially; and the three semicircular canals, placed posterolaterally in the petrous part of the temporal bone.

The vestibule is roughly oval-shaped. The medial wall (here toward the reader) forms part of the fundus of the internal meatus. Two deepened areas of unequal size are present on this wall; the posterior one, the elliptical recess, serves for reception of the utriculus (histological structure shown in Figure III–50); the anterior, smaller, rounded area, the spherical recess, receives the saccule (microscopic anatomy in Figure III–57*c*). In the latter the perforated area transmits the saccular branch of the vestibular nerve.

The bony semicircular canals are three curved tubes, each of which is continuous at two points with the space of the vestibule. The lateral, or "horizontal," canal produces the *prominentia* in the wall of the epitympanic recess. Its plane is not exactly horizontal. The other two canals run in approximately vertical planes. The superior canal stands at a right angle to the axis of the petrous pyramid; it gives rise to the *eminentia arcuata* on the anterior surface of the pyramid. The posterior canal lies almost parallel to the posterior surface of the pyramid. One of the two ends of each semicircular canal presents a flask-shaped enlargement, the osseous ampulla. The nonampullated ends of the superior and posterior canals unite to form a *crus commune.* The corresponding semicircular duct occupies the periphery of the canal (represented here by sulci between scalae).

The cochlea, or "snail," is cone-shaped with the axis placed horizontally. The base is directed towards the fundus of the internal acoustic meatus. It curls upon itself into about two and three-quarters turns. The basal turn projects into the tympanic cavity as the promontorium. The cochlear duct, like each of the semicircular ducts, occupies the outer aspect of each coil (here appearing as sulci).

In the macerated bone the space is continuous with four offsets, carried across the bone to the opposite surface of the pyramid. These appendages are the following: vestibular aqueduct, cochlear canaliculus (or aqueduct), fissula ante fenestram, and fossula post fenestram.

The histological features of these areas are illustrated in Figures III–108*a*, *b* (vestibular aqueduct); III–122*a* (cochlear aqueduct); III–90*a* and III–123*a* (fissula ante fenestram); and III–90*a* and III–123*b* (fossula post fenestram).

(From Anson, Harper, and Winch: Arch. Otolaryng., 85:497–514, 1967.)

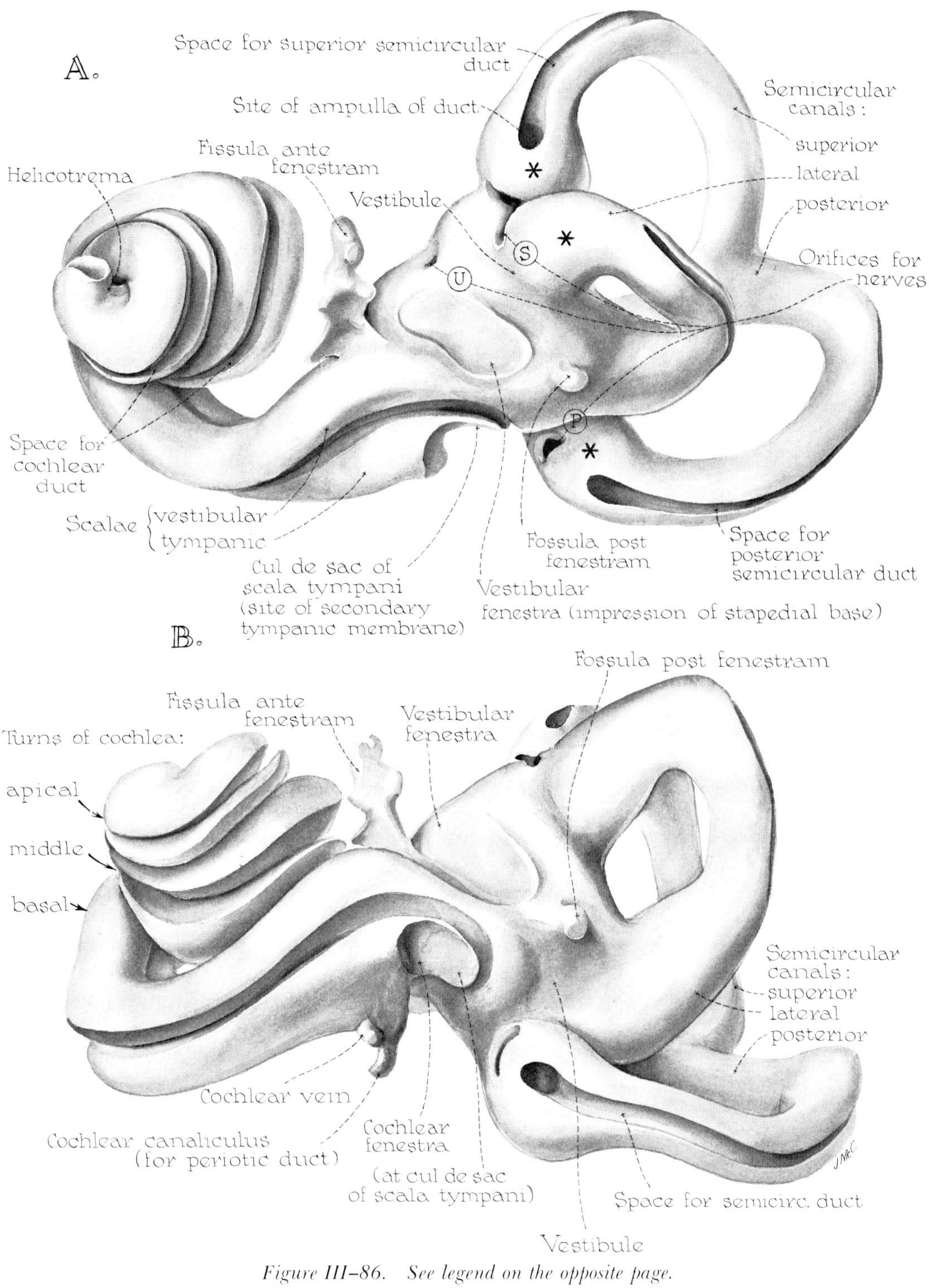

Figure III–86. See legend on the opposite page.

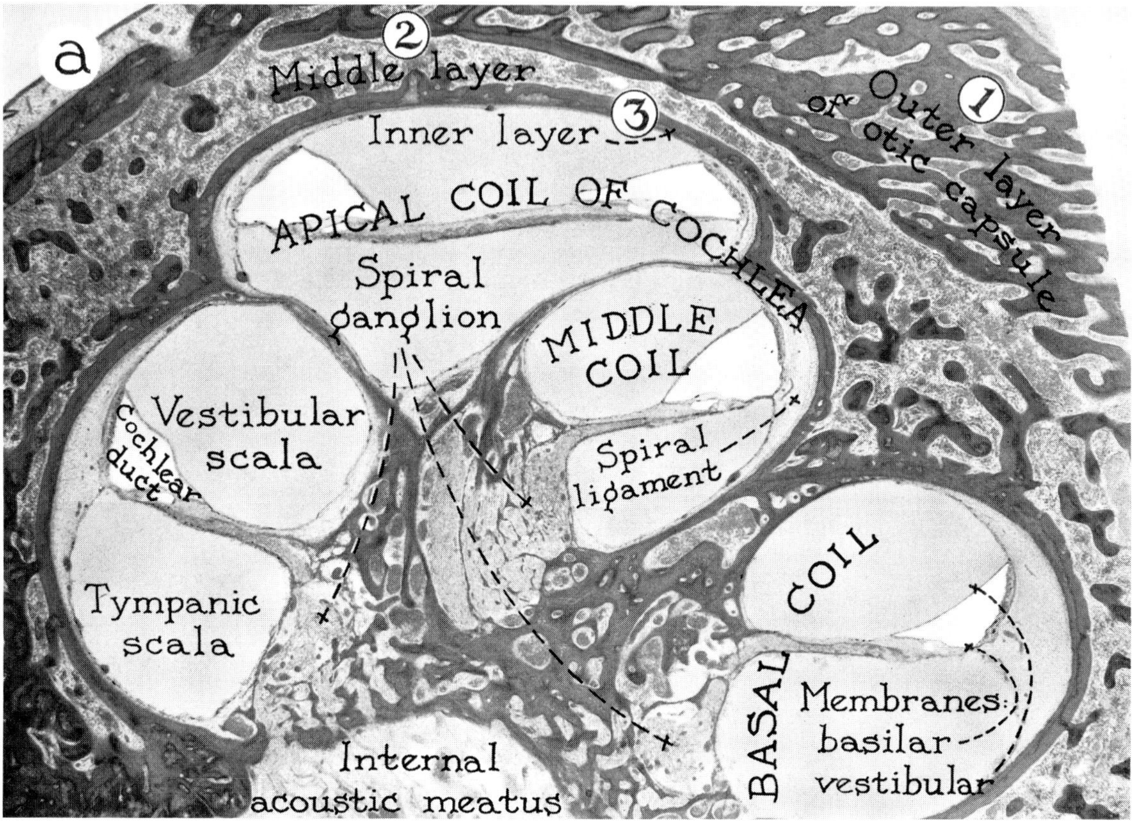

Figure III–87. OSSEOUS LABYRINTH, CONTAINED PERILYMPHATIC SYSTEM OF INTERCOMMUNICATING SPACES. *a.* NEWBORN (4-DAY PREMATURE). *b* and *c.* INFANT, 10 WEEKS OF AGE. *d.* INFANT, 6 MONTHS OLD.

a. A section through the cochlear turns; the scalae in comparison with the cochlear duct. The inner periosteal layer (at *3*) is the immediate skeletal boundary of the perilymphatic labyrinthine system. It is internal to the middle lamina (at *2*), which is invested by the outer periosteal layer (at *1*) of the trilaminar capsule (see developmental stages, Figure III–88).

Figure III–87 continues on the opposite page.

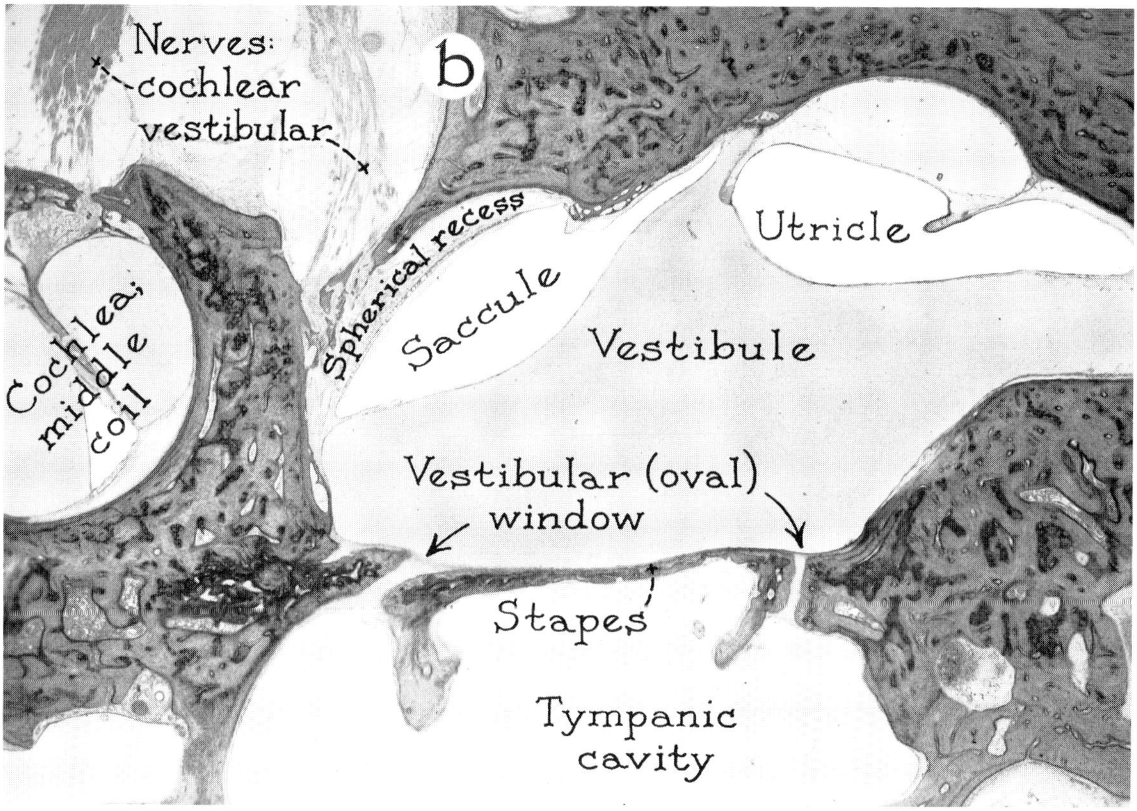

Figure III–87, Continued.

b. A section at the horizontal level of the vestibular fenestra and the vestibular division of the osseous labyrinth, demonstrating the capacity of perilymphatic space in comparison with that of the saccule and utricle.

Figure III–87 continues on the following page.

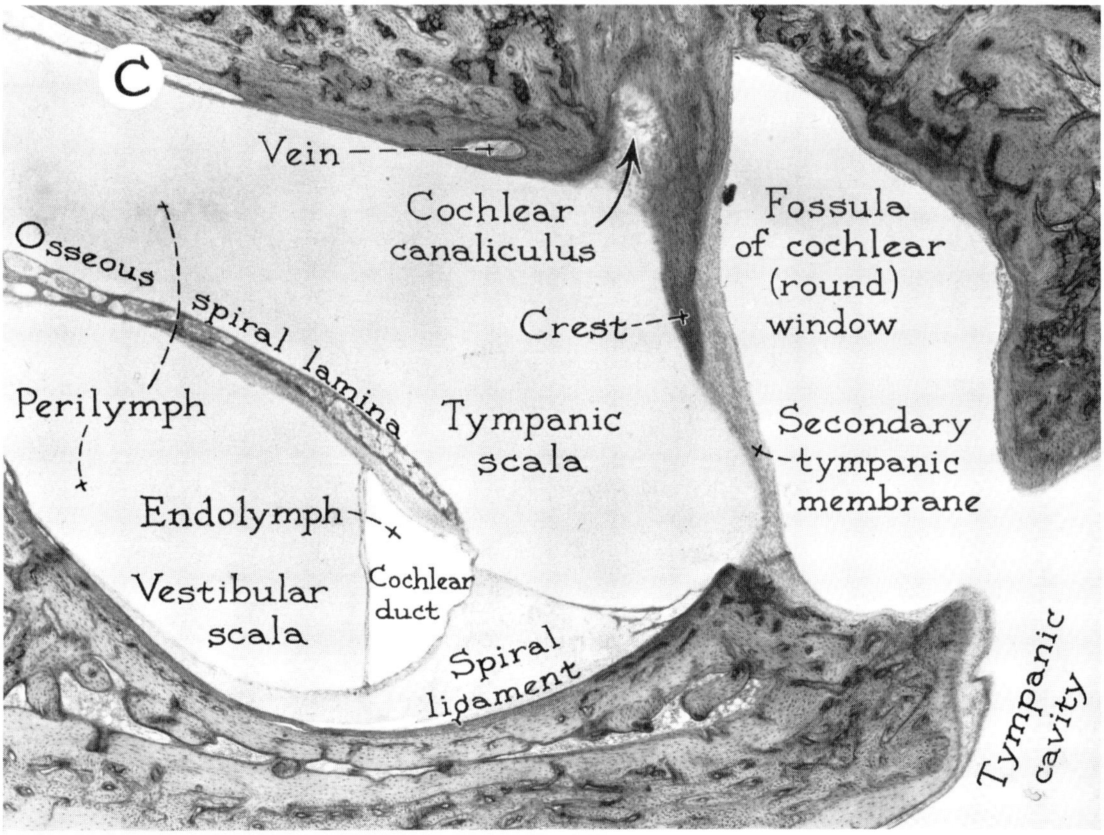

Figure III–87, Continued. OSSEOUS LABYRINTH, CONTAINED PERILYMPHATIC SYSTEM OF INTERCOMMUNICATING SPACES. *a.* NEWBORN (4-DAY PREMATURE). *b* and *c.* INFANT, 10 WEEKS OF AGE. *d.* INFANT, 6 MONTHS OLD.

c. A section through the basal turn of the cochlea, emphasizing the relatively great capacity of the tympanic scala in comparison with that of the cochlear duct.

Figure III–87 continues on the opposite page.

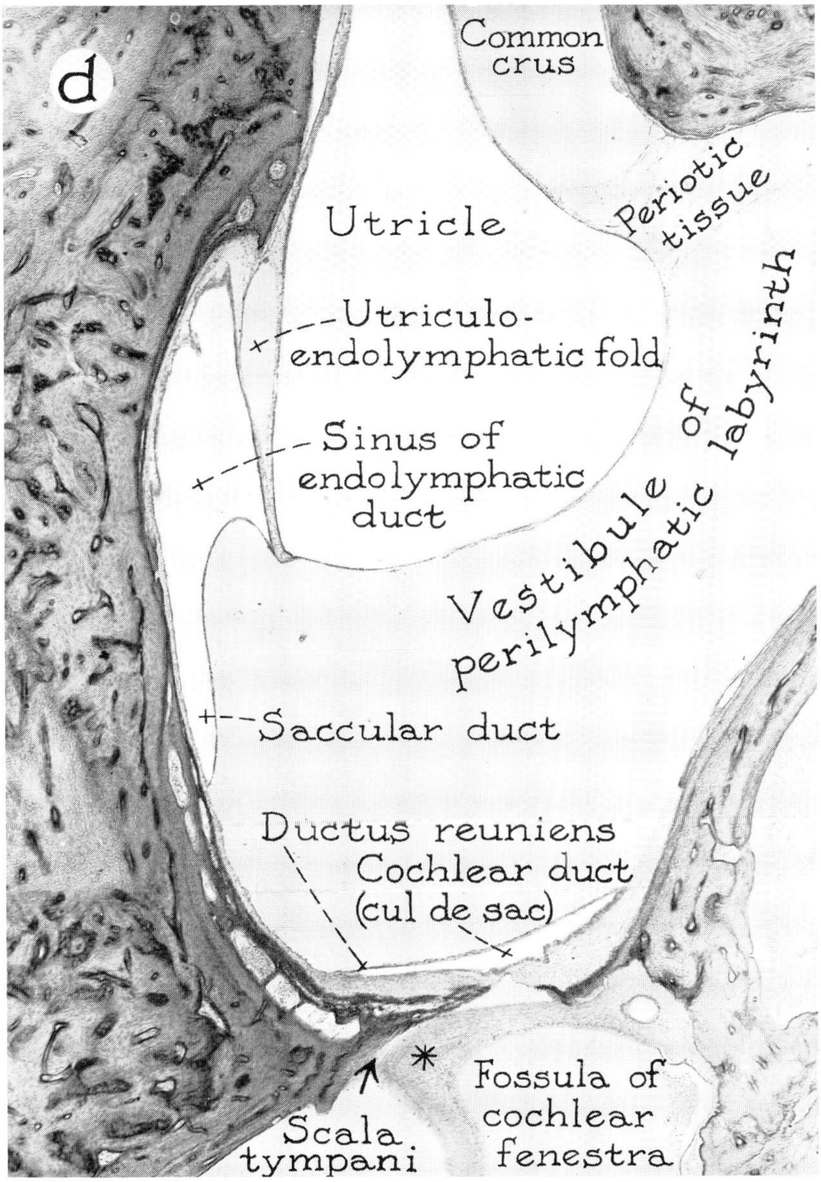

Figure III–87, Concluded.

d. A section at the level of the cochlear fenestra, demonstrating relative capacities. Asterisk indicates secondary tympanic membrane. The membrane does not have the form of a flattened diaphragm; rather, that of the flexed hand with the concavity facing the fossula.

Explanatory Note: The labyrinthine spaces have been emphasized by use of the air brush; the lumen of the membranous duct system has been whitened, the surrounding osseous labyrinth darkened.

Transverse sections, Wisconsin Collection, series as follows: *a*, 124; *b* and *c*, 83; *d*, 121. *a*, ×19; *b*, ×23; *c*, ×30; *d*, ×32.

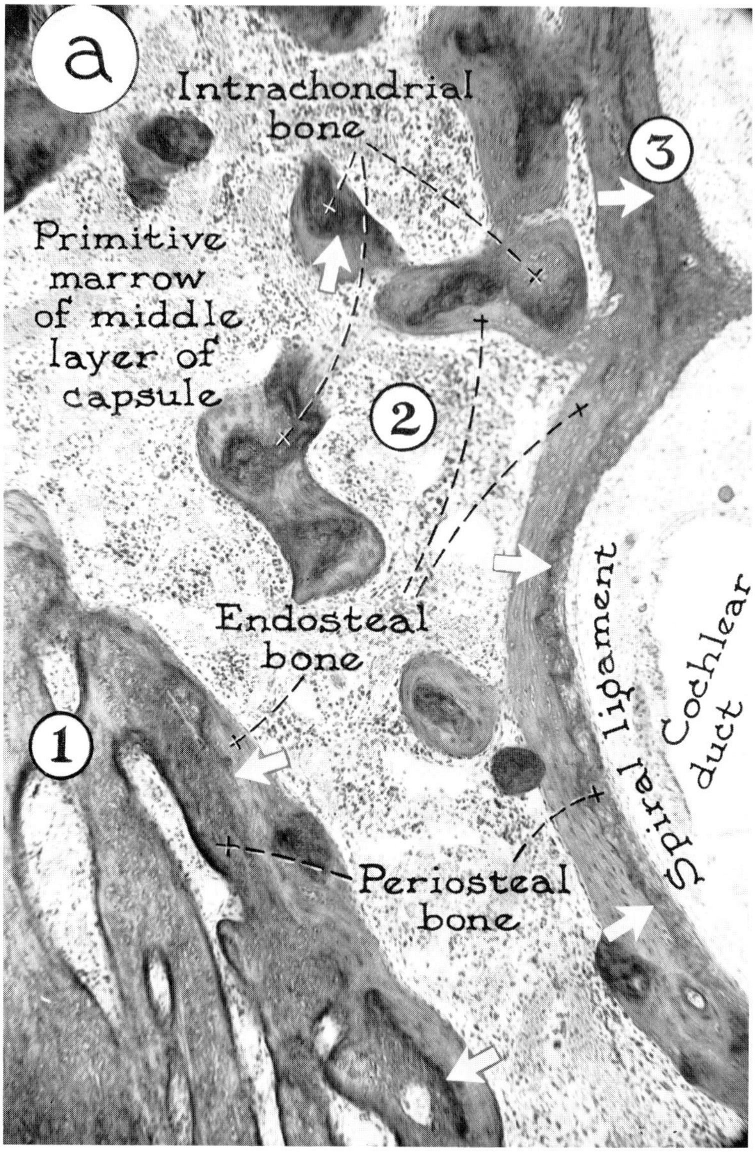

Figure III–88. OSSEOUS WALL OF THE COCHLEA: TRILAMINAR ARCHITECTURE, REPRESENTATIVE OF THE OTIC CAPSULE GENERALLY. *a*. NEWBORN (4-DAY PREMATURE). *b*. FETUS AT TERM. *c*. INFANT OF 4 MONTHS.

a. In neonatal and in late fetal specimens the immediate wall of the labyrinthine system of spaces is the maturing inner periosteal layer of bone (at *3*) to the outer surface of which endosteal bone has been deposited (to the depth indicated by the unlabeled arrows, reader's right). In the middle layer (at *2*) marrow still outbulks bone, the latter consisting of "cartilage islands" (intrachondrial bone) upon which endosteal bone has been deposited (arrow, upper middle of the field). Endosteal bone is also deposited on the inner surface of the outer periosteal layer (at *1*, to the depth of the unlabeled arrows).

b. Continuing deposition of endosteal tissue results in histological approach to a petrous consistency, with scattered areas of persisting marrow.

c. In early postnatal stages, the capsule has attained architectural maturity as the core of the *pars petrosa*.

Note: The steps in morphogenesis of the otic capsule have been followed in Part II (Figures II–5, 6, 34, 35, and 37). In addition, the same feature is illustrated in Figure III–88*c*, in order further to emphasize the extent to which the trilaminar layering of the fetal capsule (established in the 20-week stage) is retained in the *pars petrosa* of the adult ear.

Transverse sections, Wisconsin Collection, series 124, 102, and 119, respectively. *a*, ×227; *b*, ×86; *c*, ×42.

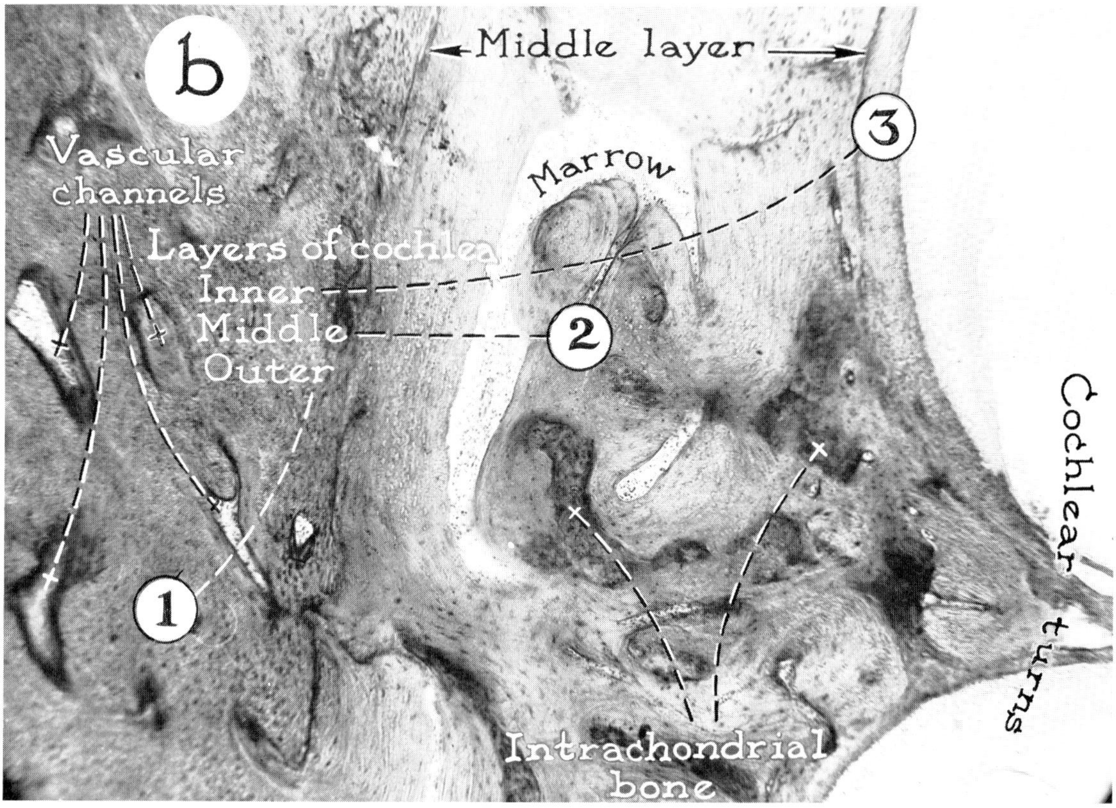

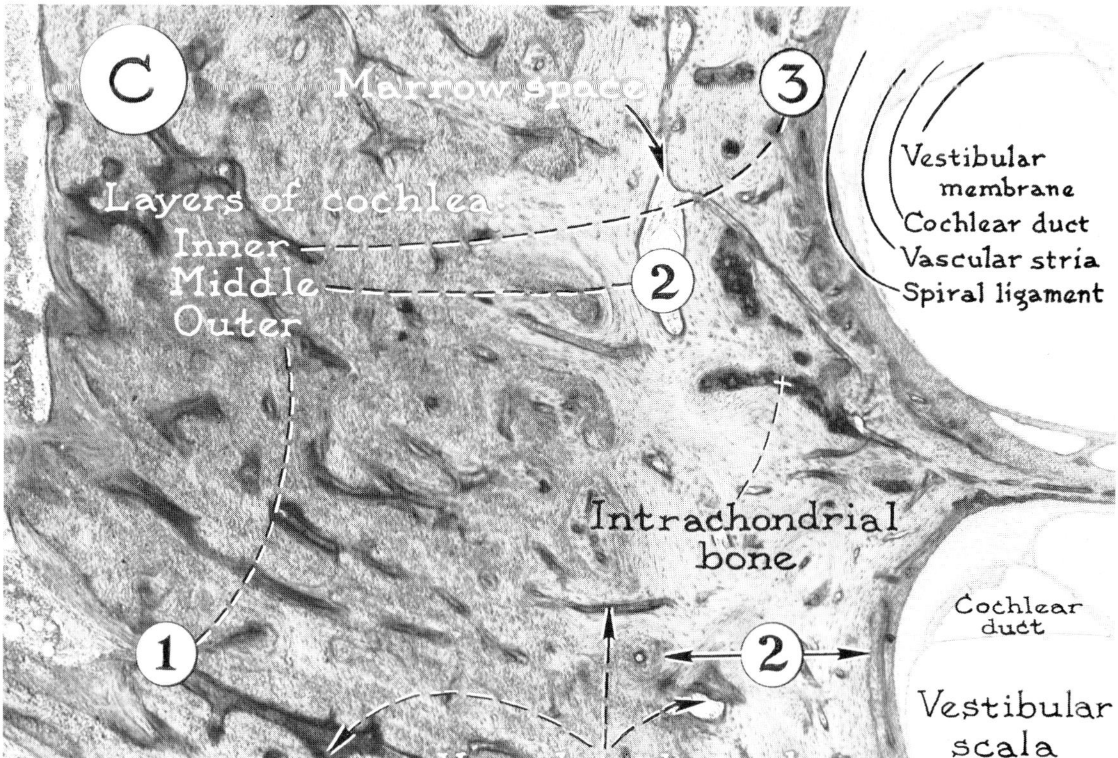

Figure III–88. See legend on the opposite page.

Figure III–89. VESTIBULAR (OVAL) WINDOW, IN RELATION TO THE COCHLEAR (ROUND) WINDOW AND TO THE FACIAL CANAL: SKELETAL PREPARATION.

The dissection now covers the entire course of the facial canal from the geniculum to the stylomastoid foramen (compare Figure III–77).

The space of the general tympanic cavity communicates with two fossulae: The oval window (closed in the natural state by the stapedial footplate) is situated in the depths of the *fossula fenestrae vestibuli*; the space of the tympanum opens into the *fossula fenestrae cochleae* (closed by the secondary tympanic membrane). The aditus of the cochlear fossula is very much narrower than that of the vestibular; their long axes are placed at an approximate right angle to each other (see Figures III–92*a, c* and III–93*a, b*).

The "shell" of bone that forms the exposed wall of the canal has been removed along its middle third (the margins of the dissected bone being indicated by unlabeled arrows). The openings in the wall communicate with vascular channels in the bone. One aperture (out of view) transmitted the stapedius muscle.

The canal follows an even curve from the horizontal segment (beginning at the geniculum) to the vertical segment (terminating at the stylomastoid foramen). The length of the canal, as here exposed, is 26 mm. Continuing in a posterior direction from the geniculum in a horizontal ridge on the labyrinthine wall of the tympanic cavity, the canal lies immediately above the vestibular (oval) window. After passing beyond the area of the mastoid antrum, the canal descends in the mastoid wall of the tympanic cavity adjacent to the air cells. It ends at the stylomastoid foramen, on the inferior surface of the temporal bone, just behind the styloid process (the latter is small in this specimen). Just inferior to the vestibular window, the labyrinthine wall projects outward as the promontory which contains the first turn of the cochlea.

Dissection by Dr. Raymond L. Warpeha.

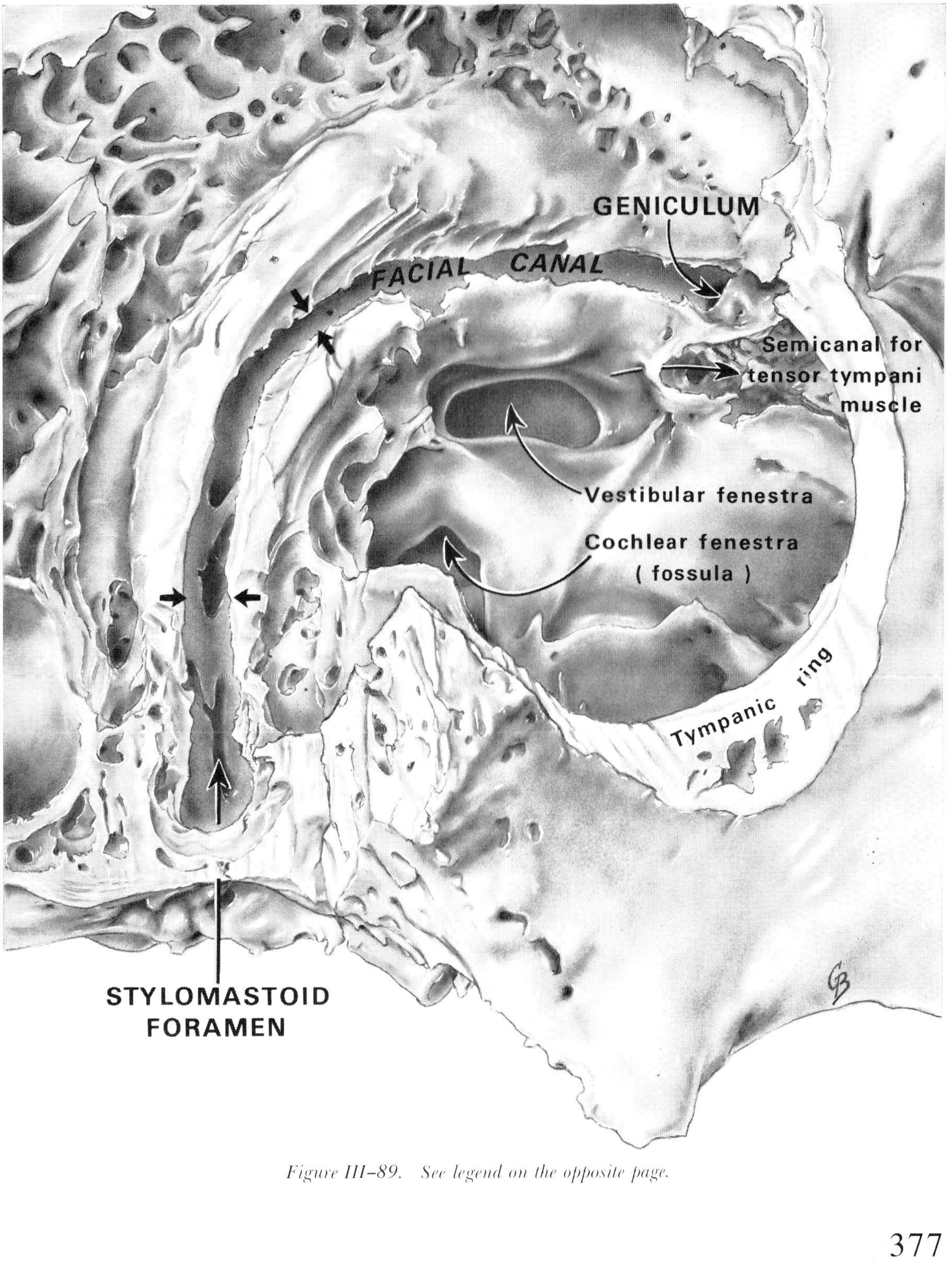

Figure III–89. See legend on the opposite page.

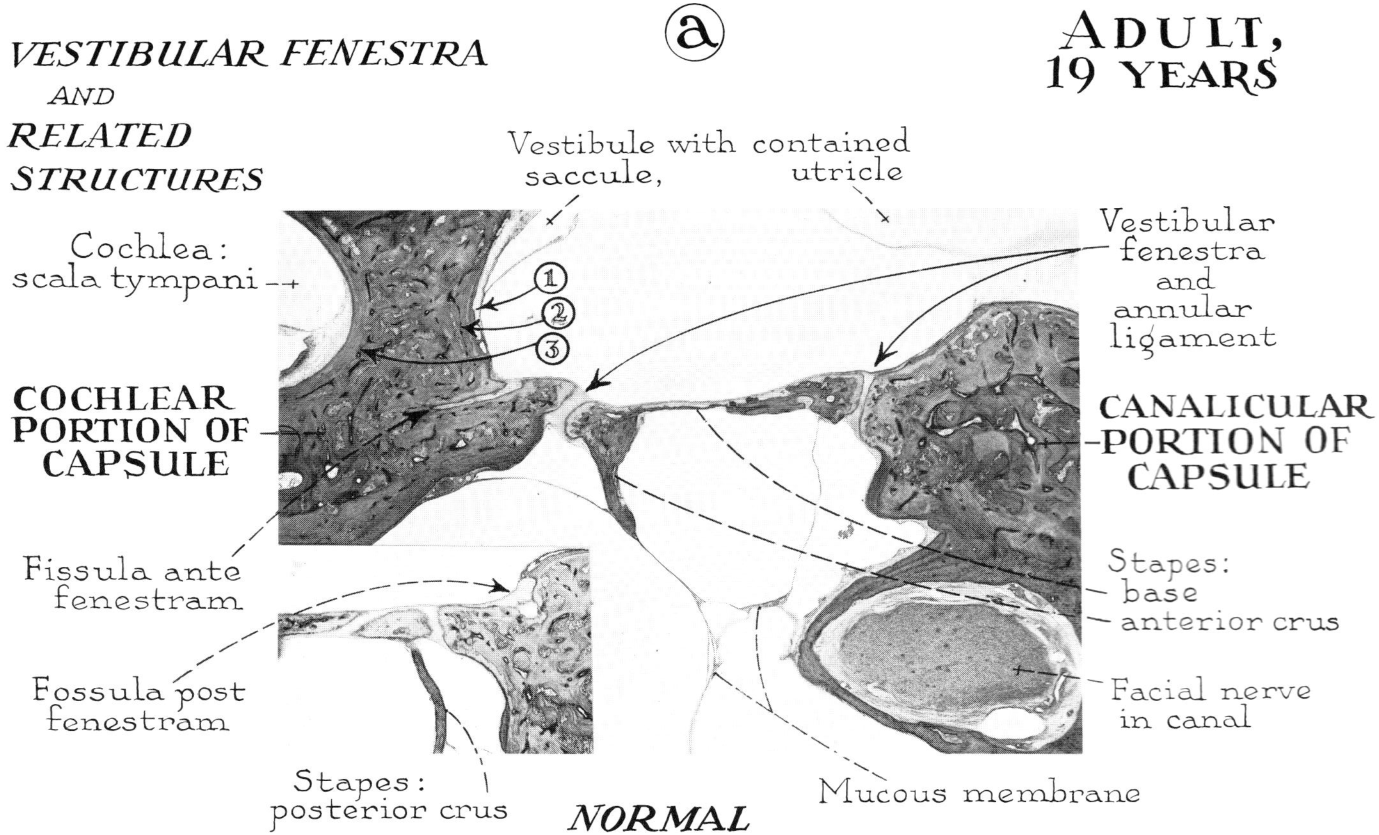

Figure III–90. AREA OF THE VESTIBULAR (OVAL) WINDOW IN HEALTH AND DISEASE. *a* MALE, 19 YEARS OLD. *b.* MALE, 65 YEARS.

a. In the normal *pars petrosa* the fissula ante fenestram is a complete transcapsular channel, the vestibular portion of which is shown in this photomicrograph. It is occupied by slightly vascular connective tissue which is continuous with the periotic tissue at the inner (vestibular) aperture and with the submucosa at the outer (tympanic) aperture. The fossula post fenestram is usually incomplete, being represented (as in this instance) only by a vestibular opening.

Figure III–90 continues on the opposite page.

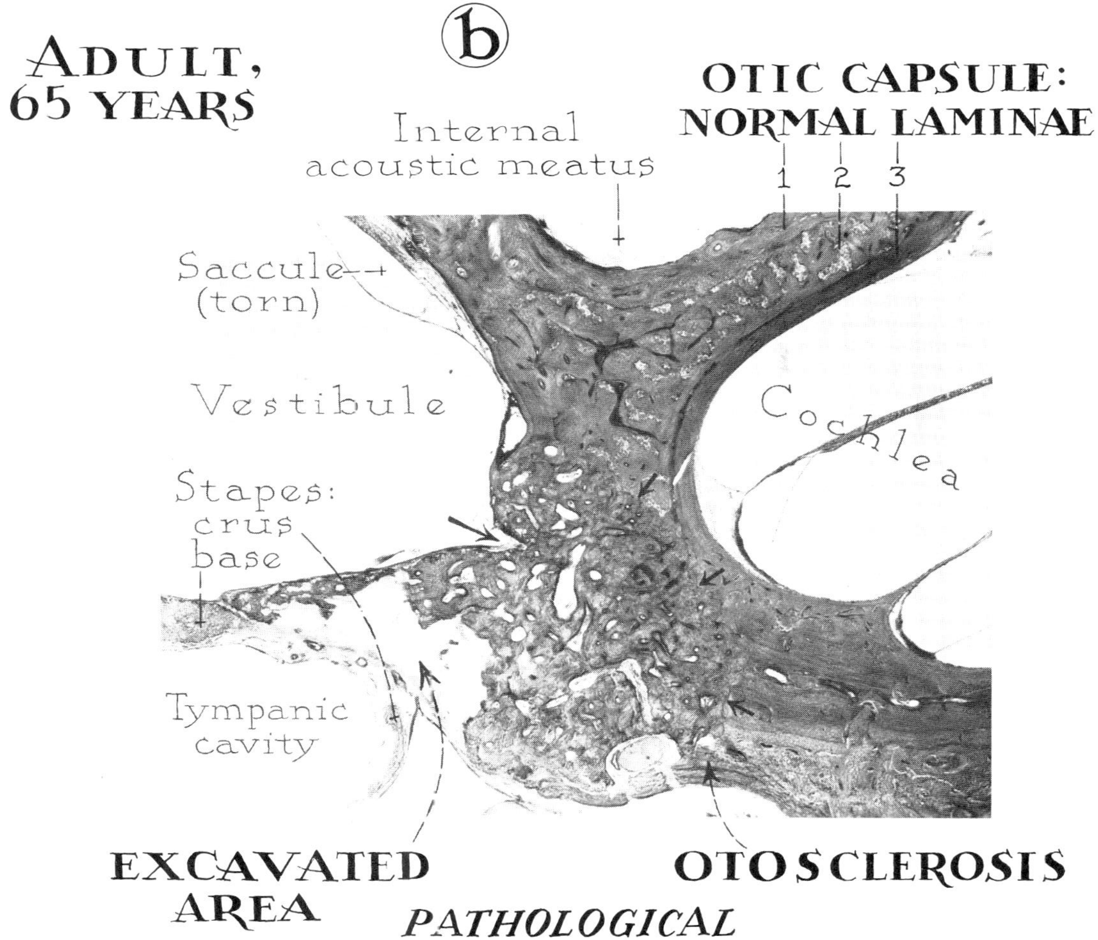

Figure III–90, Continued.

b. The fissular region – in front of the vestibular window – is the predilected site for formation of otosclerotic bone. In this case, the vestibular aperture of the fissula (at the unlabeled arrow) remained identifiable. The pathological change involved not only a replacement of normal bone of the middle layer of the otic capsule, but also destruction of the bone on the anterior wall of the window (topography and form of lesions are shown in Figures III–124*c*, III–125*c*, and III–126).

Transverse sections, Wisconsin Collection, series 29 and 47, respectively. *a*, ×39; *b*, ×28.

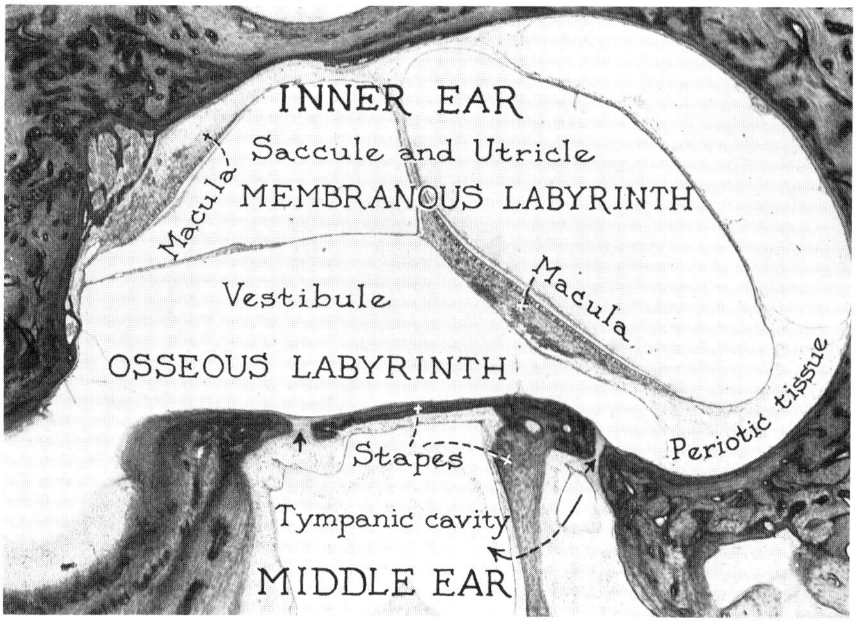

a

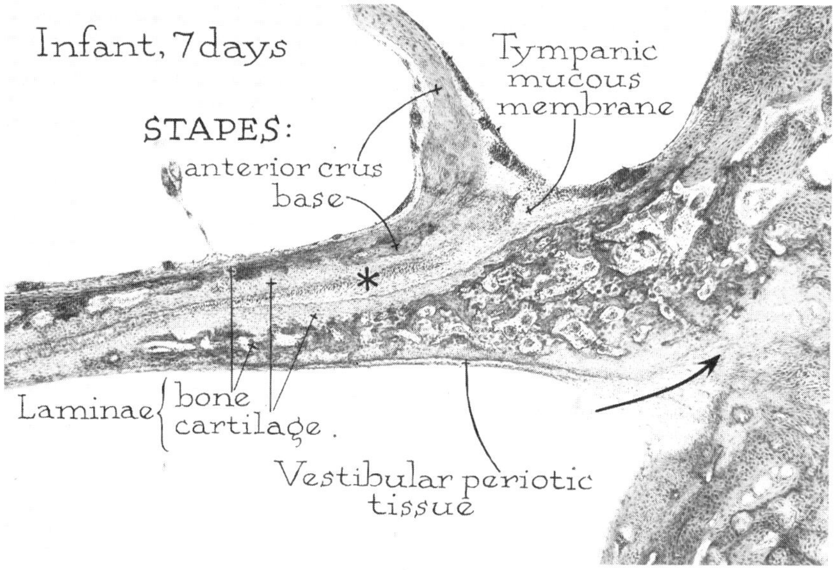

b

Figure III–91. Vestibular fenestra and stapedial base (footplate) in relation to the structures of the inner and middle ear. *a.* Infant, 6 months old. *b.* Infant, 7 days old. *c.* Male, 19 years old.

a. The stapes occupies the vestibular, or oval, window in the labyrinthine wall of the middle ear. It is held in place by the annular ligament. The stapedial base faces the saccule and utricle of the membranous duct system, separated from them by the vestibule of the osseous labyrinth (see also Figure III–47). The saccule and utricle are lodged in small depressions on the medial wall of the vestibule termed, respectively, spherical recess and elliptical recess.

b. The base, or footplate, of the stapes is two-layered (see also Figure III–25). The osseous plate, on the tympanic aspect, contains the vascular channels. It is invested by mucous membrane. The cartilaginous plate is covered by an excessively thin layer of periotic tissue, except anteriorly, where the base overrides the margin of the fenestra. In this situation, toward the cochlear part of the otic capsule, the cartilage of the stapes faces that of the fenestra. The annular ligament (at asterisk) intervenes between the two chondral laminae.

Figure III–91 continues on the opposite page.

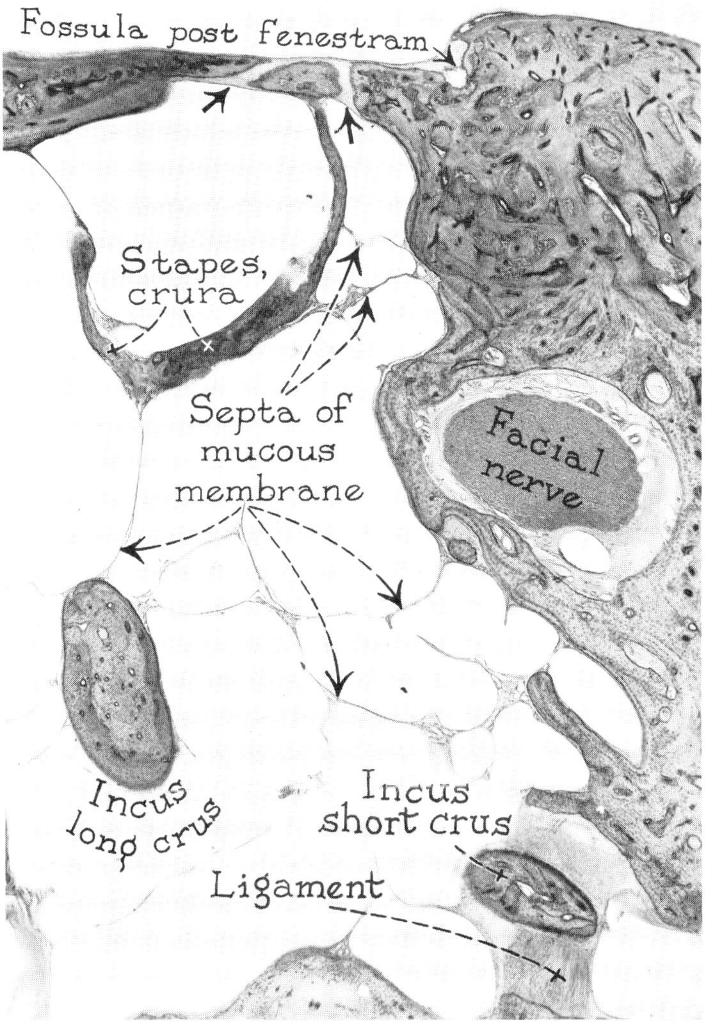

c

Figure III–91, Continued.

c. The vestibular window, when viewed from the middle ear, lies in the depths of a fossula (stapes "niche"). The jutting posterior wall of the space is formed by the facial canal, the anterior wall by the promontory of the basal cochlear coil (see Figure II–43*b*). The tissue on the vestibular surface of the stapedial base (footplate) is an excessively thin periotic layer; on the opposite, or tympanic, aspect the footplate is covered by mucous membrane. This mucosal tissue is reflected, in the form of septa, from the labyrinthine wall of the tympanic cavity to the auditory ossicles (see also Figure III–141). The vestibular (oval) window is indicated by unlabeled arrows.

Transverse sections. *a* and *c*, Wisconsin Collection, series 121 and 29, respectively. *b*, Northwestern Collection, series 5.8.36. *a*, ×29; *b*, ×45; *c*, ×20.

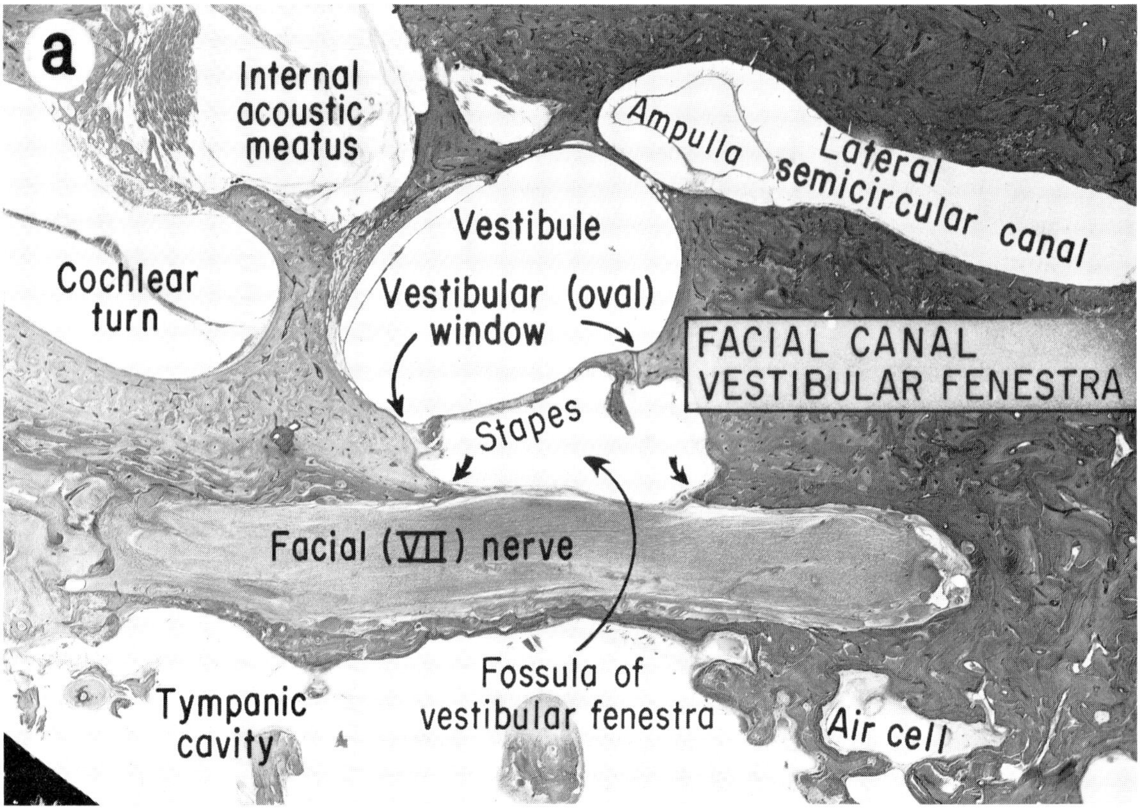

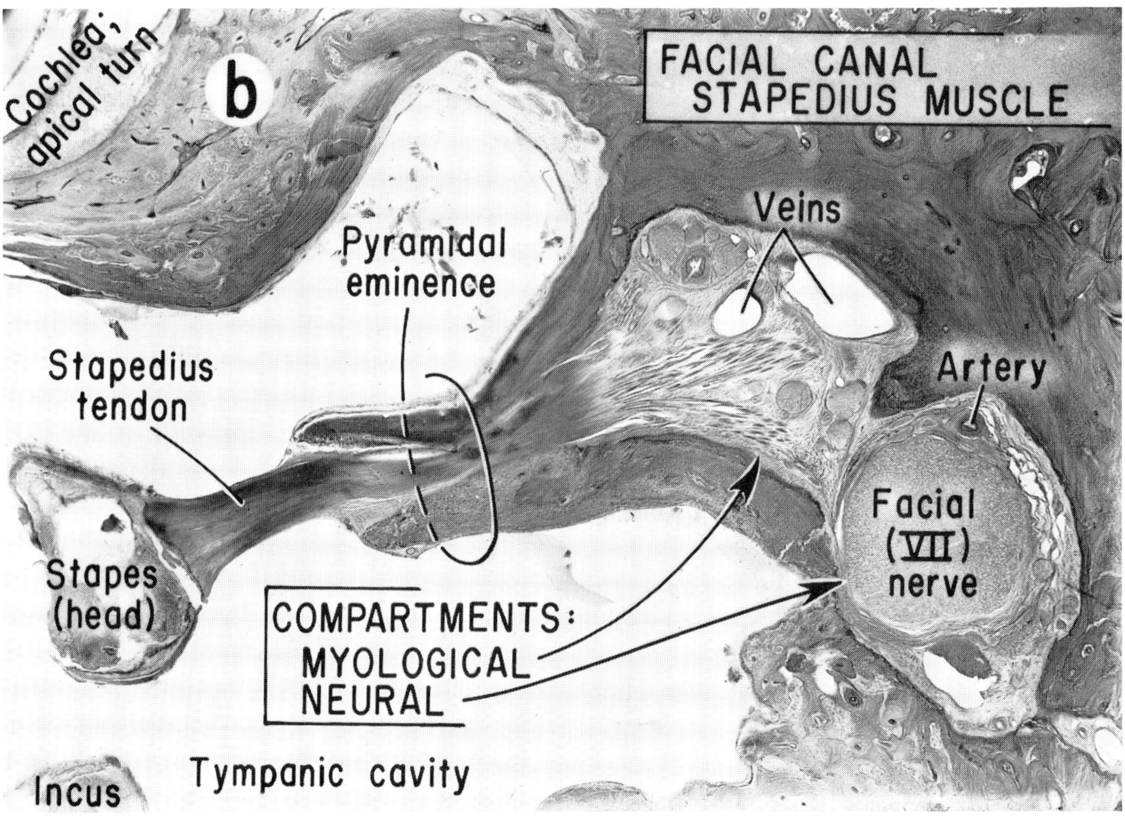

Figure III–92. See legend on the opposite page.

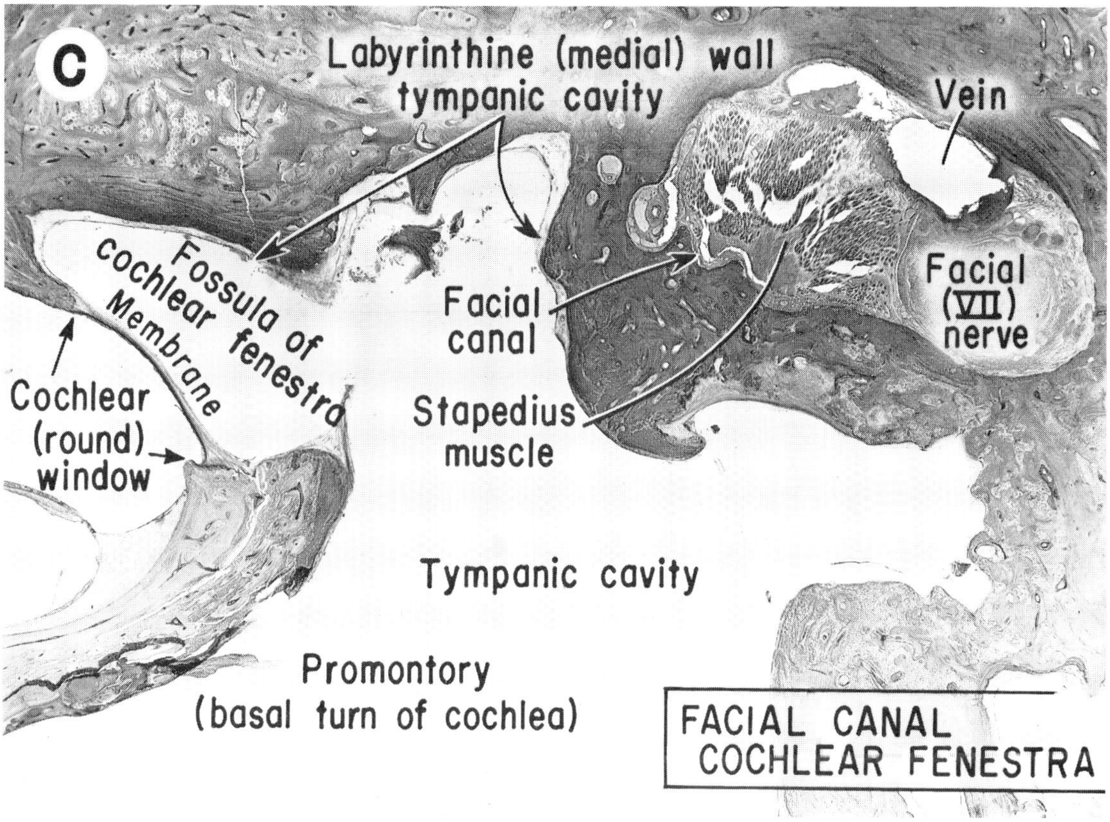

Figure III–92. VESTIBULAR AND COCHLEAR FENESTRAE: STRUCTURE AND TYMPANIC RELATIONSHIPS. MALE, 40 YEARS OF AGE.

a. Demonstrating the position of the stapedial base (footplate) as it forms the medial boundary of the fossula of the vestibular fenestra (oval window). The section passes through the cranial part of the fossula, the latter being the stapes "niche" in otological terminology. The lateral boundary of the space is the facial canal, which in this specimen is dehiscent (between unlabeled arrows) in the horizontal segment of its course.

b. In the area between the two windows, the stapedius tendon crosses the tympanic cavity from the tip of the pyramidal eminence to the head of the stapes.

c. Showing the position of the secondary tympanic membrane as it separates the fossula of the cochlear fenestra from the tympanic scala of the basal turn of the cochlea.

The fossula of the round window, directed toward the descending segment of the facial canal, leads upward, forward and medialward, toward the basal cochlear turn; the fossula of the oval window leads medialward, toward the vestibule.

Transverse sections, Wisconsin Collection, series 18. *a*, ×12; *b*, ×18; *c*, ×12.

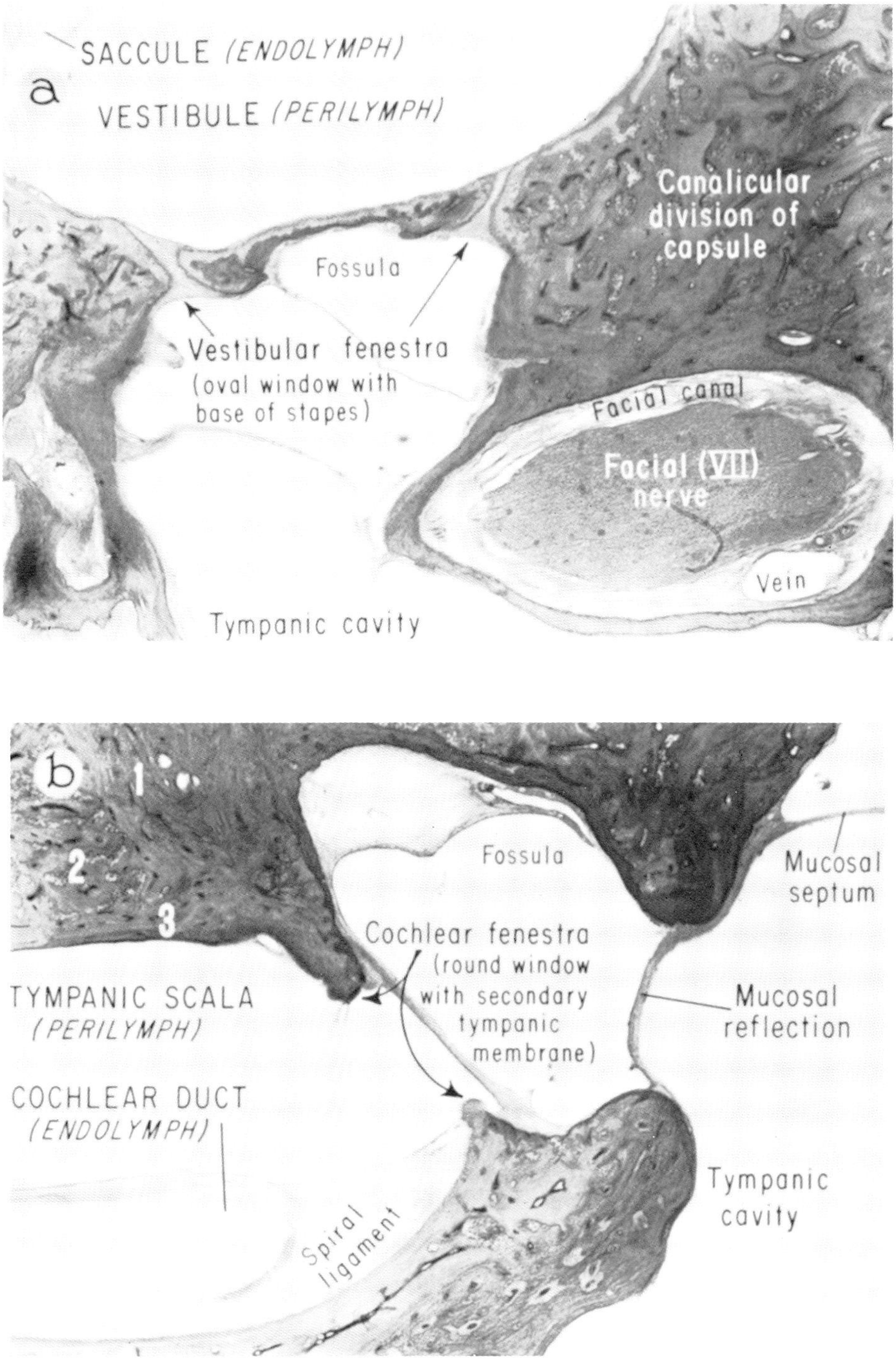

Figure III–93. VESTIBULAR AND COCHLEAR FENESTRAE WITH RELATED ANATOMY. MALE, 19 YEARS OLD.

a. The stapes occupies the window on the medial wall of the tympanic cavity, anchored to the rim by the annular ligament.

b. The secondary tympanic membrane closes the cochlear fenestra (round window); the latter is situated below the oval window in the depths of a space termed the fossula of the cochlear fenestra (see Figure III–94). The numerals indicate the layers of bone of the trilaminar capsule (see Figures II–34 and II–35).

Transverse sections, Wisconsin Collection, series 29. *a*, ×21; *b*, ×17.

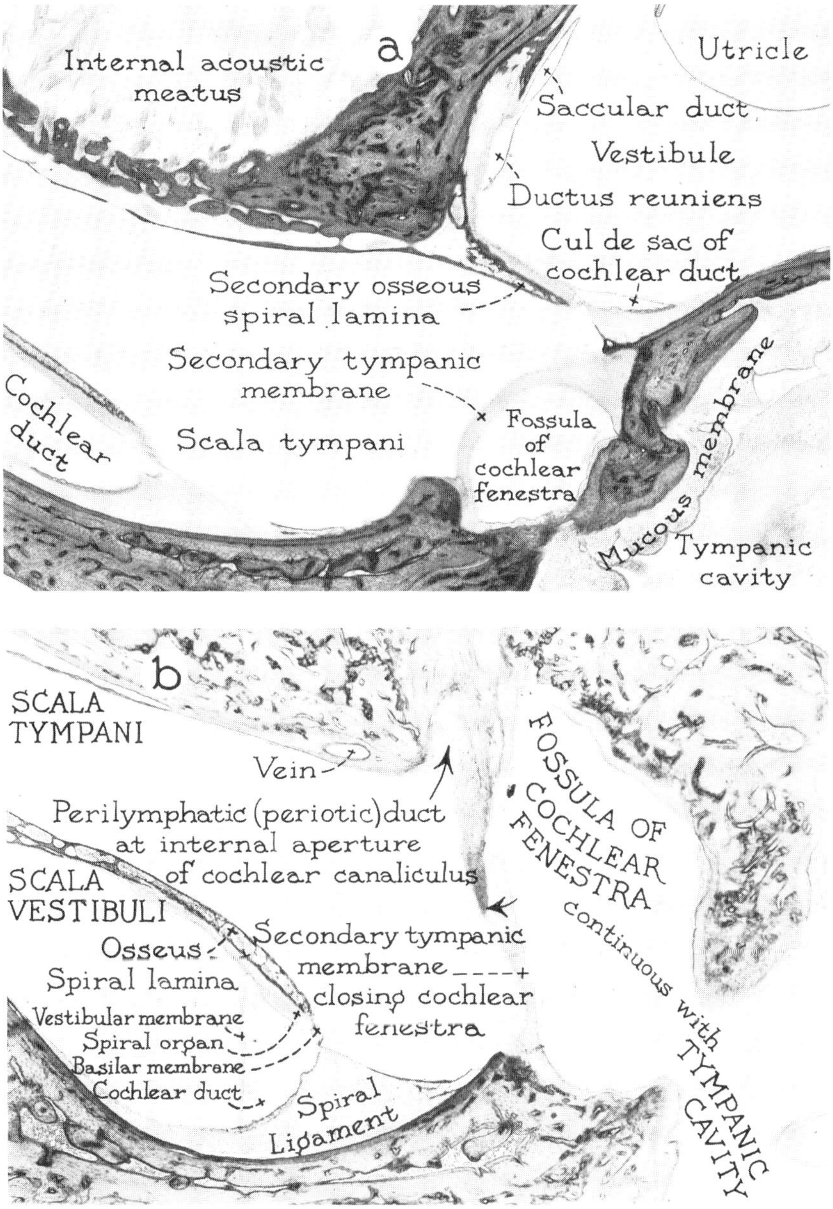

Figure III–94. Cochlear (round) window, the fossular bay of the latter, and the related structures of the inner ear in the vestibule and in the basal turn of the cochlea. *a.* Infant of 6 months. *b.* Infant of 10 weeks.

a and *b.* These sections demonstrate the fossula of the cochlear, or round, window and the secondary tympanic membrane in relation to the vestibular and cochlear parts of the membranous duct system.

The beginning of the basal coil of the cochlea produces a large projection into the tympanic cavity. Just posterior to the jutting edge of this promontory, a triangular declivity leads forward, upward, and medianward into the fossula of the cochlear fenestra (round window). In a skeletal preparation this bay, as an offset from the general tympanic cavity, opens into the basal turn of the cochlea. It is bordered by a narrow bony ridge, the *crista fenestrae cochleae* (at the unlabeled arrow in *b*). In the fresh state the secondary tympanic membrane, attached circumferentially to the crest, separates the space of the fossula from that of the *scala tympani.*

Transverse sections, Wisconsin Collection, series 121 and 83, respectively. *a*, ×20; *b*, ×30.

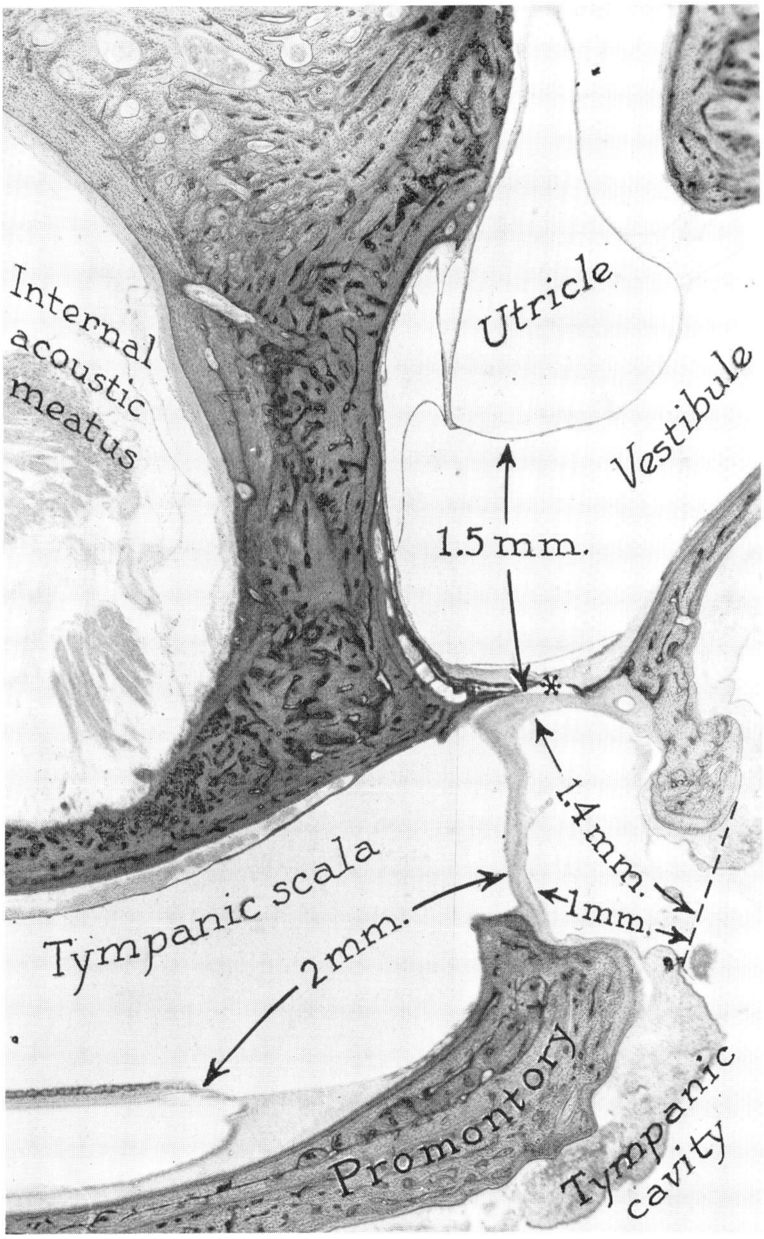

Figure III–95. Cochlear window: measurements of interdistances in the middle and inner ear. Infant of 6 months.

The distance from the *aditus* of the fossula to the membrane varies, being 1.0 mm. to 1.4 mm. in the specimen illustrated. On the cochlear side, the distance between the secondary tympanic membrane and basilar membrane of the cochlear duct is 2.0 mm. On the vestibular side the distance from the *aditus* to the utricle is approximately 3.0 mm. This means that the distance from the *aditus* to the utricle matches the distance from the *aditus* to the basilar membrane. In this area (at the asterisk) a succession of structures makes for complexity: a cul-de-sac of the tympanic scala is succeeded by a comparable diverticulum, the *caecum vestibulare* of the cochlear duct, and then by the space of the vestibule.

In the area where the vestibule is apposed to the tympanic scala, the secondary tympanic membrane does not possess the form of a stretched diaphragm. Rather, it is concave toward the middle ear, the resulting form suggesting that of a flexed hand (palm outward). It appears to be applied to the "floor" of the vestibular cecum. At other levels (for example, where the scala is related to the fossula), the membrane is flat (see Figure II–93*b*).

Transverse section, Wisconsin Collection, series 121. ×30.

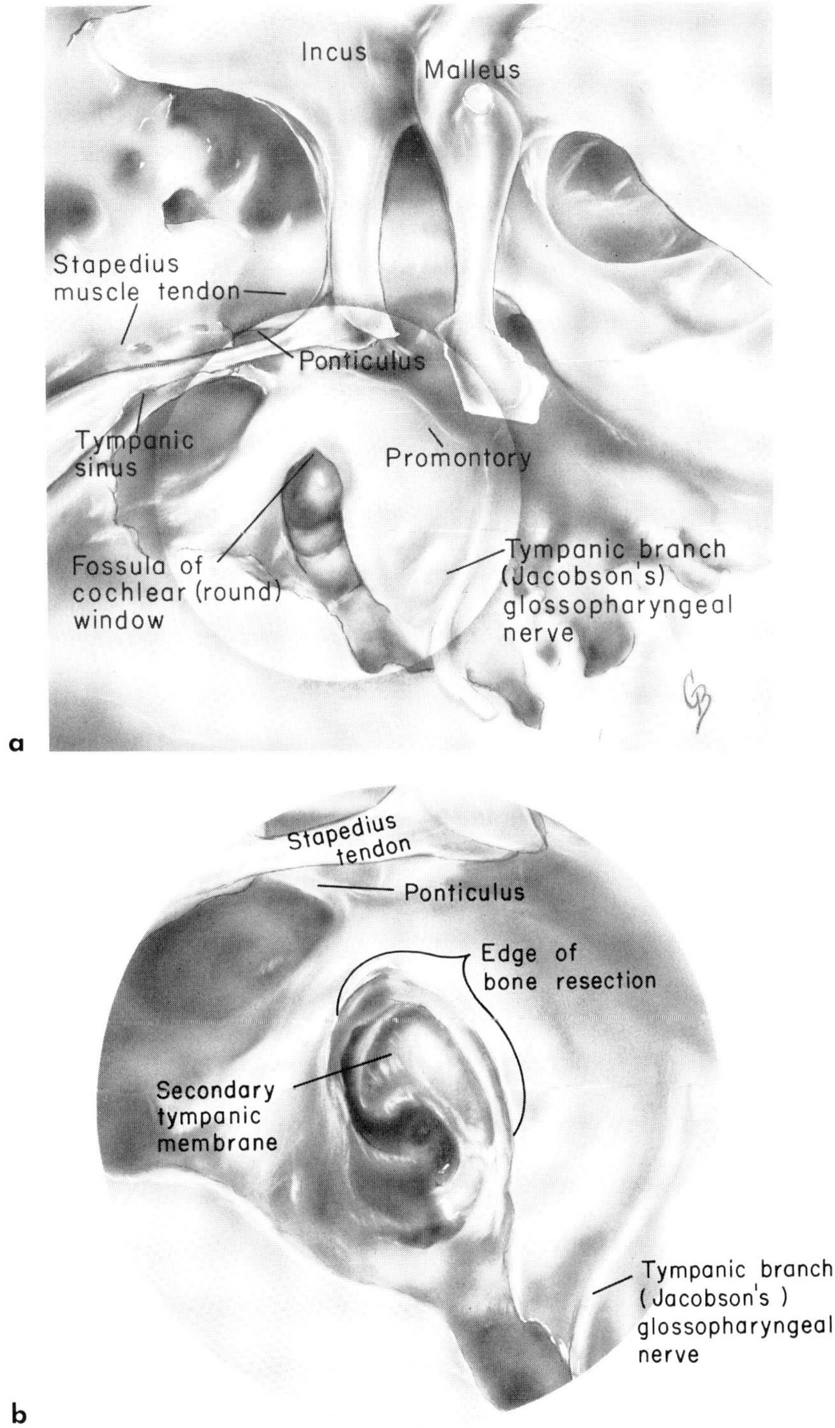

Figure III–96. FOSSULA OF THE COCHLEAR (ROUND) WINDOW: VARIATIONAL ANATOMY. UNEMBALMED SPECIMENS. EXAMPLE I, TYPICAL FORM.

a. Anatomy of the medial, or labyrinthine wall of the tympanic cavity exposed by removal of the external acoustic meatus and tympanic membrane. The area of the fossula is encircled. The external aperture has the form of a Gothic arch, which is the characteristic shape in this series of specimens (Examples I to V).

b. The area encircled in *a* is shown after the anterior and posterior margins of the aperture have been dissected away to the edge of the secondary tympanic membrane.

(From Donaldson: Arch. Otolaryng., 88:124–130, 1968.)

Figure III–96 continues on the following page.

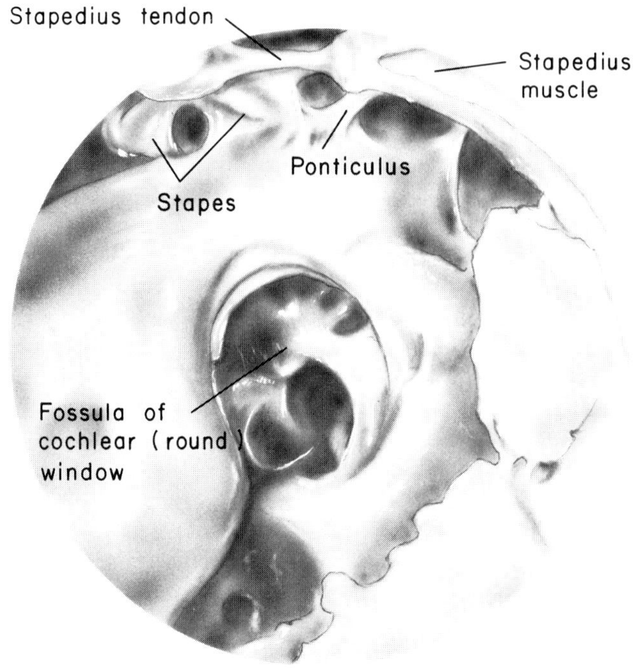

c

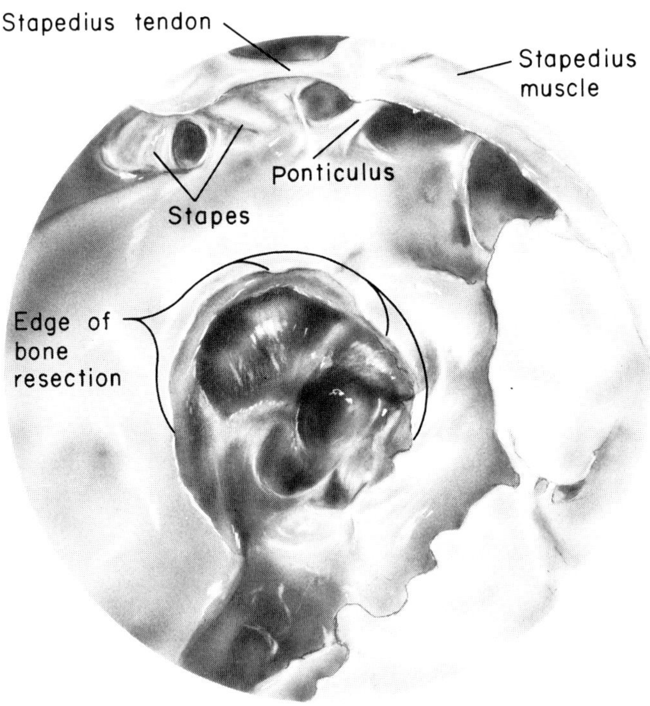

d

Figure III–96, Continued. FOSSULA OF THE ROUND WINDOW: VARIATIONAL ANATOMY. II, ATYPICAL FORM.

c. Here the aperture of the fossula is round as is that of the fenestra itself, representing a departure from the characteristic form.

d. Bone forming the margins of the aperture has been removed to a line corresponding with that of the natural edge of the secondary tympanic membrane.

(From Donaldson: Arch. Otolaryng., 88:124–130, 1968.)

Figure III–96 continues on the opposite page.

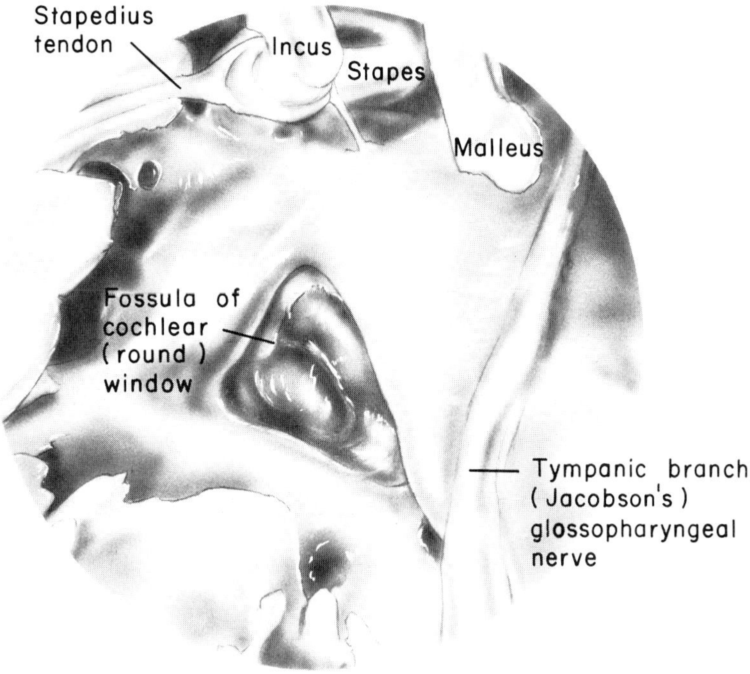

e

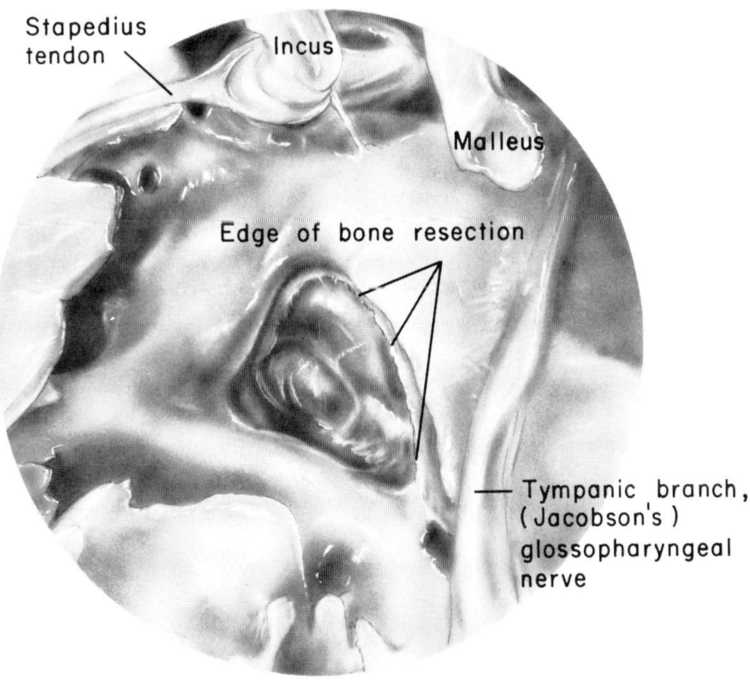

f

Fiture III–96, Continued. FOSSULA OF THE ROUND WINDOW: VARIATIONAL ANATOMY. III, ATYPICAL FORM.

e. The aperture of the fossula of the cochlear fenestra is triangular, thus differing from the common form.

f. Resection of the bone at the margin of the aperture demonstrates that it closely corresponds, in outline, to that of the membrane.

(From Donaldson: Arch. Otolaryng., 88:124–130, 1968.)

Figure III–96 continues on the following page.

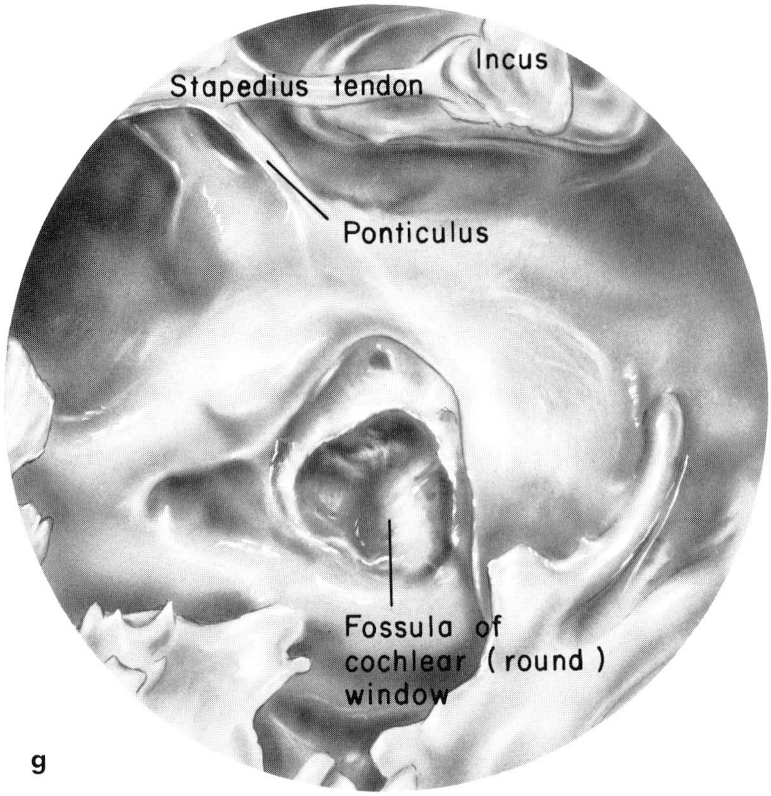

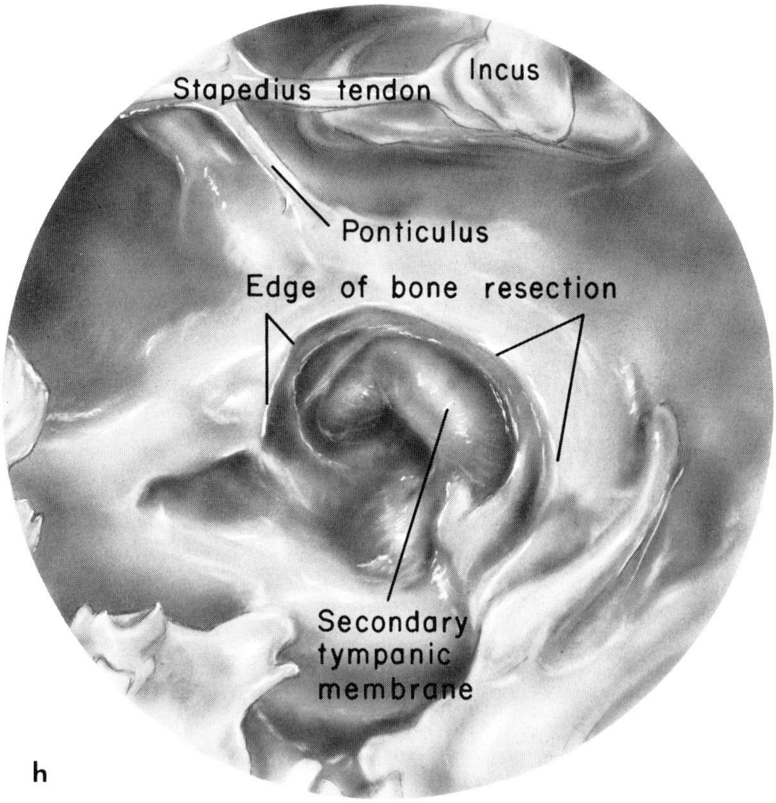

Figure III–96, Continued. FOSSULA OF THE ROUND WINDOW: VARIATIONAL ANATOMY. IV, ATYPICAL FORM.

g. An example of an aperture trapezoidal in outline. A web of tissue crosses the fossula.

h. Resection of bone to the margin of the fossula shows that, in the natural state, the secondary tympanic membrane was concealed in direct lateral view (that is, as seen through a reflected tympanic membrane).

(From Donaldson: Arch. Otolaryng., 88:124–130, 1968.)

Figure III–96 continues on the opposite page.

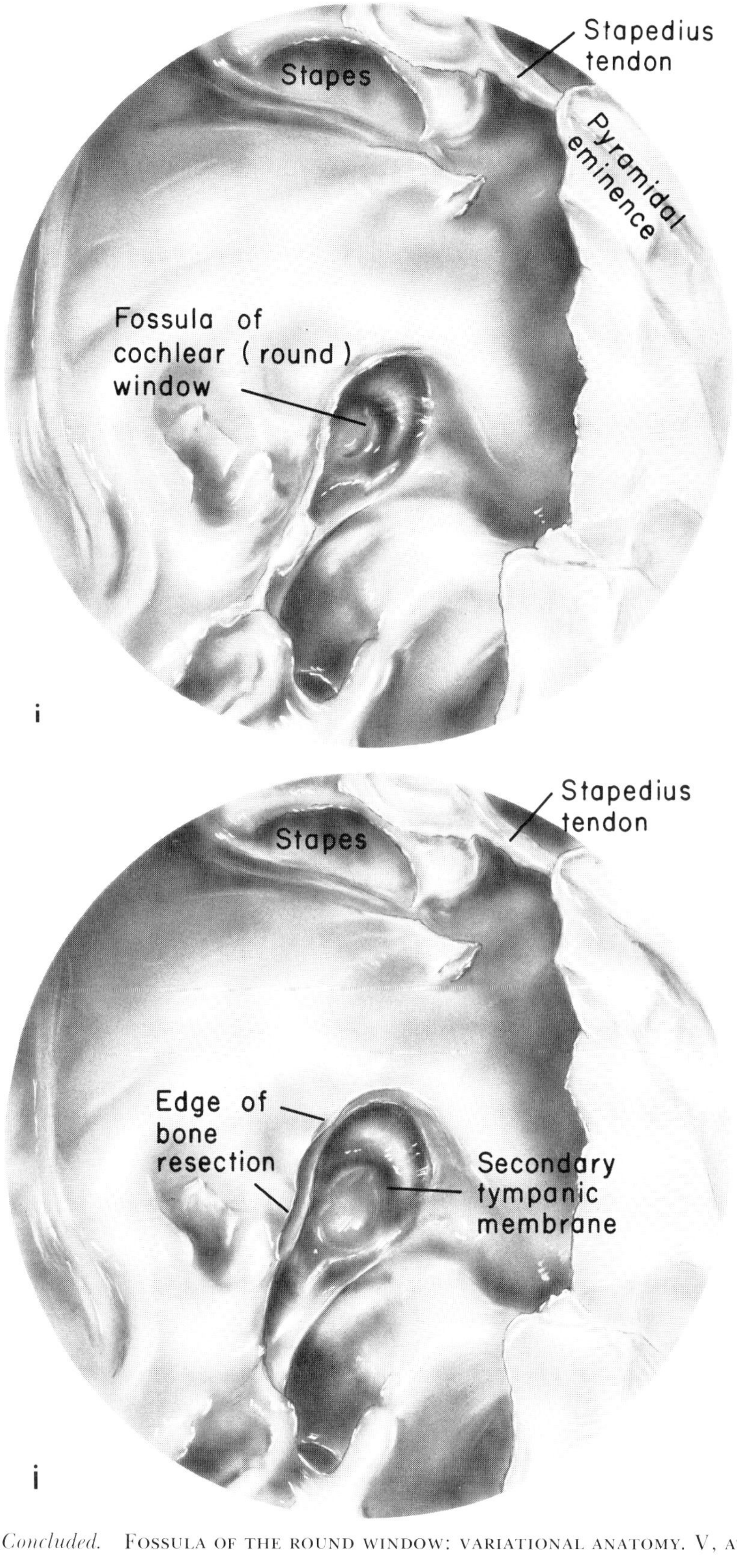

Figure III–96, Concluded. FOSSULA OF THE ROUND WINDOW: VARIATIONAL ANATOMY. V, ATYPICAL FORM.

i. The shape of the aperture of the fossula is that of an inverted droplet. Owing to height (that is, extension cranialward), it would seem that the secondary tympanic membrane would be visible in lateral view.

j. Dissection demonstrated that the membrane was actually thus exposed to the space of the tympanic cavity.

(From Donaldson: Arch. Otolaryng., 88:124–130, 1968.)

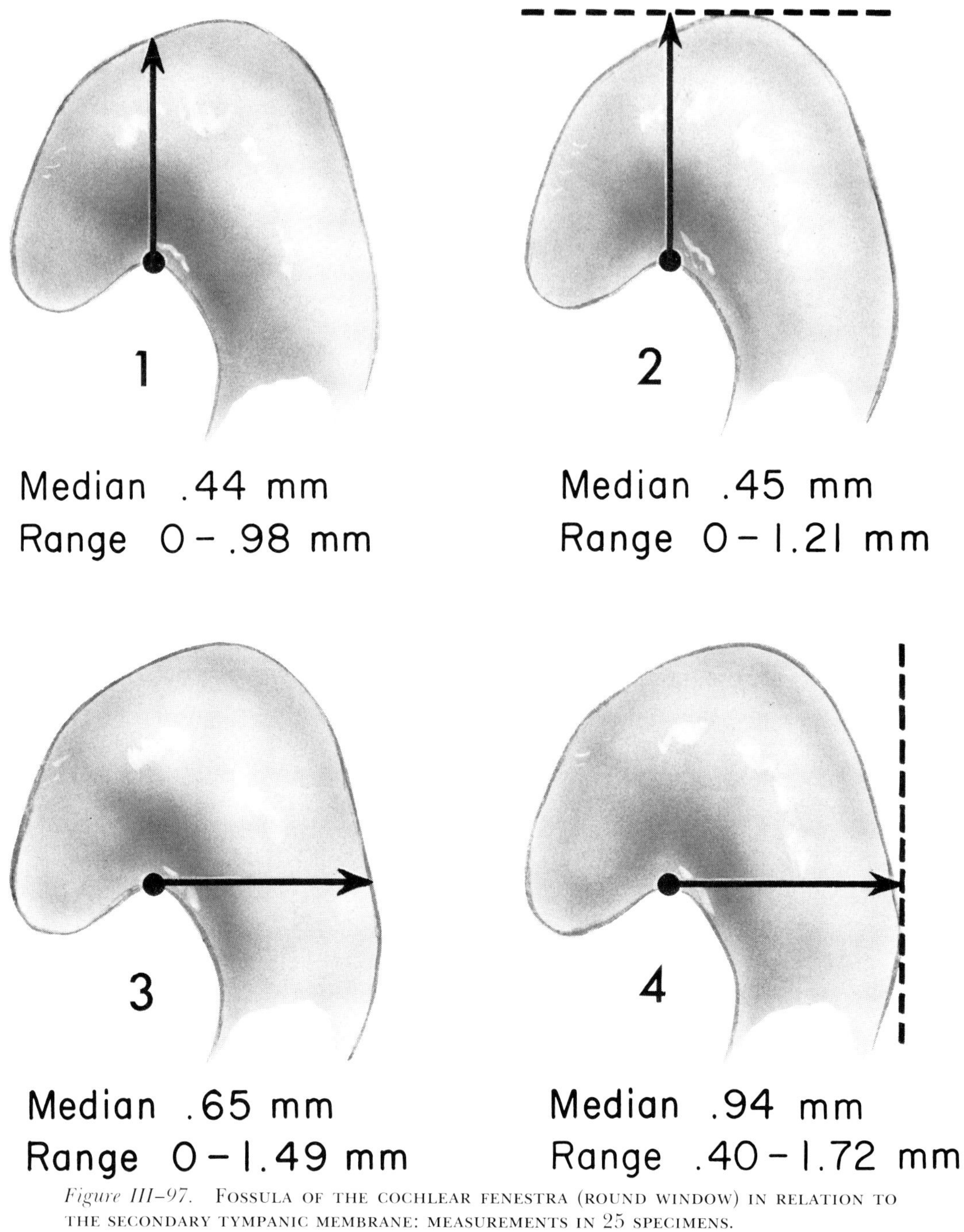

Figure III–97. FOSSULA OF THE COCHLEAR FENESTRA (ROUND WINDOW) IN RELATION TO THE SECONDARY TYMPANIC MEMBRANE: MEASUREMENTS IN 25 SPECIMENS.

The black dot in the figure indicates the reference point at the junction of the anterior and posterior margins from which measurements were made: the distance from there to the edge of the secondary tympanic membrane. The measurements recorded are the following: *1*, directly cephalad (cranialward) to the membrane; *2*, to the most superior edge of the membrane; *3*, to the latter's anterior edge; *4*, to the most anterior edge.

(From Donaldson: Arch. Otolaryng., 88:124–130, 1968.)

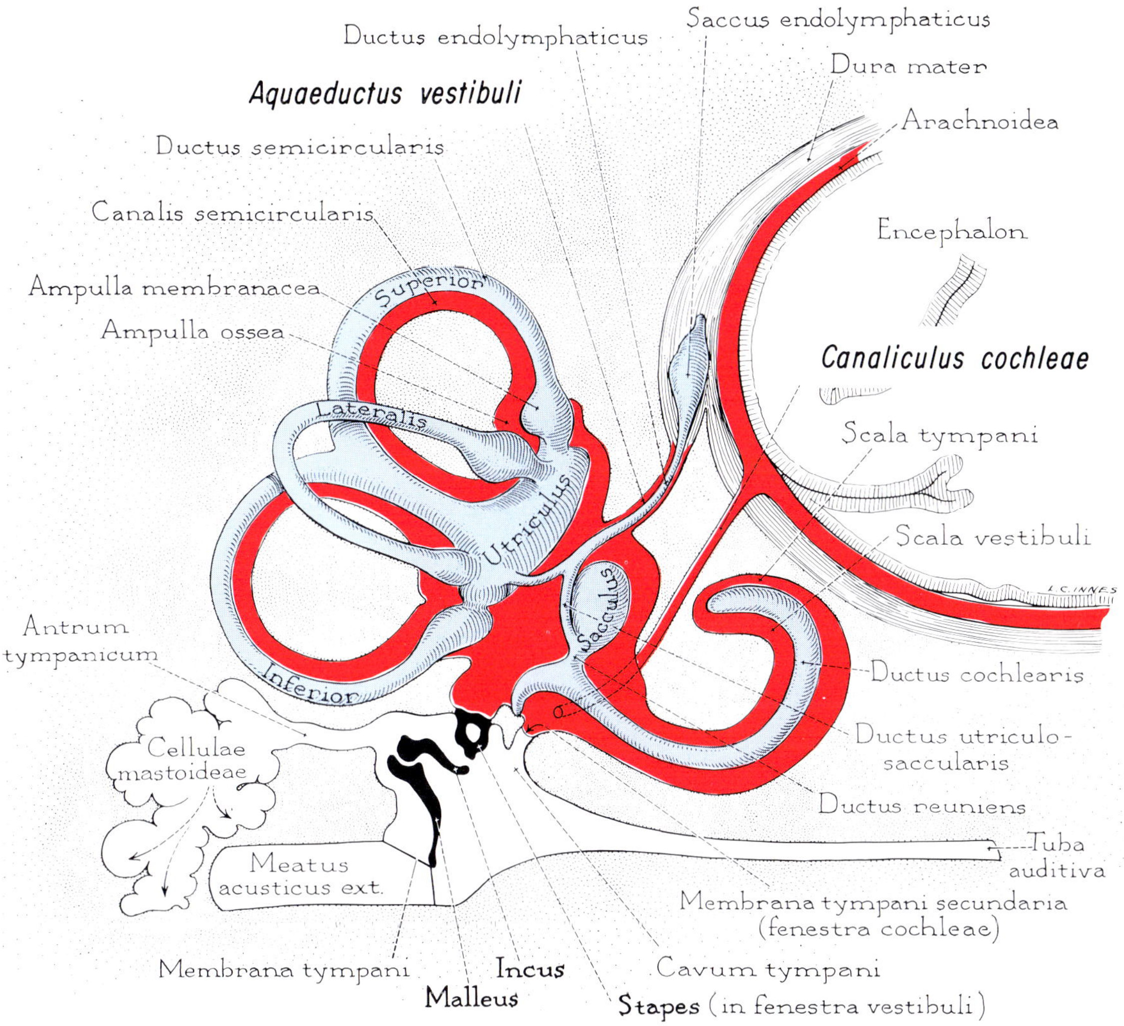

Figure III–98. Vestibular and cochlear aqueducts in relation to the labyrinthine systems for endolymph and perilymph (the latter shown in red). Schematic representation.

The vestibular aqueduct begins on the wall of the vestibular division of the labyrinth and traverses the temporal bone to terminate on the posterior surface of the pyramid (see details of anatomy in Figures III–100, III–101, III–104, and III–106). The aqueduct transmits the endolymphatic duct and the proximal part of the sac (Figures III–60 and III–104). The duct and sac are lodged in vascular connective tissue (Figures III–61*b* and III–62*b*).

The cochlear aqueduct (*canaliculus cochleae*) begins on the wall of the tympanic scala of the basal turn of the cochlea near the cochlear (round) window. It ends on the inferior surface of the pyramid (details of anatomy in Figures III–119 to III–121 and III–132). The aqueduct is occupied by relatively avascular connective tissue, continuous proximally with the tissue (termed "periotic") that lines the wall of the osseous labyrinth and distally with the arachnoid layer of the cranial meninges. The interstices among the fibers of collagen have been unfortunately termed perilymphatic "duct." Although functionally they serve as a channel of exchange between perilymph and cerebrospinal fluid, they are not to be likened to the histologically different endolymphatic duct—the latter being an epithelial tube, not a system of spaces of the kind which elsewhere in the body would serve to transmit lymph.

(From Anson, Warpeha, and Rensink: Ann. Otol., 77:583–607, 1968.)

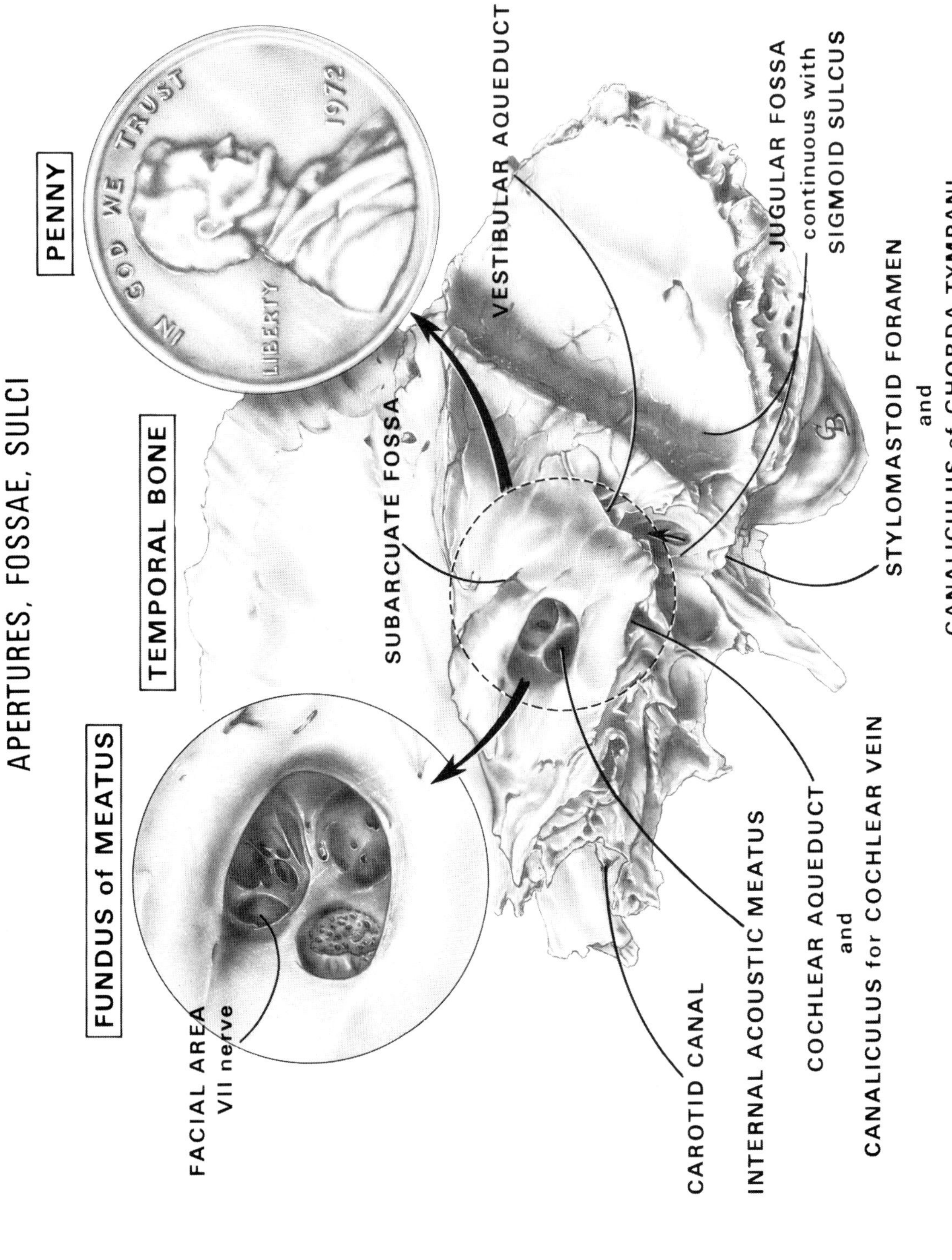

Figure III–99. See legend on the opposite page.

Figure III–99. APERTURES, SULCI, FOSSAE, AND RELATED LANDMARKS ON THE POSTERIOR AND INFERIOR SURFACES OF THE TEMPORAL BONE, EMPHASIZING THE CLOSE GROUPING OF ANATOMIC LANDMARKS IN THE AREA OF THE TWO AQUEDUCTS. *Insets.* FUNDUS AND COIN.

The area encircled is the size of a copper cent (*Inset*, upper right). In the penny-sized field, the following appear: the external apertures of the aqueducts; the opening of the subarcuate fossa; part of the sulcus for the sigmoid venous sinus; and the *porus* of the internal acoustic meatus (*Inset*, upper left).

The external aperture of the vestibular aqueduct is usually a slitlike opening, oblique in direction, that matches the adjacent margin of the sigmoid sulcus. It is, however, subject to variation in form, size, and location (see Figures III–110 to III–118). The internal aperture is a small depression on the wall of the elliptical recess of the vestibule. Between the two extremities the aqueduct follows a gently curving course through the temporal bone (see Figure III–101).

The external aperture of the cochlear aqueduct (or canaliculus) opens in a funnel-shaped expansion upon the inferior surface of the pyramid, just medianward from the jugular fossa. From the posterior surface, its presence is marked by a notch along the posterior angle of the pyramid. The notch is almost directly inferior to the pore of the internal acoustic meatus. The internal aperture is situated on the deep wall of the tympanic scala, just internal to the crest for attachment of the secondary tympanic membrane (see Figure III–94). Between the extremities, the aqueduct follows an almost straight course through the bone (see Figure III–101). The course of the canaliculus for the cochlear vein matches that of the aqueduct, from which it remains independent.

The pore of the internal acoustic meatus leads transversely and frontally into the bone, to end at the fundus (*Inset*, upper left). Areas transmit the fibers of the acoustic (vestibulocochlear) and facial nerves (see Figure III–134). The facial area marks the beginning of the intraosseous course of the facial nerve, a progress which ends at the stylomastoid foramen (see Figure III–119). Like the other apertures (described hereinafter), the meatus is subject to variation. For measurements, refer to the legend for Figure III–133.

The canaliculus of the chorda tympani in some instances is wholly independent of the facial canal, of which it is typically an offset. In such cases, the aperture opens upon the inferior aspect of the pyramid, just dorsal to the stylomastoid foramen (see Figure III–66*c*).

The subarcuate fossa is usually situated above and behind the *porus* of the meatus, near the superior angle of the pyramid. However, it is subject to variation in size, form, and position (see Figure III–127). Frequently small sulci pass between the pore and the fossa, giving evidence of close vascular relation between the two channels (see Figure III–128) or with the superior petrosal sulcus. Regularly small in the mature temporal bone, the fossa is capacious in the fetus, where its vascular content determines the course of development of the canalicular division of the otic capsule (see Figures II–37 and II–38).

Save for innervation of the stapedius muscle, the facial nerve contributes nothing directly to the function of hearing. This suggests the concept of a bone that acts as a king's highway for blood vessels and nerves that pass to areas beyond the ear. The reasonableness of this concept is strengthened by the cranial anatomy of the internal jugular vein and the internal carotid artery.

The fossa for the superior bulb of the internal jugular vein is a depression just posterior to the aperture of the cochlear aqueduct where it is continuous with the sigmoid sulcus. The fossa is highly variable in depth (see Figures III–130 to III–133).

The carotid canal is a curved channel which passes—first perpendicularly, then horizontally—forward and medialward through the pyramid. It begins in a large round foramen on the inferior surface of the bone (immediately in front of the jugular fossa), emerges near the apex of the pyramid in an irregular opening, and forms the anterior wall of the tympanic cavity (see Figure III–129). It is related to the promontory formed by the cochlea, to the semicanal for the tensor tympani muscle, and to air cells.

Note Especially: This specimen demonstrates several closely interrelated features, each of them surgically significant (see Figure III–132).

(From Anson, Donaldson, and Shilling: Ann. Otol., 81:616–631, 1972.)

Figure III–100. COCHLEAR AND VESTIBULAR AQUEDUCTS, PERILYMPHATIC AND ENDOLYMPHATIC DUCTS, AND THEIR COMPARATIVE FORM AND COURSE.

a and *c*. Semischematic drawings based upon several sections. *b* and *d*. Drawings of selected specimens of temporal bone, demonstrating the form of the external aperture.

The cochlear canaliculus begins on the wall of the tympanic scala, just internal to the crest for attachment of the secondary tympanic membrane (*a*). After traversing the bone, it terminates medial to the jugular fossa in a triangular funnel-shaped depression on the inferior surface of the petrous pyramid (*b*). This external aperture is visible from the medial aspect, in the form of a notch on the posterior angle of the bone.

The internal aperture of the vestibular aqueduct is a minute depression on the wall of the elliptical recess of the vestibule, which serves for reception of the utricle (*c*). The aqueduct passes through the bone, to end in an external aperture on the posterior surface of the pyramid (*d*).

Typically, this slitlike opening is situated about midway between the superior petrosal sulcus above and the jugular incisure below. However, variations are common, some of them being striking departures from the anatomic "normal" (Figures III–114 and III–115). The aperture, while usually oblique, may be virtually horizontal in direction; and, although in most instances it is closer to the superior angle of the pyramid than to the posterior, it may open into the sigmoid sulcus. This means, of course, that the location of the endolymphatic sac is subject to corresponding variation.

Contrary to conventional descriptions, the cochlear aqueduct does not transmit a vein; from an early fetal stage onward throughout life, the related vein is housed in a separate osseous channel. The vestibular aqueduct, unlike the cochlear, contains both arteries and veins that enter the connective tissue from canals in the surrounding bone and from the cranial meninges. Both aqueducts are occupied by connective tissue, which is as loosely textured around the endolymphatic sac as is the entire fibrous content of the cochlear aqueduct. The tissue within the two aqueducts resembles that through which fluid generally moves in other parts of the body. Two additional features are similar: the cochlear and vestibular aqueducts open internally upon the wall of the osseous labyrinth (containing the perilymph); both terminate externally through orifices on the petrous pyramid. They begin in periotic tissue and terminate in the meninges.

In the ten dissected specimens, the average diameter of the internal aperture of the cochlear aqueduct, or canaliculus, was 0.09 mm. (range, 0.05 to 0.125 mm.) and that of the external aperture, 0.83 mm. (range, 0.5 to 1.25 mm.). The average length was 11.5 mm. (range, 10.0 to 14.0 mm.). In the same specimens the average diameter of the internal aperture of the vestibular aqueduct was 0.35 mm. (range, 0.25 to 0.5 mm.) and the average length of the aqueduct, 7.1 mm. (range, 3.5 to 12.0 mm.). The external aperture, unlike the internal, almost invariably has the form of a flattened oval rather than that of a circle. In the examination of 250 gross specimens it varies from pinpoint dimensions to a width of 8.0 mm.

(From Anson, Donaldson, Warpeha, and Winch: Laryngoscope, 75:1203–1223, 1965.)

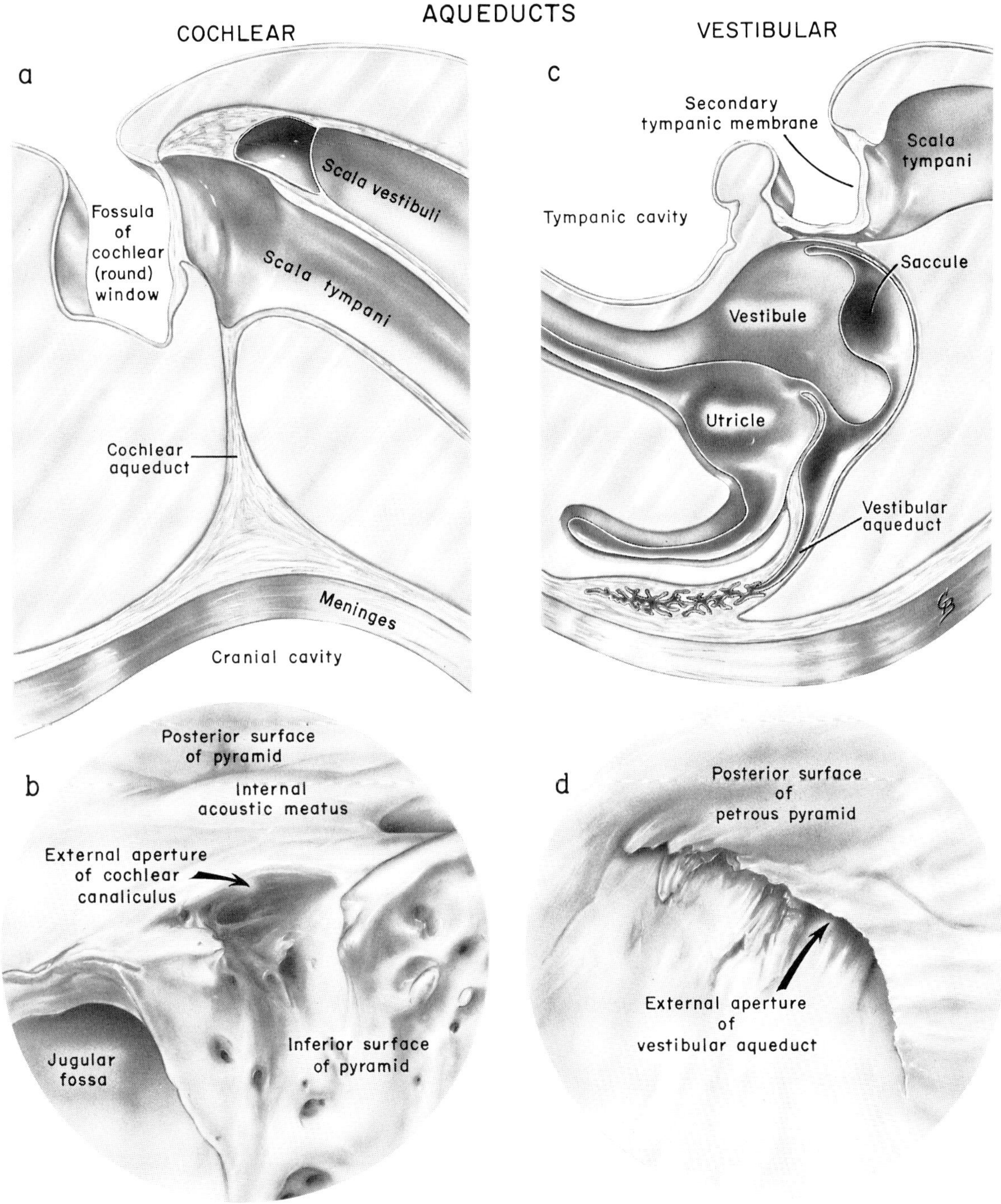

Figure III–100. See legend on the opposite page.

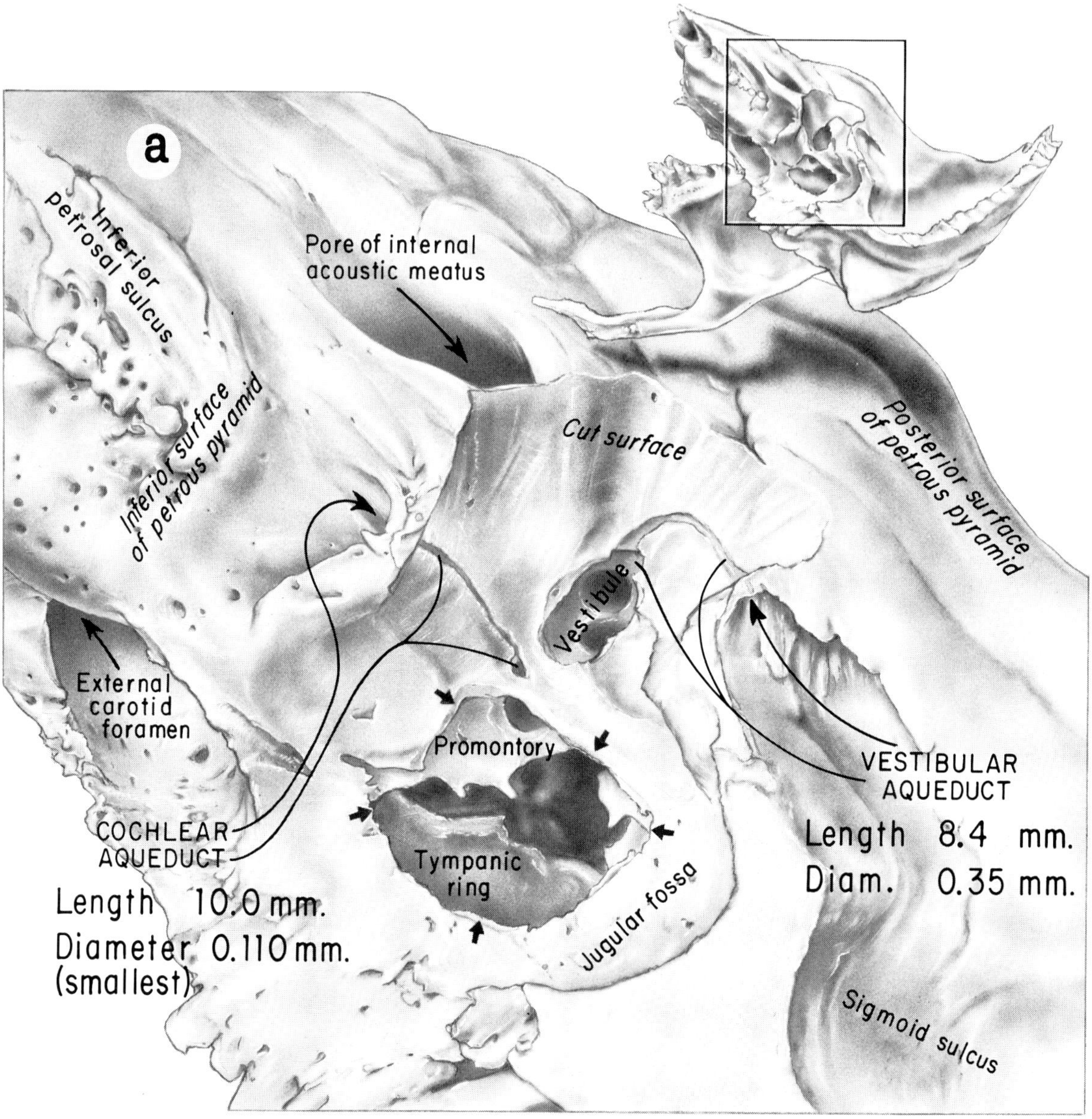

Figure III–101. Vestibular and cochlear aqueducts: three views.

a. Showing both aqueducts on the cut surface of the bone. The inset serves topographically to indicate the part of the temporal bone that is included in the main drawing. Measurements for each aqueduct are recorded. The cochlear aqueduct follows a virtually straight course; that of the vestibular aqueduct is curved (see Figures II–24*b* and III–107*c*).

Bone has been drilled away to produce an excavation in adjacent parts of the posterior and inferior surfaces of the *pars petrosa*, between the external apertures of the two aqueducts. The small unlabeled arrows point to a dehiscence in the floor of the hypotympanum which also serves as the roof of the jugular fossa. Such an osseous defect allows the bulb of the internal jugular vein to present itself immediately below the mucous membrane of the middle ear, where it may be mistaken for a glomus tumor.

Dissection by Dr. Raymond L. Warpeha.

Figure III–101 continues on the opposite page.

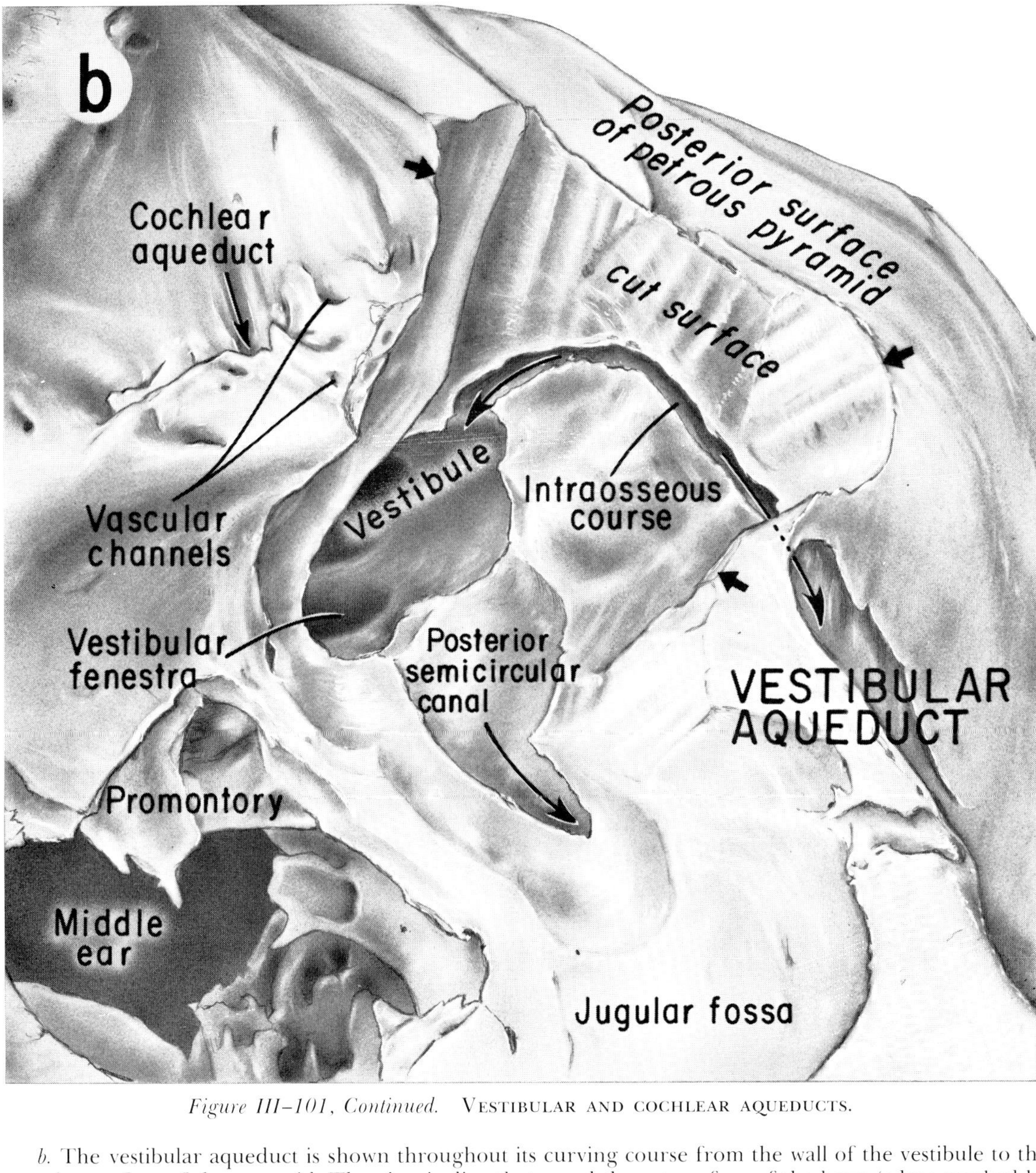

Figure III–101, Continued. VESTIBULAR AND COCHLEAR AQUEDUCTS.

b. The vestibular aqueduct is shown throughout its curving course from the wall of the vestibule to the posterior surface of the pyramid. The view is directly toward the cut surface of the bone (edges marked by arrows).

Figure III–101 continues on the following page.

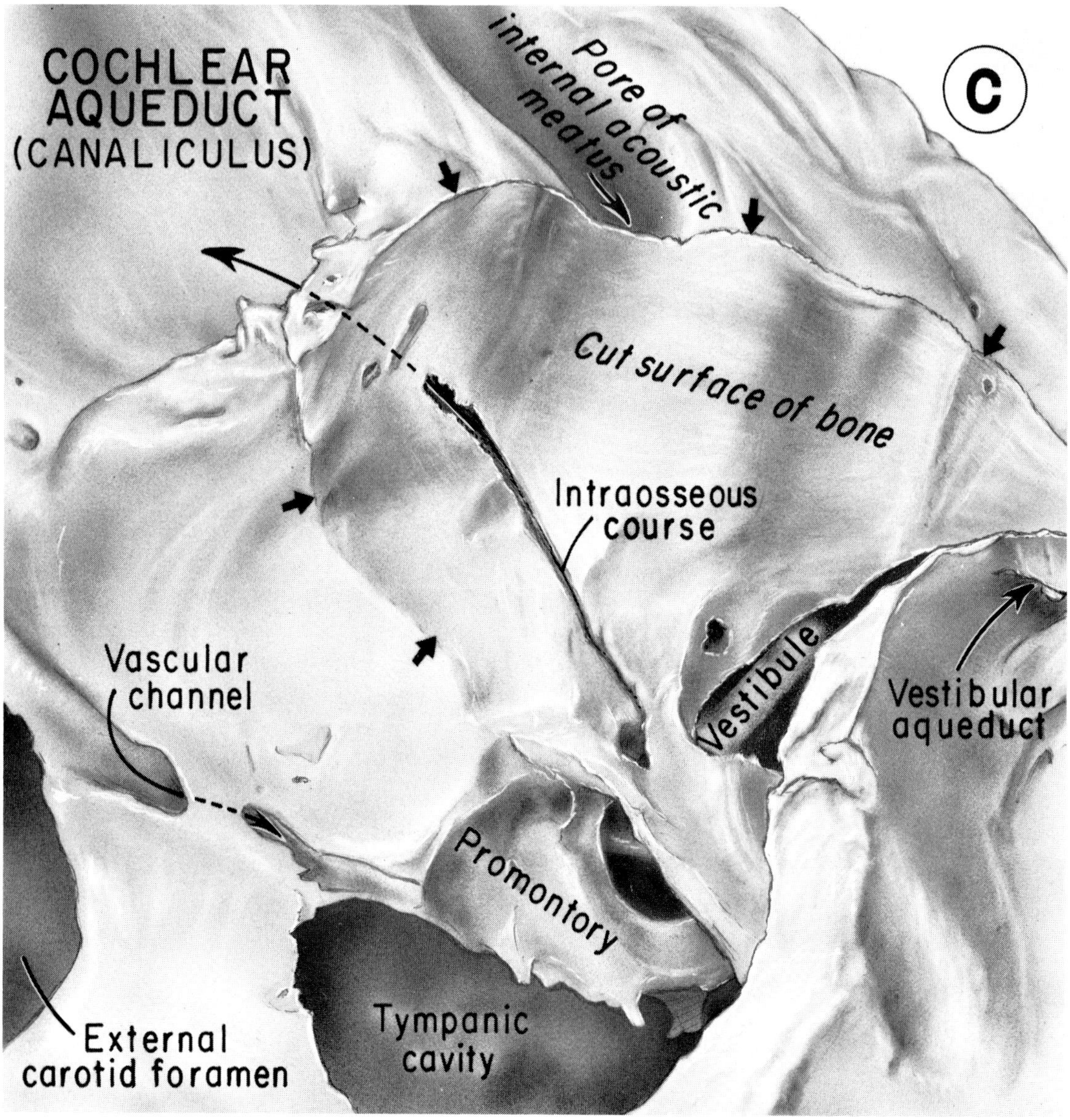

Figure III–101, Concluded. VESTIBULAR AND COCHLEAR AQUEDUCTS.

c. The cochlear aqueduct (or canaliculus) is opened from the basal coil of the cochlea to a point near its termination on the inferior surface of the pyramid. The specimen has been turned so that the view is now toward the anterior aspect of the dissected area.

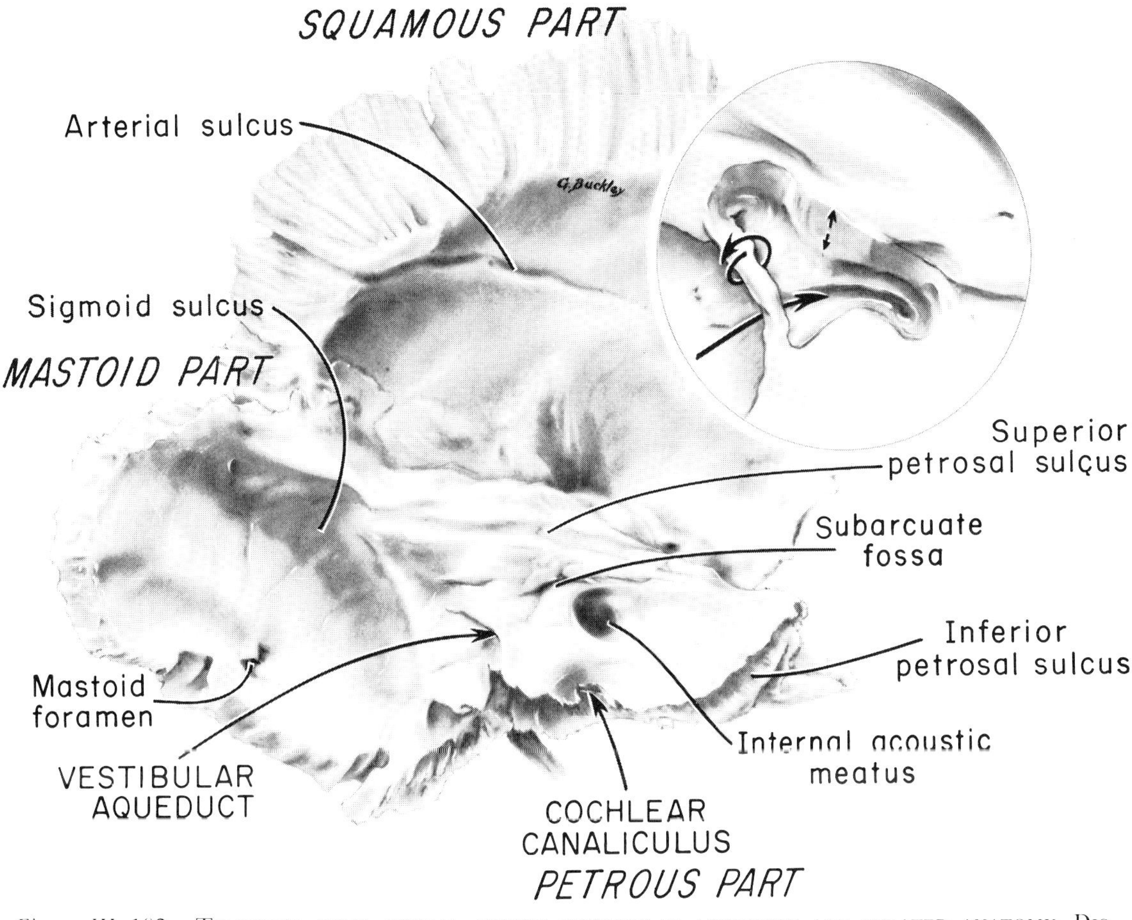

Figure III–102. Temporal bone, medial aspect: vestibular aqueduct and related anatomy. Dissection shown in the inset.

The external aperture of the vestibular aqueduct in this specimen is typical in form and size. The aperture is obliquely directed and is situated closer to the sigmoid sulcus than to the pore of the external acoustic meatus (see Figure III–118).

The distal segment of the aqueduct, exposed in the smaller illustration, is triangular in outline, with its apex directed inward. In the fresh state, this space would be occupied by the intraosseous part of the rugose endolymphatic sac (see Figure III–61 and III–62). The sac is prolonged into the posterior cranial fossa beyond the overhanging crest of the aperture (here retained for purpose of topography and encircled with arrow). At the point of apical narrowing, the sac would become continuous with the isthmus of the endolymphatic duct (Figure III–60). The depth of the overlying bone is indicated by the small unlabeled arrows. In some specimens it is excessively thin.

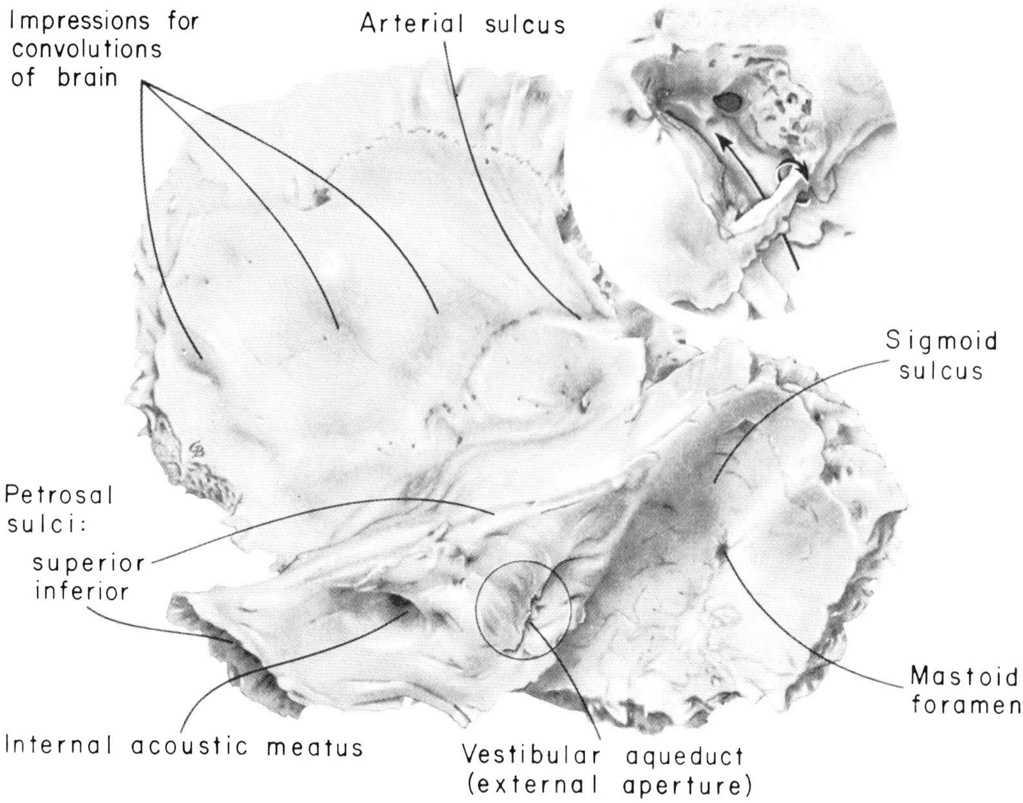

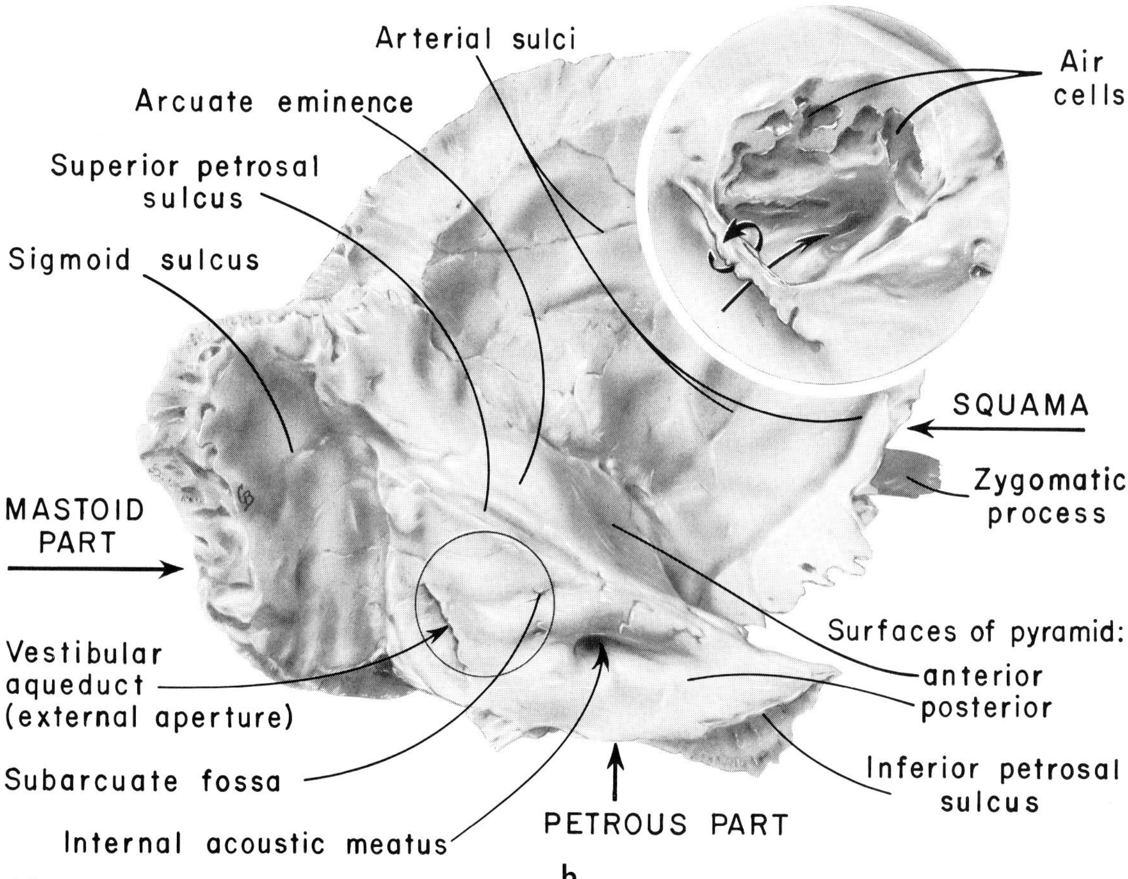

Figure III–103. See legend on the opposite page.

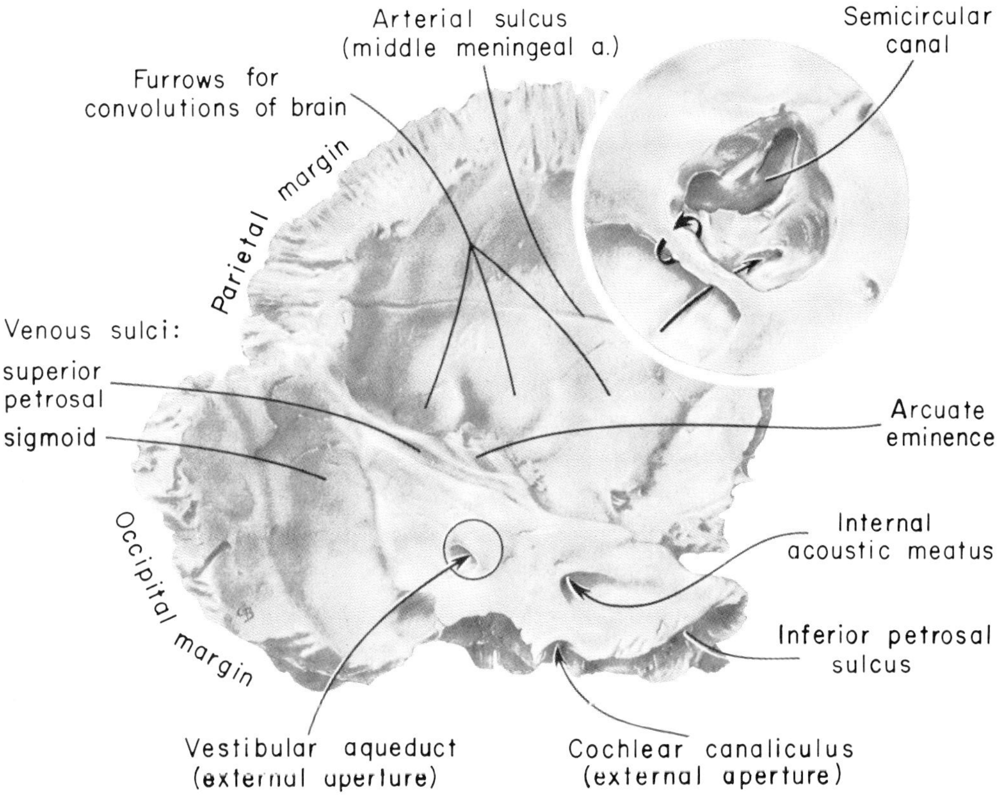

Figure III–103. Distal expanded segment and external aperture of the vestibular aqueduct: variation in the content of the immediately adjacent bone. Three selected dissections.

In each figure, for purposes of topography, a bridge of bone (enclosed in an arrow) remains on the medial border of the slitlike opening; the elongate unlabeled arrow points to the narrow segment of the aqueduct. In each instance the area enlarged in an inset is indicated by a circle in the inclusive figure.

a, b, and *insets.* The outer wall of the aperture contained marrow and air cells.

c and *inset.* The superior semicircular canal was separated from the space of the aqueduct by a very thin layer of bone (see dissection in Figure III–104).

Dissections by Dr. Raymond L. Warpeha.

(*a* from Anson, Winch, Warpeha, and Donaldson: Ann. Otol., 75:921–944, 1966; *c* from Anson, Donaldson, Warpeha, and Winch: Laryngoscope, 75:1203–1223, 1965.)

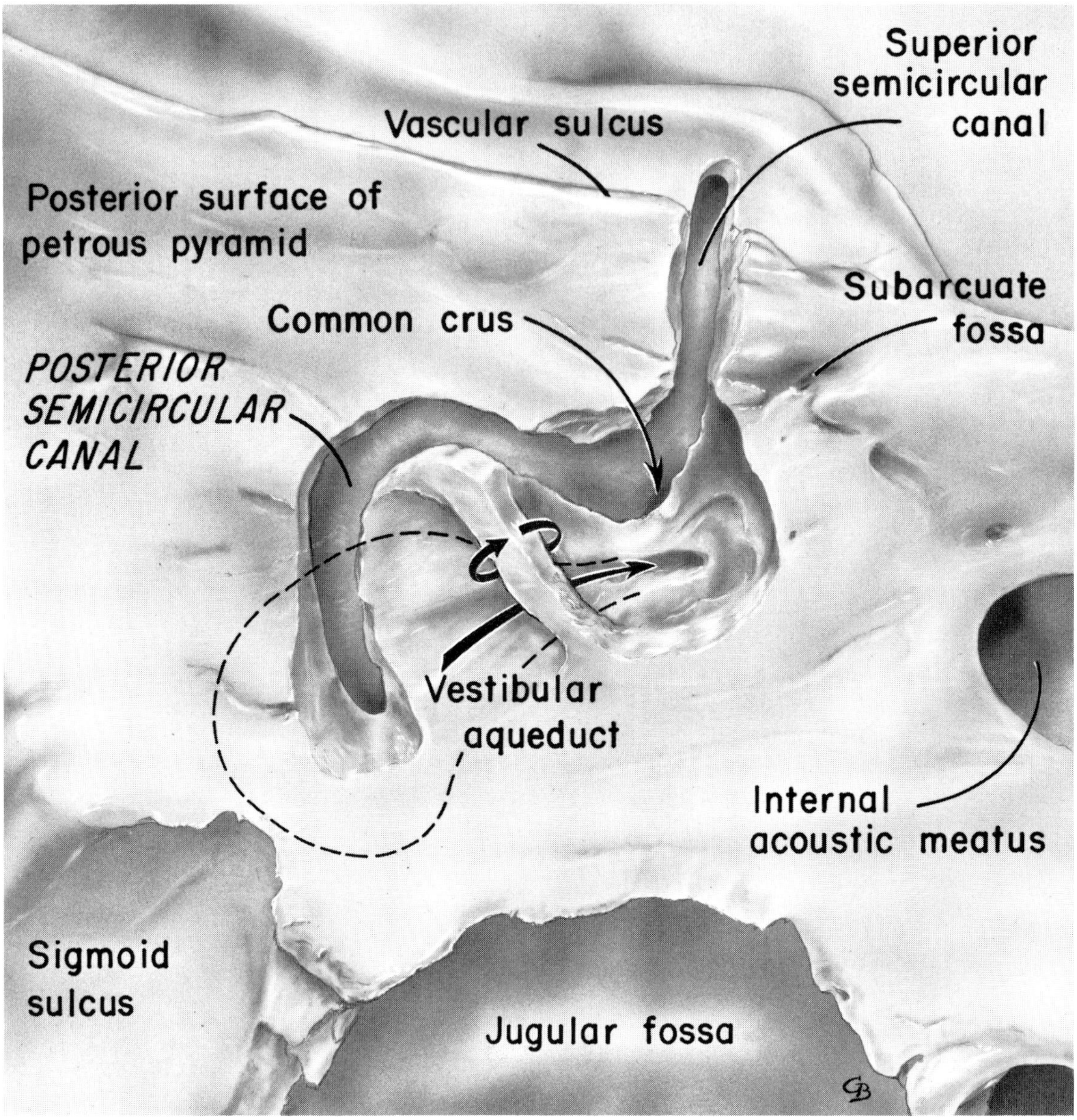

Figure III–104. VESTIBULAR AQUEDUCT, SEMICIRCULAR CANALS, AND CUSTOMARY SITE OF SURGICAL INCISION FOR APPROACH TO ENDOLYMPHATIC SAC. SPECIMEN OF LEFT TEMPORAL BONE SEEN FROM MEDIAL SIDE.

The distal segment of the vestibular aqueduct has been opened to demonstrate the continuity of its space with the fovea for reception of the endolymphatic sac. Similarly, the superior and posterior semicircular canals and common crus have been opened. For service in topography, a bridge of bone (encircled with arrow) remains at the aperture of the aqueduct. The former site of a typical endolymphatic sac is outlined by broken lines. The unlabeled arrow passes from the posterior fossa of the cranial cavity, through the external aperture of the vestibular aqueduct, and into the distal segment of the latter. The space narrows to an apex where the sac would become continuous with the duct. Typically, the cranial part of the sac extends postero-inferiorly to approach the margins of the sigmoid sulcus and the jugular fossa (Figure III–105).

Dissection by Dr. Raymond L. Warpeha.

(From Anson: Arch. Otolaryng., 89:96–110, 1969.)

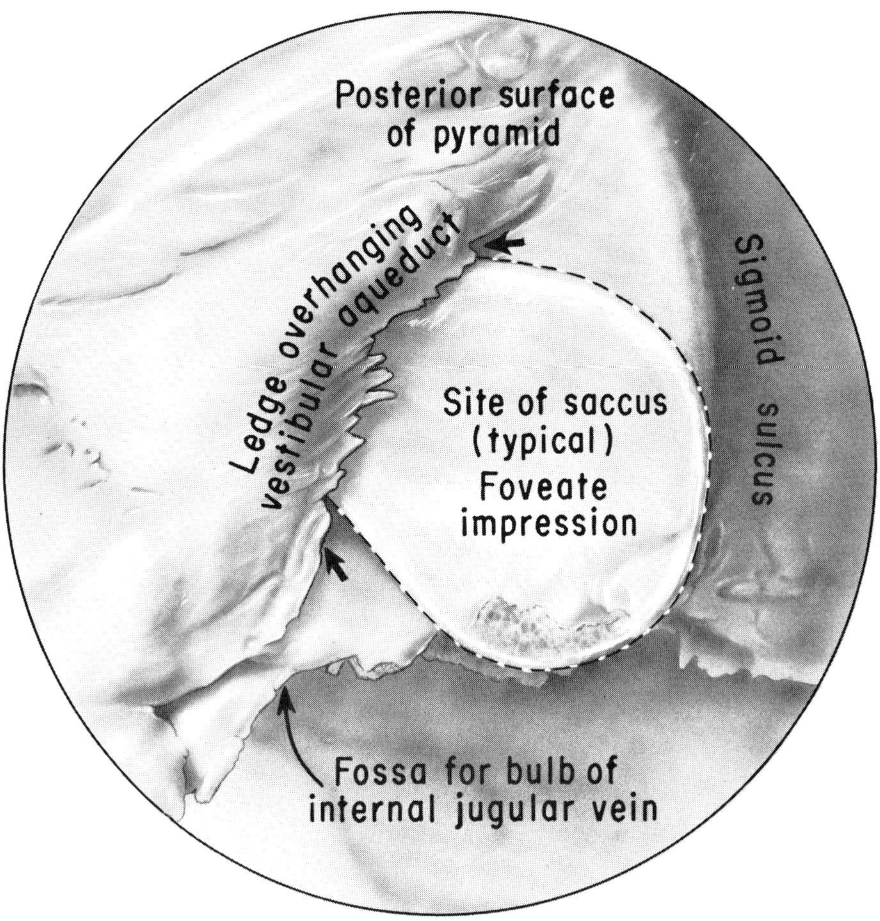

Specimen	Length, mm.	Specimen	Max. Width, mm.
2	7	1	5
2	8	4	6
2	9	8	7
4	10	7	8
6	11	7	9
5	12	2	10
5	13	1	11
1	14	30	
2	15		
1	16		
30			

Figure III–105. External aperture of the vestibular aqueduct and intradural part of the endolymphatic sac. Skeletal preparation with superimposed saccus of typical form, size, and relationships. Tabulation covers measurements on 30 injected specimens (hemisected heads, embalmed).

The sac regularly extends posteroinferiorly beyond the ledge of bone that forms the medial boundary of the external aperture of the aqueduct (margins of the latter opening indicated by unlabeled arrows), downward to or beyond the posterior angle of the pyramid. This means that it may be in contact with, or rest upon, the sigmond venous sinus (see measurements in Figure III–118).

In 20 of the 30 specimens, the range in length of the intradural part of the endolymphatic sac lay between 10 and 13 mm.; in 22, the range in width lay between 7 and 9 mm.

(From Anson, Warpeha, and Rensink: Ann. Otol., 77:583–607, 1968.)

Figure III–106. VESTIBULAR AQUEDUCT, INTERNAL ACOUSTIC MEATUS, COCHLEAR AQUEDUCT, AND RELATED ANATOMY OF THE VESTIBULAR AND CANALICULAR PARTS OF THE INTERNAL EAR. DISSECTION OF A TEMPORAL BONE, SEEN FROM THE MEDIAL SIDE.

The meatus is exposed from the pore to the fundus. The vestibular aqueduct is similarly opened from the external aperture into the posterior cranial fossa to the internal aperture on the wall of the vestibule. At the opening of each, on the posterior surface of the pyramid a bridge of bone (encircled with arrow) remains. The semicircular canals have been opened.

Measurements of the vestibular aqueduct and of a diamond burr are recorded for purposes of comparison.

Dissection by Dr. Raymond L. Warpeha.

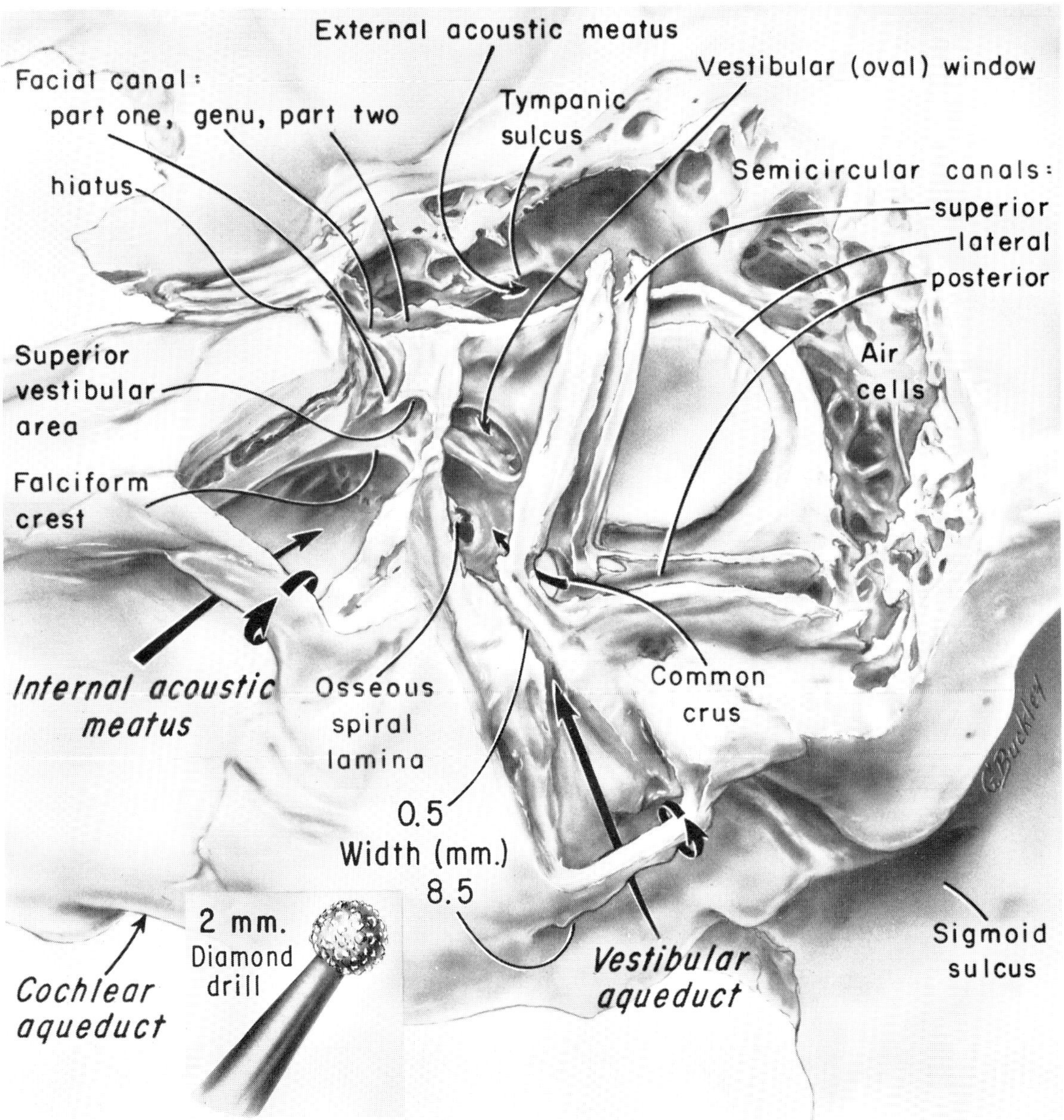

Figure III–106. See legend on the opposite page.

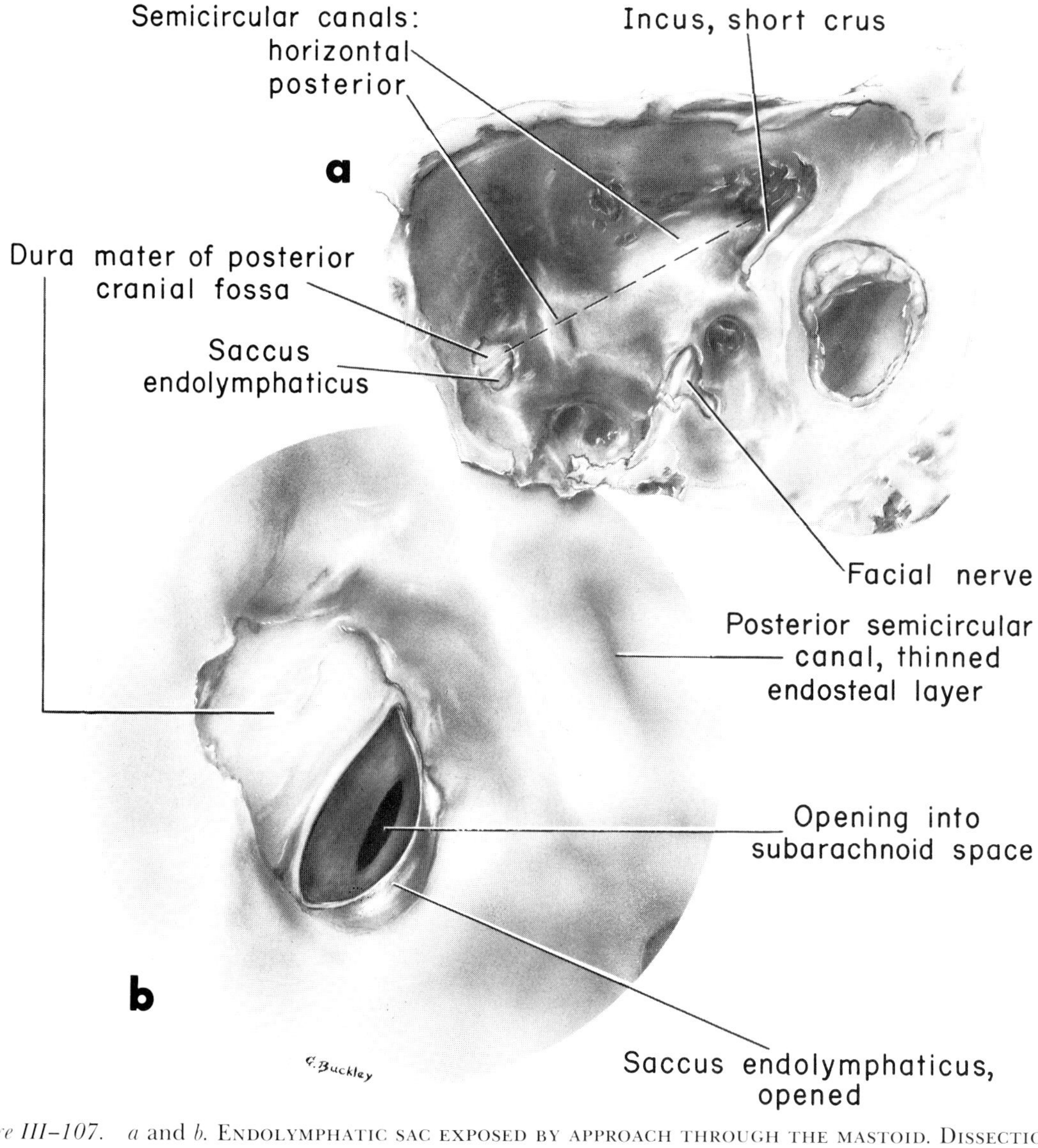

Figure III–107. *a* and *b*. ENDOLYMPHATIC SAC EXPOSED BY APPROACH THROUGH THE MASTOID. DISSECTION OF AN UNEMBALMED SPECIMEN. PROCEDURE OF WILLIAM HOUSE, M.D. *c*. THE ENDOLYMPHATIC DUCT AND SAC, INTRAOSSEOUS AND INTRADURAL PARTS. MALE, 37 YEARS OF AGE.

a. In carrying out a complete mastoidectomy, the following structures are identified: the facial nerve, the lateral (so-called horizontal) and posterior semicanals, and the sigmoid sinus. The wall of the posterior canal, acting as a serviceable topographical guide, is thinned to a "blue line." The lateral semicircular canal, in being directed lateralward as well as backward, produces the *prominentia* on the wall of the epitympanic recess. Typically, the saccus is to be found between the posterior semicircular canal and the sigmoid sinus, at or below a line drawn in the plane of the "horizontal" canal.

b. In the area of the endolymphatic sac, now shown enlarged, the inner periosteal layer of bone has been removed. An incision in the dural layer of the posterior cranial fossa exposed the sac; a cut through both walls of the sac carried the dissection into the subarachnoid space.

Figure III–107 continues on the opposite page.

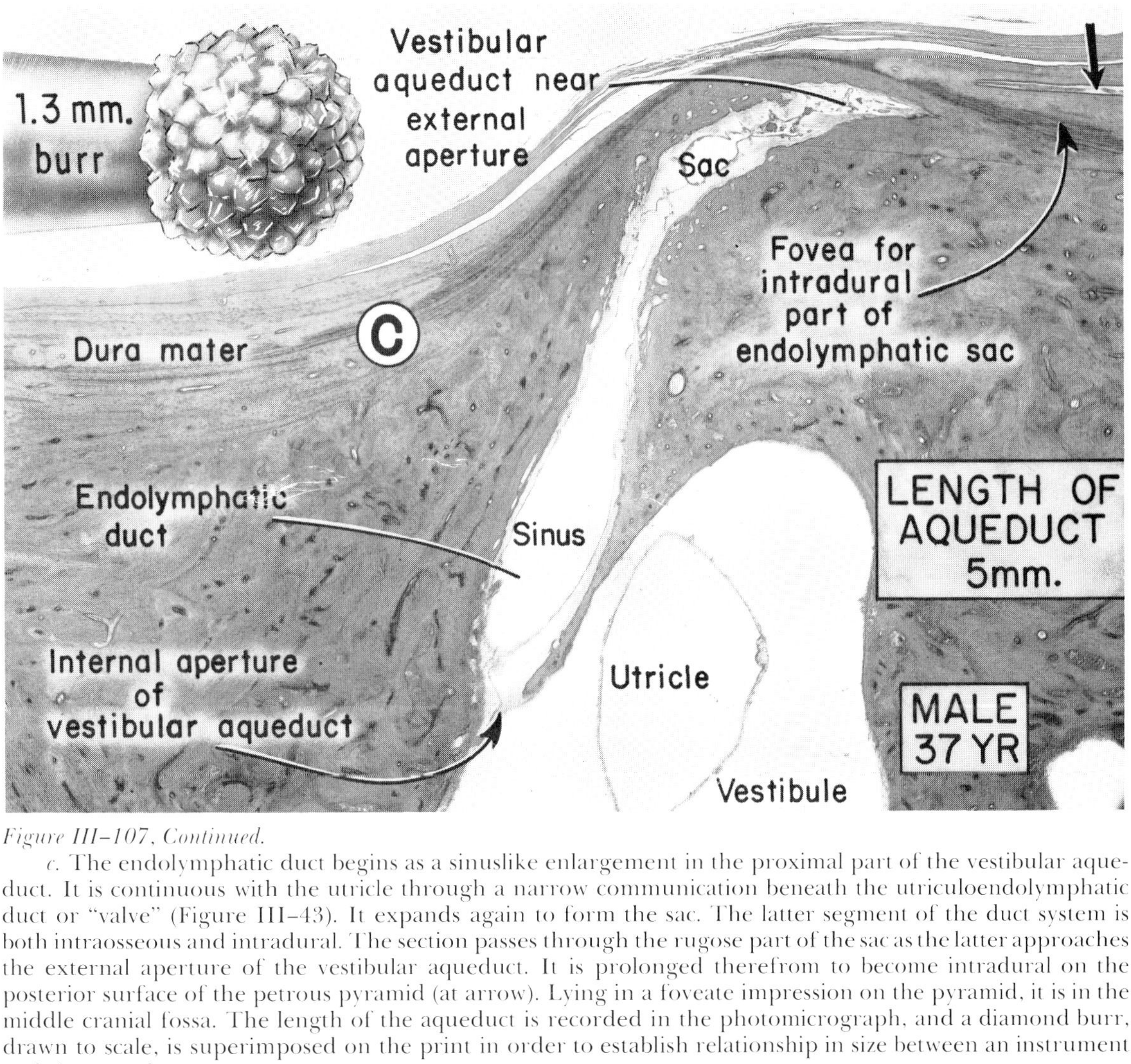

Figure III–107, Continued.

c. The endolymphatic duct begins as a sinuslike enlargement in the proximal part of the vestibular aqueduct. It is continuous with the utricle through a narrow communication beneath the utriculoendolymphatic duct or "valve" (Figure III–43). It expands again to form the sac. The latter segment of the duct system is both intraosseous and intradural. The section passes through the rugose part of the sac as the latter approaches the external aperture of the vestibular aqueduct. It is prolonged therefrom to become intradural on the posterior surface of the petrous pyramid (at arrow). Lying in a foveate impression on the pyramid, it is in the middle cranial fossa. The length of the aqueduct is recorded in the photomicrograph, and a diamond burr, drawn to scale, is superimposed on the print in order to establish relationship in size between an instrument and the aqueduct.

Transverse section, Wisconsin Collection, series 21, left temporal bone. ×21.

(*a* and *b* from Anson, Donaldson, Warpeha, and Winch: Laryngoscope, 74:480–497, 1964; *c* from Anson: Trans. Amer. Acad. Ophthal. Otolaryng., 76:108–129, 1972.)

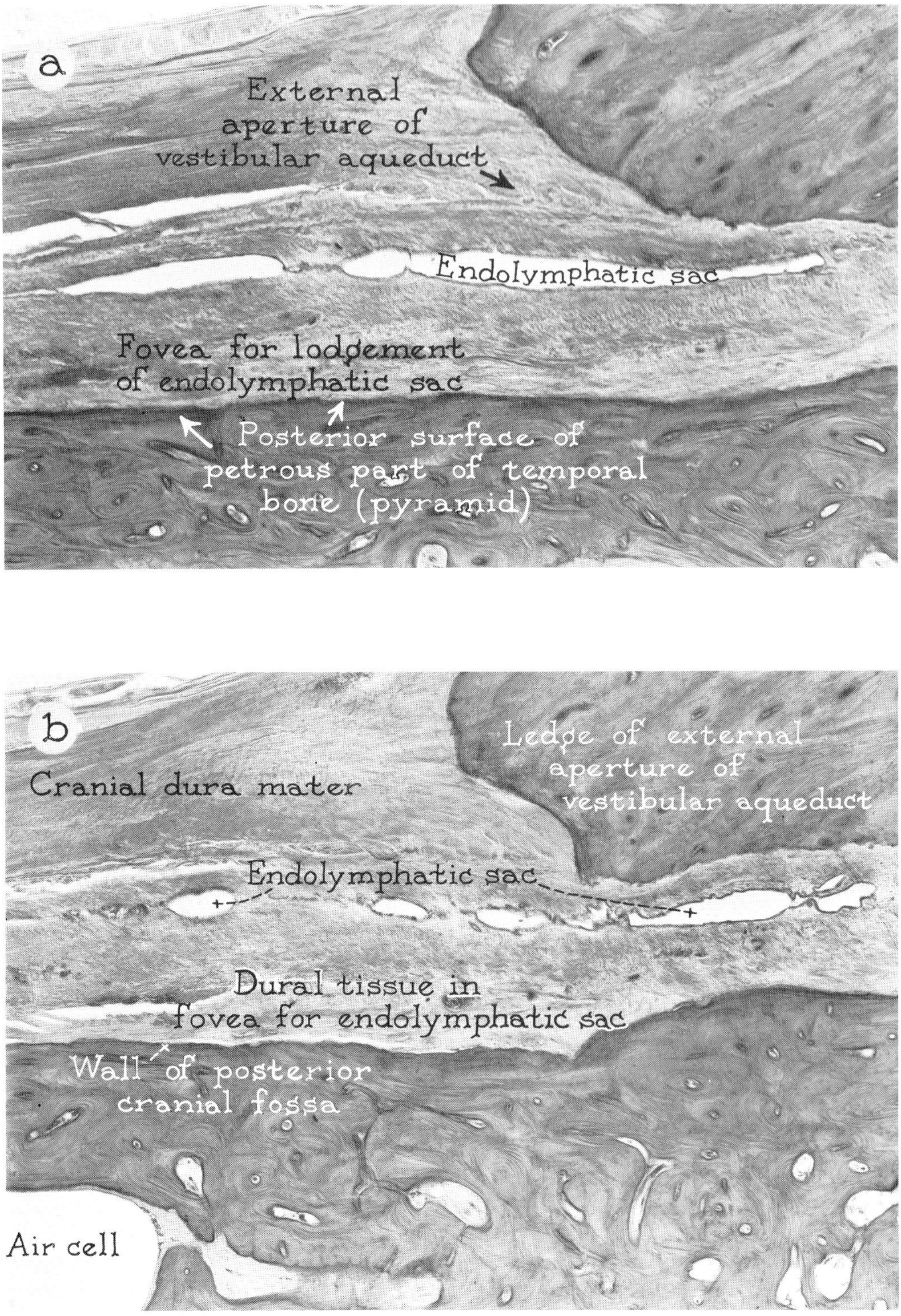

Figure III–108. See legend on the opposite page.

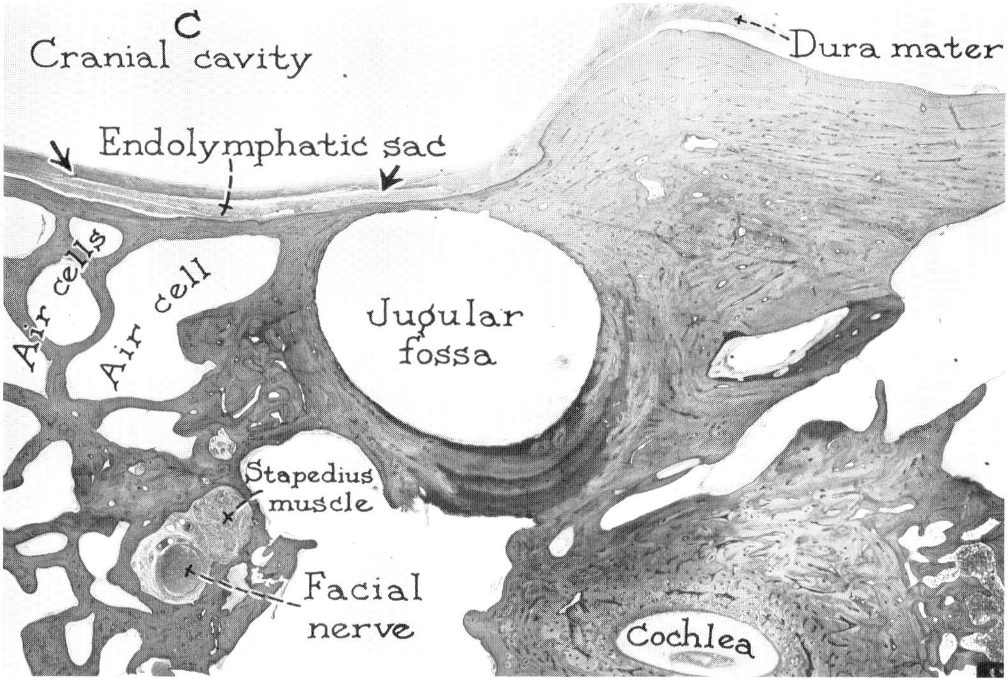

Figure III–108. Intradural portion of the endolymphatic sac: form and relationship to the external aperture of the vestibular aqueduct and to structures in the wall of the posterior cranial fossa. *a* and *b*. Female, 36 years of age. *c*. Female, 38 years old.

a. The endolymphatic duct leaves the vestibule through a small depression, the internal aperture of the vestibular aqueduct, situated on the wall of the elliptical recess (Figure III–52*b*). It courses through the bone toward the posterior surface of the petrous pyramid. Approaching the external aperture of the aqueduct, the duct becomes a flattened cecal dilatation, the endolymphatic sac. The saccus extends beyond the aperture in a duplicature of the cranial *dura mater*. In this position it occupies a fovea situated between the overhanging ledge of bone and the sigmoid sulcus (Figures III–103, III–105).

The deep relations of the sac vary. In this specimen the bone immediately subjacent to the sac is solid except for the presence of small vascular channels. Other types of relationship are shown in the following illustrations (compare with gross dissections in Figures III–103 and III–104).

b. At a different level in the same specimen the *saccus* was related to air cells.

c. In another specimen the sac, flattened in its fovea, was separated by a very thin layer of bone from the fossa for the bulb of the internal jugular vein. In still other instances the arc of the posterior semicircular canal is similarly related to the sac.

Transverse sections, Wisconsin Collection, series as follows: *a* and *b*, 40; *c*, 24. *a*, ×40; *b*, ×39; *c*, ×6.

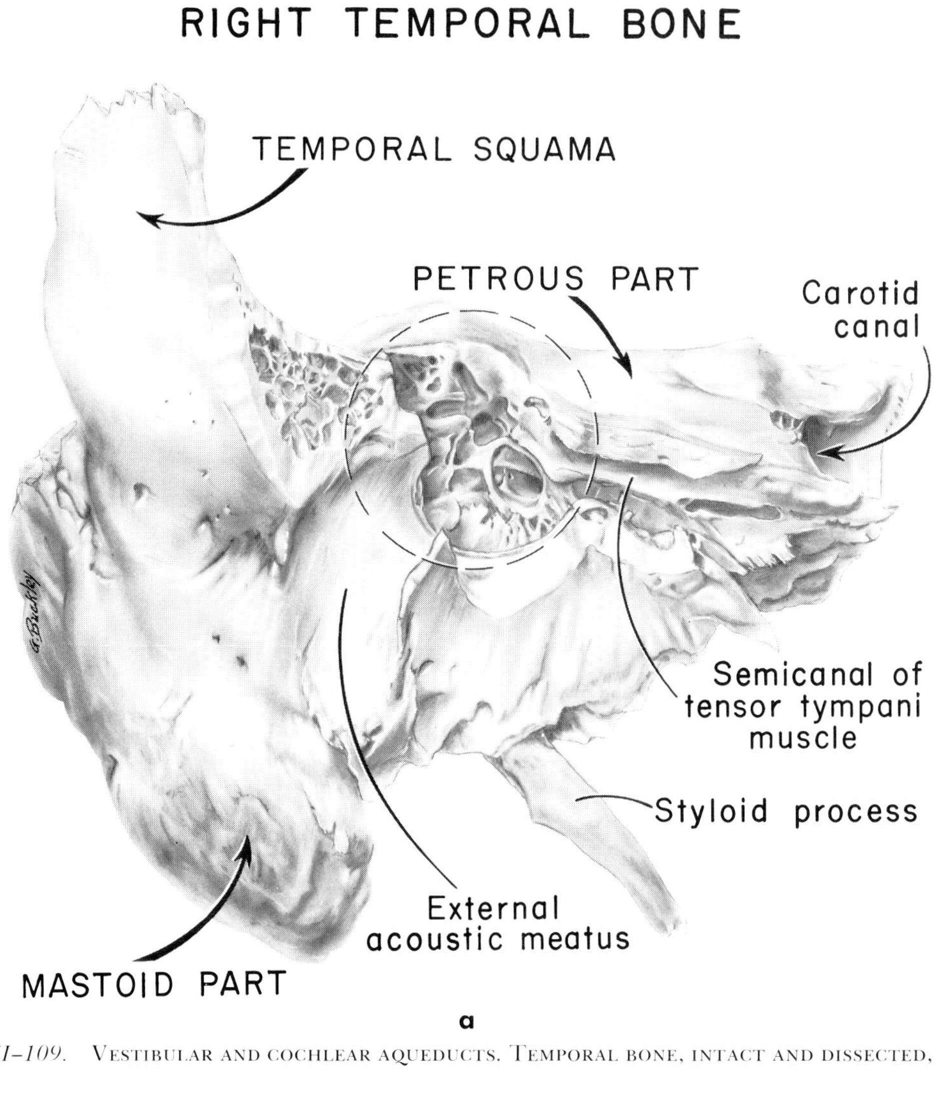

Figure III–109. Vestibular and cochlear aqueducts. Temporal bone, intact and dissected, lateral aspect.

a. Showing especially the relations of the internal apertures of the vestibular and cochlear aqueducts. The detailed anatomy of the encircled area is shown enlarged in the following figure.

b. Same specimen; detailed anatomy of the area marked in the preceding figure. After exposure of the medial wall of the middle ear, the stapes has been removed from the vestibular fenestra (oval window); the cochlear fenestra (round window) and related portion of the basal turn of the cochlea have been revealed by dissecting away the bone which forms the outer boundary of the fossula and the scalae. The cut edge of the bone is marked by small arrows; remnant of the wall, retained for service in orientation, is encircled by a single arrow.

Figure III–109 continues on the opposite page.

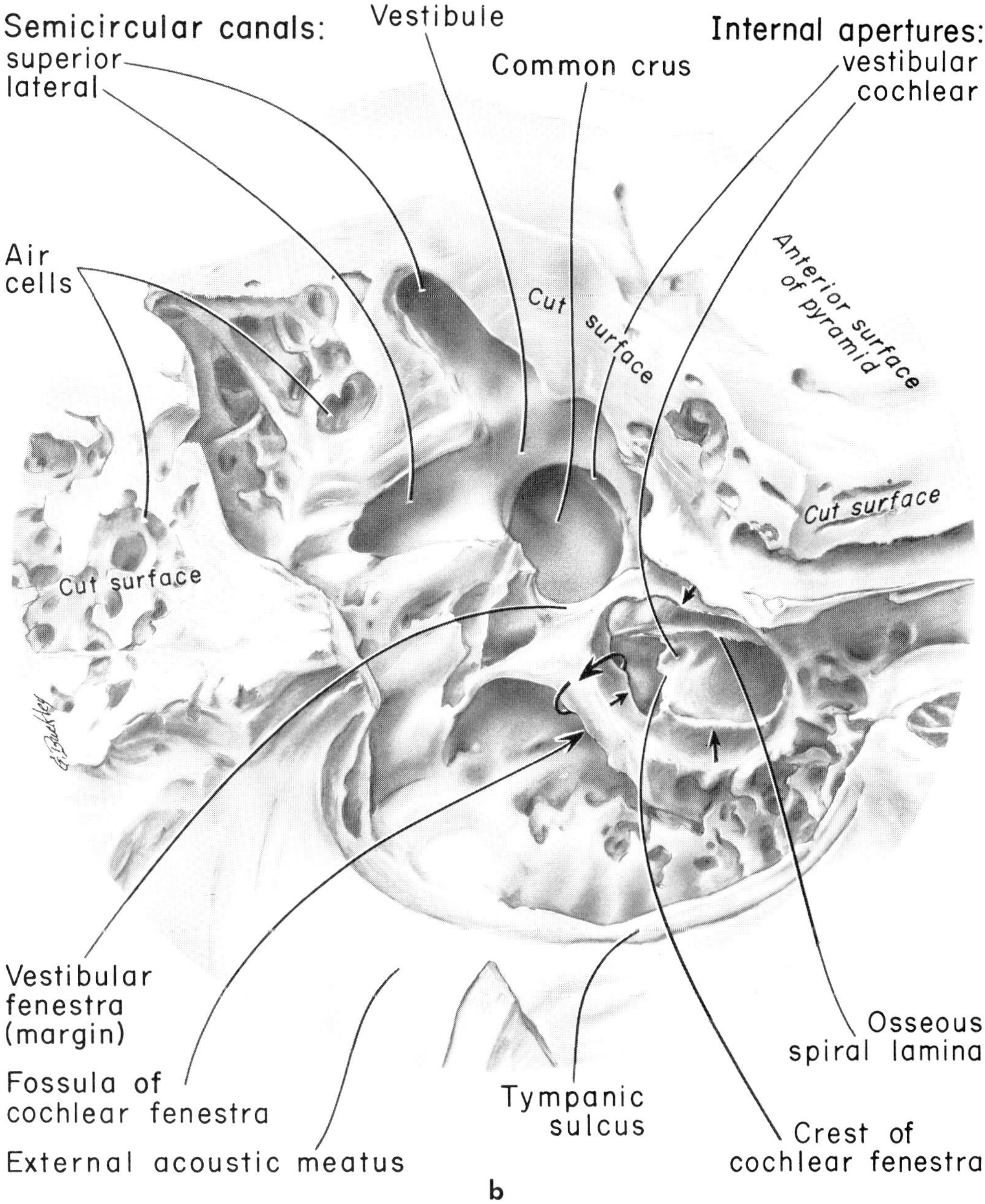

Figure III–109, Continued. VESTIBULAR AND COCHLEAR AQUEDUCTS. TEMPORAL BONE, INTACT AND DISSECTED, LATERAL ASPECT.

It is demonstrated that the internal aperture of the vestibular aqueduct opens as a small depression upon the oval *recessus ellipticus* (for reception of the utricle) on the anterior wall of the vestibule of the osseous labyrinth. The external aperture is a slit-shaped opening on the posterior surface of the pyramid which usually descends with a lateral inclination toward the jugular incisure.

The internal aperture of the cochlear aqueduct (or canaliculus) is a minute opening situated on the wall of the tympanic scala just beneath the osseous spiral lamina and close to the crest for attachment (in the fresh state) of the secondary tympanic membrane (see Figures III–94 and II–40*e*). The external aperture ends in the depths of a funnel-shaped depression on the inferior surface of the petrous pyramid between the jugular fossa and the external carotid foramen (see Figures III–119 and III–132).

The dissection also shows the following related features of the middle ear and internal ear: tympanic sulcus, semicanal for the tensor tympani muscle, superior and lateral semicircular canals, orifice of the fossula of the cochlear fenestra, external acoustic meatus, and the tympanic air cells. In the natural state the secondary tympanic membrane, attached to the crest of the cochlear fenestra (here partially removed), separates the space of the fossula from the tympanic scala.

Dissection by Dr. Raymond L. Warpeha.

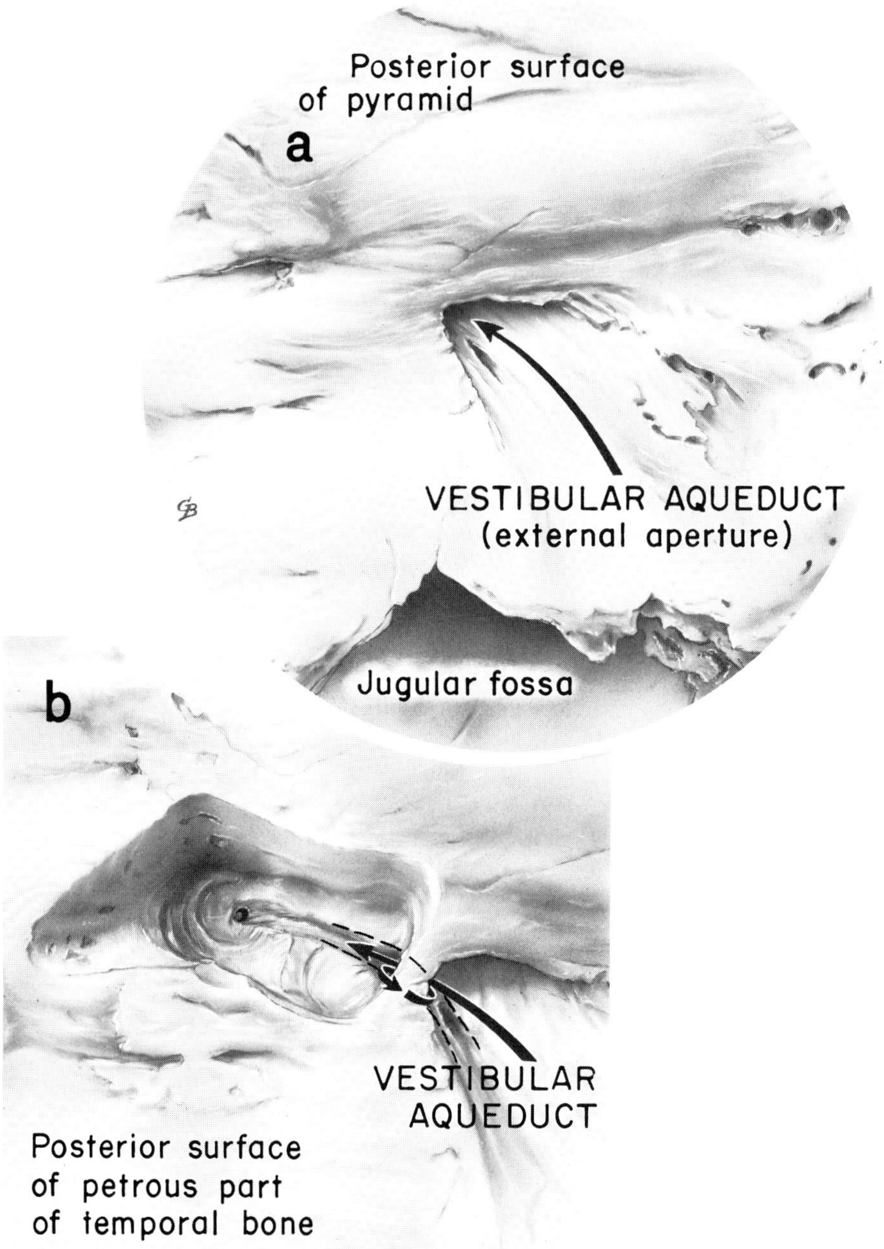

Figure III–110. EXTERNAL APERTURE OF THE VESTIBULAR AQUEDUCT: SELECTED EXAMPLES. SPECIMEN INTACT AND DISSECTED.

a. An aperture of unusually small size.

b. The dissection reveals a distal segment (of the aqueduct) that does not expand as it ends at the external aperture. For topographical service, a bridge of bone (encircled) remains at the aperture.

Explanatory Note: In using the burr to expose the distal segment of the vestibular aqueduct (dissections in *b* of Figures 110 to 116), a swath wider than that of the subjacent aqueduct is cut in the bone proximal to the aperture. In the drawing, then, the space of the aqueduct (margins indicated by broken lines) appears as a furrow (the true aqueduct) on the "floor" of the wider excavation.

Dissection by Dr. Raymond L. Warpeha.

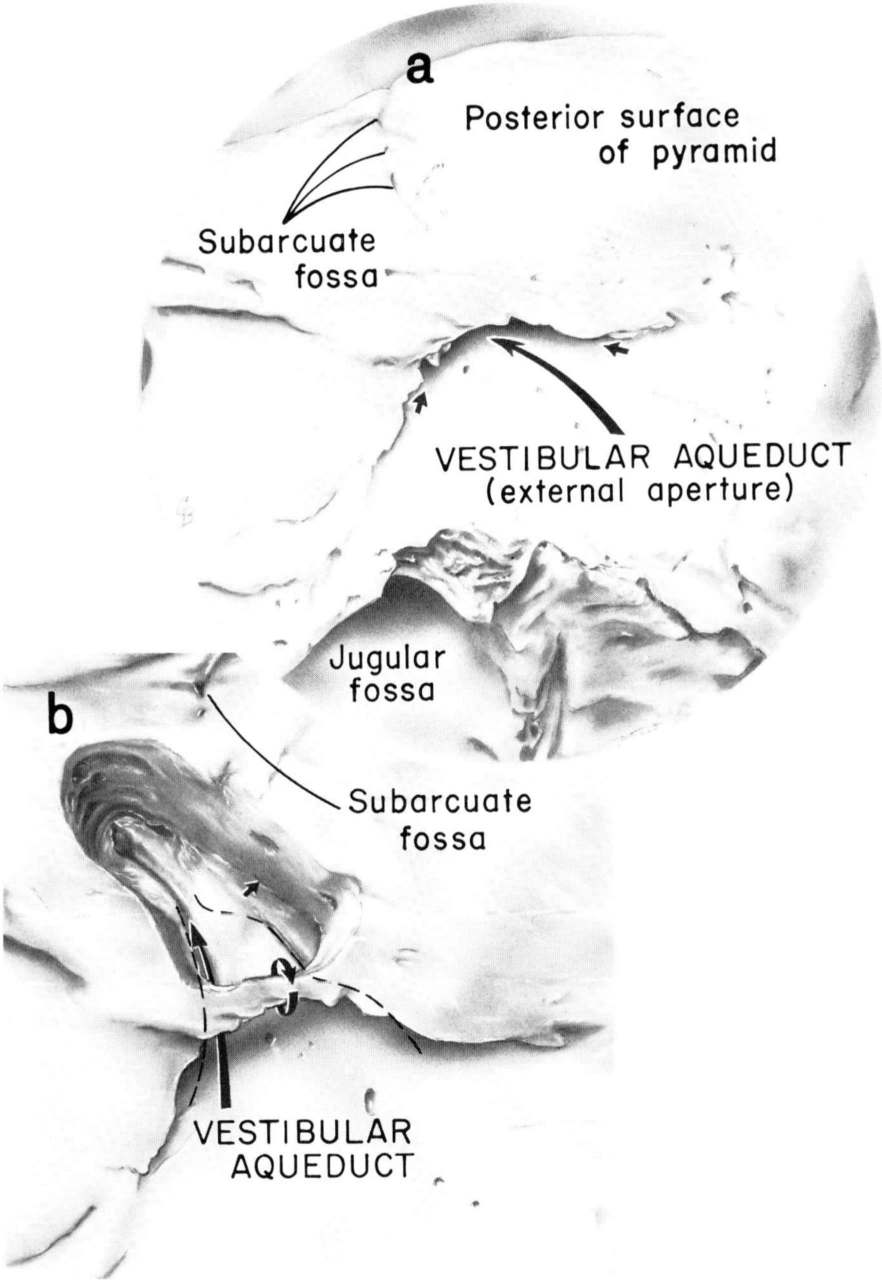

Figure III–111. External aperture of the vestibular aqueduct: examples, continued. Specimen intact and dissected.

a. The ledge of bone that overhangs the aperture is semilunar in outline. The margins are indicated by unlabeled arrows. The subarcuate fossa consists, atypically, of the three openings.

b. The distal segment of the aqueduct is typically triangular in outline. Inward, the apical part becomes continuous with the narrowed segment which, in the fresh state, transmits the isthmus of the endolymphatic duct (see Figures III–60 and II–22*e*).

Dissection by Dr. Raymond L. Warpeha.

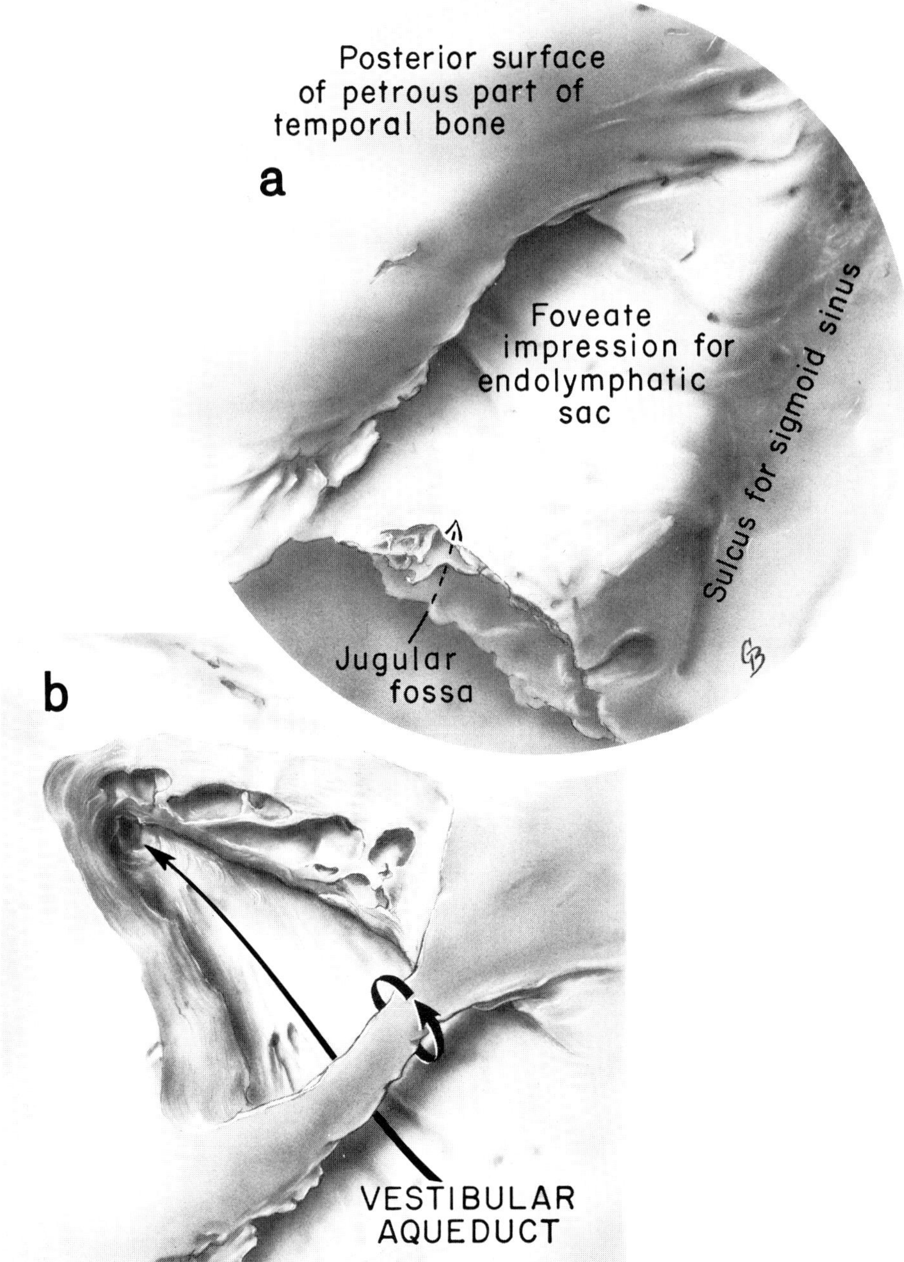

Figure III–112. External aperture of the vestibular aqueduct: examples, continued. Specimen, intact and dissected.

a. The prominent obliquely-directed ledge of bone overarches a capacious external aperture; the latter opens upon a relatively broad fovea for reception of the intradural part of the endolymphatic sac. In such a specimen, a sac of typical size would touch, or possibly overlie, the internal jugular vein or the sigmoid venous sinus.

b. The bone that forms the wall of the aqueduct regularly contains spaces (of the kind here exposed) occupied by air cells (see Figures III–103*b* and III–108*b, c*).

Dissection by Dr. Raymond L. Warpeha.

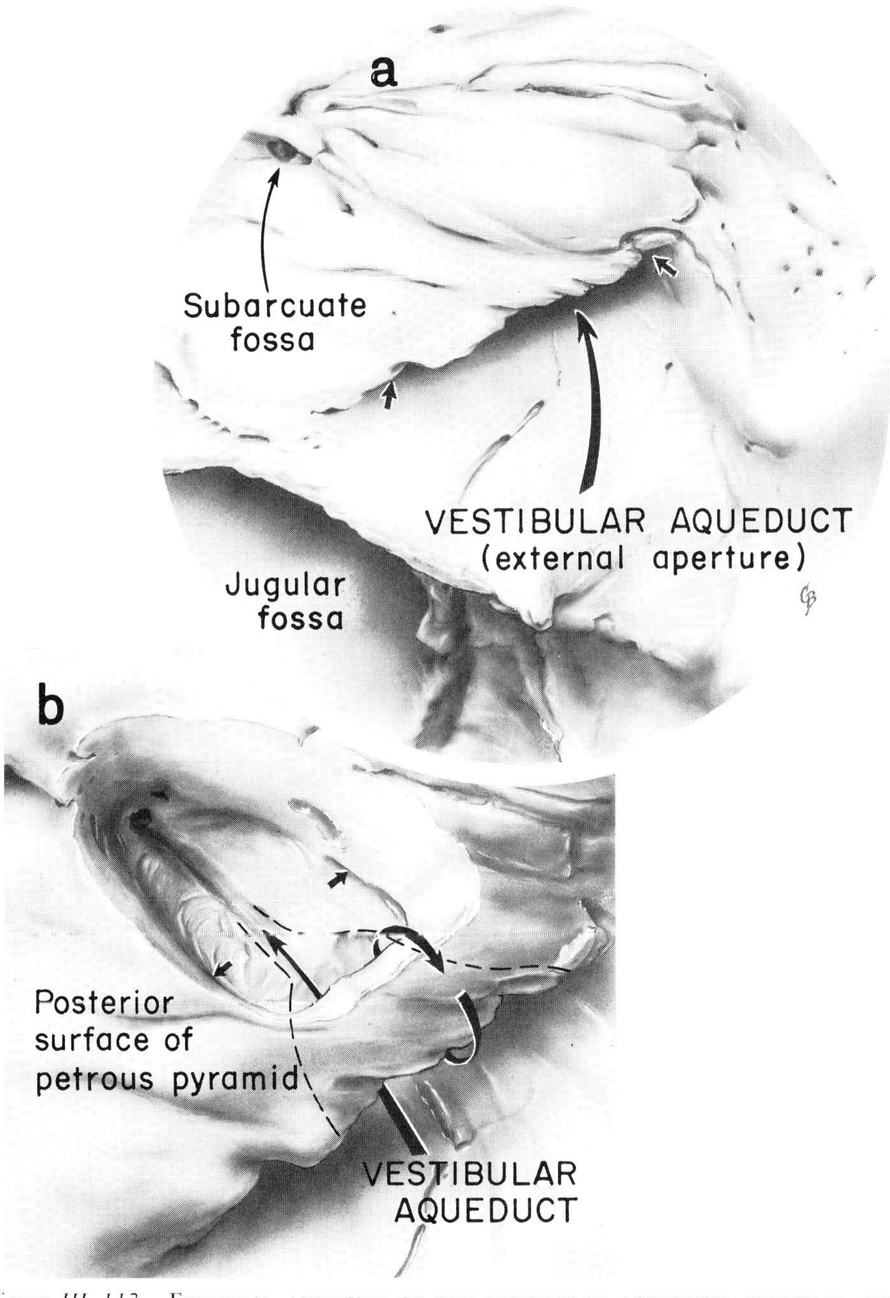

Figure III–113. EXTERNAL APERTURE OF THE VESTIBULAR AQUEDUCT: EXAMPLES, CONTINUED. SPECIMEN INTACT AND DISSECTED.

a. An example of an elongate aperture, the boundaries of which are indicated by the unlabeled arrows. The posterior surface of the bone is marked by sulci and apertures which, in the natural state, transmitted dural blood vessels to or from the subarcuate fossa, vestibular aqueduct, superior petrosal sulcus, and lesser openings into the bone. Sulci are also present in the bone of the fovea. They carry vessels that contribute to the vascular supply of the *saccus* (see Figures III–61, III–62, and III–114*a*).

b. Bone has been removed (to the tips of the unlabeled arrows) to expose the distal segment of the vestibular aqueduct. Here, as is typically the case, it is triangular in outline (as indicated by the broken line), with the apex directed inward.

Dissection by Dr. Raymond L. Warpeha.

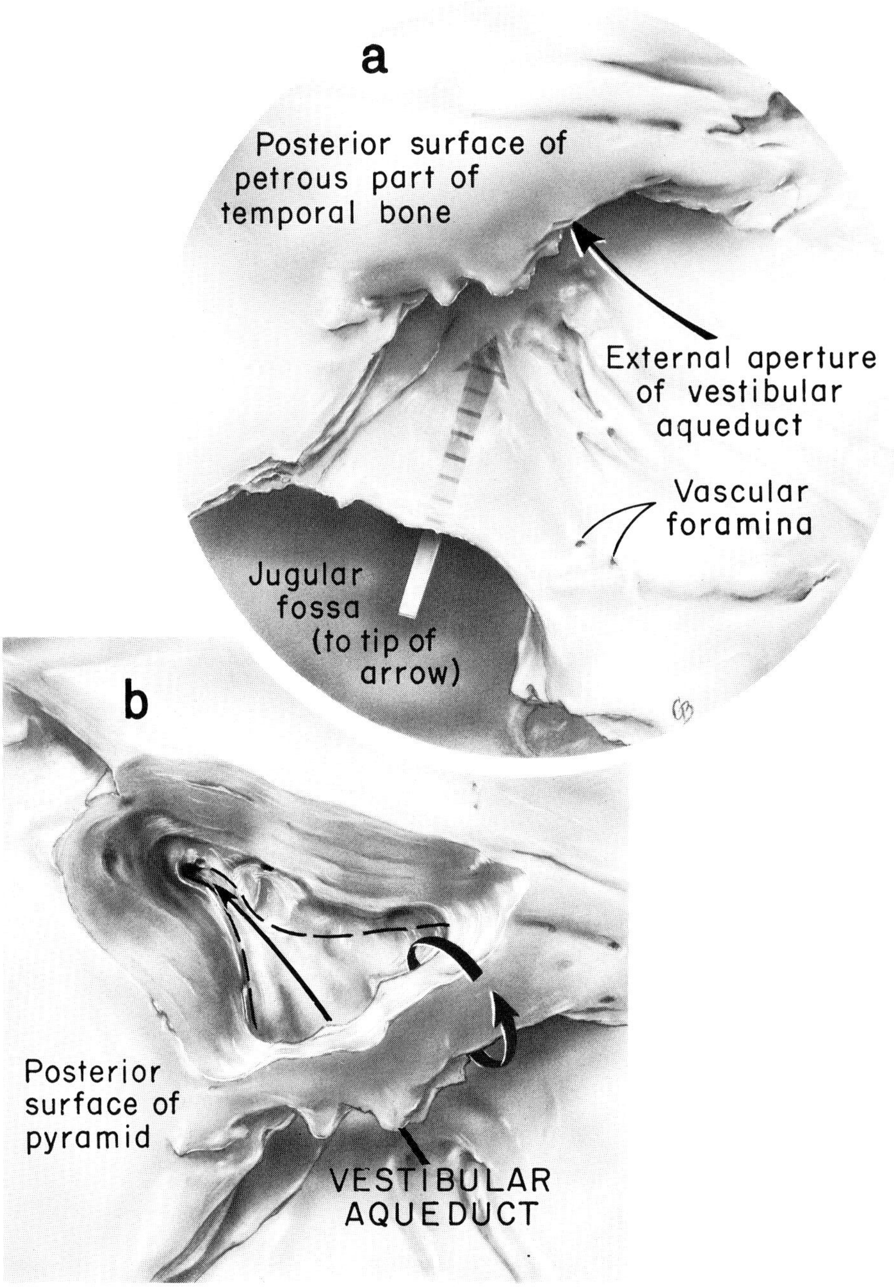

Figure III–114. EXTERNAL APERTURE OF THE VESTIBULAR AQUEDUCT: EXAMPLES, CONTINUED. SPECIMEN INTACT AND DISSECTED.

a. Here the aperture is similar to that in the preceding figure. However, its relationship to the fossa for the internal jugular vein is strikingly different; the foveate area for reception of the endolymphatic sac is separated from a deep jugular fossa by a plate of bone so thin as to be translucent (see section in Figure III–108*c*). The roof of the fossa may be dehiscent (see Figure III–132). In such instances the fossa (with the superior bulb of the internal jugular vein) is separated from the space of the tympanic cavity merely by mucous membrane.

b. The distal segment of the vestibular aqueduct possesses the typical triangular form (margins indicated by broken lines).

Dissection by Dr. Raymond L. Warpeha.

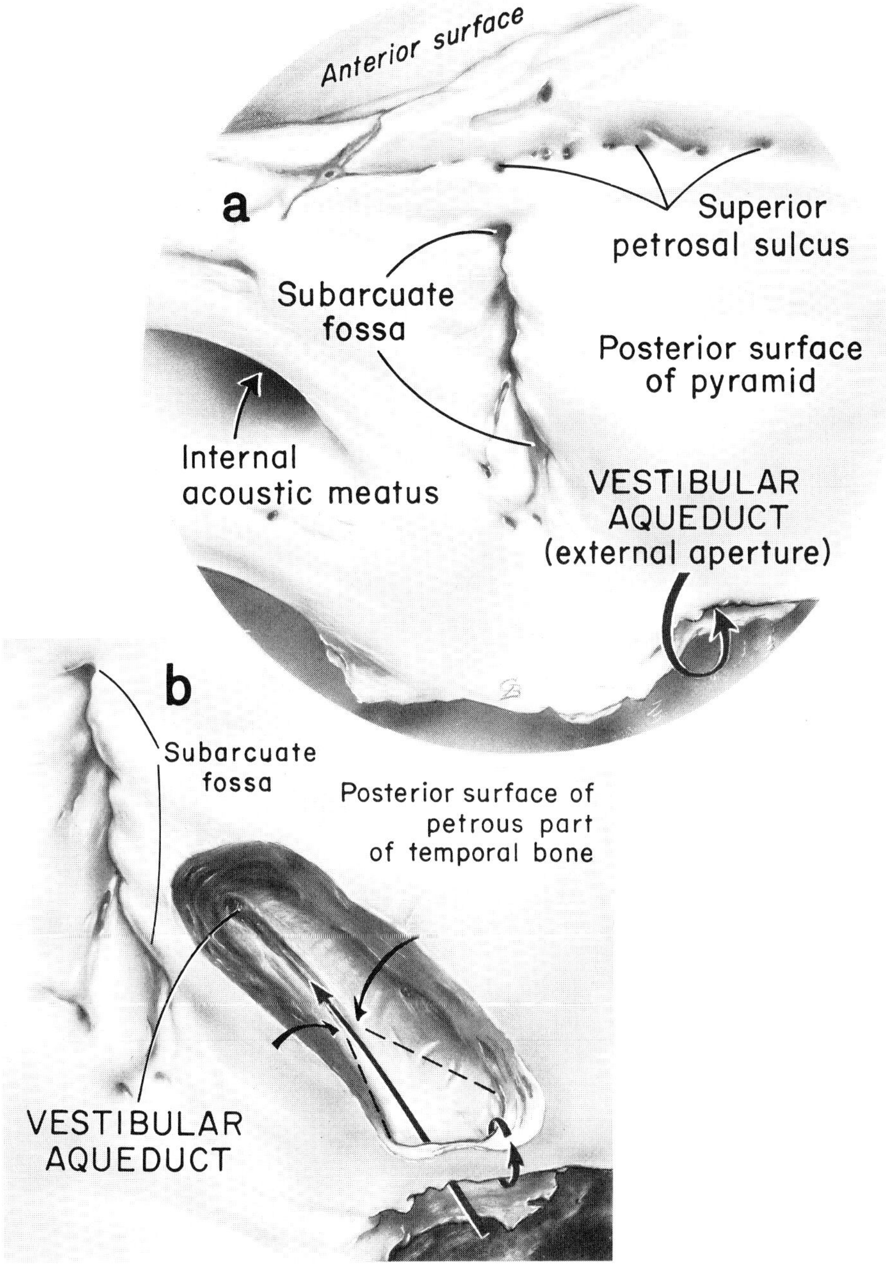

Figure III–115. External aperture of the vestibular aqueduct: examples, continued. Specimen intact and dissected.

a. An aperture of very unusual location in the presence of a subarcuate fossa of exceptional size, form, and position. The fossa occupies the customary position of the external aperture of the vestibular aqueduct, the latter opening being situated at the angle of junction of the posterior and inferior surfaces of the petrous pyramid.

b. The vestibular aqueduct is typical in form despite its unusual position. It passes inward (in the direction of the elongate arrow) to change from a triangle-shaped distal segment into a narrow part (at the point marked by the curved arrows). In the natural state the widened part of the aqueduct would be occupied by the sac, the narrow portion by the isthmus of the endolymphatic duct (see diagram in Figure II–22*e*).

Dissection by Dr. Raymond L. Warpeha.

Figure III–116. VESTIBULAR AQUEDUCT; EXTERNAL APERTURE AND DISTAL EXPANDED SEGMENT, TOGETHER WITH SURGICAL MILLS: EXAMPLES, CONCLUDED.

a. The external aperture (at *1*) in relation to the fossa for the bulb of the internal jugular vein. Emissary apertures are indicated by unlabeled arrows. They transmit dural blood vessels of small size that supply both the bone and the saccus. The thin ledge of bone over the external aperture is prolonged into the fovea of the saccus.

b. The same specimen dissected to demonstrate the triangular form of the distal segment and the way in which it meets the fovea for the saccus. The ridge (at *2*) continues widely in both directions beyond the limits of the true aperture (at *1* in *a*).

c. Burrs shown at a magnification matching that of the dissection in *b.*

Dissection by Dr. Raymond L. Warpeha.

(From Anson, Warpeha, and Rensink: Ann. Otol., 77:583–607, 1968.)

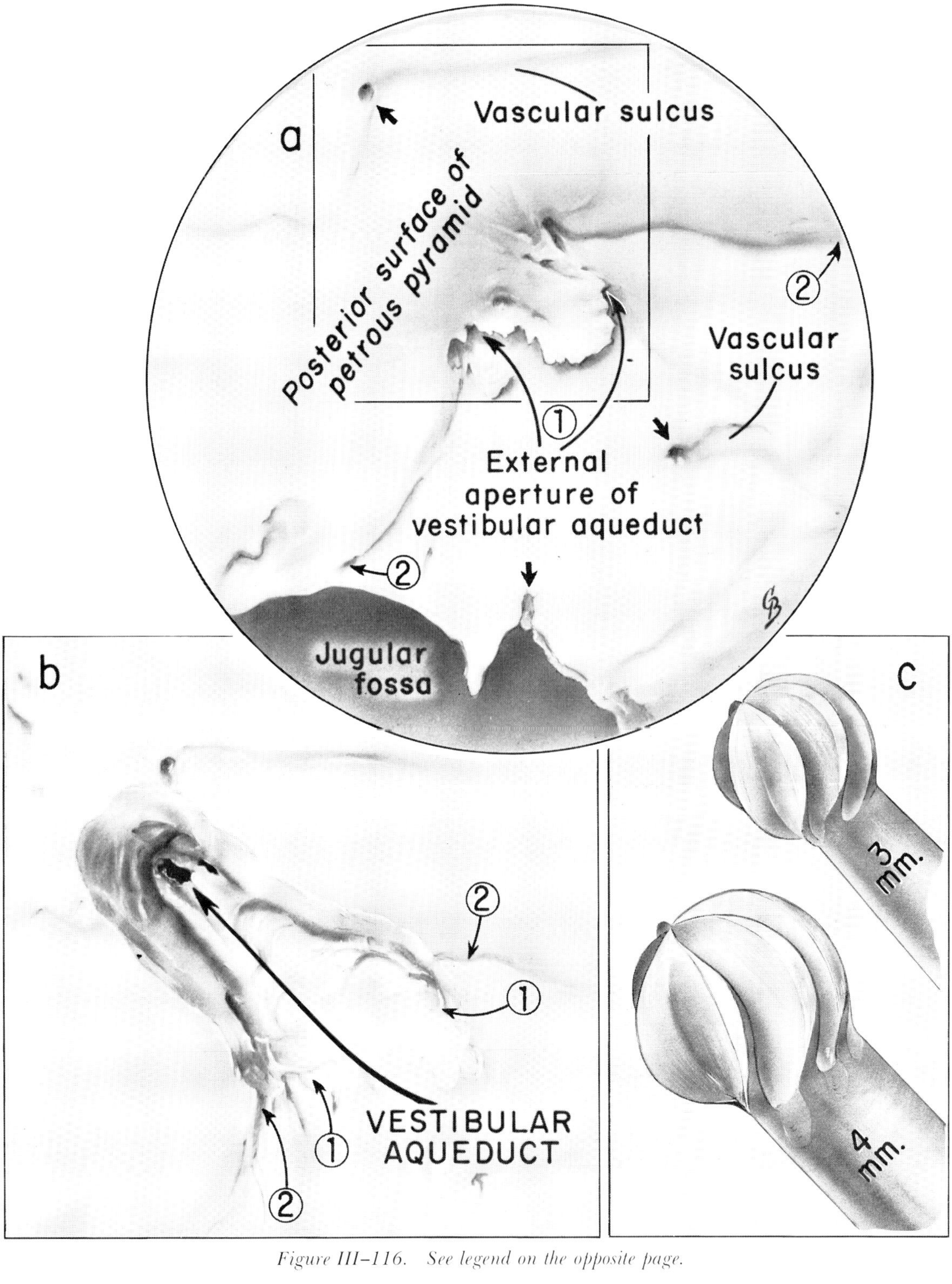

Figure III–116. See legend on the opposite page.

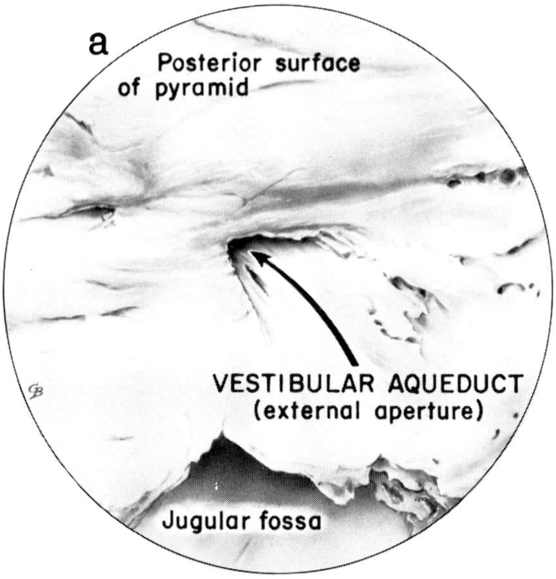

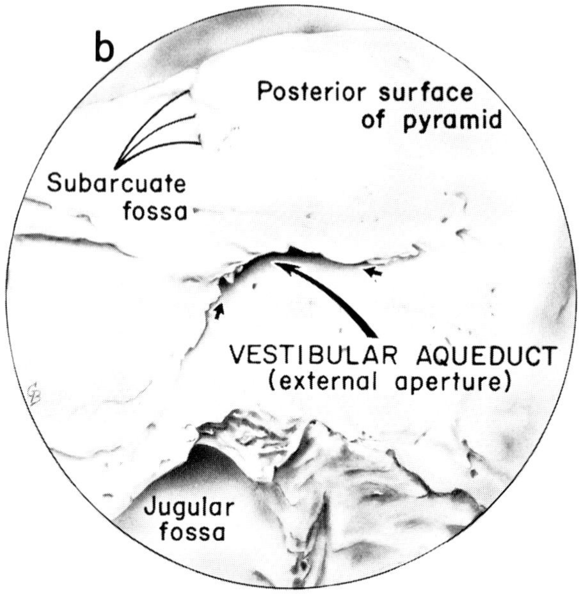

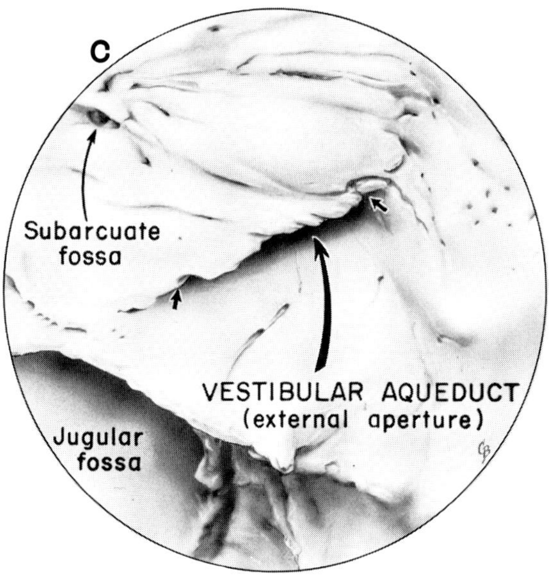

APERTURE

	Specimen	Width, mm.
	3	0.5
	7	1
90%	35	2
90%	51	3
90%	71	4
90%	49	5
90%	19	6
	5	7
	6	8
	2	9
	2	10
	250	

Figure III–117. VESTIBULAR AQUEDUCT: VARIATION IN FORM AND SIZE OF THE EXTERNAL APERTURE.

a. An example of small aperture (as in Figure III–110*a*). Small openings (unlabeled) transmits vessels of dural location into the bone.

b. An aperture of usual form and width (margins indicated by the small arrows). The subarcuate fossa consists of three small openings in the bone (Figure III–111*a*).

c. An aperture typically oblique in direction, but of width greater than average (Figure III–113*a*).

The tabulation shows that the width in 250 specimens varied between 0.5 mm. and 10 mm., and in the preponderant number of cases (90 per cent) it measured between 2 mm. and 6 mm.

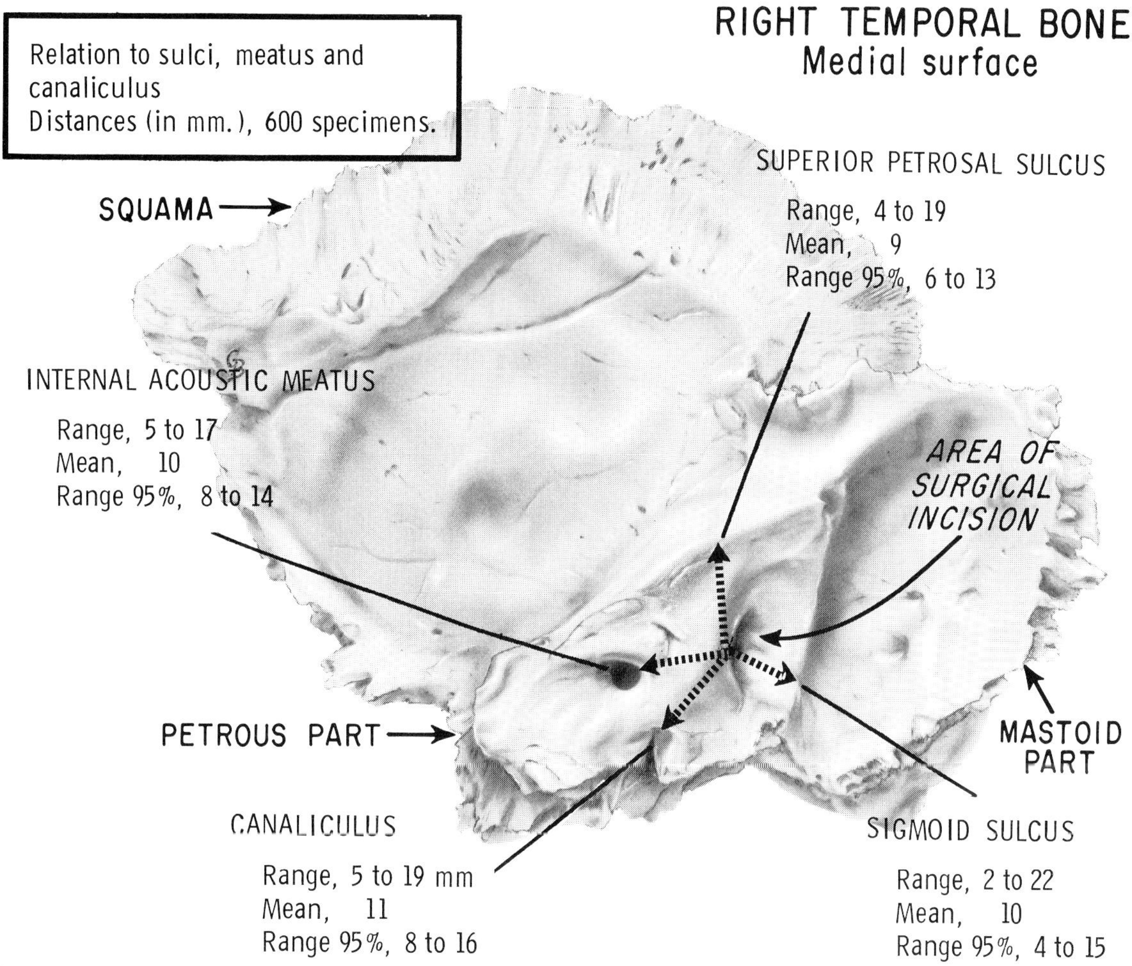

Figure III–118. Posterior surface of the pyramid, with data on variational anatomy of the external aperture of the vestibular aqueduct in 600 consecutive specimens.

The measurements (maximum, minimum, mean) are recorded for distances intervening between the center of the aperture and near margin of each of the following openings or sulci: superior petrosal sulcus, pore of the internal acoustic meatus, subarcuate fossa, sigmoid sulcus, and external aperture of the cochlear aqueduct (or canaliculus) which appears as a notch on the posterior angle of the pyramid.

The leader from the label *Area of Surgical Incision* points to the foveate impression for reception of the intradural segment of the endolymphatic sac. It would be exposed in the shunt-procedure of Dr. William F. House. The saccus would be exposed from the lateral aspect in mastoid approach (see Figure III–107).

The example here pictured would be regarded as typical. However, variations are common, some of them representing striking departures from the anatomic "norm" (see Figures III–110 to III–117).

Figure III–119. THE FORM, POSITION, AND RELATIONS OF THE EXTERNAL APERTURE OF THE COCHLEAR CANALICULUS (OR AQUEDUCT). LEFT TEMPORAL BONE, VIEWED FROM BELOW.

The external aperture of the cochlear canaliculus, or aqueduct, is situated on the inferior surface of the petrous pyramid. It begins in a three-sided impression, the medial aspect of which appears as a notch at the junction of the posterior and inferior surfaces of the pyramid. Like the corresponding aperture of the vestibular aqueduct, it is subject to considerable variation.

On the inner ear side the relationships of the cochlear canaliculus to other structures are relatively simple; they are many and complex on the inferior aspect. Numerous foramina and canaliculi open upon this lower surface. They will now be described.

The external carotid foramen is a circular opening of the canal for transmission of the internal carotid artery (see III–138*d*), accompanied by the internal carotid plexus of sympathetic nerves. Within the canal one or two minute ostia lead into the caroticotympanic canaliculi, to transmit communicating twigs between the internal carotid and tympanic plexuses and to convey an artery to the tympanum.

The petrosal fossula is situated on the summit of the carotid ridge between the carotid canal and the jugular fossa. This small depression leads into the minute tympanic canaliculus that transmits the tympanic branch of the glossopharyngeal nerve (Jacobson's nerve) and a small branch from the ascending pharyngeal artery. The fossula itself lodges the petrosal ganglion of the glossopharyngeal nerve.

The stylomastoid foramen is situated at the base of the styloid process. It is the external orifice of the canal for the facial nerve and the stylomastoid branch of the posterior auricular artery (a vessel important despite its small size). Within the canal the artery gives off branches to the mastoid cells, the stapedius muscle and tendon, and part of the tympanic membrane. Sometimes the auricular branch of the vagus nerve is transmitted by the stylomastoid foramen.

The jugular fossa is an elliptical depression situated posterior to the carotid ridge. It forms the anterolateral part of the bony wall of the jugular foramen in which is contained the dilation at the commencement of the internal jugular vein. The fossa is continuous with the sigmoid sulcus. In addition, the jugular foramen contains the inferior petrosal sinus, the glossopharyngeal nerve (with its superior ganglion), the vagus nerve (with the jugular ganglion) and the accessory nerve. On the lateral wall of the jugular fossa is situated a minute foramen, the mastoid canaliculus, for the entrance of the auricular branch of the vagus (Arnold's nerve) into the interior of the petrous part of the temporal bone.

(From Anson, Donaldson, Warpeha, and Winch: Laryngoscope 75:1497–1517, 1965.)

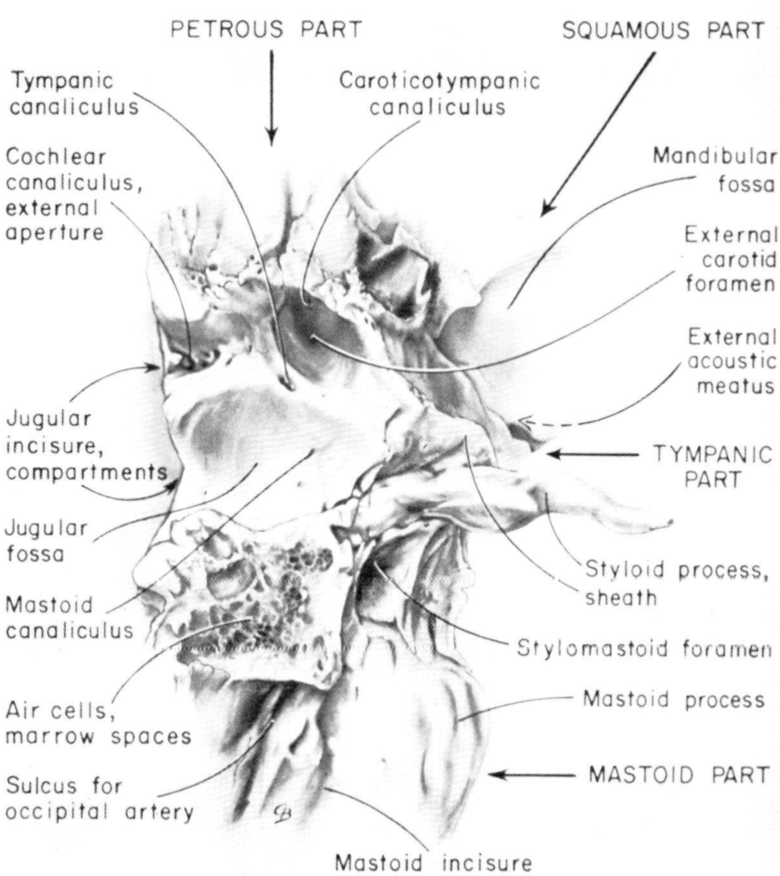

Figure III–119. See legend on the opposite page.

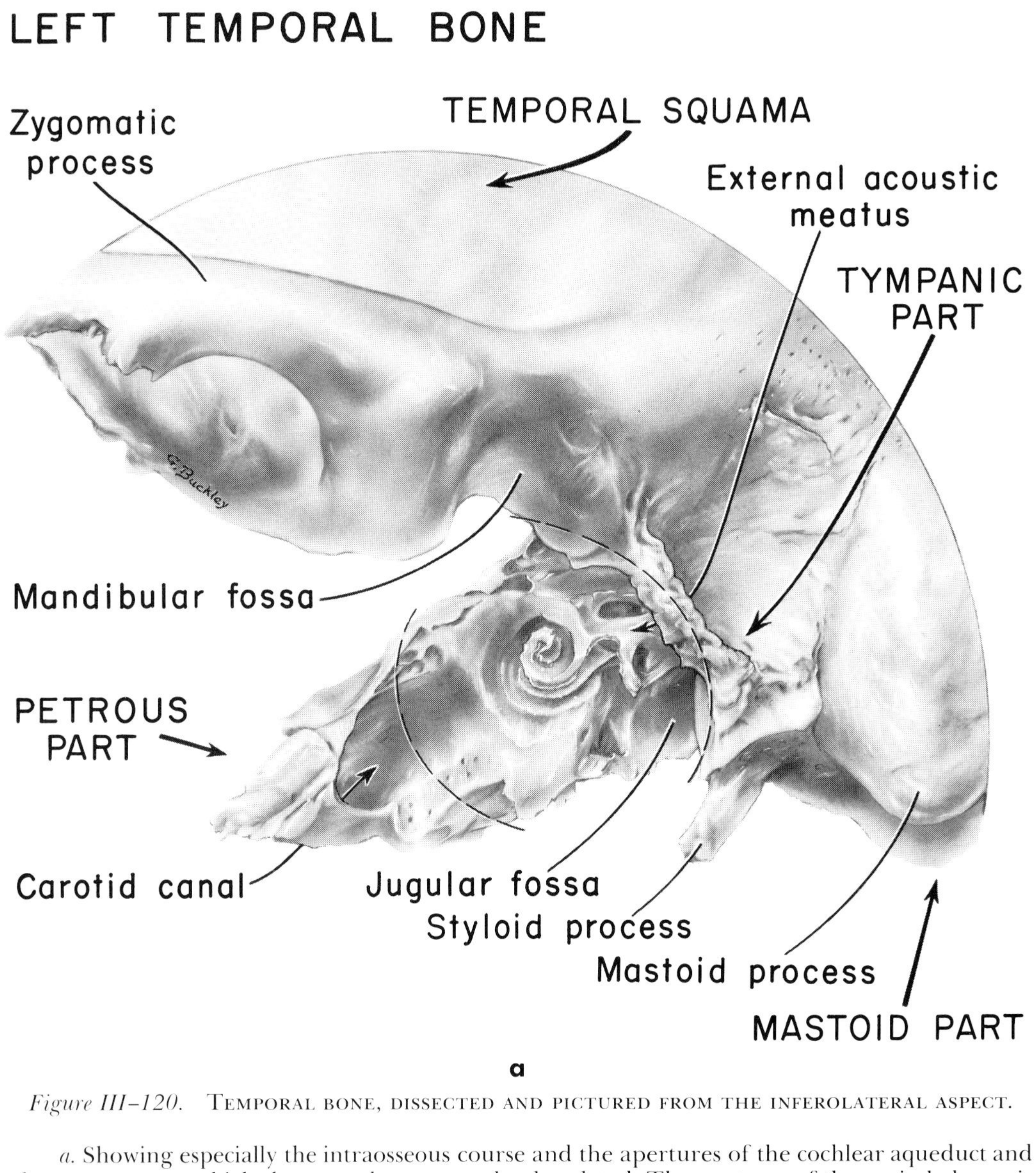

Figure III–120. Temporal bone, dissected and pictured from the inferolateral aspect.

a. Showing especially the intraosseous course and the apertures of the cochlear aqueduct and the structures to which the several parts are closely related. The anatomy of the encircled area is shown in detail in the following figure.

Figure III–120 continues on the opposite page.

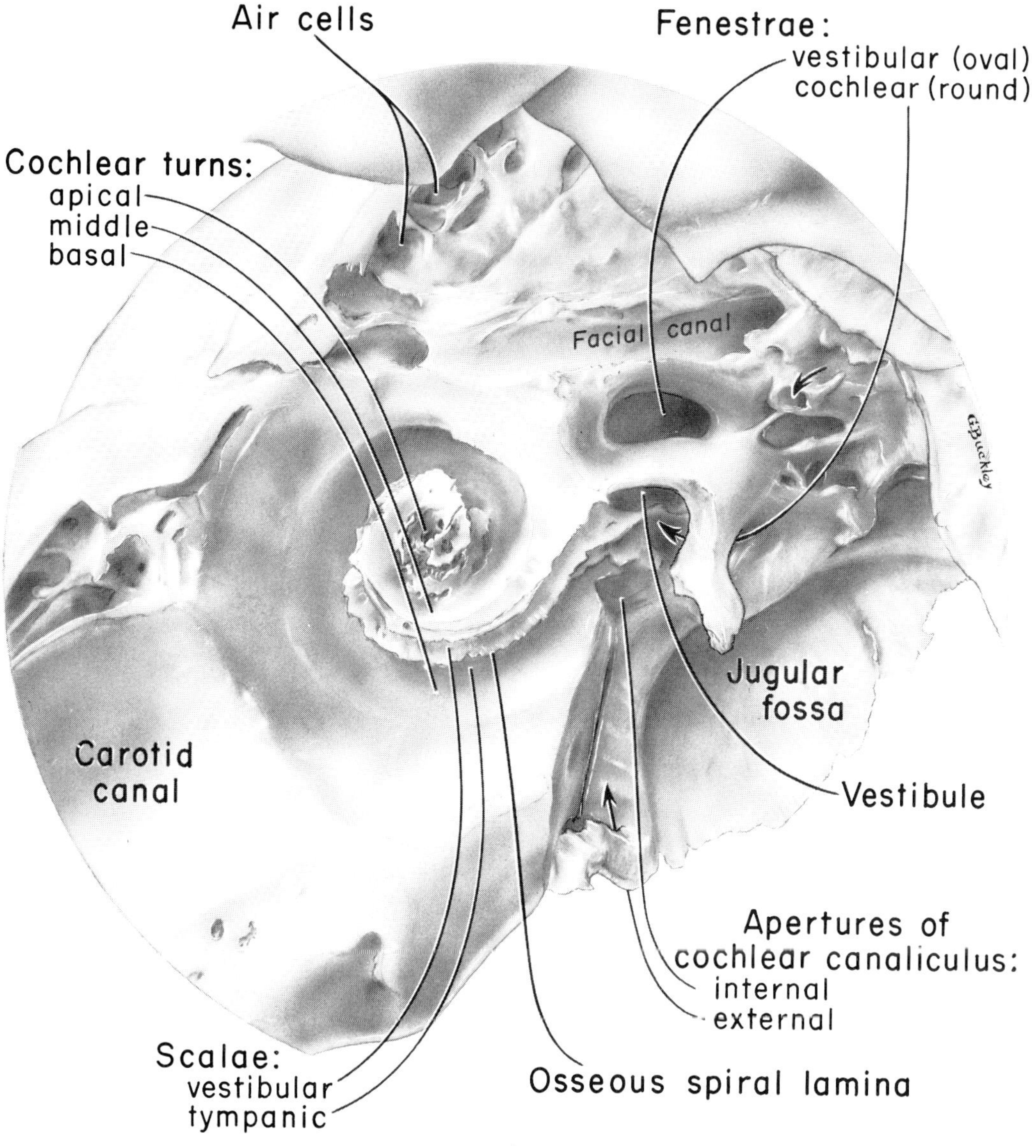

b

Figure III–120, Continued. TEMPORAL BONE, DISSECTED AND PICTURED FROM THE INFEROLATERAL ASPECT.

b. Same specimen, depicting in detail the anatomy of the cochlear aqueduct. The aqueduct (canaliculus) has been opened from the external aperture on the inferior surface of the petrous pyramid to the internal aperture on the wall of the *scala tympani.* The external opening is marked by a bridge of bone beneath which the leader passes. The internal opening is situated on the cochlear side of the *crista* for attachment of the secondary tympanic membrane along the circumference of the cochlear fenestra (round window). The window is exposed by removal of the bone of the tympanic (lateral) wall of the *fossula fenestra cochleae* (through which latter the arrow passes). The relation of the internal aperture is further established by exposing both scalae of the cochlea.

The following anatomical structures are also shown: the facial canal (opened) in its horizontal course, from the *geniculum canalis facialis* toward the *eminentia pyramidalis* (at unlabeled arrow); the vestibular fenestra (oval window), from which the stapes has been removed; the carotid canal (opened). The external acoustic meatus is beyond the area pictured (to the reader's right); the rim is shown in the preceding figure for purposes of topography.

Dissection by Dr. Raymond L. Warpeha.

(From Anson, Donaldson, Warpeha and Winch: Laryngoscope, 74:945–966, 1964.)

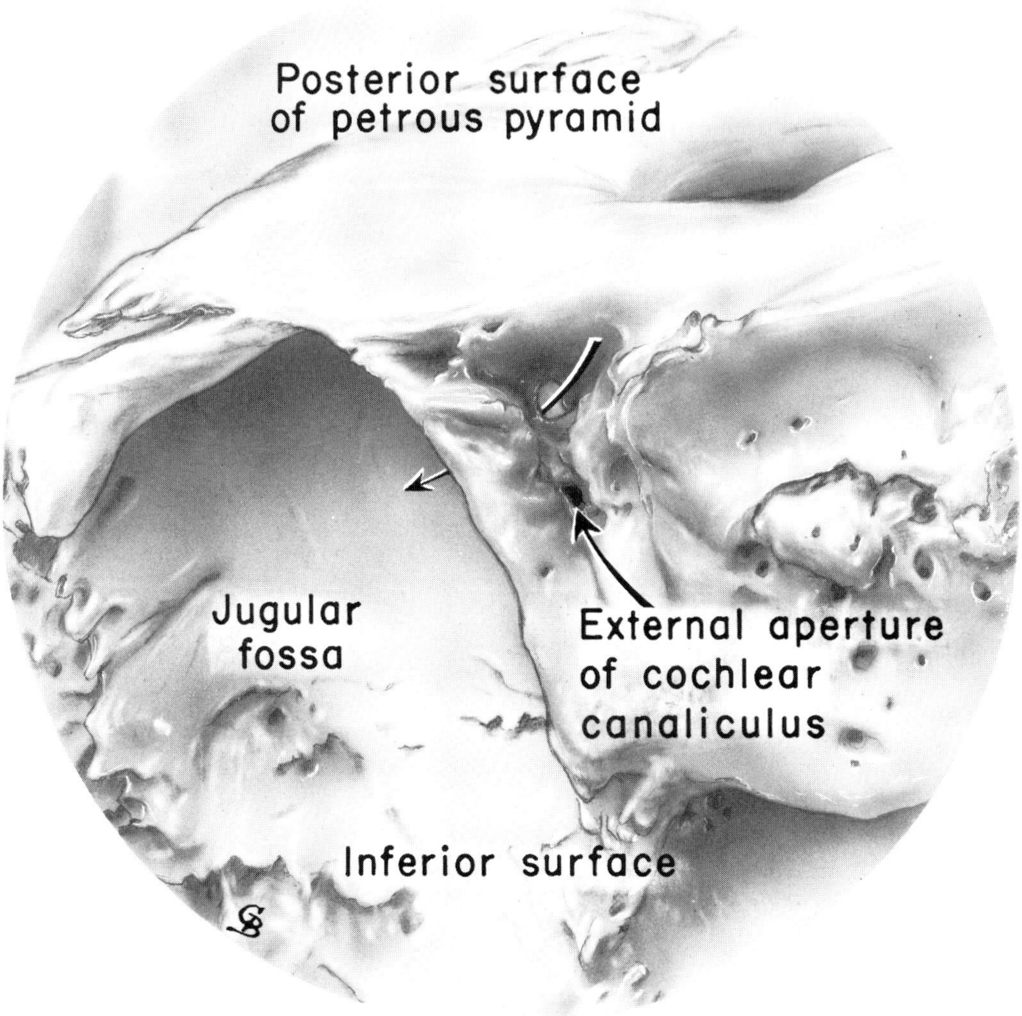

a

Figure III–121. External aperture of the cochlear canaliculus: its form and immediately related venous, neural, and arterial channels. Left temporal bone, inferomedial view.

a. The external aperture of the cochlear canaliculus appears in the depths of an infundibuliform depression on the inferior surface of the petrous pyramid. In being situated near the posterior angle of the latter, the depression appears as a notch when the bone is viewed from the medial side. Its posterior wall is also a boundary of the fossa for the bulb of the jugular vein. In this specimen a communication occurred between the two spaces (traversed by the unlabeled arrow). The external carotid foramen is lateral and anterior to the canaliculus; the *porus* of the internal acoustic meatus is superior to it, on the posterior surface of the petrous pyramid.

Figure III–121 continues on the opposite page.

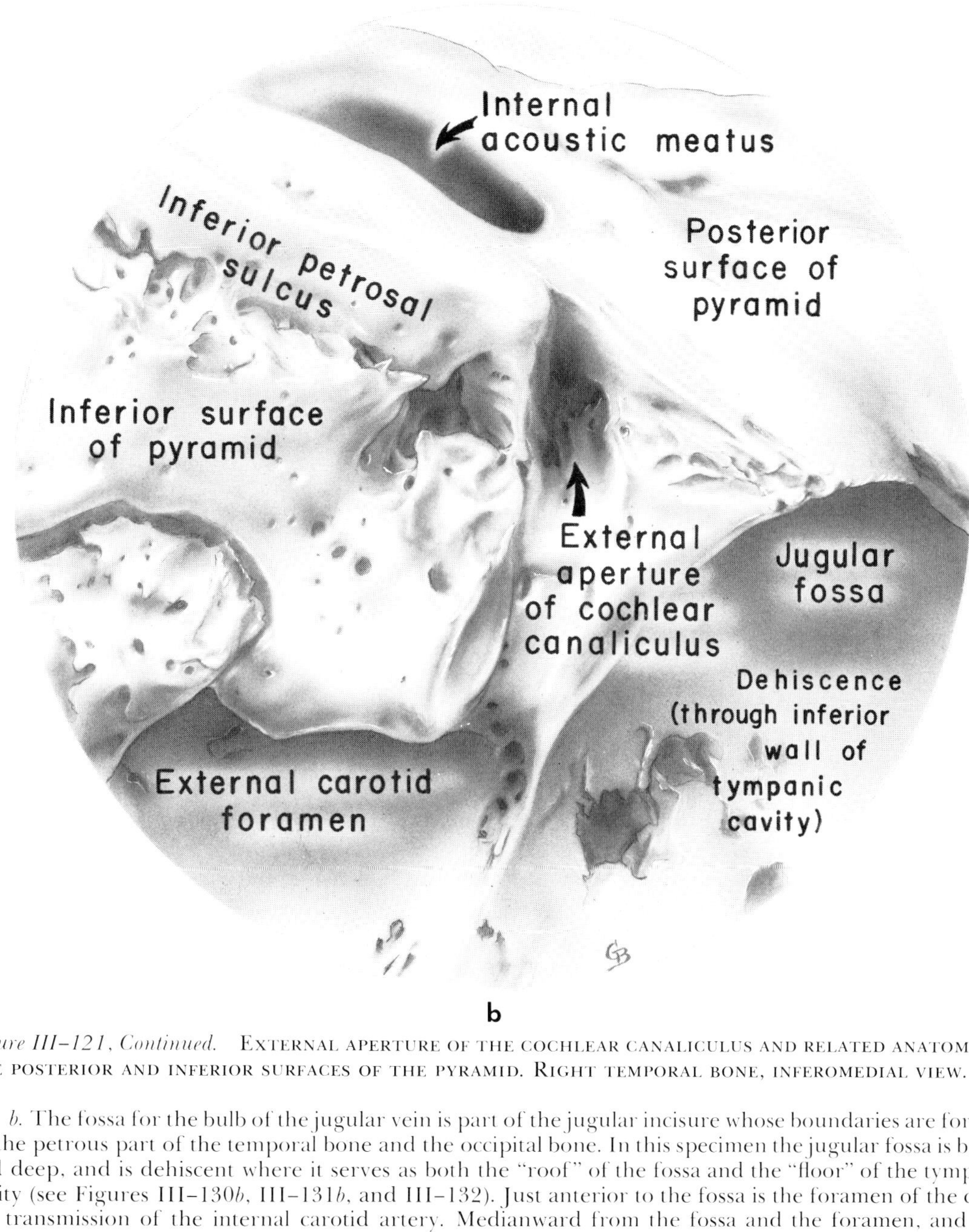

b

Figure III–121, Continued. EXTERNAL APERTURE OF THE COCHLEAR CANALICULUS AND RELATED ANATOMY ON THE POSTERIOR AND INFERIOR SURFACES OF THE PYRAMID. RIGHT TEMPORAL BONE, INFEROMEDIAL VIEW.

b. The fossa for the bulb of the jugular vein is part of the jugular incisure whose boundaries are formed by the petrous part of the temporal bone and the occipital bone. In this specimen the jugular fossa is broad and deep, and is dehiscent where it serves as both the "roof" of the fossa and the "floor" of the tympanic cavity (see Figures III–130*b*, III–131*b*, and III–132). Just anterior to the fossa is the foramen of the canal for transmission of the internal carotid artery. Medianward from the fossa and the foramen, and in a location between them, the external aperture of the cochlear canaliculus (aqueduct) opens into a triangular funnel-shaped depression. In the fresh state the channel contains tissue that constitutes the perilymphatic, or periotic, duct.

The aperture is situated at the posterior angle of the pyramid and appears as a notch when the temporal bone is viewed from the medial side (see Figures I–3 and I–4). Anterior to the aperture is seen the inferior petrosal sulcus, to the formation of which the basilar part of the occipital bone also contributes. The area is foraminous for passage of vessels of emissary type from the interior of the petrous pyramid to the inferior petrosal venous sinus (see dissection in Figure III–132). Just above the notch for the external aperture of the canaliculus are located the pore of the internal acoustic meatus and the small orifice of the subarcuate fossa (see Figures III–127 and III–128).

(From Anson, Donaldson, Warpeha, and Winch: Laryngoscope, 75:1203–1223, 1965.)

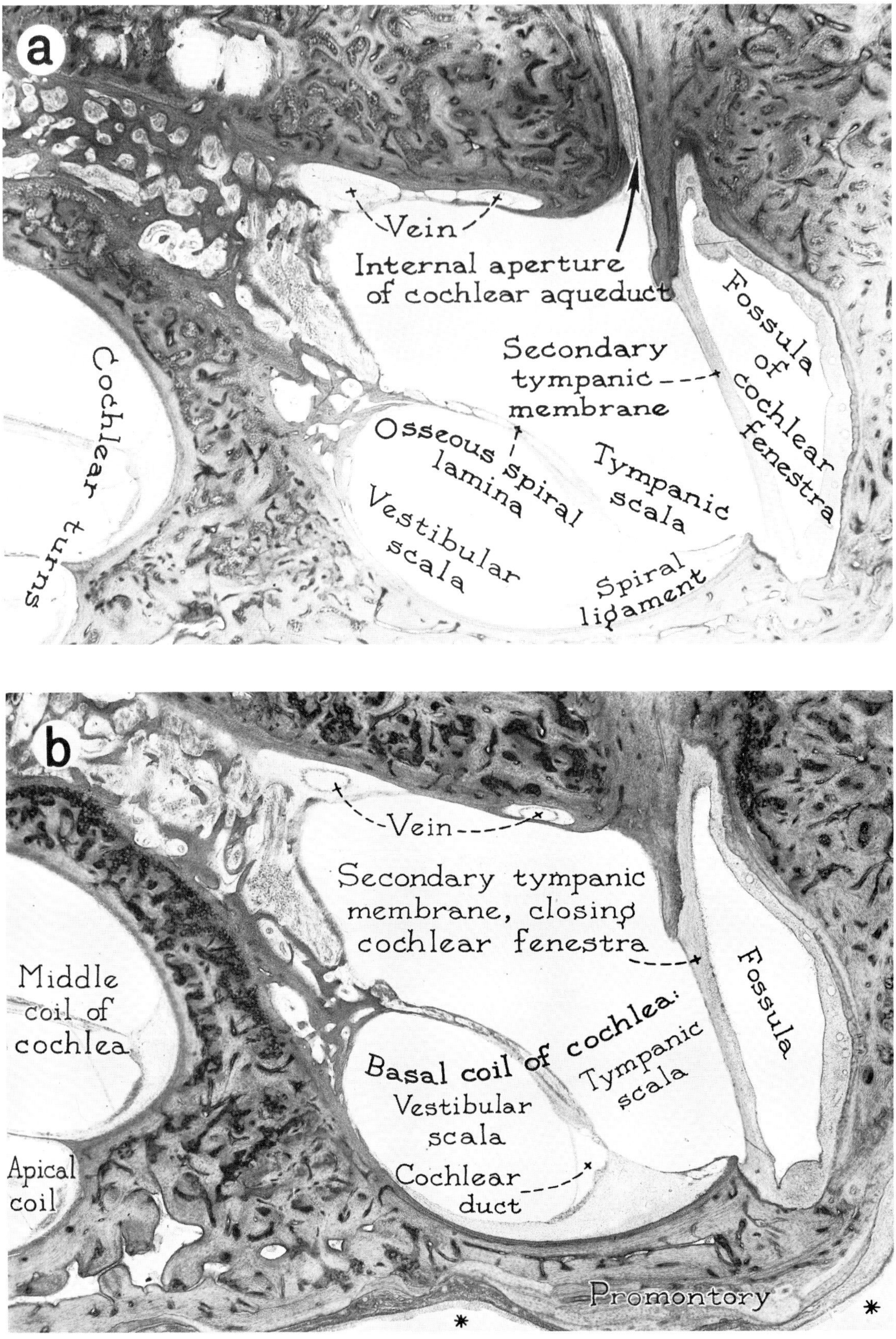

Figure III–122. See legend on the opposite page.

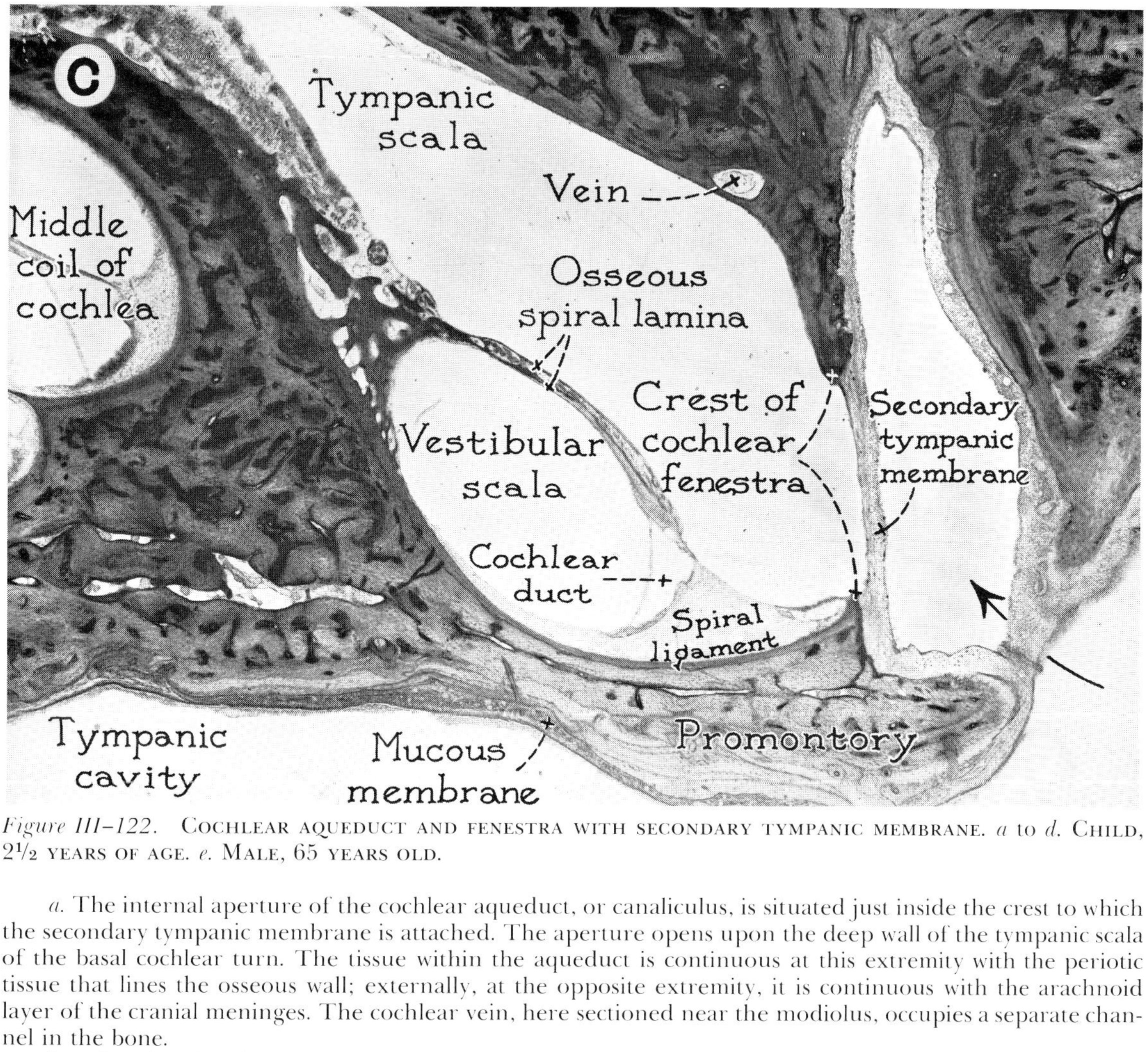

Figure III–122. COCHLEAR AQUEDUCT AND FENESTRA WITH SECONDARY TYMPANIC MEMBRANE. *a* to *d*. CHILD, 2½ YEARS OF AGE. *e*. MALE, 65 YEARS OLD.

a. The internal aperture of the cochlear aqueduct, or canaliculus, is situated just inside the crest to which the secondary tympanic membrane is attached. The aperture opens upon the deep wall of the tympanic scala of the basal cochlear turn. The tissue within the aqueduct is continuous at this extremity with the periotic tissue that lines the osseous wall; externally, at the opposite extremity, it is continuous with the arachnoid layer of the cranial meninges. The cochlear vein, here sectioned near the modiolus, occupies a separate channel in the bone.

b and *c*. Showing the cochlear vein as it courses from the modiolus toward the cochlear (round) window. It will terminate on the inferior surface of the pyramid near the external aperture of the cochlear aqueduct. The secondary tympanic membrane lies on the deep wall of a fossula, the space of which is an offset (at arrow in *c*) of the general tympanic cavity (indicated by asterisk in *b*).

Figure III–122 continues on the following page.

Figure III–122, Continued. COCHLEAR AQUEDUCT AND FENESTRA WITH SECONDARY TYMPANIC MEMBRANE. *a* to *d*. CHILD, $2\frac{1}{2}$ YEARS OF AGE. *e*. MALE, 65 YEARS OLD.

d. The external aperture of the aqueduct on the inferior surface of the pyramid. The space left after stripping away the leptomeninges was occupied by arachnoid. The interstices among its fibrils constitute the so-called perilymphatic (or periotic) "duct."

e. Demonstrating the cochlear aqueduct in a large segment of its course from the wall of the tympanic scala to the inferior surface of the pyramid (see specimen in Figures III–101*c* and III–109).

Transverse sections, Wisconsin Collection, series 88 and 47. *a*, ×26; *b*, ×26; *c*, ×23; *d*, ×24; *e*, ×20.

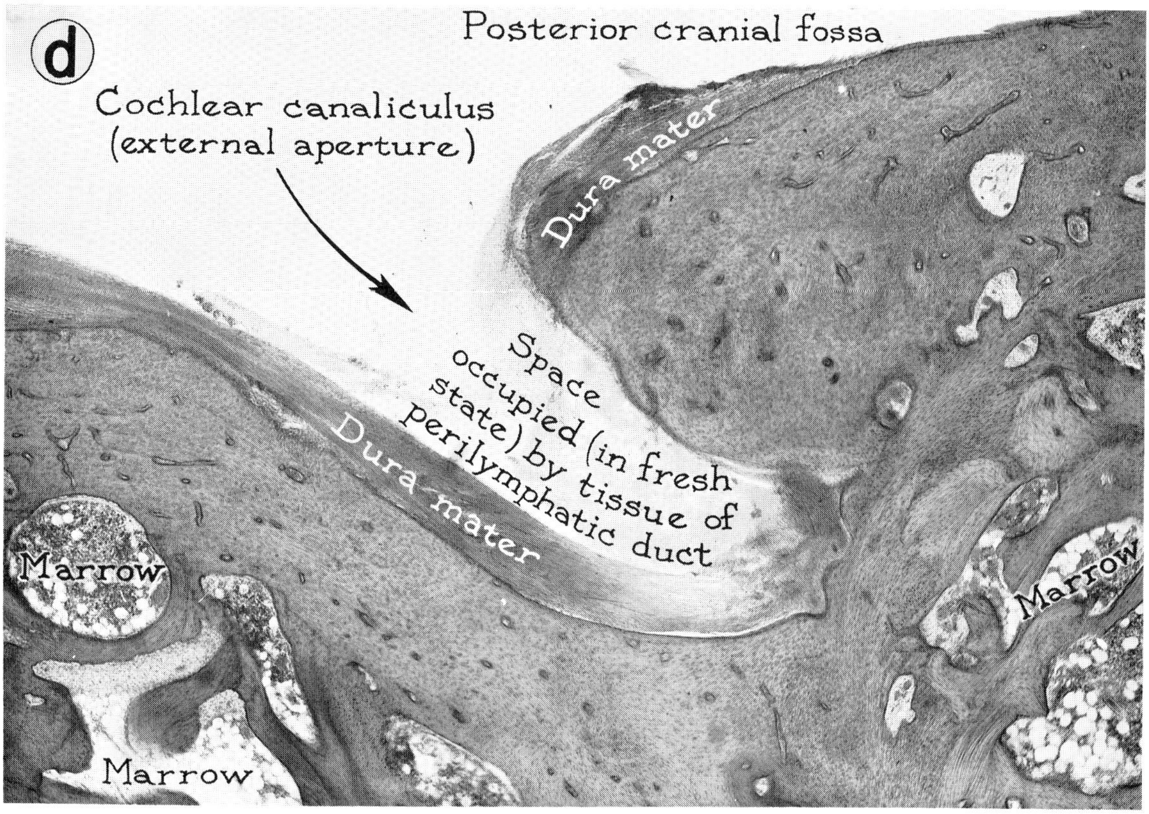

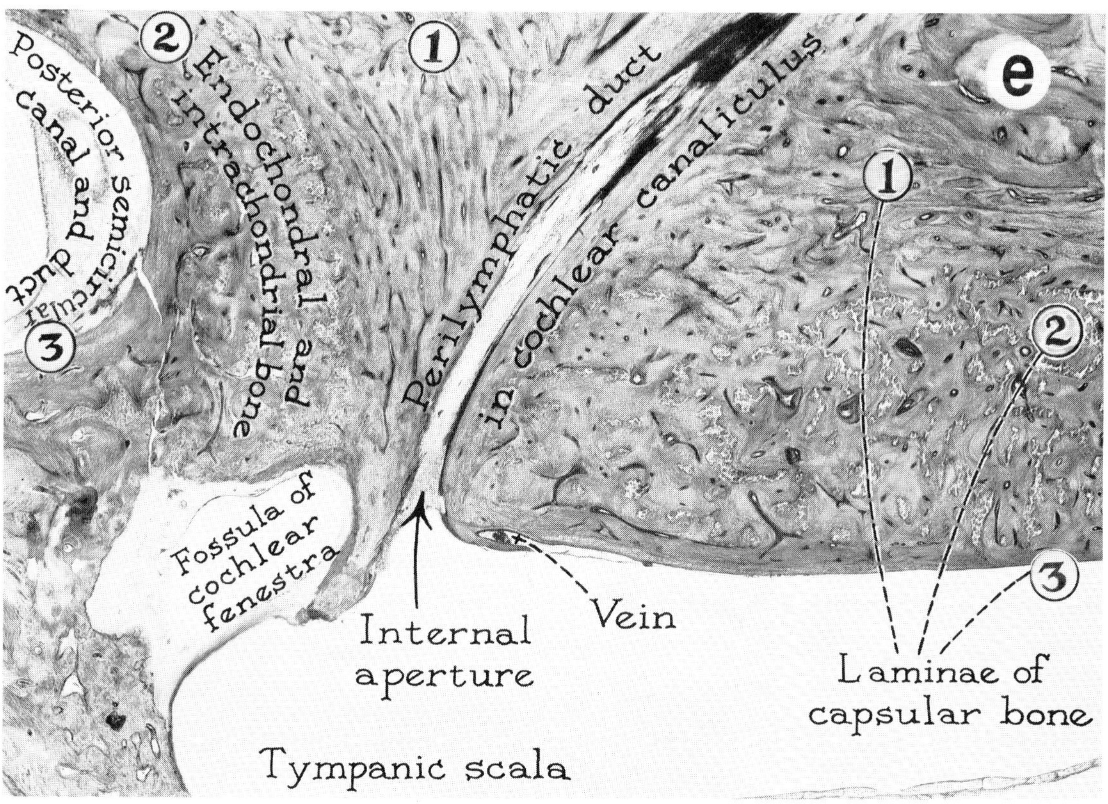

Figure III–122, Concluded. See legend on the opposite page.

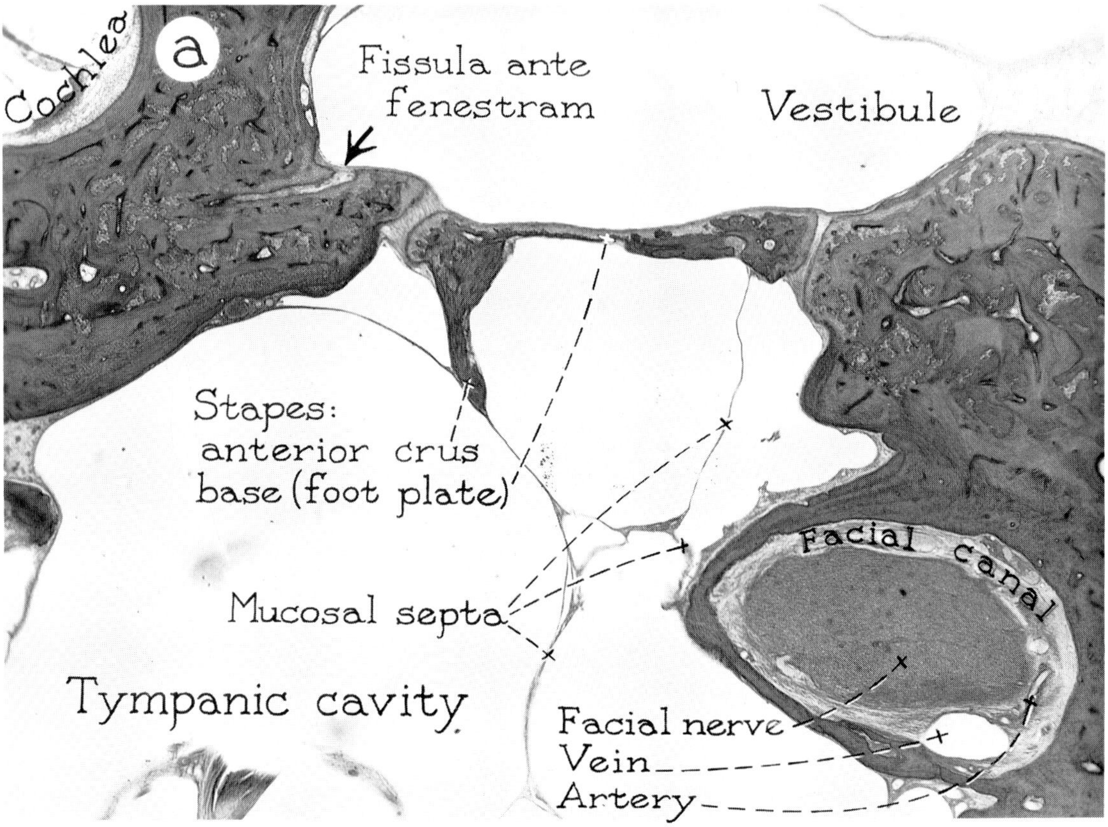

Figure III–123. FISSULA ANTE FENESTRAM AND FOSSULA POST FENESTRAM. MALE, 19 YEARS OF AGE.

a. The fissular tract situated anterior to the vestibular fenestra, shown with its inner aperture situated just anterior to the rim of the window. The normal fibrous content may be replaced by cartilage (Figure III–124*b*) or by otosclerotic bone (Figures III–124*c* and III–126).

Figure III–123 continues on the opposite page.

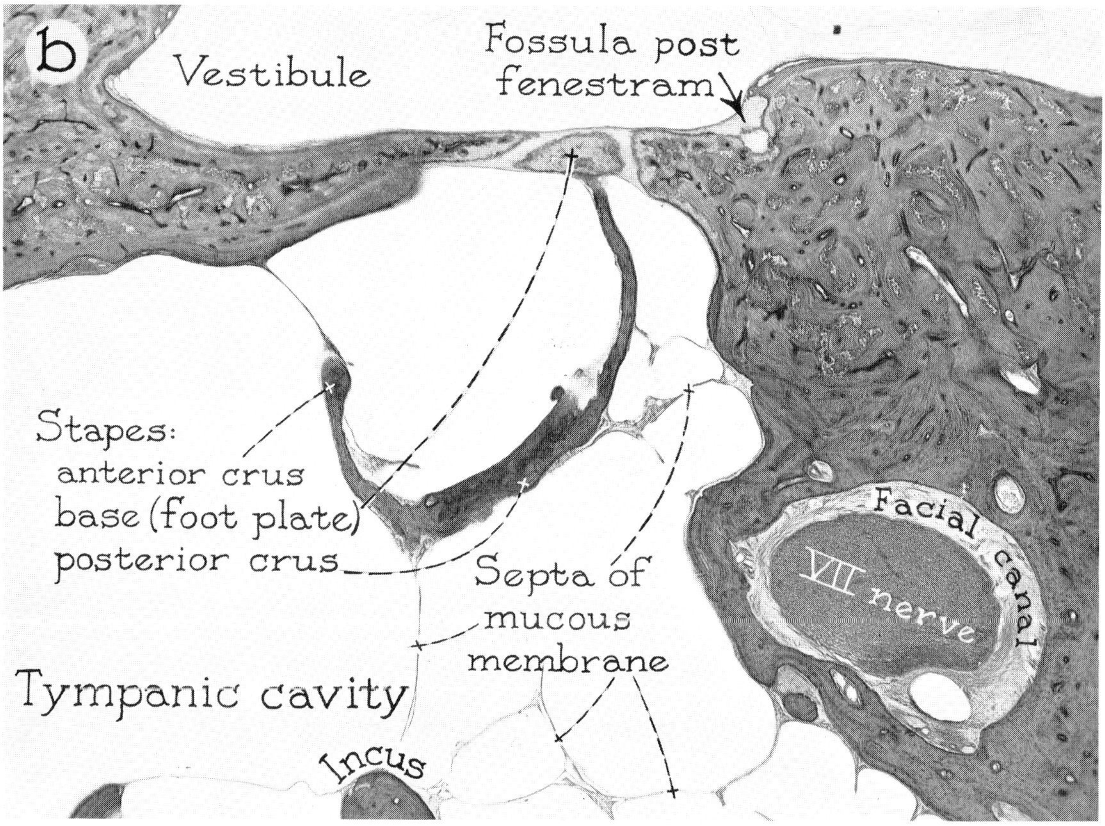

Figure III–123, Continued. Fissula ante fenestram and fossula post fenestram. Male, 19 years of age.

b. The fossular channel, posterior to the window, here (as is typically the case) represented only by a vestibular aperture. In some individuals it is absent.

Transverse sections, Wisconsin Collection, series 29. *a*, ×20; *b*, ×18.

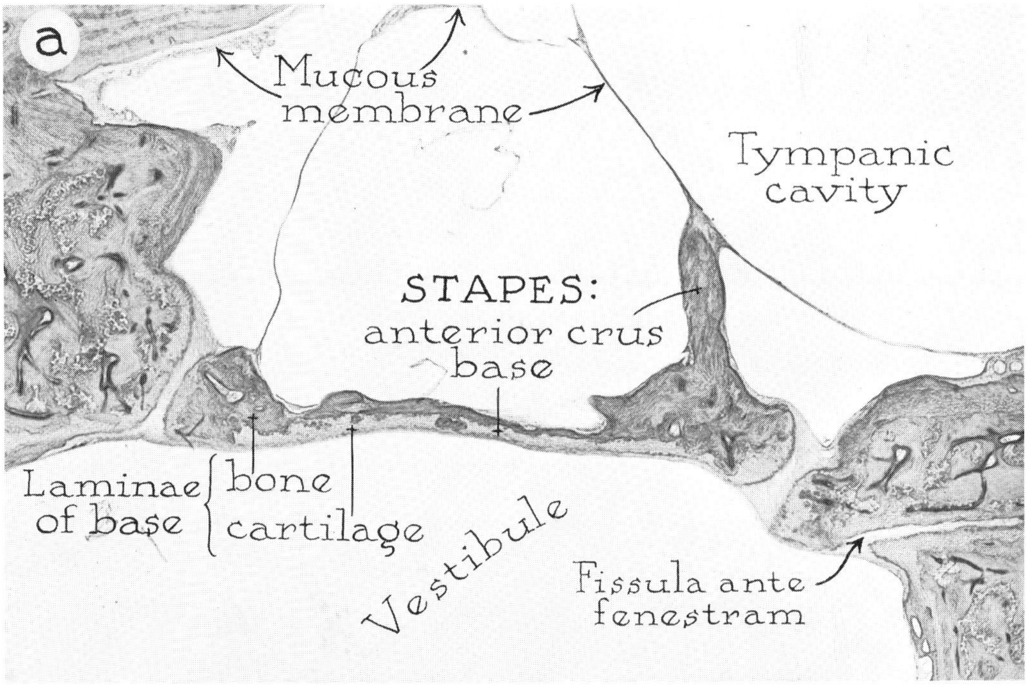

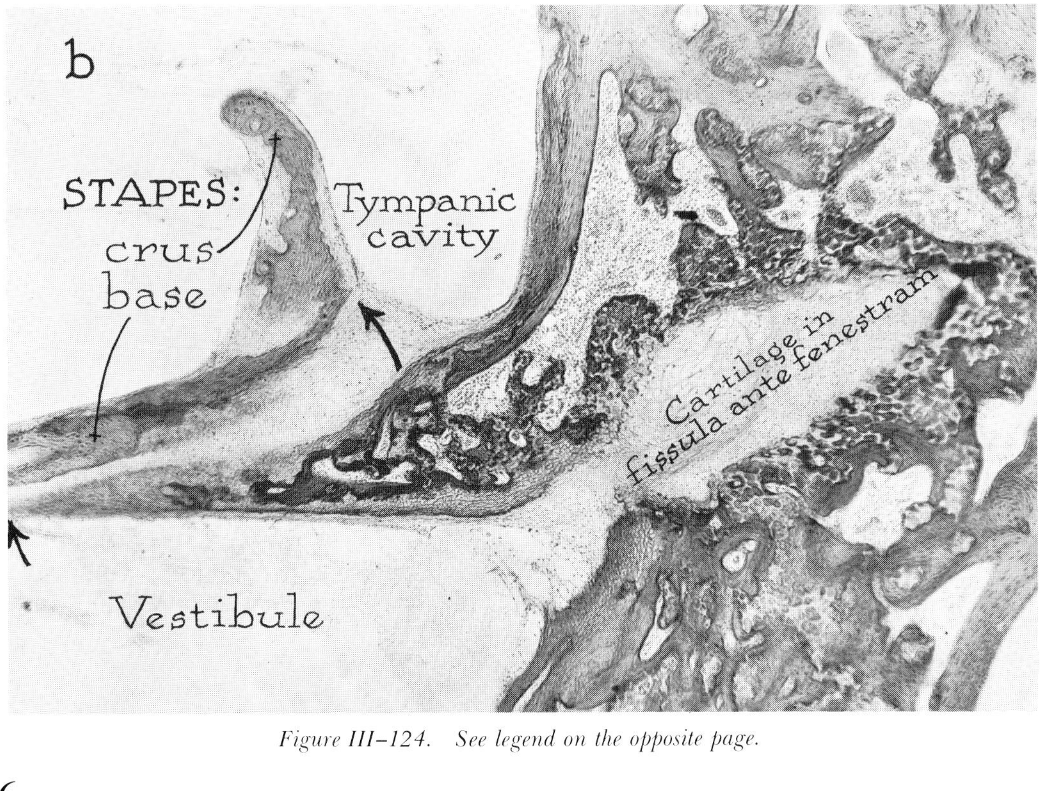

Figure III–124. See legend on the opposite page.

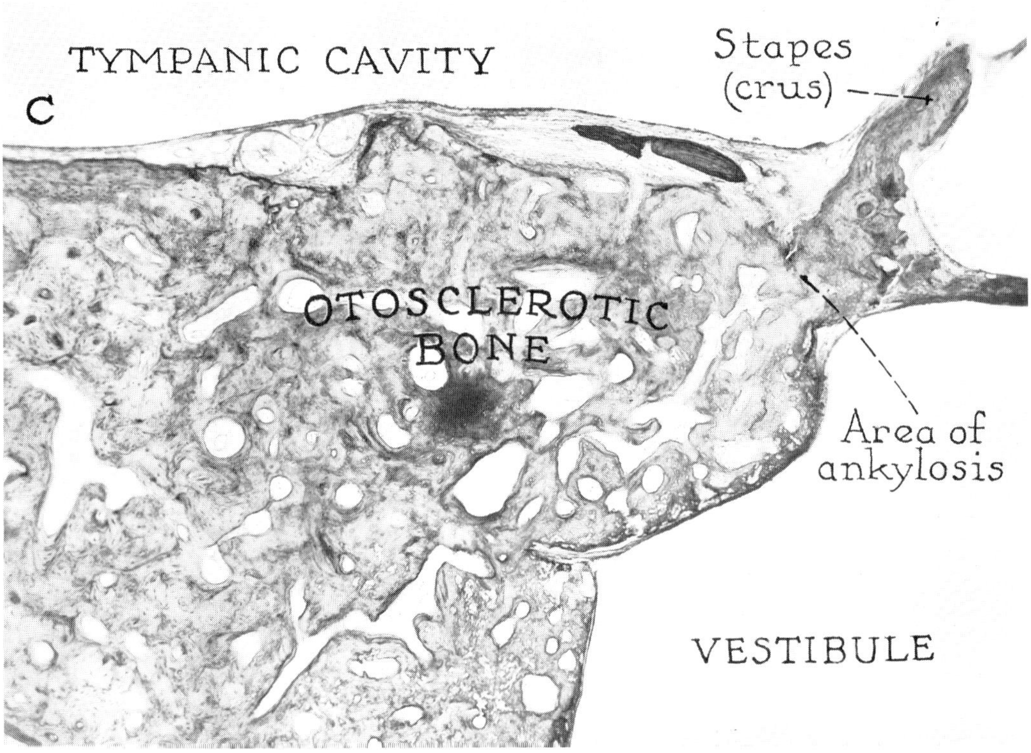

Figure III–124. FISSULAR TRACT ACROSS THE ANTEFENESTRAL REGION OF THE TEMPORAL BONE: NORMAL, ABERRANT, AND PATHOLOGICAL FORM AND CONTENTS. IN EACH INSTANCE THE VESTIBULAR EXTREMITY IS PICTURED. *a.* MALE, 19 YEARS OLD. *b.* CHILD, 2 YEARS OF AGE. *c.* AGE UNRECORDED.

a. Typically, as here shown, the *fissula ante fenestram* appears histologically as a fibrous stripe in the otic capsule. Its content is continuous medially with the periotic tissue of the vestibule and laterally with the submucosa on the medial (labyrinthine) wall of the tympanic cavity. A thin perichondrial layer immediately surrounds the loose connective tissue of the fissula. Apparently activity in this layer accounts for the normal reduction in caliber of the channel in later life, and for the aberrant formation of chondromatous masses that are frequently encountered in late fetal and early postnatal specimens (see following figure).

b. A chondroma occupies the vestibular segment of the fissular tract. It is continuous with the cartilage that regularly lines the vestibular (oval) window and is carried therefrom, for a variable distance, into the fissula. The cartilage faces similar tissue on the inner (vestibular) surface of the stapedial base (or footplate). At this anterior segment of the fenestral rim the stapes overrides the margin of the window (through the area indicated by the arrows).

c. In this specimen pathological bone occupies the antefenestral area, obliterating the *fissula ante fenestram.*

Transverse sections, Wisconsin Collection, series as follows: *a*, 29; *b* and *c*, unrecorded.

Figure III–125. FISSULA ANTE FENESTRAM: ABNORMAL CONTENTS IN PART OR ALL OF THE FISSULAR TRACT. PHOTOGRAPHS OF RECONSTRUCTIONS PREPARED BY THE BORN WAX-PLATE METHOD.

a. A cartilage mass, cranial to the level to the tympanic extremity of the fissula ante fenestram, is continuous with the connective tissue which, in the normal way, occupies the fissula between the tympanic and vestibular apertures.

b. The cartilage mass completely obliterates the space of a spacious fissula. Small unlabeled arrows indicate some of the numerous areas where the cartilage is related to vascular channels in the surrounding bone.

c. An area of chondromatous tissue is continuous with normal connective tissue inferiorly and with otosclerotic bone superiorly. A tympanic extremity is lacking.

(Adapted from Bast and Anson: The Temporal Bone and the Ear. Springfield, Charles C Thomas, 1949.)

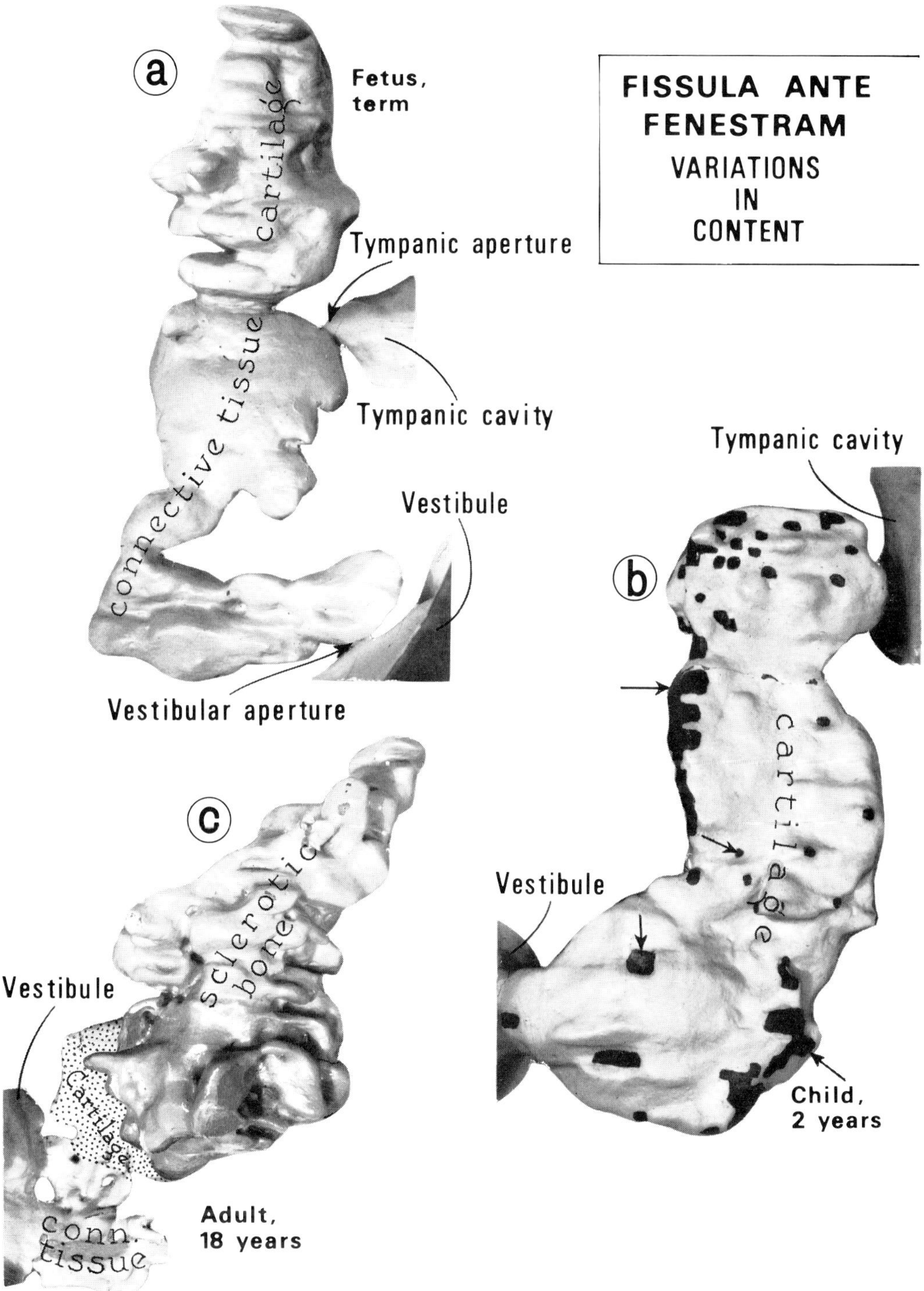

Figure III-125. See legend on the opposite page.

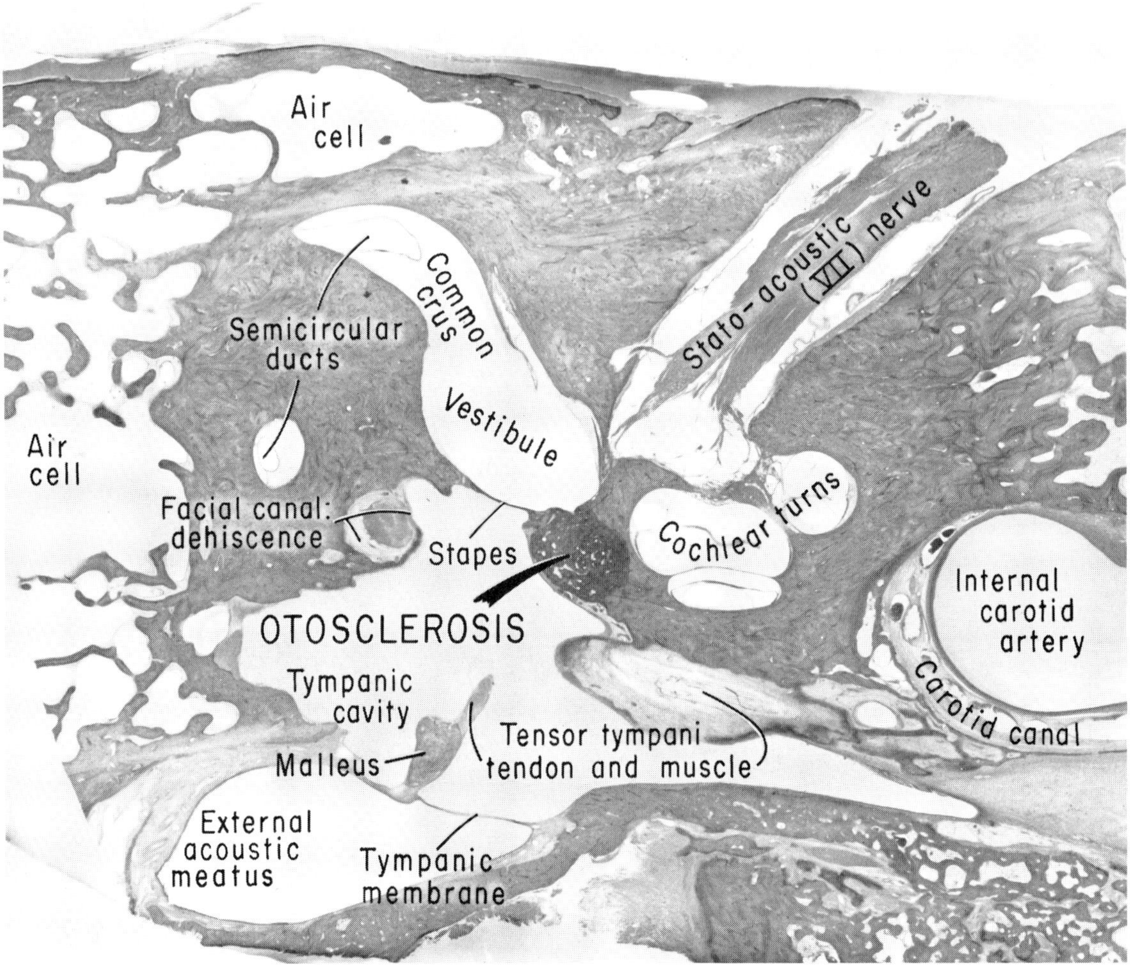

Figure III–126. Temporal bone: pathology (otosclerosis). Male, 54 years of age.

An otosclerotic lesion occupies the customary site of the fissula ante fenestram. This demonstrates also a congenital defect in the form of an incomplete facial canal (see Figure III–70). At a more cranial level, the otosclerotic tissue forms three-fourths of the circumference of the facial canal (Figure III–85).

At this favorable topographical level in the otological series, the following additional features are demonstrated: the location of the facial canal in the mastoid wall of the tympanic cavity; the tensor tympani muscle in the semicanal and tendon at the attachment to the malleus; the statoacoustic (vestibulocochlear) nerve at the point of separation into vestibular and cochlear divisions; the carotid canal in relation to the cochlea; and the superior semicircular duct in relation to the air cells situated close to the meninges on the posterior surface of the pyramid (see also Figure III–70).

Courtesy of Dr. C. M. Kos.

Transverse section, University of Iowa Collection, series 583.R. ×4.

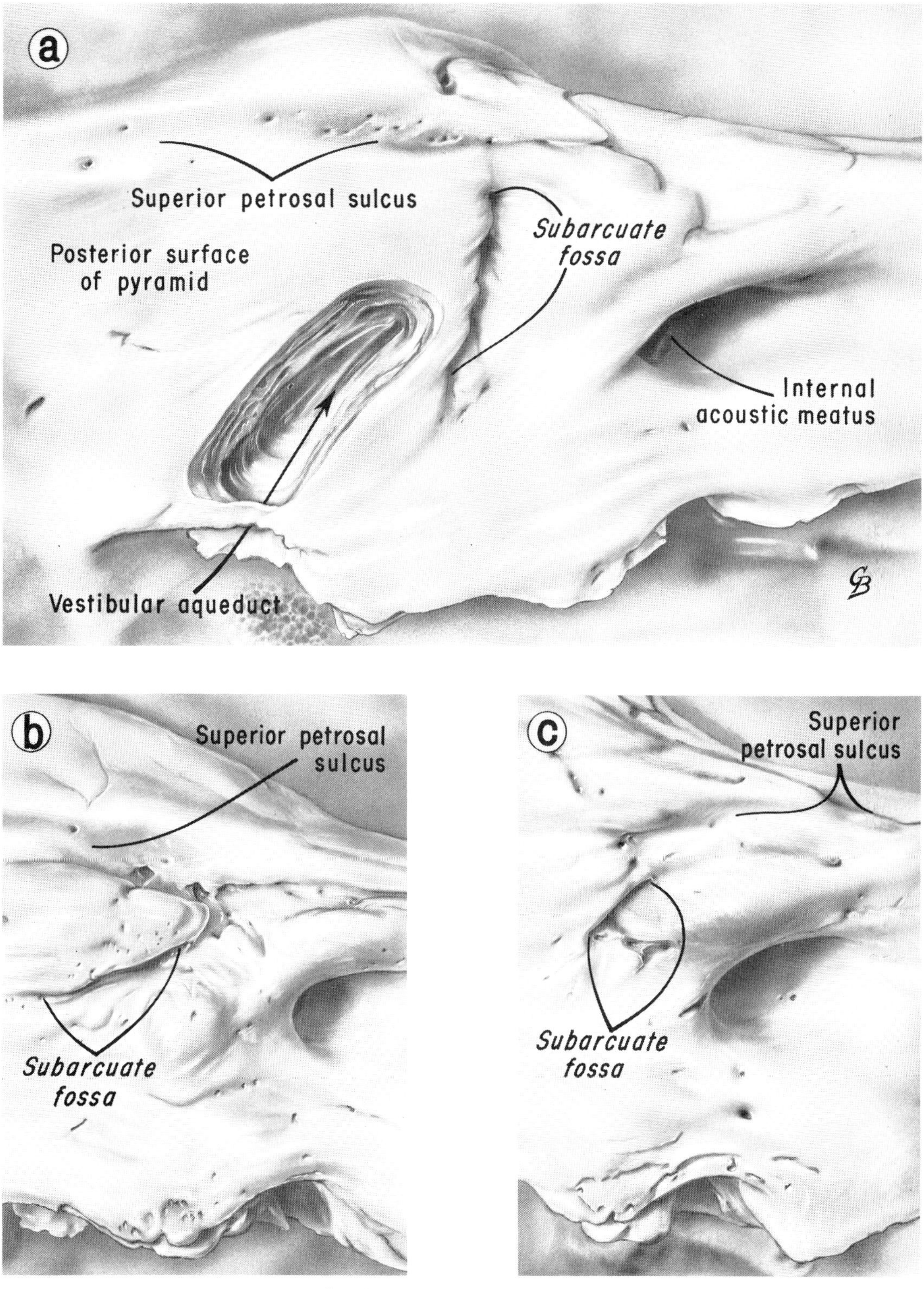

Figure III–127. SUBARCUATE FOSSA: SELECTED EXAMPLES.

a. The fossa is an elongate slit occupying the customary position of the external aperture of the vestibular aqueduct. The latter terminates at the posterior angle of the pyramid. The distal segment of the aqueduct has been opened. It narrows upon passing inward (at point of the arrow).

b and *c.* Here the fossae are larger than average. Each is related to other vascular channels either near those of the superior petrosal sulcus (in *b*) or to others on the posterior surface of the pyramid (in *c*).

Dissection by Dr. Raymond L. Warpeha.

(From Anson: Trans. Amer. Acad. Ophthal. Otolaryng., 73:17–38, 1969.)

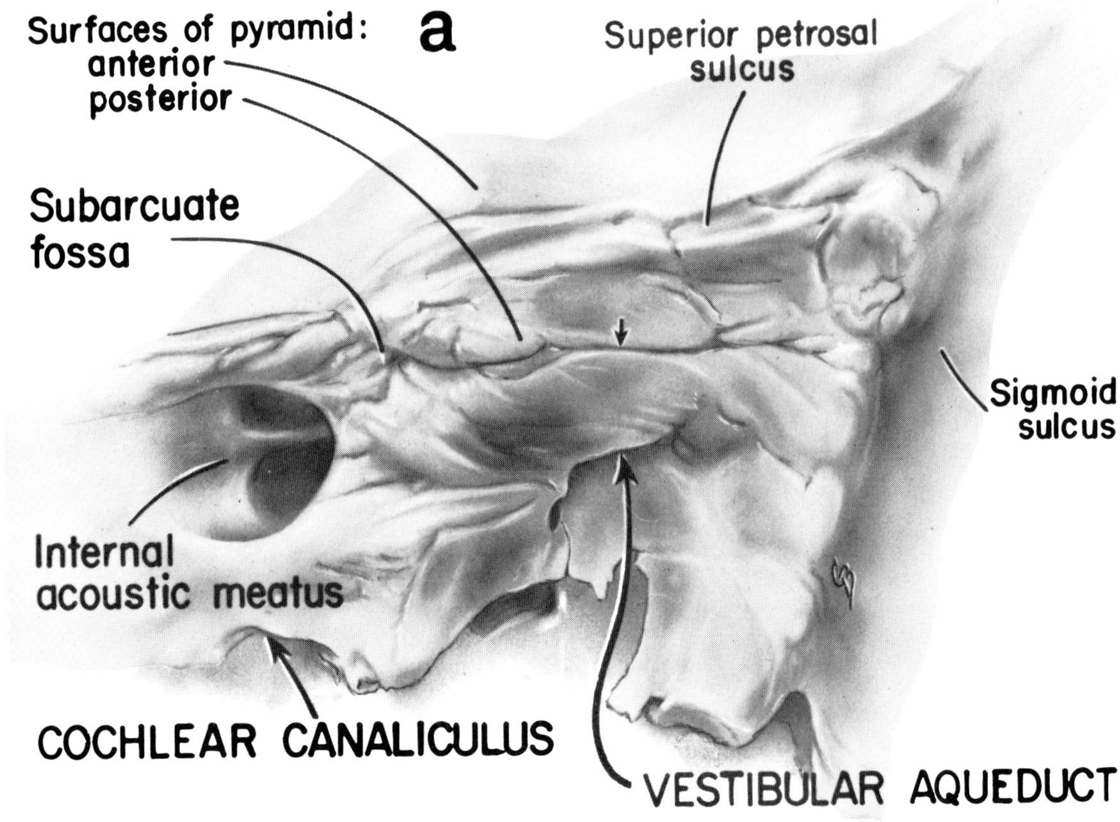

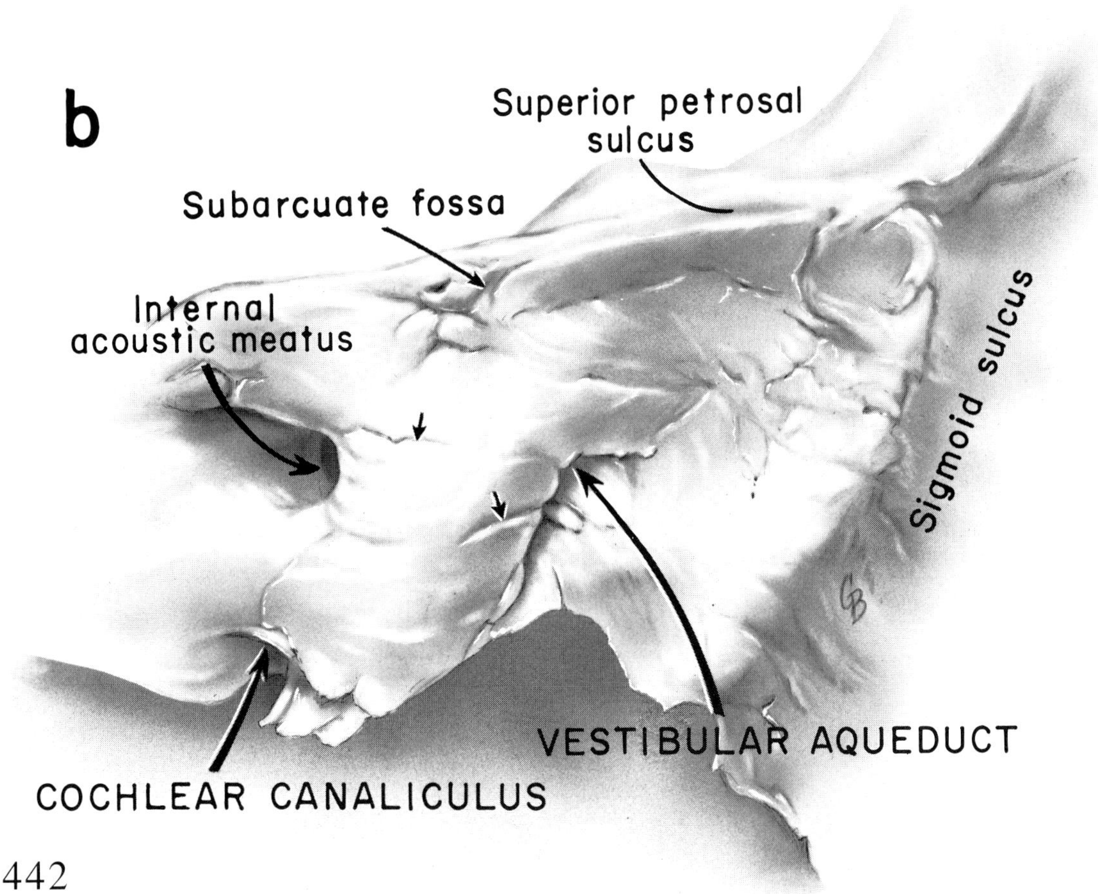

Figure III–128. See legend on the opposite page.

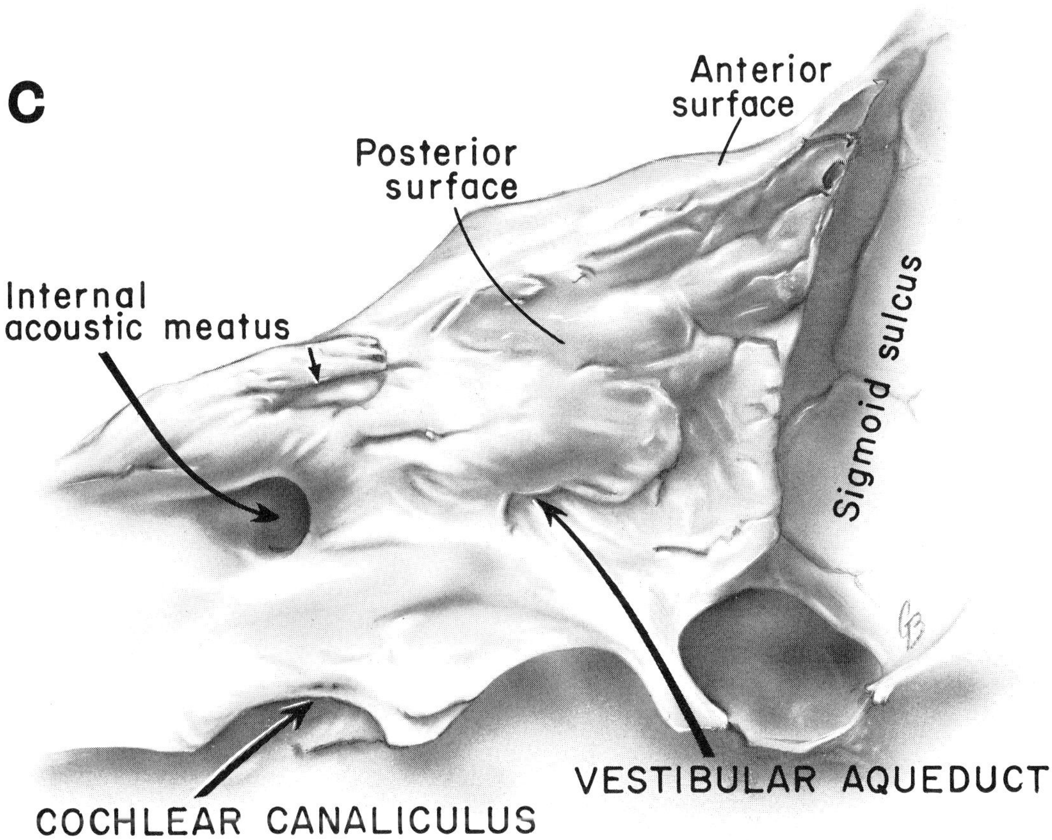

Figure III–128. Subarcuate fossa and related structures: variational anatomy. Selected examples.

The subarcuate fossa is typically a small opening into the bone on the posterior surface of the pyramid above and behind the pore of the internal acoustic meatus. It lies just below the superior angle of the petrous part of the temporal bone. Large in fetal stages and in the newborn, it may be but slightly indicated in the adult. It attains maximum dimensions in the 5-month fetus, gradually diminishes in caliber thereafter (see Figures II–37*a*, *b* and II–38). The fossa transmits offsets of the internal auditory artery and vein and may communicate with meningeal blood vessels. It is highly variable in form, position, and dimensions (see also Figure III–127).

a. An example of fossa continuous with an elongate vascular sulcus (at unlabeled arrow) which extended backward to the sigmoid sulcus and communicated above with the superior petrosal sulcus.

b. A small fossa confluent with the superior petrosal sulcus. Small sulci carry meningeal blood vessels into the vestibular aqueduct and the internal acoustic meatus.

c. An inconspicuous fossa (at arrow) which lacks connection with vascular sulci. The specimens also serve to demonstrate variation in the following: the size and angulation of the internal acoustic meatus (widely open in *a*, small in *b* and *c*); the form of the notch at the posterior angle of the bone, leading to the external aperture of the cochlear aqueduct on the inferior surface.

Note: Small sulcate impressions are indicated by unlabeled arrows. The absence of sulci on the surface of the bone does not of necessity indicate regional want of meningeal vessels of dissectible size; they may be limited to a course in the overlying dural layer.

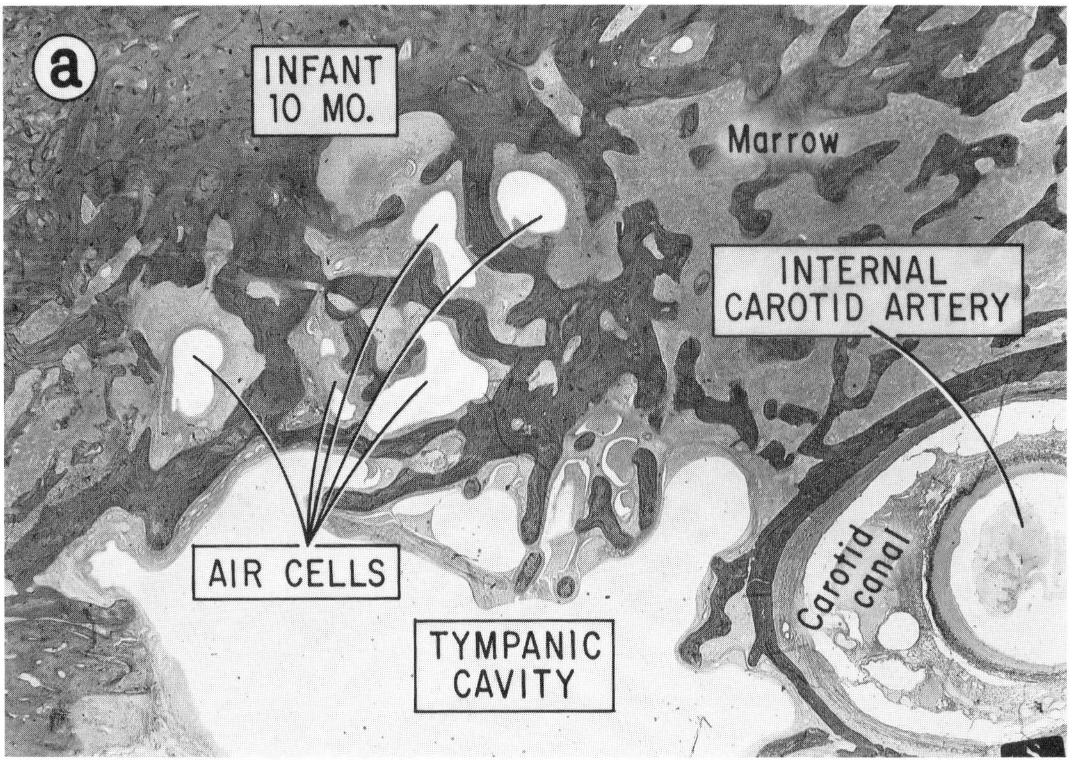

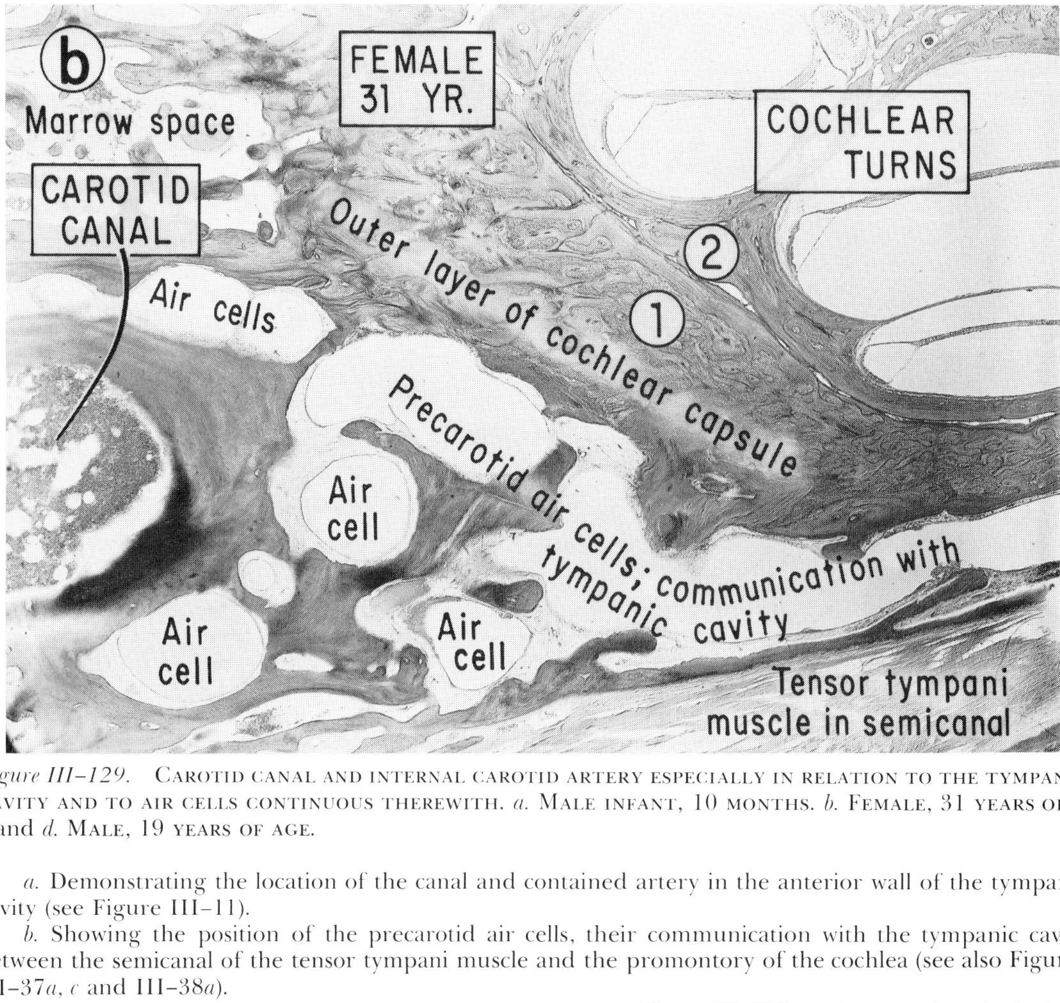

Figure III–129. Carotid canal and internal carotid artery especially in relation to the tympanic cavity and to air cells continuous therewith. *a.* Male infant, 10 months. *b.* Female, 31 years old. *c* and *d.* Male, 19 years of age.

a. Demonstrating the location of the canal and contained artery in the anterior wall of the tympanic cavity (see Figure III–11).

b. Showing the position of the precarotid air cells, their communication with the tympanic cavity between the semicanal of the tensor tympani muscle and the promontory of the cochlea (see also Figures III–37*a*, *c* and III–38*a*).

Figure III–129 continues on the opposite page.

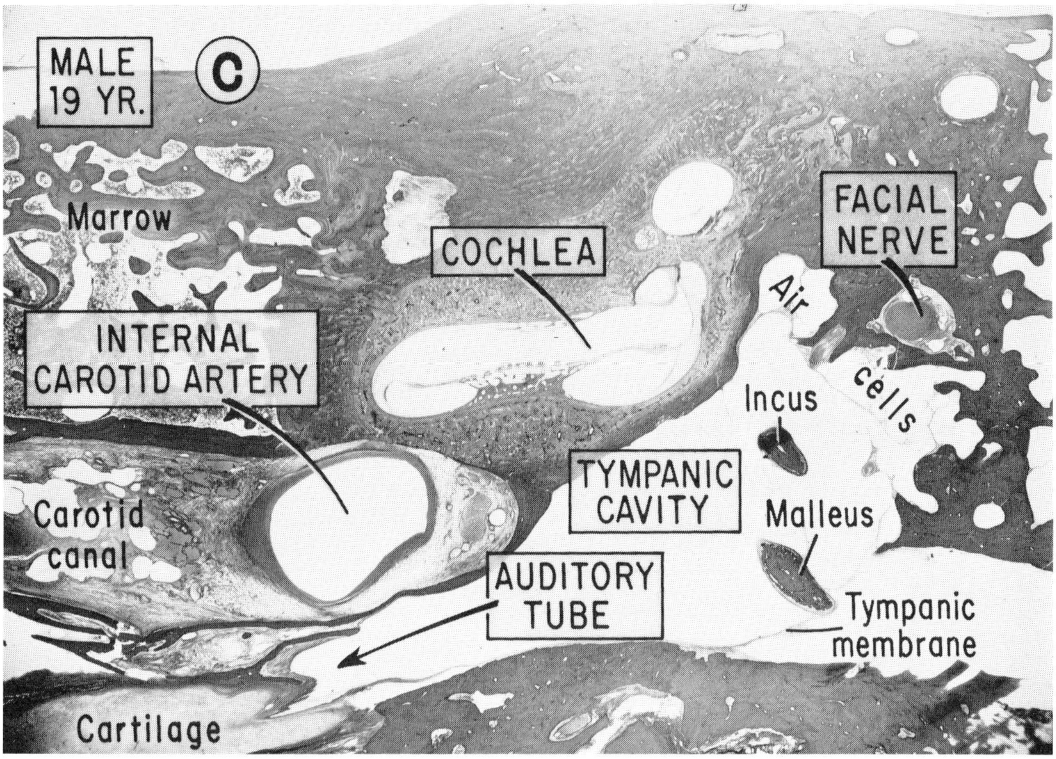

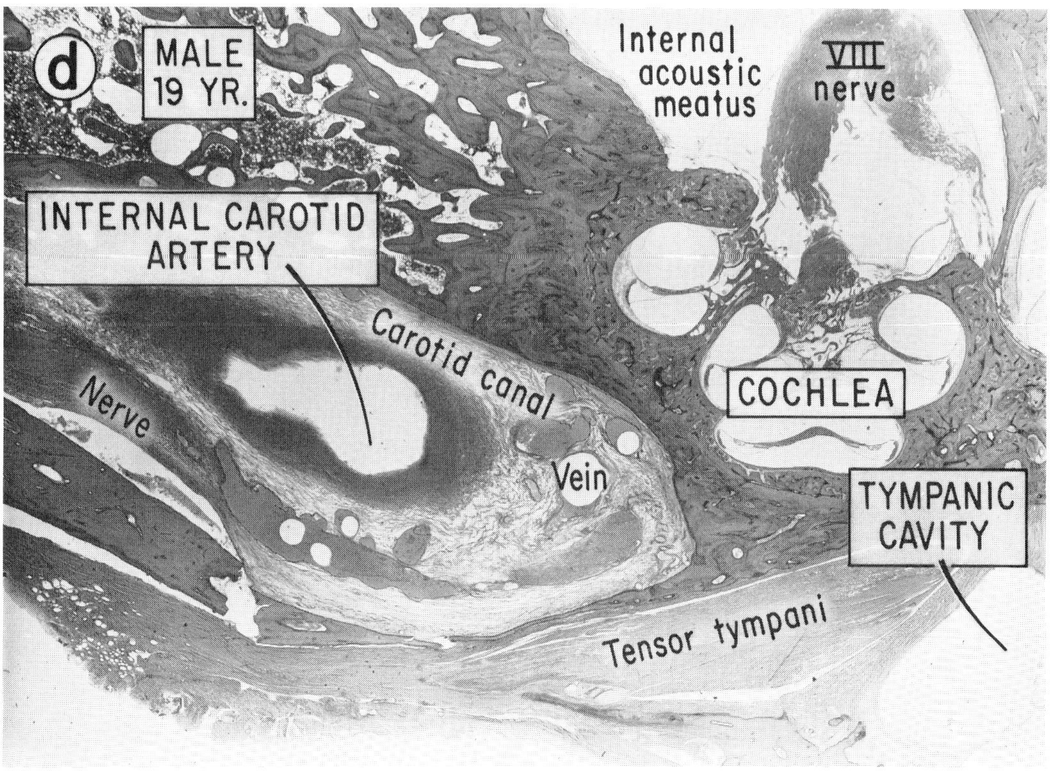

Figure III–129, Continued. Carotid canal and internal carotid artery especially in relation to the tympanic cavity and to air cells continuous therewith. *a.* Male infant, 10 months. *b.* Female, 31 years old. *c* and *d.* Male, 19 years of age.

c and *d.* Illustrating the anatomical relationships of the carotid canal as it occupies the anterior wall of the tympanic cavity.

Transverse sections, Wisconsin Collection, series as follows: *a*, 97; *b*, 3; *c* and *d*, 29. *a*, right temporal bone; *b*, *c*, and *d*, left temporal bones. *a*, ×12; *b*, ×15; *c*, ×5; *d*, ×7.

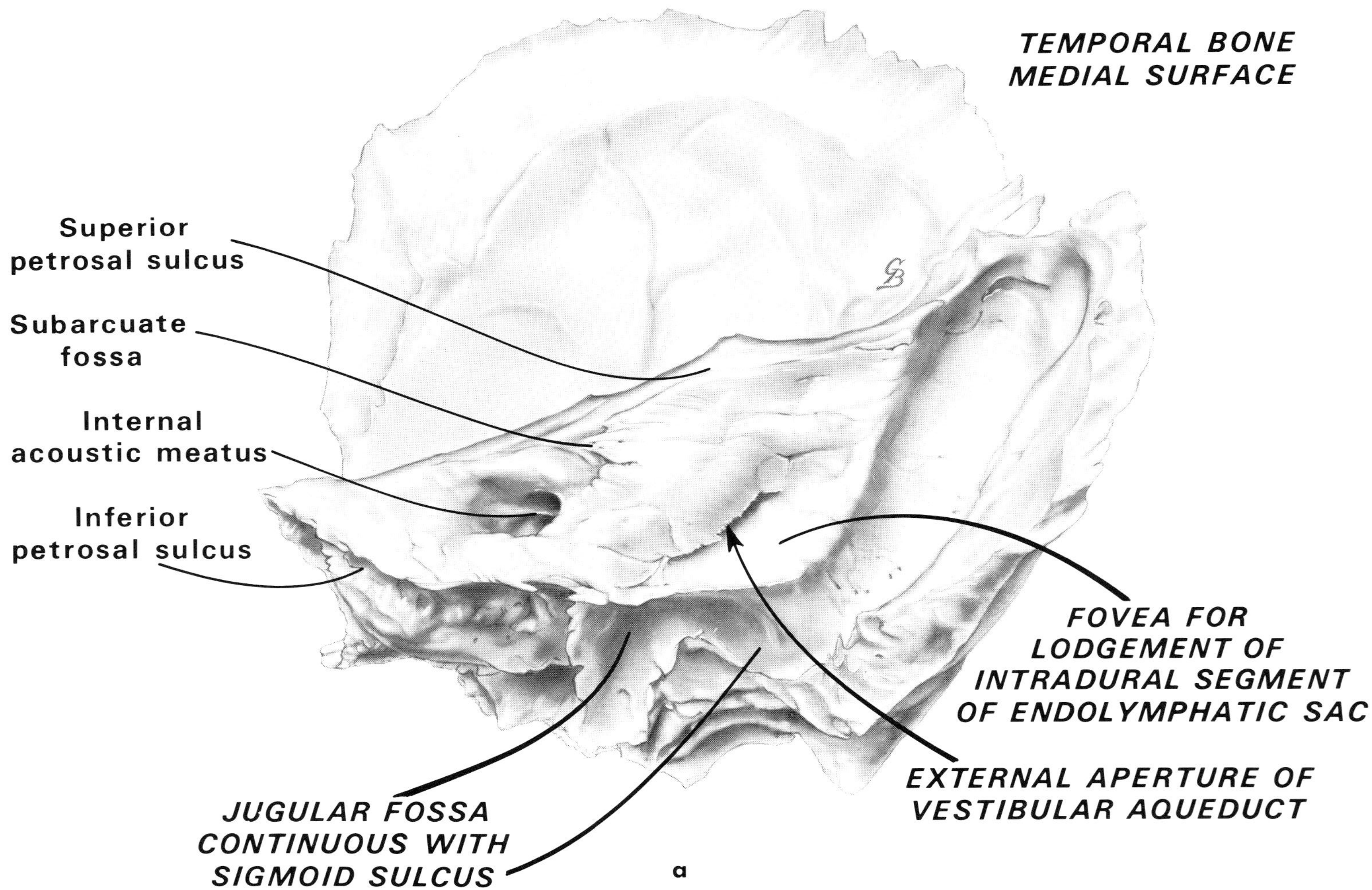

Figure III–130. Jugular fossa and related sulci and apertures: variational anatomy. Two Examples.

a. A specimen in which the jugular fossa is prominently continuous with the sigmoid part of the transverse sinus.

Figure III–130 continues on the opposite page.

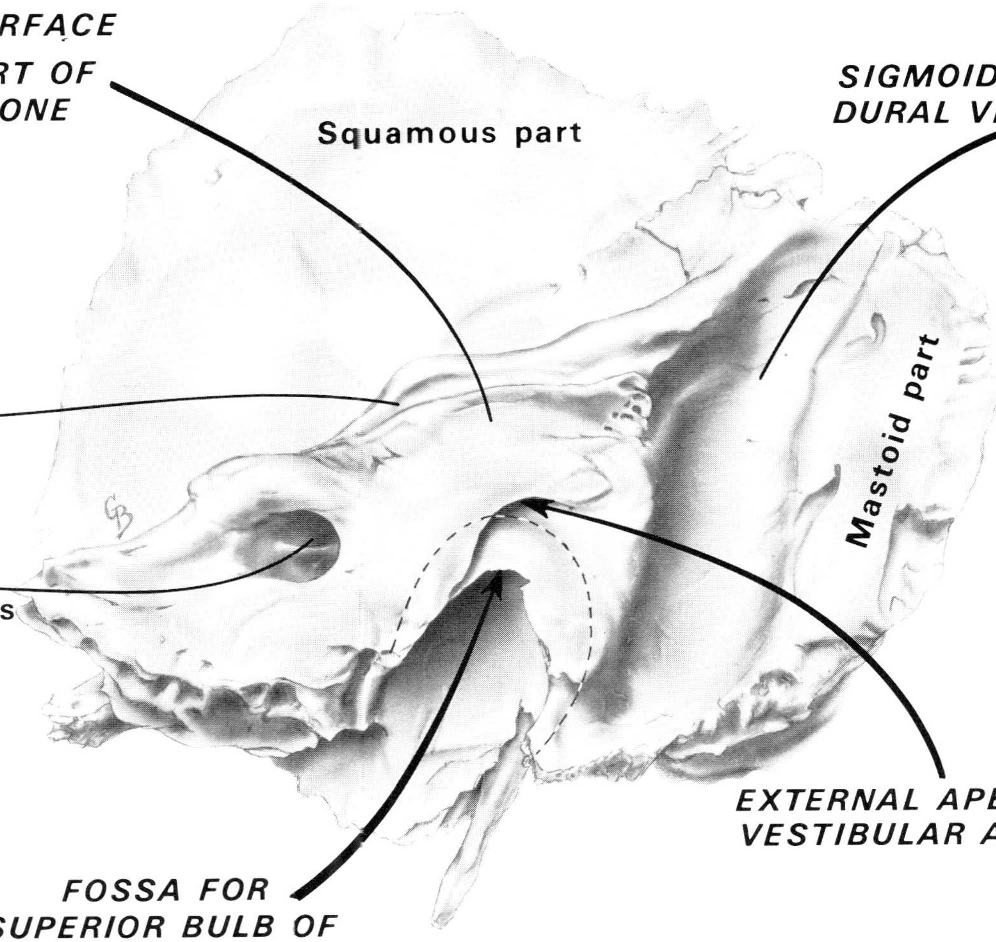

Figure III–130, Continued.

b. An example of a deep jugular fossa, to the height of the broken line. A mere pellicle of bone (in the area indicated by the dotted line) separated the jugular bulb from the intradural segment of the endolymphatic sac. The space of the fossa is exposed by dissection (to the points indicated by the arrows). In such cases the superior bulb of the internal jugular vein intervenes between the endolymphatic sac and the mastoid cavity (see Figure III–107).

(From Anson: Trans. Amer. Acad. Ophthal. Otolaryng., 76:108–129, 1972.)

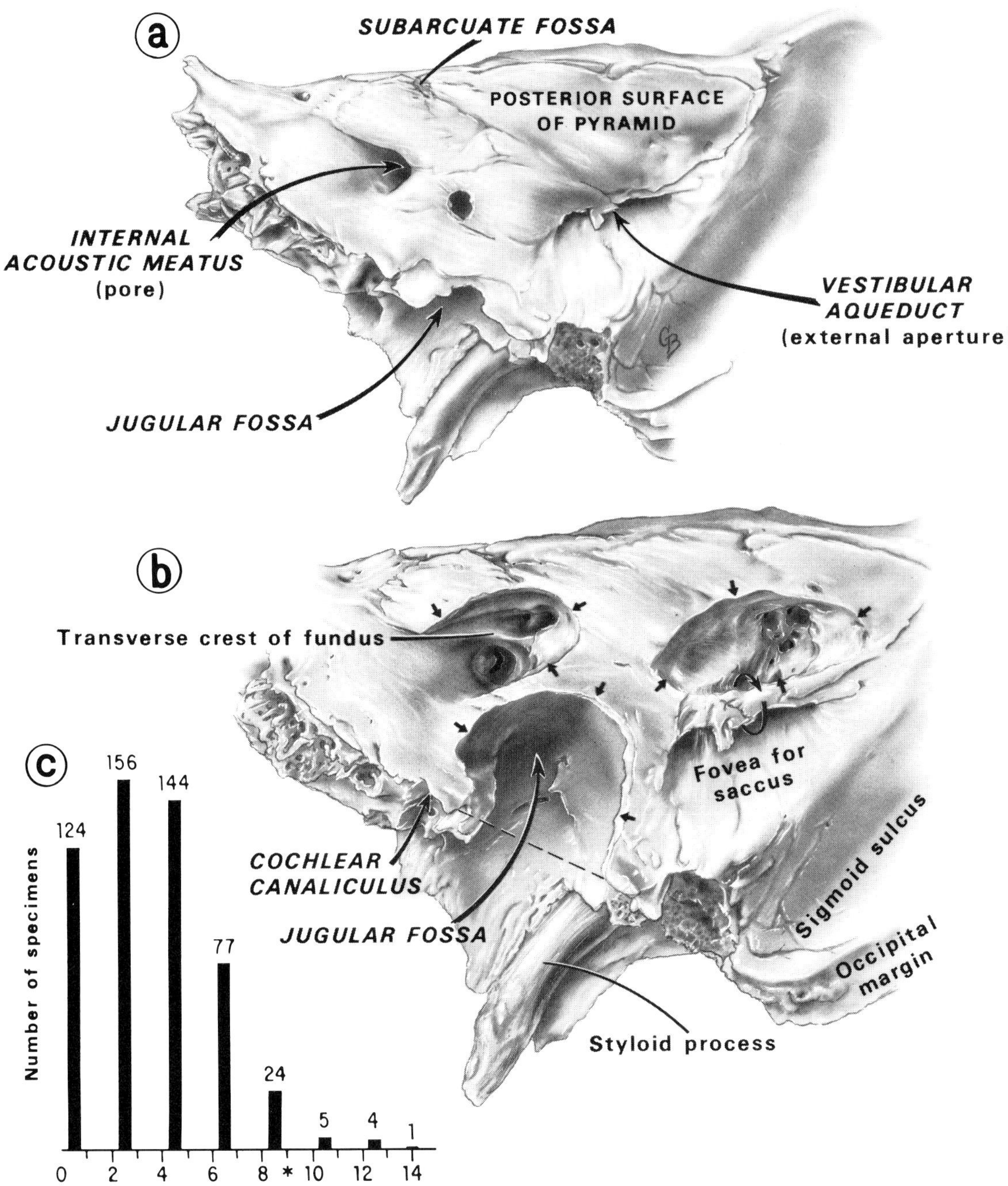

Figure III–131. Jugular fossa and related openings, together with data on variational anatomy. Right temporal bone.

a and *b*. The location of the jugular fossa brings the contained superior bulb of the jugular vein into close relationship with the following: seventh and eighth nerves and internal auditory vessels (in the internal acoustic meatus); the endolymphatic duct and sac (in the vestibular aqueduct and the fovea distal to the external aperture of the aqueduct); the vessels of the subarcuate fossa; and the sigmoid venous sinus as the latter continues into the jugular bulb.

Figure III–131 continues on the opposite page.

Figure III–131, Continued.

The jugular fossa on the inferior surface of the pyramid, posteromedial to the external carotid foramen (see Figure III–138*d*) is separated from the posterior cranial fossa by a thin plate of bone (intact in *a*, removed in *b*). In some specimens the fossa is broadly continuous with the sigmoid sulcus (see Figure III–133*a*).

The internal acoustic meatus begins on the posterior surface of the pyramid in a transversely oval opening (the pore); it runs inward in a transverse plane to a lateral end at the fundus. The pore is bounded by a sharp posterior (lateral) and blunt anterior (medial) boundary. This aperture varies in size and form, just as the long axis of the meatus varies in inclination. In some instances, configuration and direction are such that the fundus is in view when the observer directly faces the posterior surface of the pyramid. The fundus is divided into upper and lower parts by a horizontally disposed sharp-edged ridge, the transverse crest, which divides the entire wall into areas for the facial nerve and the divisions of the acoustic (vestibulocochlear) nerve (see Figure III–134). The aperture appears in *a*; the fundus is exposed in *b* by removal of bone around the pore (to the lines marked by the unlabeled arrows).

The subarcuate fossa, lying just below the superior petrosal suclus, communicates with the latter by minute furrows. Whereas these communications are inconspicuous in the present instances, they may be strikingly prominent in others (see Figure III–139*a*), sometimes passing downward and forward to the internal acoustic meatus and downward and backward to the external aperture of the vestibular aqueduct and to the sigmoid sulcus (Figure III–128*b*). Rarely are similar connections made, across the anterior surface of the pyramid, with the sulcus for the middle meningeal vessels on the medial surface of the temporal squama. Infrequent, too, are cases in which the furrowing continues into the mastoid part of the temporal bone toward the aperture for the mastoid emissary vein.

It would be expected that downward-coursing sulci would be found toward the notch on the posterior angle of the pyramid which marks the site (on the inferior surface) of the cochlear canaliculus and the neighboring aperture of the channel for the cochlear vein. These seem to be wanting. The canaliculus ends in a funnel-shaped depression between the external carotid foramen and the jugular fossa (see Figures III–119 and III–121*a*).

The jugular fossa may thus be regarded as a convenient landmark, with structures occupying sulci or apertures in three directions therefrom: posterolateralward, the sigmoid sulcus; anteromedialward, the cochlear canaliculus; and superiorly, the vestibular aqueduct, subarcuate fossa and internal acoustic meatus—in that order from behind in a forward direction.

The blood vessels (which in cranial *dura mater* produce the furrows described above) constitute a major source of supply to the bone along which they course. The presence of numerous ostia along the "floor" of each sulcate depression attests to their importance as serving a "diploic" function.

c. The jugular fossa is subject to great variation in size. Not infrequently its height is so great that this space of the tympanic cavity is greatly reduced (as it is in the present specimen). The danger that results from encroachment on the space of the tympanum is further increased when the "roof" of the fossa is dehiscent (see Figure III–121*b*). Then nothing more substantial than mucous membrane would intervene between the bulbous vein and the instrument employed in middle ear surgery.

In 535 consecutively studied adult temporal bones, the jugular fossa measured between 0 and 14 mm. in height. In some instances the surface was flat. In the specimen chosen for illustration, the depth was 9 mm. (location indicated by the asterisk).

Note: It is important to recognize the difference between the superficial and deep relationships of aqueducts, fossae and sulci. Two examples will serve to establish this point: the pore of the internal acoustic meatus and the entrance to the jugular fossa are separated by a considerable distance in the undissected specimen (*a*), but the fundus of the meatus and the "roof" of the fossa are close together; the fossa for reception of the endolymphatic sac is relatively near the jugular fossa, but the vestibular aqueduct (continuing inward from the fovea) courses away from the fossa. Briefly, differing inclination is an anatomical feature of importance in surgical approach to the interior of the petrous part of the temporal bone.

Dissection by Dr. Bruce B. Shilling.

(From Anson: Trans. Amer. Acad. Ophthal. Otolaryng., 76:108–129, 1972).

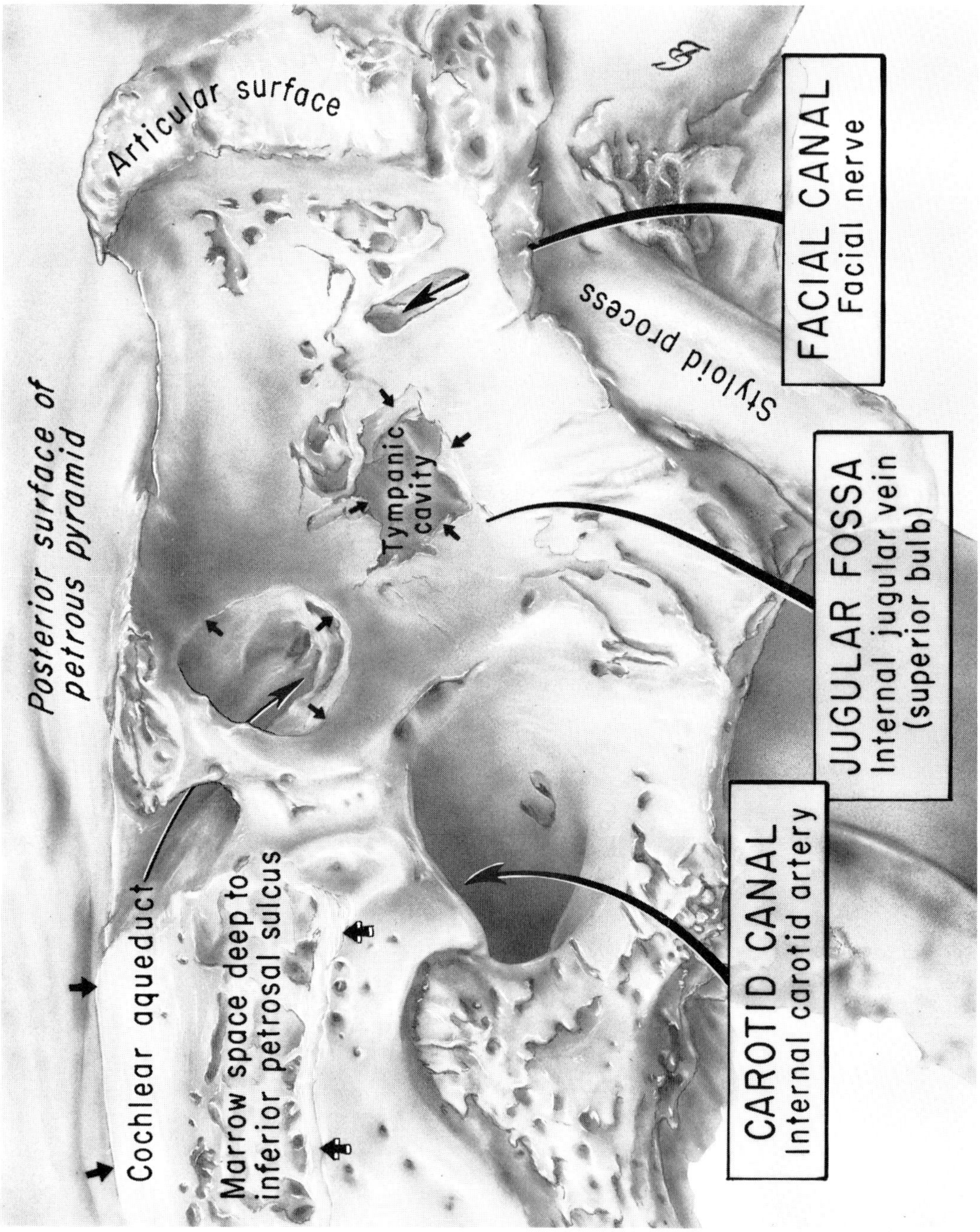
Articular surface
Posterior surface of petrous pyramid
Tympanic cavity
Styloid process
FACIAL CANAL
Facial nerve
JUGULAR FOSSA
Internal jugular vein (superior bulb)
CAROTID CANAL
Internal carotid artery
Cochlear aqueduct
Marrow space deep to inferior petrosal sulcus

Figure III–132. JUGULAR FOSSA AND RELATED ANATOMY: TEMPORAL BONE SEEN FROM BELOW. DISSECTION OF A SKELETAL PREPARATION.

The thin roof of the jugular fossa was dehiscent (at arrows). The course of the facial canal is demonstrated as it occupies the posterior wall of the fossa. The external carotic foramen lies anterior to the fossa. Communications between the inferior petrosal sulcus and the interior of the *pars petrosa* are shown by removal of bone (to the points of the arrows).

Note Especially: This specimen demonstrates several closely interrelated features, each of them surgically significant. They concern the anatomy of the following: the jugular fossa, the external aperture of the vestibular aqueduct, the fovea for the endolymphatic sac, and the facial canal.

The jugular fossa is exceptionally large. On the "roof" there is an area of dehiscence, meaning that the superior bulb of the internal jugular vein was, in that local area, separated from the middle ear cavity merely by mucous membrane.

The medial wall of the fossa is also dehiscent; thus, the vein was separated from the endolymphatic sac solely by the investing *dura mater* as the sac lay in the foveate impression on the posterior surface of the pyramid. The posterior wall is also dehiscent where normally bone would complete the facial canal. The facial nerve would have been in contact with the vein. The stylomastoid foramen was separated from the space of the jugular fossa by a slender bridge of bone.

Dissection by Dr. Raymond L. Warpeha.

(After Anson, Harper, and Winch: Third Symposium on the Role of the Vestibular Organs in Space Exploration, NASA SP-152, pp. 259–288. Washington, D.C., U.S. Government Printing Office, 1968.)

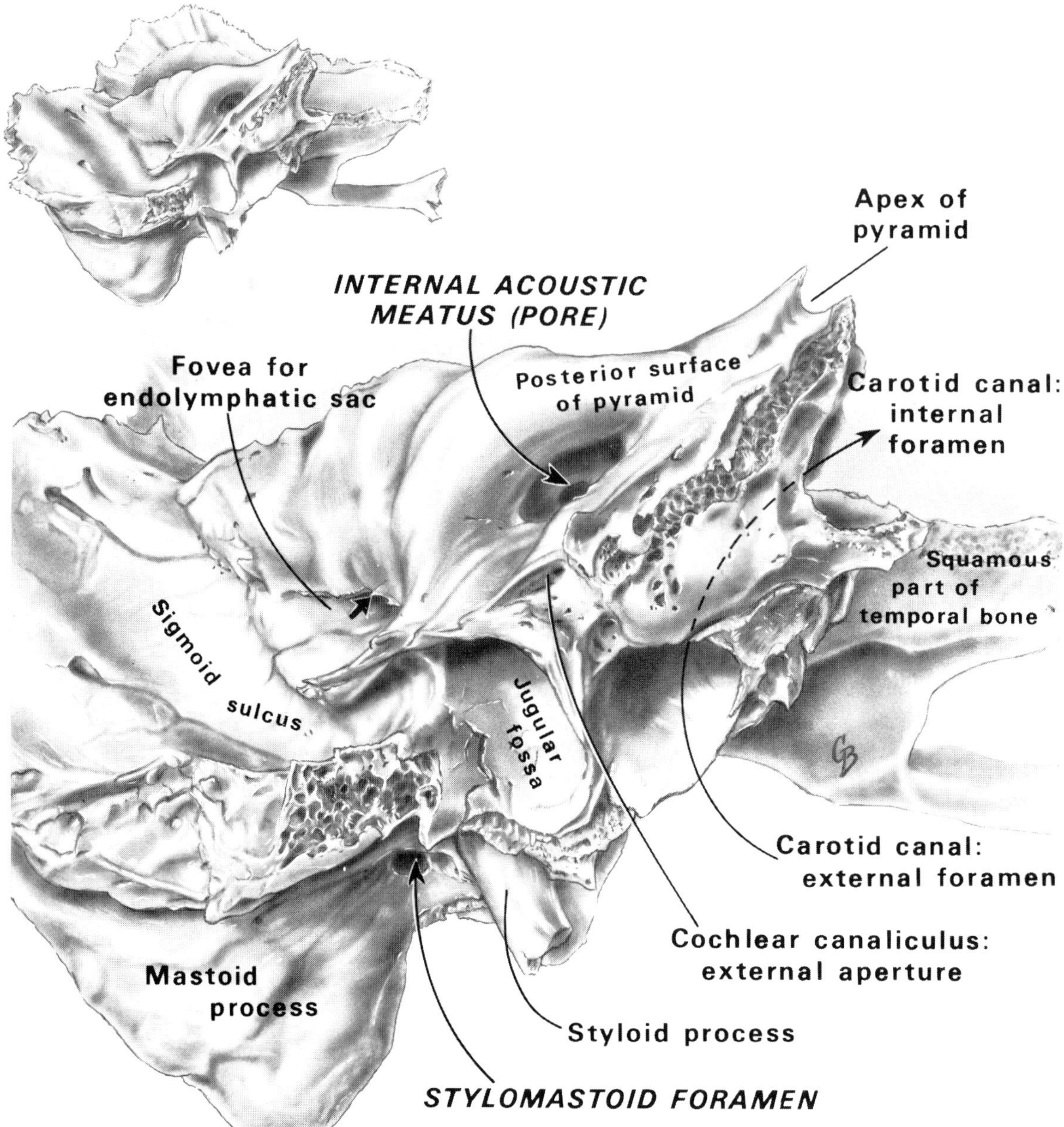

Figure III–133. INTERNAL ACOUSTIC MEATUS AND RELATED ANATOMY. *a.* ON THE POSTERIOR AND INFERIOR SURFACES OF THE PYRAMID.

a. On the posterior surface of the pyramid are seen both the fovea for reception of the saccus at the external aperture of the vestibular aqueduct and the pore of the internal acoustic meatus, marking the beginning of the course of the facial nerve through the temporal bone. On the inferior surface appear the jugular fossa (continuous with the sigmoid sulcus), the external carotid foramen and the stylomastoid foramen (of the facial canal), and the external aperture of the cochlear aqueduct. *Inset.* Entire specimen.

In 75 skeletal preparations of adult temporal bone (meaning those freed of all soft tissue), the *porus* was measured in vertical dimension. This measurement (height of aperture) was as follows: 2 mm. in 7 specimens, 3 mm. in 24, 4 mm. in 35, and 5 mm. in 9. Measurement of the horizontal dimension (width) would be unreliable, since a definite anterior margin does not exist (the medial wall passing insensibly into the posterior surface of the pyramid).

In the same lot of specimens, the depth of the meatus was taken (that is, the distance from *porus* to *fundus*). This measurement was as follows: 5 mm. in 2 specimens, 6 mm. in 2, 7 mm. in 10, 8 mm. in 19, 9 mm. in 14, 10 mm. in 18, 11mm. in 2, 12 mm. in 4, and 13 mm. in 4. Thus, in 61 of the 75 specimens (80 per cent), the range was between 7 and 10 mm.

Figure III–133 continues on the opposite page.

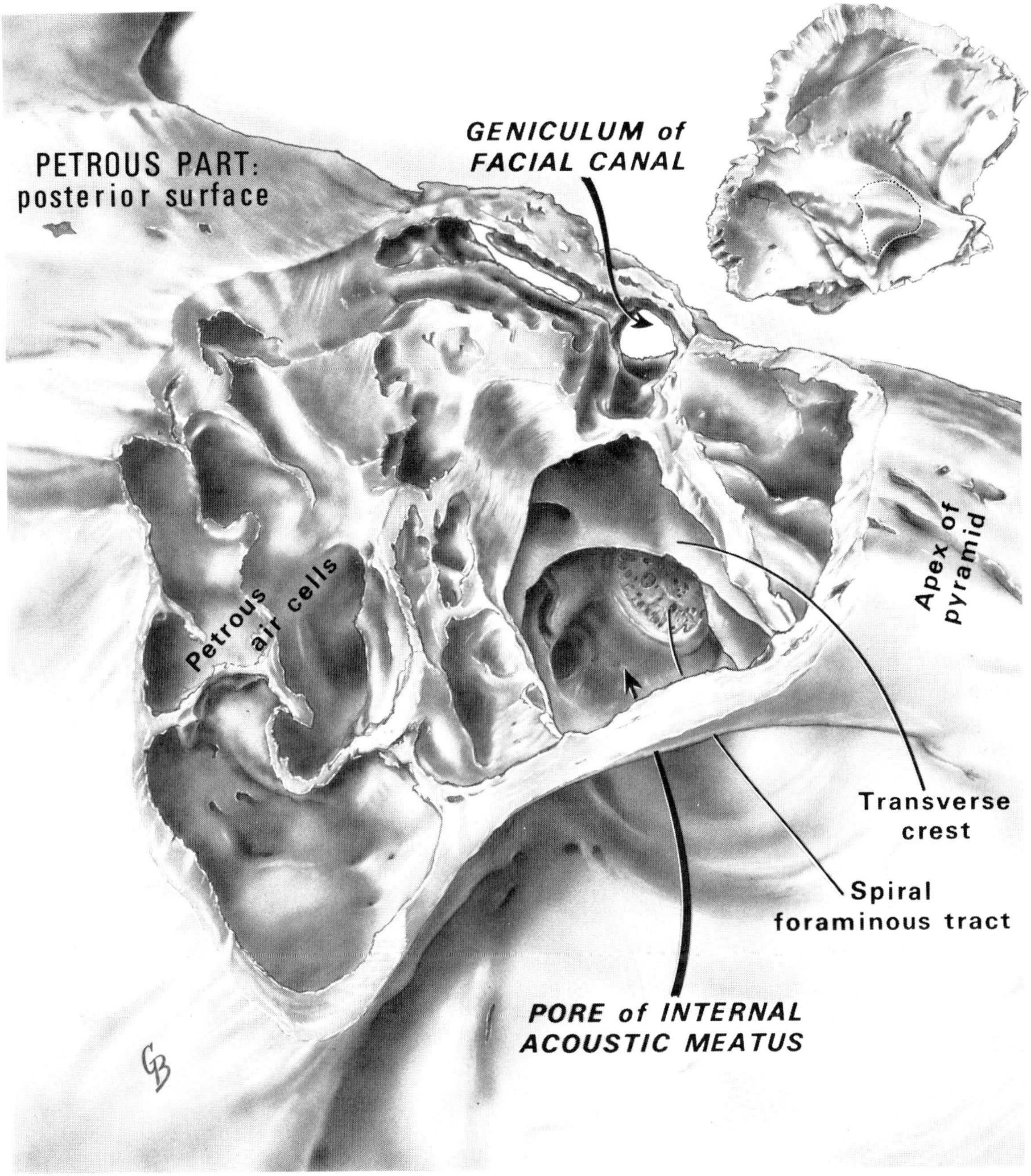

b

Figure III–133, Continued. INTERNAL ACOUSTIC MEATUS AND RELATED ANATOMY. *b.* DISSECTED SPECIMEN VIEWED FROM THE MEDIAL SIDE AND FROM SLIGHTLY ABOVE.

b. From the posterior surface the facial and related areas of the fundus are exposed by removal of the "roof" of the internal acoustic meatus. *Inset.* The dissected area is marked on the drawing of the entire specimen.

The location of the medial end of the meatus is indicated by the rim of bone remaining at the pore. The lateral end, the fundus of the meatus, is closed by a plate of bone which is also in large part the medial wall of the vestibule and cochlea. The facial area of the fundus (for passage of the seventh nerve) is situated above a transverse crest and adjacent to the vestibular area (for transmission of the upper terminal branch of the vestibular nerve). The related openings, below the crest, are the following: spiral foraminous tract (cochlear nerve); inferior vestibular area (saccular nerve); and singular foramen (posterior ampullary nerve). From the anterior surface of the pyramid the geniculum of the facial canal has been exposed by local removal of the overlying bone. The dissections of the two areas described above serve to demonstrate the route by which the facial nerve passes from the cranial cavity to the labyrinthine wall of the tympanic cavity (see also Figures III–72 and III–140).

The air cells in this highly pneumatized temporal bone are situated in front of, behind, and above the internal acoustic meatus and the facial canal.

Dissection by Dr. Raymond L. Warpeha.

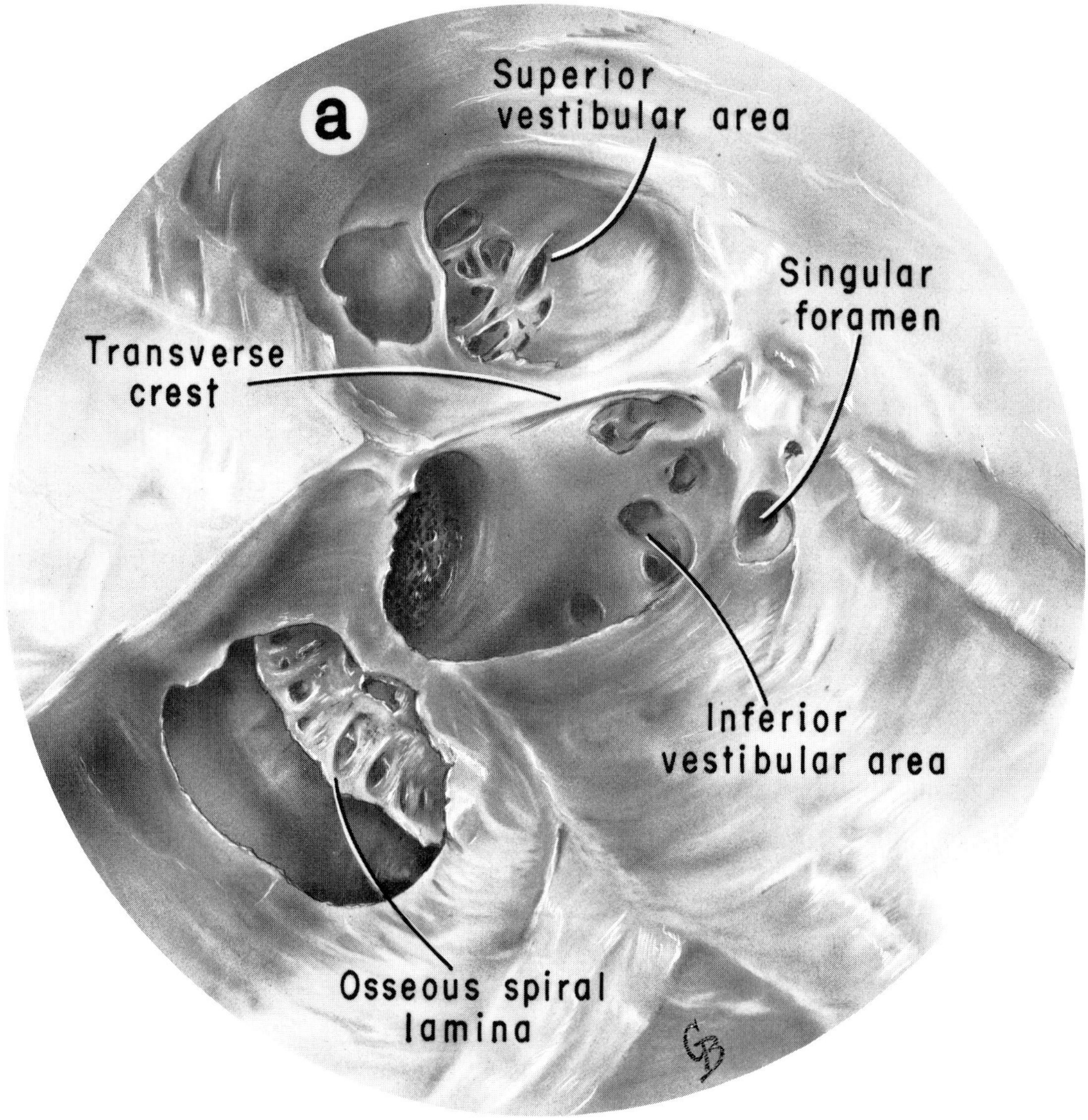

Figure III–134. FUNDUS OF INTERNAL ACOUSTIC MEATUS, RIGHT EAR. *a.* DEMONSTRATING THE OPENINGS IN THE FUNDUS OF THE INTERNAL ACOUSTIC MEATUS.

a. The internal acoustic meatus is a short canal coursing nearly transversely and frontally. The lumen varies with the individual. It begins medially in a transversely oval opening, the internal acoustic pore, bounded by a sharp lateral and blunt medial margin; the lateral end, the fundus or floor, is closed by a bony plate which is in large part also the medial wall of the vestibule and cochlea. It is divided into an upper and a lower area by a horizontal sharp ridge, the transverse crest. The upper, smaller area, in an anterior depression, the area of the facial nerve, contains the internal opening of the facial canal (*Fallopii*); a posterior funnel-shaped depression, the superior vestibular area, contains several delicate openings of small canals which conduct the branches of the upper terminal ramus of the vestibular nerve to the superior cribrose macula of the vestibule. The lower, larger area presents a rounded depression in front, the cochlear area. Here begins the spiral foraminous tract: a broad spiral band of variably sized openings, curved like the cochlea. These foramina carry the bundles of the cochlear nerve directly to the basal turn or through the longitudinal canals of the modiolus to the middle and apical turns. In the posterior part of the inferior area, close below the *crista transversa*, lies an area with small openings, the inferior vestibular area, which conducts the bundles of the saccular nerve through small canaliculi to the middle cribrose macula of the vestibule; and somewhat medianward and behind it is to be found a single large opening, the singular foramen, through which the posterior ampullary nerve passes through a longer, delicate canaliculus to the inferior cribrose macula.

Dissection by Dr. Raymond L. Warpeha.

Figure III–134 continues on the opposite page.

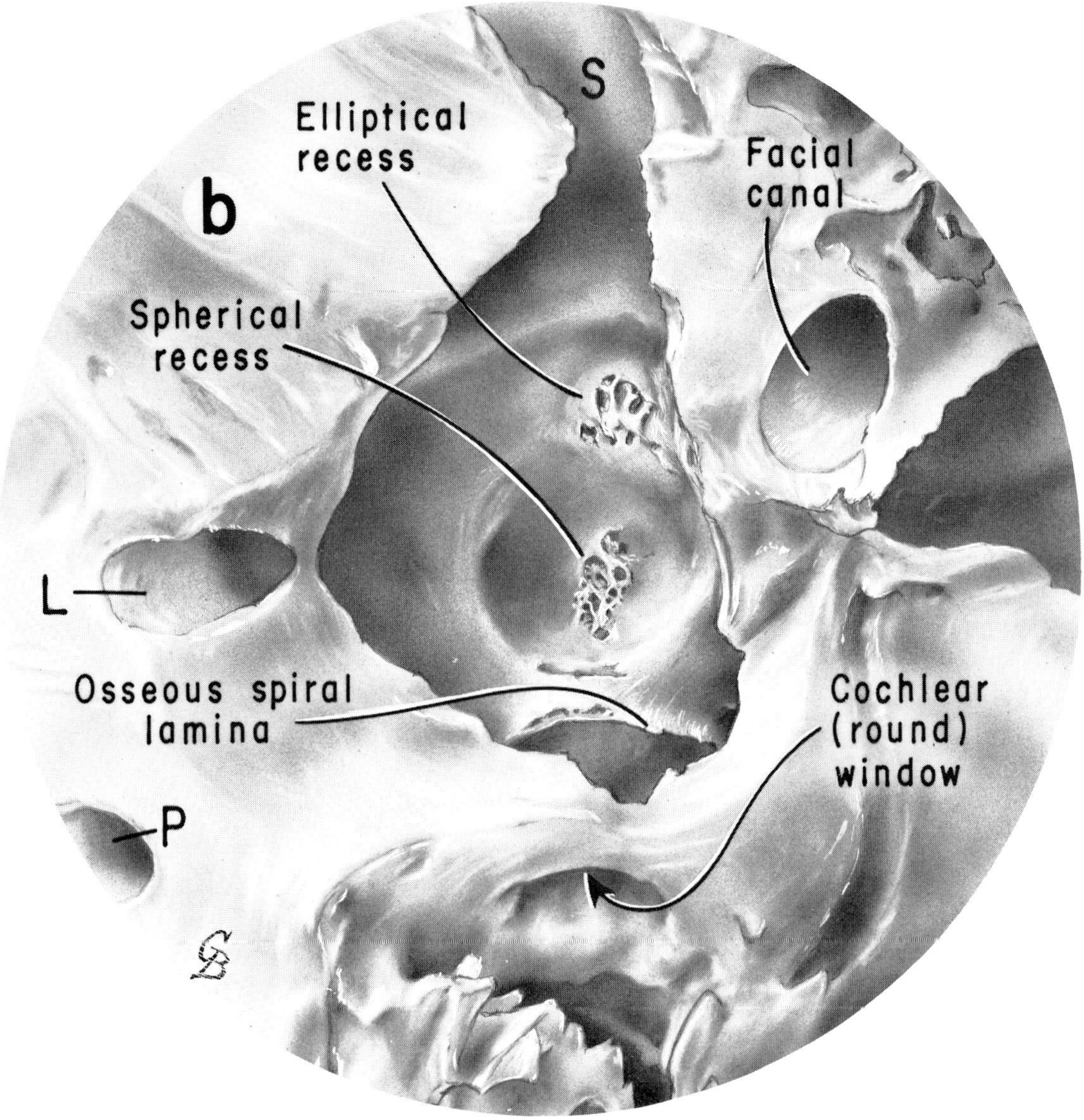

Figure III–134, Continued. VESTIBULE: MEDIAL WALL, RIGHT EAR. *b.* SAME SPECIMEN SHOWN IN THE PRECEDING FIGURE.

b. The tympanic cavity was first exposed; then bone of the labyrinthine wall of the tympanum was removed to expose, in the area of the vestibular (oval) window, the vestibule and semicircular canals with which it communicates. Natural bone remains inferiorly in the region of the cochlear (round) window. Abbreviations: *S*, *L*, and *P*; superior, lateral, and posterior semicircular canals, respectively.

The bony plate that forms the wall of the fundus of the internal acoustic meatus is in large measure the medial wall of the vestibule and the cochlea. The vestibular (superior and inferior) areas of the fundus find corresponding groupings of minute foramina called the cribrose maculae, in the depths of the elliptical and spherical recesses. These two deepened areas of the vestibule are separated by a delicate ridge, the vestibular crest.

The elliptical recess serves for reception of the utricle. It also contains a small depression, the internal aperture of the vestibular aqueduct. It is oval in form and posterosuperior in position. The spherical recess receives the saccule; its location is anteroinferior to that of the elliptical recess. The elliptical recess contains a small perforated zone, the superior cribrose macula, in which open the minute foramina of the superior vestibular area of the fundus (for transmission of the fibers of the utricular nerve). Similarly, on the wall of the spherical recess appear the foramina of the middle cribrose area, continuous with the inferior vestibular area (through which the fibers of the saccular nerve reach the vestibule).

Dissection by Dr. Raymond L. Warpeha.

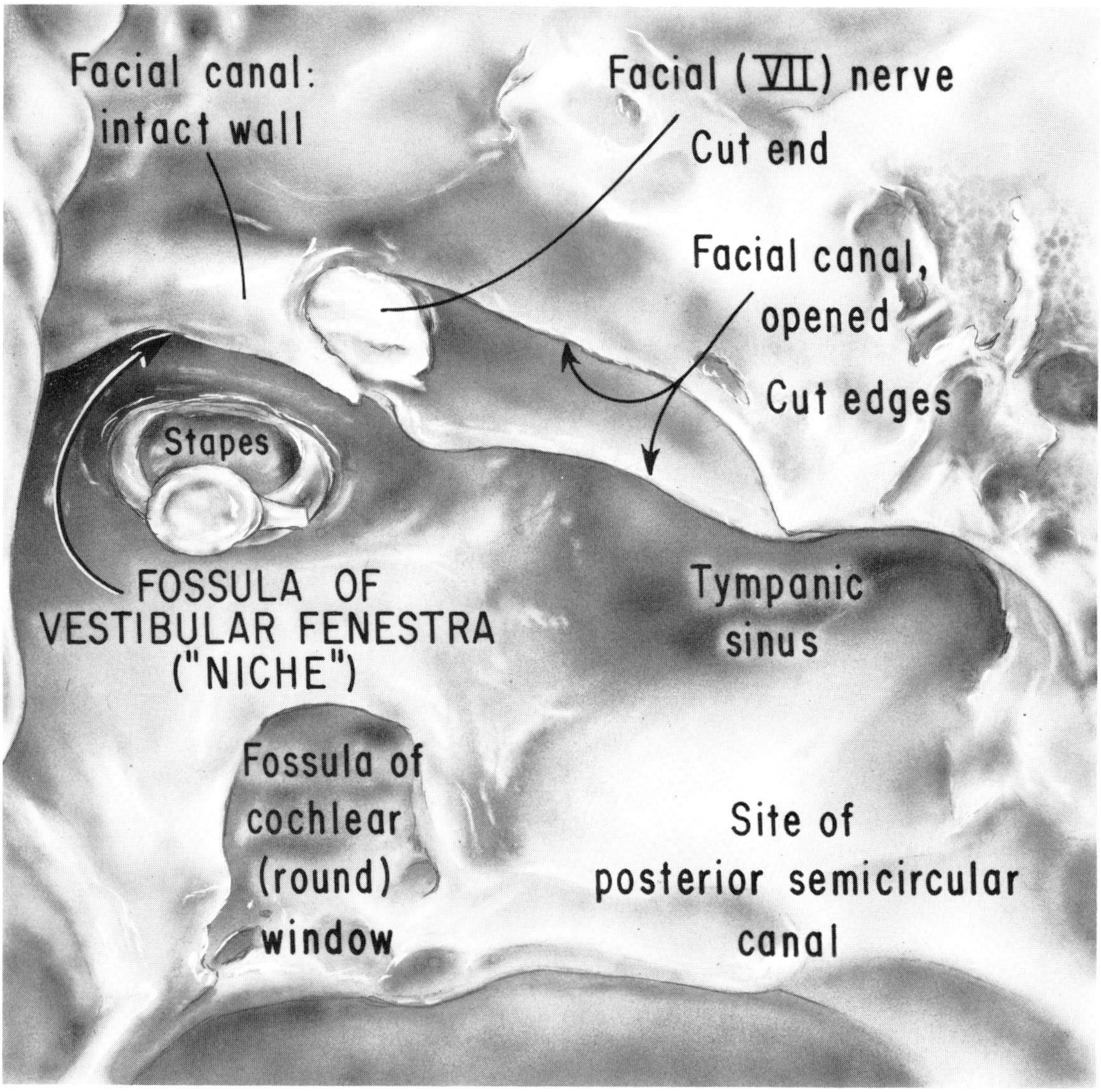

Figure III–135. FACIAL CANAL AND RELATED ANATOMICAL STRUCTURES ON THE LABYRINTHINE WALL OF THE TYMPANIC CAVITY.

Dissection of an unembalmed specimen; the facial canal has been opened, the nerve transected.

The facial canal, in coursing posteriorly from the geniculum, passes above the vestibular fenestra. In this situation, the canal forms the "roof" of a fossula which opens below into the tympanic cavity proper and behind into a large tympanic sinus.

Immediately below the vestibular fenestra lies the promontory, a projection due to the beginning of the basal turn of the cochlea. Next below, and in a slightly posterior direction, the wall of the promontory leads, at a sharp declivity, into a triangular space, the fossula of the cochlear fenestra. The fossula, in turn, leads forward and medialward into the cochlear fenestra (or round window) which opens into the tympanic scala of the basal turn of the cochlea. The inclination and depth of the fossula are such that the secondary tympanic membrane is out of view as the labyrinthine wall is seen in surgical approach from the external acoustic meatus. Above the prominence of the facial canal (as the latter overarches the stapes) the space of the tympanic cavity is continued as the epitympanic recess.

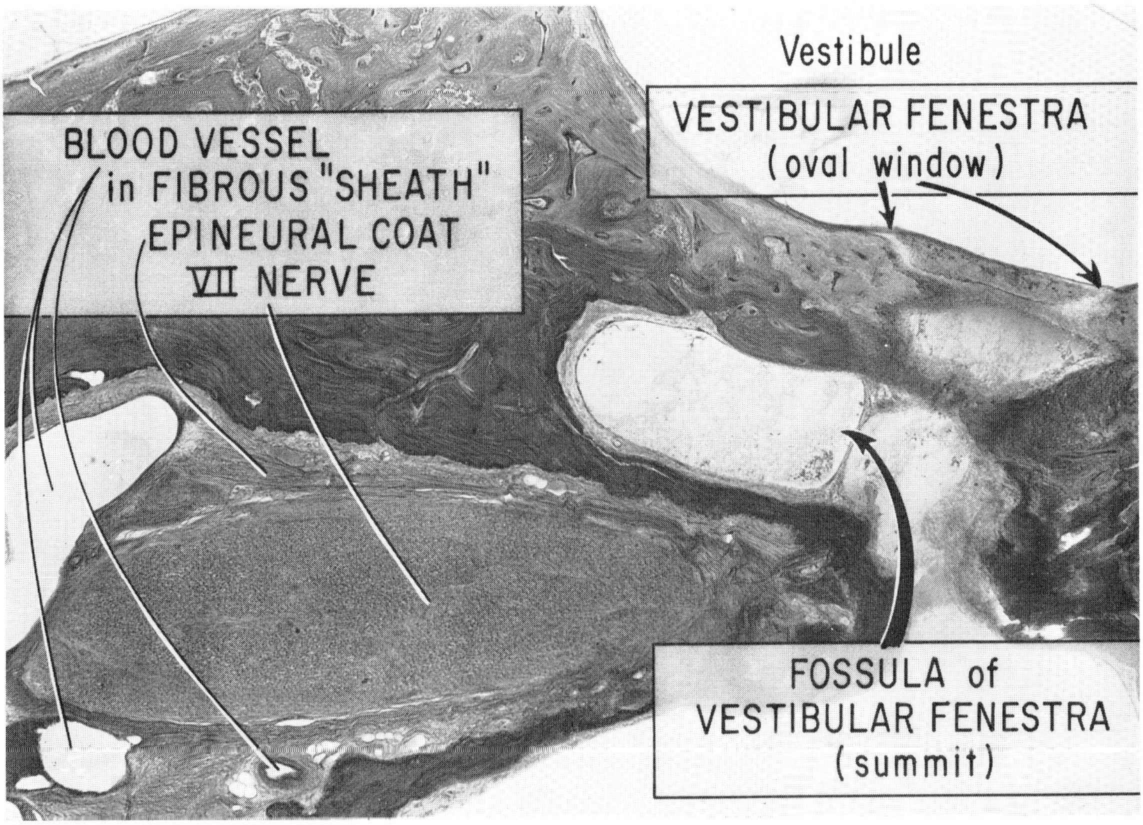

Figure III–136. FACIAL CANAL, FACIAL NERVE, AND RELATED STRUCTURES. MALE, 57 YEARS OF AGE.

At the facial area of the fundus of the internal acoustic meatus (above the transverse crest), the facial nerve is transmitted to the geniculum of the facial canal. Therefrom, the canal passes horizontally backward, arching over the vestibular fenestra and the stapes. In this location, the canal forms the lateral wall of a cul-de-sac of the general tympanic cavity, termed the fossula of the vestibular fenestra (or stapes "niche" in everyday otological usage). At the horizontal level here pictured, the canal is in the labyrinthine wall of the tympanic cavity, between the cochlea and the vestibule. Even in this proximal segment of its course, the canal contains large blood vessels in addition to the nerve (see Figure III–78*b*).

Distal to the area shown in the present section, the canal turns caudalward (downward) in an even curve to the stylomastoid foramen. In its descent, the canal occupies the mastoid (posterior) wall of the tympanic cavity (see Figure III–11). Within the canal, vascularity grows progressively richer, the fibrous sheath of the nerve histologically more definite.

In this specimen the osseous wall is complete. However, cases of dehiscence are common. The fault in the wall may occur at any level (see Figure III–84).

Transverse section, Wisconsin Collection, series 32 R. ×22.

Figure III–137. MAJOR ROUTES OF BLOOD SUPPLY TO THE PETROUS PART OF THE TEMPORAL BONE ON THE POSTERIOR AND INFERIOR SURFACES.

The following channels through which blood vessels reach the labyrinths within the petrous part of the temporal bone are shown: internal acoustic meatus (*b*), subarcuate fossa (*c*), and vestibular aqueduct (*e*). The site of the external aperture of the cochlear canaliculus, or aqueduct (*d*), on the inferior surface of the bone is visible in this view as a notch at the posterior angle (*a*). The channel for the cochlear vein reaches the inferior surface near the aperture of the cochlear canaliculus.

(From Anson, Harper, and Winch: Third Symposium on the Role of the Vestibular Organs in Space Exploration, NASA SP-152, pp. 259–288. Washington, D.C., U.S. Government Printing Office, 1968.)

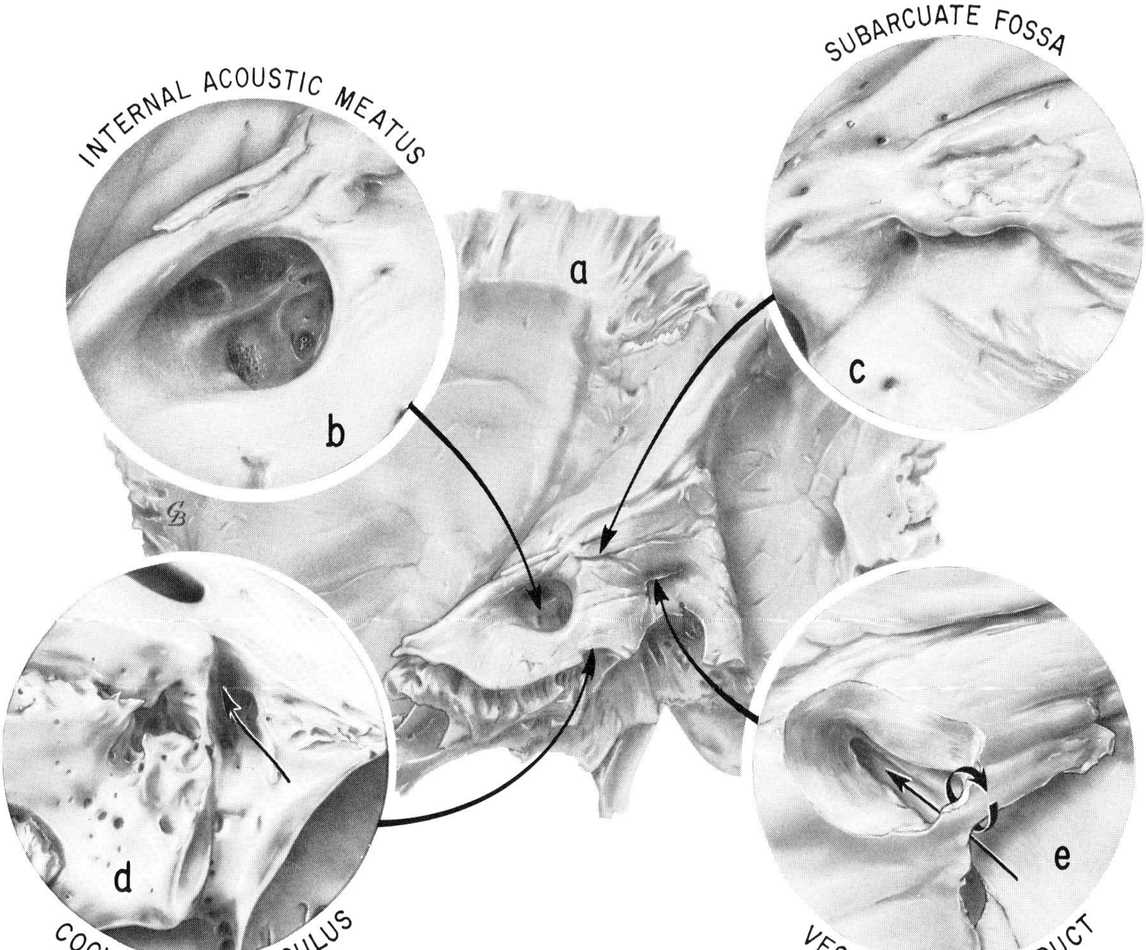

Figure III–137. See legend on the opposite page.

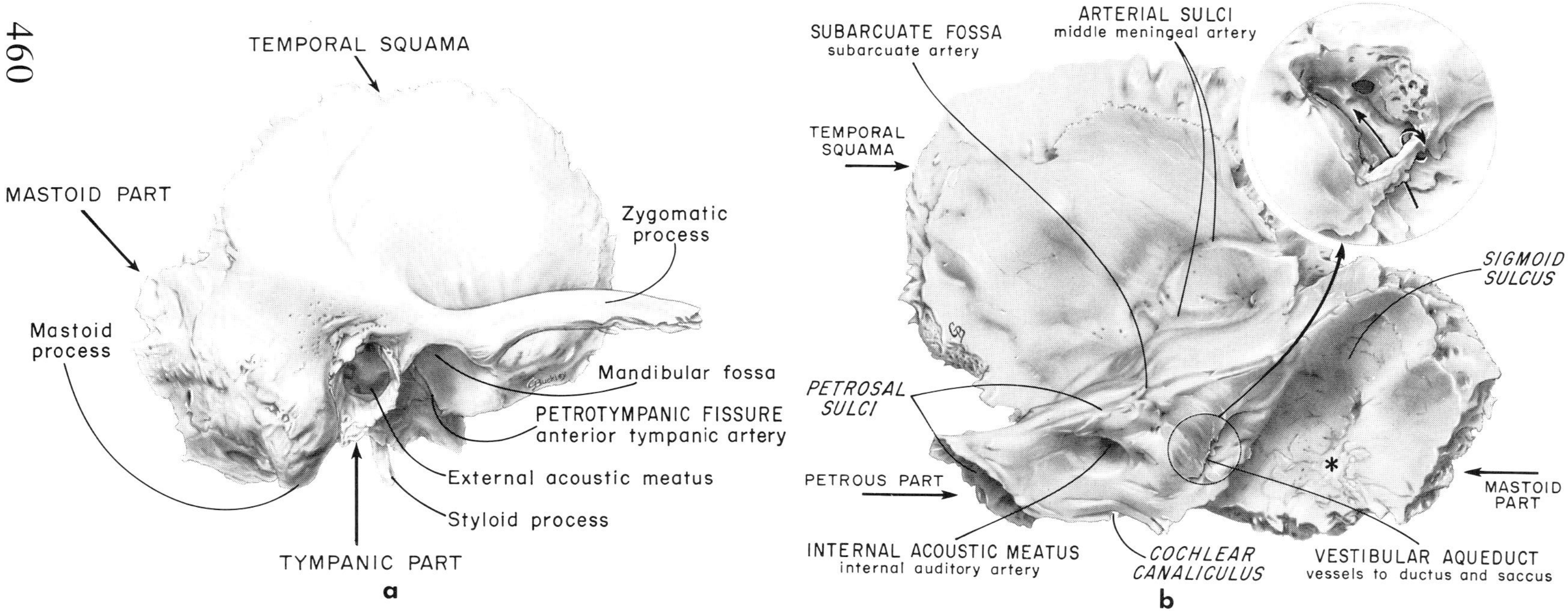

Figure III–138. Blood supply of the temporal bone. Specimen shown in lateral, medial, anterior, and inferior views.

a. Lateral Surface. The petrotympanic fissure transmits the anterior tympanic branch of the maxillary from the external division of the common carotid; upon reaching the middle ear, it ramifies in the mucous membrane and anastomoses with tympanic vessels of other sources.

b and *c. Medial and Anterior Surfaces.* The vertebral branch of the subclavian artery, upon leaving the transverse foramen in the atlas, enters the cranial cavity through the foramen magnum. It unites with the vessel of the opposite side to form the unpaired basilar artery, of which the internal auditory is one branch. The latter artery goes lateralward with the facial and vestibulocochlear nerves, to course through the internal acoustic meatus to the cochlea. At the porus of the meatus a very small branch is sent to the subarcuate fossa for supply of the canalicular part of the petrous pyramid.

The external aperture of the vestibular aqueduct, situated posterior to the opening of the meatus, receives small vessels from the meningeal branch of the occipital artery. The latter is a branch of the external carotid; it ascends through the jugular foramen (with the vein) in *dura mater* of the posterior cranial fossa.

In a medial view of the temporal bone is also seen the petrosquamous fissure, through which the superior tympanic branch of the middle meningeal artery reaches the bone. The middle meningeal, a branch of the maxillary (the latter from the external carotid), reaches the cranial cavity by passing through the foramen spinosum.

On the anterior surface of the petrous pyramid is seen the hiatus of the facial canal. In addition to the nerve, it transmits the superficial petrosal ramus of the middle meningeal artery. This vessel anastomoses with the stylomastoid branch of the posterior auricular.

Figure III–138 continues on the opposite page.

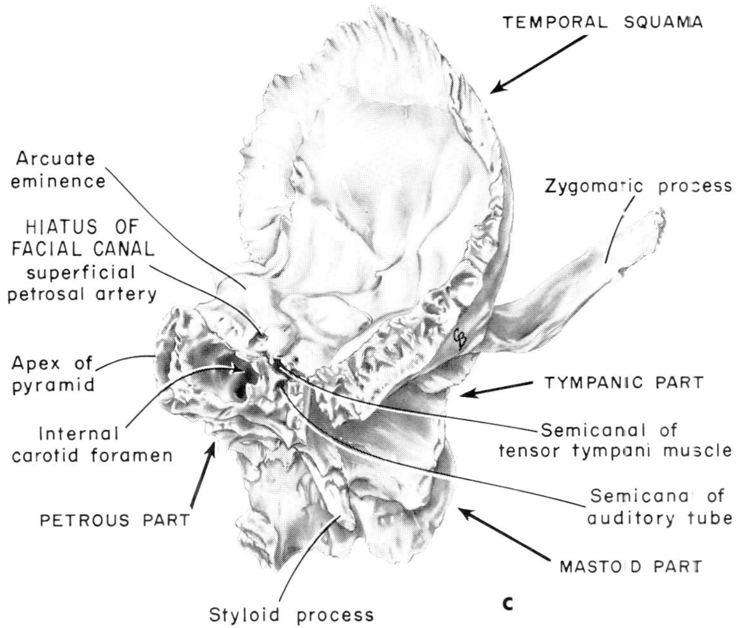

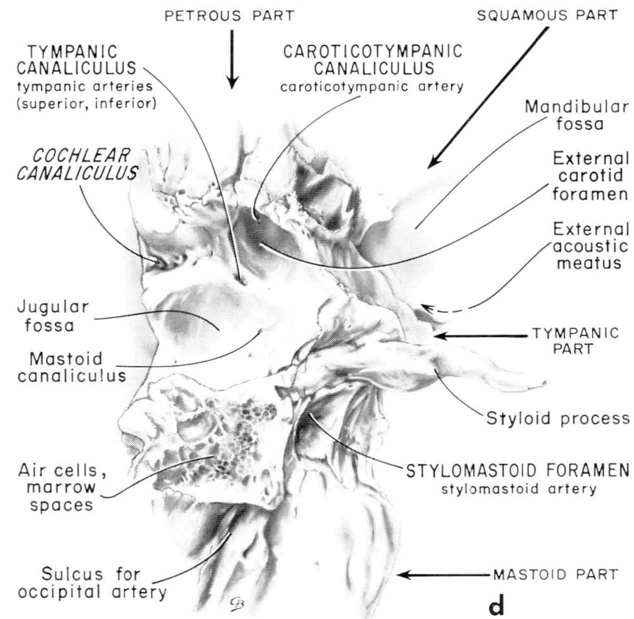

Figure III–138, Continued. BLOOD SUPPLY OF THE TEMPORAL BONE. SPECIMEN SHOWN IN LATERAL, MEDIAL, ANTERIOR, AND INFERIOR VIEWS.

Veins, additional to those accompanying the arteries of the same name, are received from the bone by the superior and inferior sulci and the sigmoid sulcus.

d. Inferior Surface. In the wall of the carotid canal a small foramen (or foramina) of the caroticotympanic canaliculus transmits a similarly named artery into the middle ear. The branches anastomose on the promontory with those from the maxillary and middle meningeal.

The stylomastoid branch of the posterior auricular (from the external carotid) ascends through the facial canal to the canaliculus of the chorda tympani, through which it reaches the middle ear as the posterior tympanic artery. It anastomoses with the superficial petrosal branch of the middle meningeal.

The inferior tympanic branch of the ascending pharyngeal (the latter from the external carotid) passes from the petrosal fossula and tympanic canaliculus into the middle ear, where its twigs contribute to the plexus on the promontory.

It is evident, then, that most of the vessels are tympanic; they contribute to a plexus that is richest in the mucous membrane of the promontory. Some of these vessels give off branches to the auditory ossicles and to the tympanic membrane. Additionally, the outermost layer of bone on the labyrinthine wall of the tympanic cavity receives a lesser supply. As histological examinations of sectioned temporal bones show, the supply is virtually limited to the middle ear and its contents. An account of the progress of ossification, in its effect on the blood supply of the cochlea, may be traced in a series of steps beginning with that of the fetus in the third month of intrauterine life (see Figure II–50).

(From Anson, Winch, Warpeha, and Donaldson: Ann. Otol., 75:921–944, 1966.)

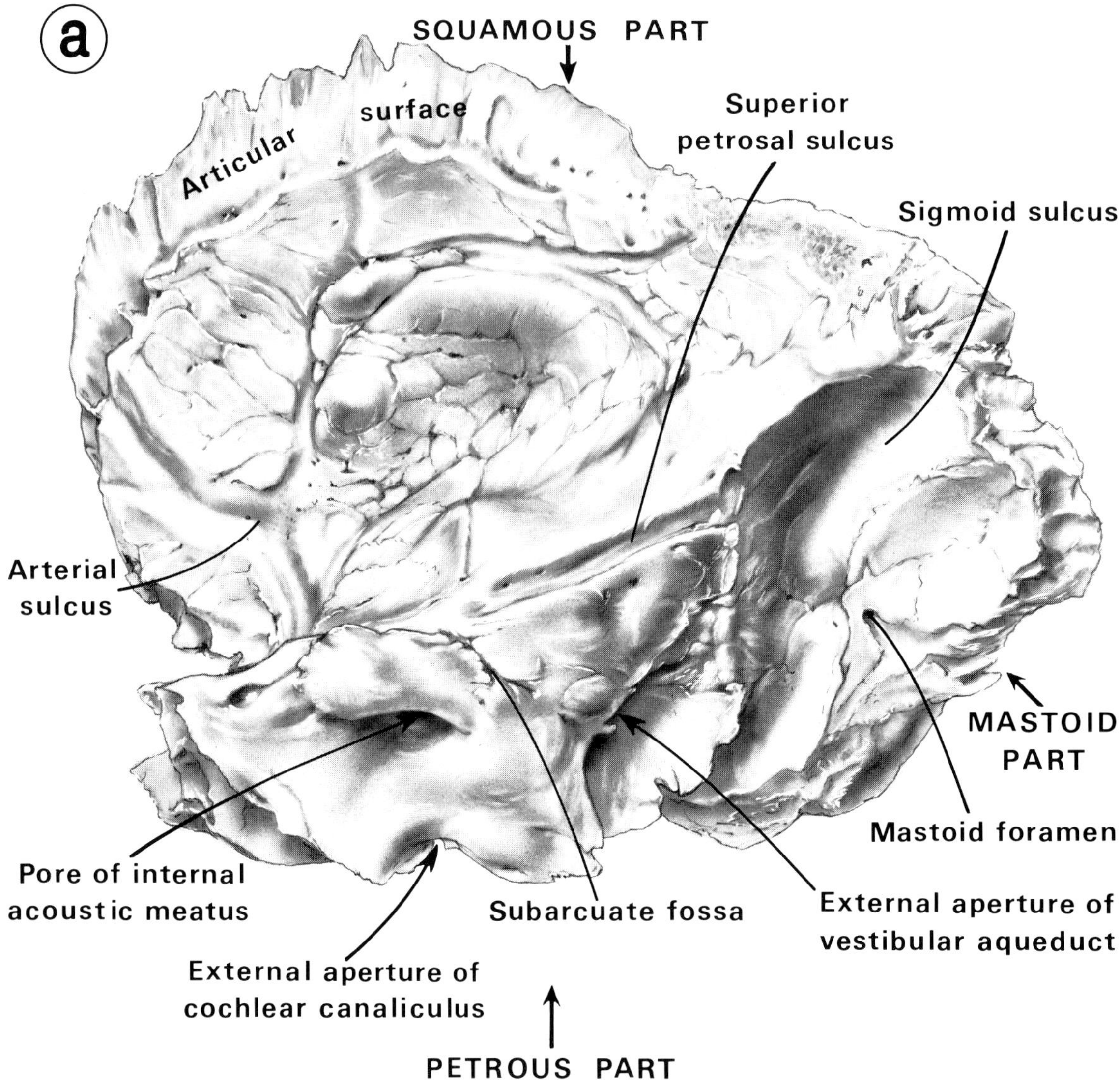

Figure III–139. VASCULAR ROUTES TO THE RIGHT TEMPORAL BONE. *a.* MEDIAL VIEW. *b.* SUPERIOR VIEW.

Deep sculpturing of the surface renders this specimen exceptionally useful in a review of the meningeal course of arteries and veins that supply the several parts of the temporal bone.

The middle meningeal artery, from the internal maxillary, ascending from the *foramen spinosum* is distributed inside the skull in arterial sulci to the frontal, parietal and temporal regions. On the temporal squama the artery follows an arching course paralleling the line of the parietotemporal suture. Branches arising from both sides in arborescent fashion diminish in caliber as they spread. Along the way radicles, entering minute foramina in the bone, reach the diploic tissue. Corresponding veins, after communicating with dural sinuses, converge upon the *foramen spinosum.*

Differing from the richness of vascular supply to the cerebral surface of the squama, the adjacent anterior surface of the petrous part of the temporal bone is almost devoid of blood vessels. Lacking prominent sulci, the meningeal surface of the pyramid presents an almost marblelike appearance.

Figure III–139 continues on the opposite page.

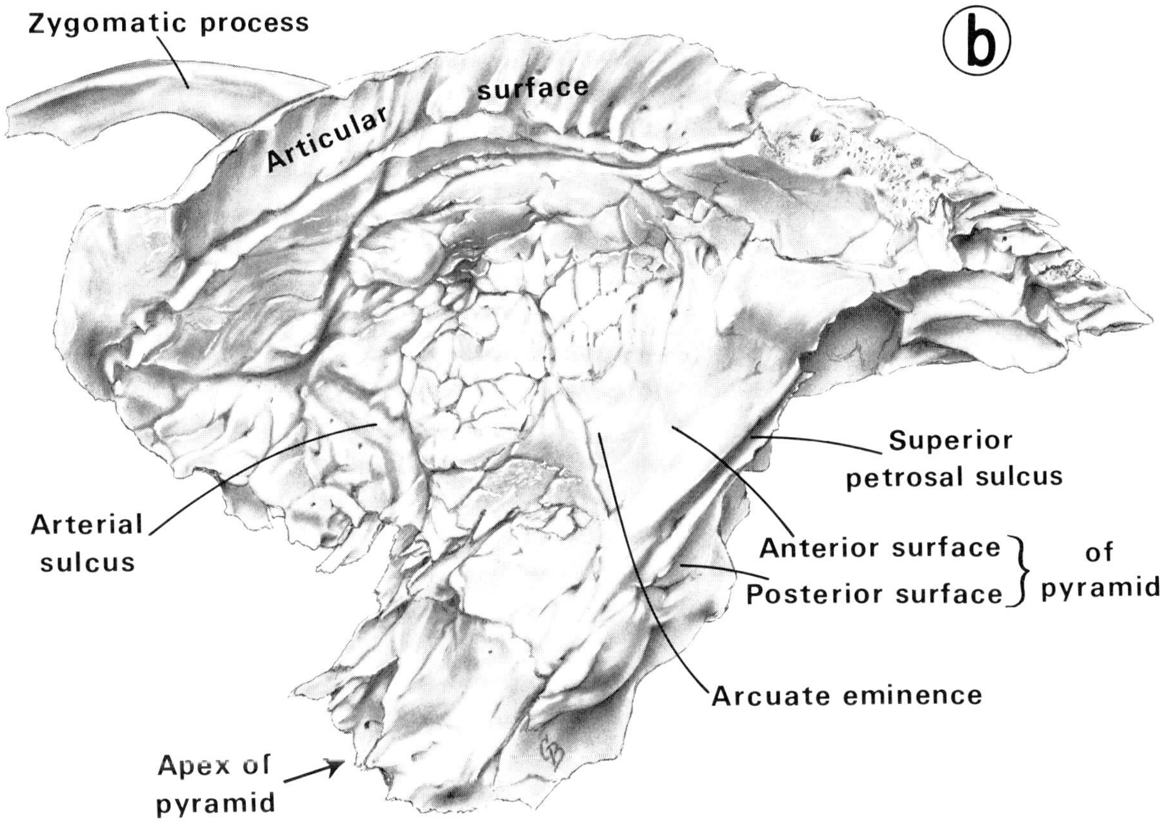

Figure III–139, Continued.

On the posterior surface of the pyramid, branches of the internal auditory artery (from the basilar) enter the vestibular aqueduct and the subarcuate fossa, their course usually being marked by delicate sulci (see Figure III–128*a* to *c*). Otherwise, the sculpturing is caused by dural venous channels, the superior petrosal sulcus along the superior angle of the pyramid, the inferior petrosal sinus along the posterior angle. The former vein ends in the sigmoid part of the transverse sinus; the latter usually terminates in the bulb of the internal jugular vein (see Figure III–130).

The sigmoid sulcus, housing the sinus, is a deep groove on the medial surface of the mastoid part of the bone. It describes an S-shaped figure, curving from above and behind, downward and forward. In some specimens, the "floor" of the sigmoid sulcus is marked by a delicate sculpturing, recording the presence (in the fresh state) of veins in a vermiculate pattern of distribution.

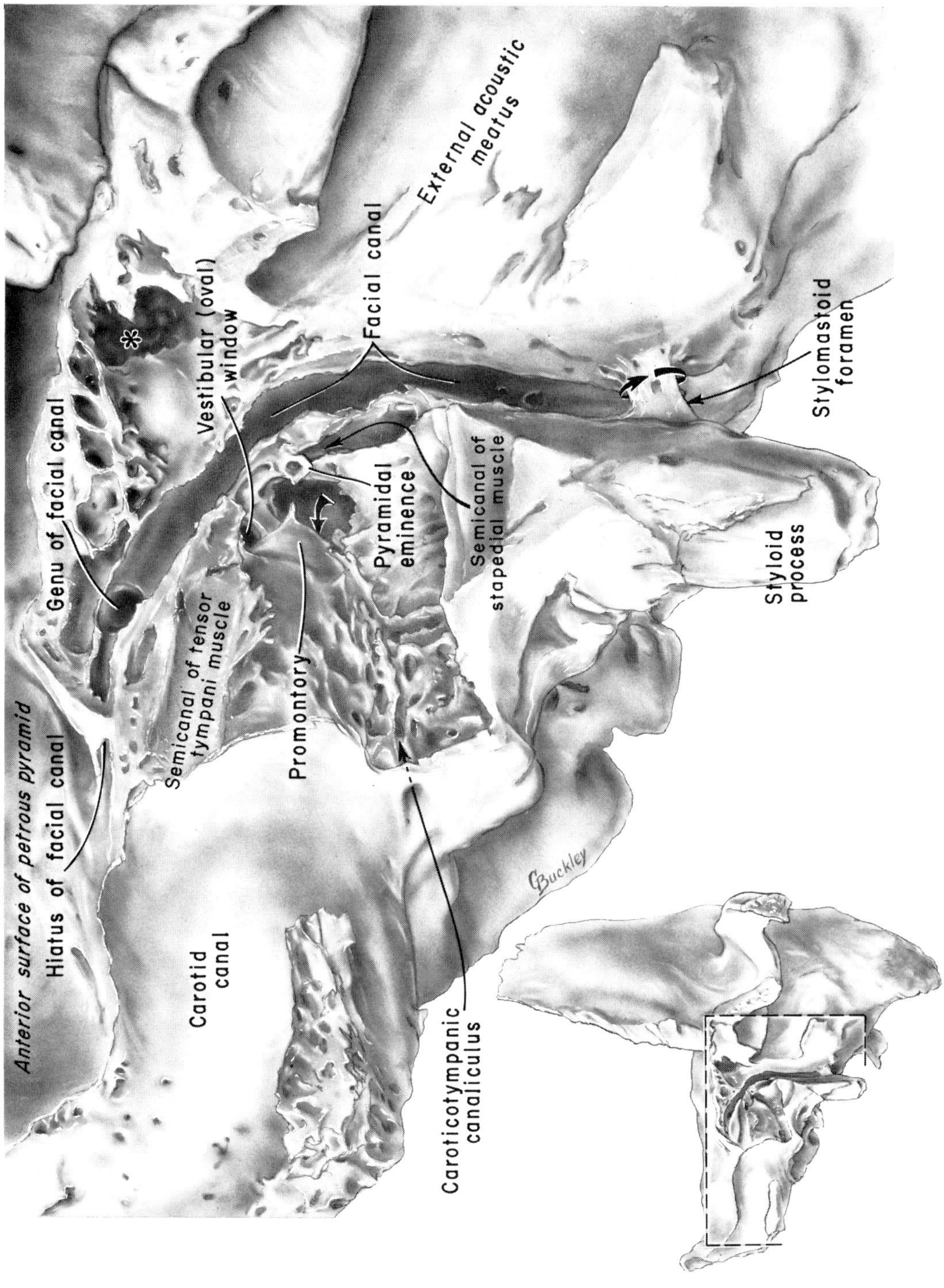
Anterior surface of petrous pyramid
Hiatus of facial canal
Carotid canal
Semicanal of tensor tympani muscle
Promontory
Caroticotympanic canaliculus
Genu of facial canal
Vestibular (oval) window
Facial canal
External acoustic meatus
Pyramidal eminence
Semicanal of stapedial muscle
Styloid process
Stylomastoid foramen

Figure III–140. ROUTES OF BLOOD SUPPLY TO THE PETROUS PART OF THE TEMPORAL BONE ON THE MEDIAL (OR LABYRINTHINE) WALL, SHOWING FIVE OF THE SEVERAL ROUTES FOLLOWED BY VESSELS THAT CONTRIBUTE TO THE TYMPANIC PLEXUS.

The arterial supply of the petrous part of the temporal bone involves branches of the subclavian artery, as well as the external and internal carotid (see discussion of the arteries that ascend in the neck, page 189). At the neck these give off branches that enter the following foramina, canals, or fissures: foramen magnum, stylomastoid foramen, petrosquamous fissure, petrotympanic fissure, jugular foramen, vestibular aqueduct, caroticotympanic canaliculus (in the carotid canal), tympanic canaliculus (in the fossula petrosa), hiatus of the facial canal, and small openings that make up the subarcuate fossa.

In addition to these, the minute channel for transmission of the cochlear vein is to be added (as it follows the general course of the cochlear canaliculus, but remains separate therefrom). Otherwise, the veins accompany arteries of the same name.

The vessels in the mucous membrane that covers the walls of the tympanic cavity are named for their position (anterior, posterior, superior, and inferior). The posterior tympanic artery, a branch of the stylomastoid (the latter from the posterior auricular), leaves the facial canal through the canaliculus of the *chorda tympani.* The superior tympanic, from the middle meningeal (the latter a branch of the internal maxillary), goes through the tympanic canaliculus (in the cochleariform process) to the promontory. The inferior tympanic, from the ascending pharyngeal, also enters the middle ear through the same canaliculus to ramify on the promontory. The anterior tympanic, from the internal maxillary, enters the middle ear through the petrotympanic fissure. The caroticotympanic canaliculus transmits small branches of the same name, derived from the internal carotid artery. The natural orifice of the stylomastoid foramen is marked by a remnant of the wall (encircled with arrow). The asterisk indicates the mastoid antrum. The unlabeled arrow indicates the general area of the tympanic sinus. The dissections also demonstrate the subdivisions of the facial canal.

Dissection by Dr. Raymond L. Warpeha.

(From Anson, Harper, and Winch: Third Symposium on the Role of the Vestibular Organs in Space Exploration, NASA SP-152, pp. 259–288. Washington, D.C., U.S. Government Printing Office, 1968.)

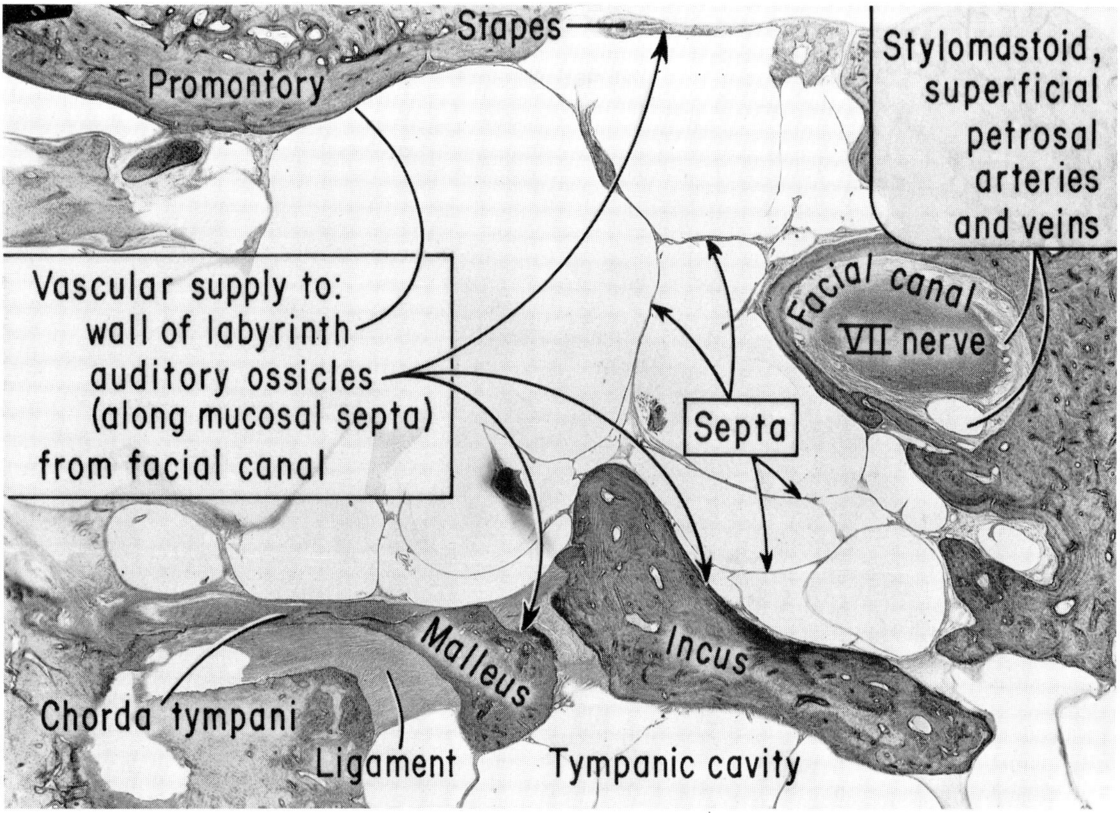

Figure III–141. VASCULAR ANATOMY OF THE TYMPANIC CAVITY. MALE, 19 YEARS OF AGE.

This illustration demonstrates the importance of the canal as a conduit for blood vessels of tympanic (middle ear) distribution.

The stylomastoid and superficial petrosal arteries and veins in the canal (noted, upper right) contribute to the tympanic plexus which supplies the labyrinthine wall, auditory ossicles and tympanic membrane (noted, middle left). Distribution is accomplished through the septa of the mucous membrane, which behave as would minute mesenteries in carrying blood vessels through connective tissue between epithelial layers. (See also Figures III–22*b*, III–26*b*, III–65*e*, and III–90*a*.)

Transverse section, Wisconsin Collection, series 29. ×13.

SELECTED READINGS

Ades, H., Angelborg, C., Bredberg, G., Engstrom, H., Stahle, J., and Sugar, J.: Inner ear studies. Acta Oto-Laryngologica, Supplement 301, 1972.

Alberti, P.: The blood supply of the long process of the incus and the head and neck of the stapes. Journal of Laryngology and Otology, 79:964–970, 1965.

Amjad, A., Starke, J., and Scheer, A.: Tympanofacial recess in the human ear. Archives of Otolaryngology, 88:131–137, 1968.

Anson, B. J.: An Atlas of Human Anatomy, 2nd ed. Philadelphia, W. B. Saunders Co., 1963, Sections II and III.

Anson, B. J.: Organ of hearing and equilibrium, Chapter 10, Part II, in Anson, B. J. (Ed.): Morris' Human Anatomy, 12th ed. New York, Blakiston Division, McGraw-Hill Book Company, 1966.

Anson, B. J.: Developmental anatomy of the ear, Chapter 1, in Paparella, M. M., and Shumrick, D. A. (Eds.): Otolaryngology, I. Philadelphia, W. B. Saunders Co., 1973.

Anson, B. J., and Bast, T. H.: Development of the otic capsule of the human ear. Illustrated in atlas series. Quarterly Bulletin, Northwestern University Medical School, 32:157–172, 1958.

Anson, B. J., and Bast, T. H.: Development of the Stapes of the human ear. Illustrated in atlas series. Quarterly Bulletin, Northwestern University Medical School, 33:44–59, 1959.

Anson, B. J., and Bast, T. H.: Development of the incus of the human ear. Illustrated in atlas series. Quarterly Bulletin, Northwestern University Medical School, 33:110–119, 1959.

Anson, B. J., Harper, D. G., and Warpeha, R. L.: Surgical anatomy of the facial canal and facial nerve. Annals of Otology, Rhinology and Laryngology, 72:713–734, 1963.

Atkins, J.: Anatomy of the facial triangle. Journal of Laryngology and Otology, 85:583–586, 1971.

Axelsson, A.: The vascular anatomy of the cochlea in the guinea pig and in man. Acta Oto-Laryngologica, Supplement 243, 1968.

Ballance, C. A.: Essays on the Surgery of the Temporal Bone. 2 vols. London, The Macmillan Company, 1919.

Bast, T. H.: Ossification of the capsule in human fetuses. Carnegie Contributions to Embryology, 21:53–82, 1930.

Bast, T. H.: Blood supply of the otic capsule of a 150 mm. (CR) human fetus. Anatomical Record, 48:141–151, 1931.

Beck, C.: Vergleichende Anatomie des Ohres. Anatomie des Ohres. Histologie des Ohres. Biochemie des Ohres. Z. Hals. Nas. Ohrenheilk., Bd. III/1:30–147, 1965.

Bellucci, R. J., and Wolff, D.: The Incus, normal and pathological. Archives of Otolaryngology, 83:413–421, 1966.

Bernstein, L.: Congenital absence of the oval window. Archives of Otolaryngology, 83:533–537, 1966.

Binns, P. M., and Riano, A.: Facial nerve homografts. Archives of Otolaryngology, 95:342–345, 1972.

Blatt, I. M., and Freeman, J. A.: Bell's palsy III: Further observations on the pathogenesis of Bell's palsy and the results of chorda tympani neurectomy. Transactions of the American Academy of Ophthalmology and Otolaryngology, 73:420–438, 1969.

Blevins, C. E.: Innervation of the tensor tympani muscle of the cat. American Journal of Anatomy, 113:287–301, 1963.

Blevins, C. E.: Studies on the innervation of the stapedius muscle of the cat. Anatomical Record, 149:157–171, 1964.

Bolz, E., and Lim, D.: Morphology of the stapediovestibular joint. Acta Oto-Laryngologica, 73:10–17, 1972.

Borghesan, C.: Anatomic relationship between limbus spiralis and tectorial membrane. Practica Oto-Rhino-Laryngologica, 31:129–135, 1969.

Bredberg, G., Engstrom, H., and Ades, H.: Cellular pattern and nerve supply of the human organ of Corti. Archives of Otolaryngology, 82:462–469, 1965.

Brownson, R. J., and Marovitz, W. F.: Scanning microscopy of normal human ossicles. Laryngoscope, 82:355–372, 1972.

Bull, T. R.: Taste and the chorda tympani. Journal of Laryngology and Otology, 79:479–493, 1965.

Cameron, D., Jennings, E., and Rannie, I.: Oxytalan fibres in the human tympanic membrane. Journal of Laryngology and Otology, 84:1235–1239, 1970.

Caparosa, R., and Klassen, D.: Congenital anomalies of the stapes and facial nerve. Archives of Otolaryngology, 83:420–421, 1966.

Cheatle, A. H.: Some Points in the Surgical Anatomy of the Temporal Bone from Birth to Adult Life. London, J. & A. Churchill Ltd., 1907.

Dass, R., Grewal, B. S., and Thapar, S. P.: Human stapes and its variations – I. General features. Journal of Laryngology and Otology, 80:11–25, 1966.

Dass, R., Grewal, B. S., and Thapar, S. P.: Human stapes and its variations – II. Footplate. Journal of Laryngology and Otology, 80:471–480, 1966.

Dass, R., Grewal, B. S., and Thapar, S. P.: Human stapes and its variations – III. Influence of age and sex. Journal of Laryngology and Otology, 80:1023–1037, 1966.

Dohlman, G. F.: Secretion and absorption of endolymph. Annals of Otology, Rhinology and Laryngology, 73:708–723, 1964.

Dohlman, G. F.: The shape and function of the Cupula. Journal of Laryngology and Otology, 83:43–53, 1969.

Durcan, D., Shea, J., and Sleeckx, J.: Bifurcation of the facial nerve. Archives of Otolaryngology, 86:619–631, 1967.

Duvall, A., and Rhodes, V.: Reissner's membrane. Archives of Otolaryngology, 86:143–151, 1967.

Engstrom, H., Ades, H., and Hawkins, J.: Structure and functions of the sensory hairs of the inner ear. Journal of the Acoustical Society of America, 34:1356–1363, 1962.

Fisch, U., and Esslen, E.: Total intratemporal exposure of the facial nerve. Pathologic findings in Bell's palsy. Archives of Otolaryngology, 95:335–341, 1972.

Flisberg, K., and Zsigmond, M.: The size of the mastoid air cell system. Acta Oto-Laryngologica, 60:23–29, 1965.

Garcia-Ibanez, J., and Iurato, S.: Anatomical study of the otosclerotic stapedial footplate. Archives of Otolaryngology, 90:410–417, 1969.

Gasser, R.: The development of the facial nerve in man. Annals of Otology, Rhinology and Laryngology, 76:37–56, 1967.

Goodhill, V.: Stapes Surgery for Otosclerosis. New York, Hoeber Medical Division, Harper & Row, Publishers, 1961.

Graves, G. O., and Edwards, L. F.: The eustachian tube. A review of its descriptive, microscopic, topographic and clinical anatomy. Archives of Otolaryngology, 39:359–397, 1944.

Guild, S. R.: Observations upon the structure and normal contents of the ductus and saccus endolymphaticus in the guinea-pig. American Journal of Anatomy, 39:1–56, 1927.

Guild, S. R.: Correlations of histologic observations and the acuity of hearing. Acta Oto-Laryngologica, 17:207–249, 1932.

Guild, S. R.: II. Normal and pathological anatomy of the petrous pyramid. Annals of Otology, Rhinology and Laryngology, 44:1011–1035, 1935.

Guilford, F. R., and Anson, B. J.: Osseous fixation of the malleus. Transactions of the American Academy of Ophthalmology and Otolaryngology, 71:398–407, 1967.

Gundersen, T.: Congenital malformations of the stapes footplate. Archives of Otolaryngology, 85:171–176, 1966.

Hall, G., Pulec, J., and Rhoton, A.: Geniculate ganglion anatomy for the otologist. Archives of Otolaryngology, 90:568–571, 1971.

Hansen, C.: Vascular anatomy of the human temporal bone. Annals of Otology, Rhinology and Laryngology, 79:269–273, 1970.

Hanson, J. R., and Anson, B. J.: Development of the malleus of the human ear. Illustrated in atlas series. Quarterly Bulletin, Northwestern University Medical School, 36:119–137, 1962.

Hanson, J. R., Anson, B. J., and Strickland, E. M.: Branchial sources of the auditory ossicles in man, Part II. Observations on embryonic stages from 7 mm. to 28 mm. (CR length). Archives of Otolaryngology, 76:200–215, 1962.

Hawkins, J. E., and Johnsson, L.: Light microscopic observations of the inner ear in man and monkey. Annals of Otology, Rhinology and Laryngology, 77:608–628, 1968.

Hitselberger, W. E., and House, W. F.: Surgical approaches to acoustic tumors. Archives of Otolaryngology, 84:286–291, 1966.

Hogg, I. D., Stephens, C. B., and Arnold, G. E.: Theoretical anomalies of the stapedial artery. Annals of Otology, Rhinology and Laryngology, 81:860–870, 1972.

Hoshino, T., and Paparella, M.: Middle ear muscle anomalies. Archives of Otolaryngology, 94:235–239, 1971.

Hough, J. V. D.: Malformations and anatomical variations seen in the middle ear during the operation for mobilization of the stapes. The Laryngoscope, 68:1337–1379, 1958.

House, W. F.: Transtemporal bone microsurgical removal of acoustic neuromas. Archives of Otolaryngology, 80:597–756, 1964.

Hovelacque, A.: Nerf-facial, in Anatomie des nerfs craniens et rachidiens et du système grand sympathique chez l'homme. 2 V. Paris, Gaston Doin et Cie, 1927.

Igarashi, M.: Dimensional study of the vestibular apparatus. The Laryngoscope, 77:1806–1817, 1967.

Igarashi, M., and Alford, B.: Cupula, cupular zone of otolithic membrane, and tectorial membrane in the squirrel monkey. Acta Oto-Laryngologica, 68:420–426, 1969.

Johnsson, L.: Degenerative changes and anomalies of the vestibular system in man. The Laryngoscope, 81:1682–1694, 1971.

Johnsson, L.: Reissner's membrane in the human cochlea. Annals of Otology, Rhinology, and Laryngology, 80:425–439, 1971.

Johnsson, L.: Cochlear blood vessel pattern in the human fetus and postnatal vascular involution. Annals of Otology, Rhinology and Laryngology, 81:22–40, 1972.

Johnsson, L., and Hawkins, J. E.: A direct approach to cochlear anatomy and pathology in man. Archives of Otolaryngology, 85:599–613, 1967.

Johnsson, L., and Hawkins, J. E.: Vascular changes in the human inner ear associated with aging. Annals of Otology, Rhinology and Laryngology, 81:364–376, 1972.

Kawabata, I., and Paparella, M.: Fine structure of the round window membrane. Annals of Otology, Rhinology and Laryngology, 80:13–26, 1971.

Kawabata, I., and Ishii, H.: Fiber arrangement in the tympanic membrane. Acta Oto-Laryngologica, 72:243–254, 1971.

Kitamura, T., Togawa, K., Tsukamoto, K., and Naito, J.: Extratemporal facial nerve surgery. Archives of Otolaryngology, 95:369–375, 1962.

Körner, O.: Das Septum petro-squamasum (mastoideum) und seine klinische Bedeutung. Z. Hals. Nas. Ohrenheilk., 17:137–140, 1926–27.

Kraus, P., and Ziv, M.: Incus fixation due to congenital anomaly of chorda tympani. Acta Oto-Laryngologica, 72:358–360, 1971.

Lawrence, M.: The double innervation of the tensor tympani. Annals of Otology, Rhinology and Laryngology, 71:705–718, 1962.

Lawrence, M.: Fluid balance in the inner ear. Annals of Otology, Rhinology and Laryngology, 74:486–499, 1965.

Lawrence, M.: Blood flow through the basilar membrane capillaries. Acta Oto-Laryngologica, 71:106–114, 1971.

Leonard, J., and Alexander, D.: Anatomic variations in the area of the oval window. Archives of Otolaryngology, 87:48–55, 1968.

Lim, D. J.: Three dimensional observations of the inner ear with the scanning electron microscope. Acta Oto-Laryngologica, Supplement 255, 1969.

Lim, D. J.: Fine morphology of the tectorial membrane. Archives of Otolaryngology, 96:199–215, 1972.

Lindeman, H., Ades, H., Bredberg, G., and Engstrom, H.: The sensory hairs and the tectorial membrane in the development of the cat's organ of Corti. Acta Oto-Laryngologica, 72:229–242, 1971.

Litton, W., Krause, C., Anson, B., and Cohen, W.: The relationship of the facial canal to the annular sulcus. The Laryngoscope, 79:1584–1604, 1969.

Lupin, A.: The relationship of the tensor tympani and tensor palati muscles. Annals of Otology, Rhinology and Laryngology, 78:792–796, 1969.

Maran, A. G. D.: Persistent stapedial artery. Journal of Laryngology and Otology, 79:971–975, 1965.

Mazzoni, A.: Internal auditory canal arterial relations at the porus acusticus. Annals of Otology, Rhinology and Laryngology, 78:797–814, 1969.

Mazzoni, A.: The subarcuate artery in man. The Larygoscope, 80:69–79, 1970.

Mazzoni, A., and Hansen, C.: Surgical anatomy of the arteries of the internal auditory canal. Archives of Otolaryngology, 91:128–135, 1970.

Mazzoni, A.: Internal auditory artery supply to the petrous bone. Annals of Otology, Rhinology and Laryngology, 81:13–21, 1972.

McCabe, B. F.: The quick component of nystagmus. The Laryngoscope, 75:1619–1646, 1965.

Meltzer, P. E.: The mastoid cells: Their arrangement in relation to the sigmoid portion of the transverse sinus. Archives of Otolaryngology, 19:326–335, 1934.

Nomura, Y., and Hiraide, F.: Cochlear blood vessel. Archives of Otolaryngology, 88:231–237, 1968.

Ogura, Y., and Clemis, J.: A study of the gross anatomy of the human vestibular aqueduct. Annals of Otology, Rhinology, and Laryngology, 80:813–825, 1971.

Palva, T., and Palva, A.: Size of the human mastoid air cell system. Acta Oto-Laryngologica, 62:237–251, 1966.

Palva, T.: Cochlear aqueducts in infants. Acta Oto-Laryngologica, 70:83–94, 1970.

Papangelou, L.: Study of the human internal auditory canal. The Laryngoscope, 82:617–624, 1972.

Proctor, B.: The development of the middle ear spaces and their surgical significance. Journal of Laryngology and Otology, 78:631–648, 1964.

Proctor, B.: Surgical anatomy of the posterior tympanum. Annals of Otology, Rhinology and Laryngology, 78:1026–1040, 1969.

Pulec, J. L.: Total decompression of the facial nerve. The Laryngoscope, 76:1015–1028, 1966.

Richany, S. F., Anson, B. J., and Bast, T. H.: The ear and temporal bone: Development and adult structure, Chapter 1, in Coates, G. M., Schenck, H. P., and Miller, M. V. (Eds.): Otolaryngology, Vol. 1. New York, Hoeber Medical Division, Harper & Row, Publishers, 1969.

Ritter, F., and Lawrence, M.: A histological and experimental study of cochlear aqueduct patency in the adult human. The Laryngoscope, 75:1224–1233, 1965.

Sando, I., Black, F. O., and Hemenway, W. G.: Spatial distribution of vestibular nerve in internal auditory canal. Annals of Otology, Rhinology and Laryngology, 81:305–314, 1972.

Sarto, H., Ruby, R., and Schuknecht, H.: Course of the sensory component of the nervux intermedius in the temporal bone. Annals of Otology, Rhinology and Laryngology, 79:960–966, 1970.

Sarto, H., Igarashi, M., Alford, B., and Guilford, F.: Anatomical measurement of the sinus tympanum. Archives of Otolaryngology, 94:418–425, 1971.

Schuknecht, H. F. (Ed.): Otosclerosis, a Henry Ford Hospital International Symposium. Boston, Little, Brown and Company, 1962.

Sellers, L. M., and Anson, B. J.: Anatomical observations on the round window by Antonio Scarpa. Archives of Otolaryngology, 75:2–45, 1962.

Shambaugh, G. E., Jr.: Cytology of the internal ear, in Cowdry (Ed.): Special Cytology, 2nd ed., Vol. 3. New York, Paul B. Hoeber, 1932.

Shambaugh, G. E., Jr.: Surgery of the Ear, 2nd ed. Philadelphia, W. B. Saunders Co., 1967.

Shimada, T., and Lim, D.: The fiber arrangement of the human tympanic membrane: A scanning electron microscopic observation. Annals of Otology, Rhinology and Laryngology, 80:210–217, 1971.

Silverstein, H.: Biochemical studies of the inner ear fluids in the cat. Annals of Otology, Rhinology and Laryngology, 75:48–63, 1966.

Smith, C. A.: Capillary areas of the membranous labyrinth. Annals of Otology, Rhinology and Laryngology, 63:435–447, 1954.

Smith, C. A., and Dempsey, E. W.: Electron microscopy of the organ of Corti. American Journal of Anatomy, 100:337–368, 1957.

Smith, C. A., and Sjöstrand, F. S.: Structure of the nerve endings on the external hair cells of the guinea pig cochlea as studied by serial sections. Journal of Ultrastructure Research, 5:523–556, 1961.

Smith, C.: Electron microscopy of the inner ear. Annals of Otology, Rhinology and Laryngology, 77:629–643, 1968.

Smyth, G., Kerr, A., and Goodey, R.: Current thoughts on combines approach tympanoplasty, Part III. Technical aspects of posterior tympanotomy. Journal of Laryngology and Otology, 85:1013–1029, 1971.

Steffen, T.: Vascular anomalies of the middle ear. The Laryngoscope, 78:171–197, 1968.

Stelter, G. P., Bast, T. H., and Anson, B. J.: The developmental and adult anatomy of the air-cells in the petrous part of the temporal bone. Quarterly Bulletin, Northwestern University Medical School, 34:23–37, 1960.

Strickland, E. M., Hanson, J. R., and Anson, B. J.: Branchial sources of the auditory ossicles in man, Part I. Archives of Otolaryngology, 76:100–122, 1962.

Wiberg, A.: Function of the Chorda Tympani before and after Operation for Clinical Otosclerosis. The University of Umea Department of Otorhinolaryngology, Umea, Sweden, 1971.

Williams, H. L.: Latent or dormant disease in the pneumatic cell tracts of the temporal bone. Transactions of the American Academy of Ophthalmology and Otolaryngology, 70:545–558, 1966.

Wilmot, T.: Hereditary conductive deafness due to incus-stapes abnormalities and assocated with pinna deformity. Journal of Laryngology and Otology, 84:469–479, 1970.

Wolff, D., and Bellucci, R. J.: The histopathology observed in fifty biopsied stapedes. Transactions of the American Academy of Ophthalmology and Otolaryngology, 64:540–553, 1960.

Wolff, D., and Bellucci, R. J.: Otosclerosis: Multiple manifestations of its basic pathology. Archives of Otolaryngology, 79:571–593, 1964.

Work, W. P., and Proctor, C. A.: The otologist and first branchial cleft anomalies. Annals of Otology, Rhinology and Laryngology, 72:548–562, 1963.

Wright, J. W., Jr., and Taylor, C. E.: Facial nerve abnormalities revealed by polytomography. Archives of Otolaryngology, 95:426–430, 1972.

Wright, J., Taylor, C., and McKay, D.: Variations in the course of the facial nerve as illustrated by tomography. The Laryngoscope, 77:717–733, 1967.

Zechner, G., and Altmann, F.: Histological studies on the human endolymphatic duct and sac. Practica Oto-Rhino-Laryngologica, 31:65–83, 1969.

INDEX

In this index *italic* page numbers indicate illustrations; those in ***boldface*** indicate that the structure is the principal subject of the illustration. Note that page numbers between 15 and 149 refer to developmental anatomy.